ADVANCES IN PROSTAGLANDIN AND THROMBOXANE RESEARCH
VOLUME 6

Advances in Prostaglandin and Thromboxane Research

Series Editors:
Bengt Samuelsson and Rodolfo Paoletti

Vol. 8: Advances in Prostaglandin and Thromboxane Research, *edited by B. Samuelsson, P. W. Ramwell, and R. Paoletti,* 609 pp., 1980.

Vol. 7: Advances in Prostaglandin and Thromboxane Research, *edited by B. Samuelsson, P. W. Ramwell, and R. Paoletti,* 606 pp., 1980.

Vol. 6: Advances in Prostaglandin and Thromboxane Research, *edited by B. Samuelsson, P. W. Ramwell, and R. Paoletti,* 600 pp., 1980.

Vol. 5: Methods in Prostaglandin Research, *edited by J. C. Frölich,* 256 pp., 1978.

Vol. 4: Prostaglandins and Perinatal Medicine, *edited by F. Coceani and P. M. Olley,* 432 pp., 1978.

Vol. 3: Prostaglandins and Phospholipases, *edited by C. Galli, G. Galli, and G. Porcellati,* 224 pp., 1978.

Vol. 2: Advances in Prostaglandin and Thromboxane Research, *edited by B. Samuelsson and R. Paoletti,* 1028 pp., 1976.

Vol. 1: Advances in Prostaglandin and Thromboxane Research, *edited by B. Samuelsson and R. Paoletti,* 506 pp., 1976.

Advances in Prostaglandin and Thromboxane Research
Volume 6

Editors

Dr. Bengt Samuelsson

Professor
Department of Chemistry
Karolinska Institute
Stockholm, Sweden

Dr. Peter W. Ramwell

Professor
Department of Physiology and
Biophysics
Georgetown University Medical
Center
Washington, D.C.

Dr. Rodolfo Paoletti

Professor and Director
Institute of Pharmacology
and Pharmacognosy
University of Milan
Milan, Italy

Raven Press ■ New York

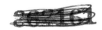

Raven Press, 1140 Avenue of the Americas, New York, New York 10036

Made in the United States of America

International Standard Book Number 0-89004-452-X
Library of Congress Catalog Card Number 79-66833

Preface

This set of volumes (6 to 8) of the *Advances in Prostaglandin and Thromboxane Research* series is based on papers presented at the Fourth International Prostaglandin Conference held in Washington, D.C. on May 28–31, 1979. It was an exciting conference which clearly showed the vitality of this broad area of research and its impact in both basic research and clinical medicine. Initial sections review the biochemistry, physiology, and pharmacology of prostaglandins and their derivatives with discussions of lipoxygenases, endoperoxides, phospholipases, and synthetase inhibition and thromboxane antagonists.

The discovery of a new group of biologically highly potent compounds, the leukotrienes (SRS), was reported during the meeting. The leukotrienes illustrate once again the enormous potential of arachidonic acid as a precursor of biologically important structures.

Sections on cardiology, circulation, and respiration review prostaglandin effects of heart function, pulmonary and systemic vasculature, platelets, and hemodynamics. Sections on the kidney review renal aspects of hypertension, diuresis, and renal pathology, and discussions of shock and trauma interrelate.

Subsequent sections deal with the involvement of prostaglandins in endocrinology, reproductive physiology, obstetrics and gynecology, neonatology, hematology, gastroenterology, inflammation, and inflammatory diseases such as arthritis, neurology, growth and tissue development, and nutrition. In addition, extensive sections deals with current laboratory and clinical research methods.

We hope that these volumes on prostaglandins and related compounds will serve as reference work for medical researchers and clinicians involved in the areas described above.

We are especially indebted to members of the Washington Organizing Committee and the secretariat and would like to cite the invaluable assistance of J. Fletcher, F. Gurch, N. Schoene, M. Kaliner, W. Criss, R. Bryant, M. Bailey, N. Coulter, and Y. Zachrisson.

The conference was sponsored by Georgetown University Medical Center, Washington, D.C., and the Lorenzini Foundation, Milan, Italy.

We also gratefully acknowledge the support for this conference from: the National Institute of Arthritis, Metabolism and Digestive Diseases; National Cancer Institute; National Institute of Allergy and Infectious Diseases, National Heart, Lung and Blood Institute; National Institute of Child Health and Human Development, Fogarty International Center, NIH; Science and Education Administration, U.S. Department of Agriculture; Bureau of Biologics, Food and Drug Administration; Bureau of Drugs, Food and Drug Administration; Naval

Medical Research and Development Command; Office of Naval Research; Geron-X; Upjohn; Wellcome; and Ono-Parke Davis-May Baker.

To ensure rapid publication of the proceedings, the authors were strongly urged to deliver the manuscripts during the meeting. We are grateful to the authors for their prompt submission of the papers and to Dr. Alan Edelson of Raven Press for arranging technical editorial review of the papers during the conference. This arrangement has made early publication possible.

The Editors

Contents of Volume 6

Introduction

1 Leukotrienes: A New Group of Biologically Active Compounds
B. Samuelsson, P. Borgeat, S. Hammarström, and R. C. Murphy

19 Recent Studies on the Chemical Synthesis of Eicosanoids
E. J. Corey, H. Niwa, J. R. Falck, C. Mioskowski, Y. Arai, and A. Marfat

27 Enzymes Involved in the Formation and Further Transformations of
Prostaglandin Endoperoxides
*Shozo Yamamoto, Shiro Ohki, Nubuchika Ogino, Takao Shimizu, Tani-
hiro Yoshimoto, Kikuko Watanabe, and Osamu Hayaishi*

35 Metabolism of the Prostaglandins and Thromboxanes
*John A. Oates, L. Jackson Roberts II, Brian J. Sweetman, Richard N.
Maas, John F. Gerkens, and Douglass F. Taber*

43 Prostacyclin in the Cardiovascular System
S. Moncada and J. R. Vane

61 Mechanism Underlying the Inhibition of Platelet Aggregation by Eicosa-
pentaenoic Acid and Its Metabolites
*Philip Needleman, Howard Sprecher, Mark O. Whitaker, and Angela
Wyche*

69 Assay Methods for Prostaglandins and Thromboxanes
Elisabeth Granström

77 Inflammation: The Role of Peroxidase-Derived Products
*F. A. Kuehl, Jr., J. L. Humes, E. A. Ham, R. W. Egan, and H. W.
Dougherty*

87 Clinical Applications
Marc Bygdeman

Lipoxygenases

95 Isolation of Glucose-Sensitive Platelet Lipoxygenase Products from
Arachidonic Acid
Robert W. Bryant and J. Martyn Bailey

101 The Role of the Arachidonate Lipoxygenase Pathway in Blood Platelet
Aggregation
C. E. Dutilh, E. Haddeman, and F. ten Hoor

vii

107   An Expoxy–Hydroxy Product from Arachidonate
      Irene C. Walker, R. L. Jones, P. J. Kerry, and N. H. Wilson

111   Study on the Property and Inhibition of Human Platelet Arachidonic
      Acid 12-Lipoxygenase
      F. F. Sun, J. C. McGuire, D. P. Wallach, and V. R. Brown

115   Interrelationships of SRS-A Production and Arachidonic Acid Metabo-
      lism in Human Lung Tissue
      J. L. Walker

121   Potentiation of SRS-A Release from Guinea Pig Chopped Lung by Sub-
      strates for Arachidonate Lipoxygenase
      Priscilla J. Piper, J. R. Tippins, H. R. Morris, and G. W. Taylor

125   Further Studies on the Inactivation of Slow Reacting Substance of Ana-
      phylaxis (SRS-A) by Lipoxidase
      Pierre Sirois

Endoperoxides

129   Chemical and Enzymic Conversions of the Prostaglandin Endoperoxide
      PGH$_2$
      D. H. Nugteren and E. Christ-Hazelhof

139   Characterization of Prostaglandin$_2$ Synthetase
      F. J. van der Ouderaa, M. Buytenhek, and D. A. van Dorp

145   Mechanism of Oxygen Activation Involved in the Prostaglandin Synthe-
      tase Mechanism
      Peter J. O'Brien and Anver D. Rahimtula

149   Mechanism of Xenobiotic Cooxygenation Coupled to Prostaglandin H$_2$
      Biosynthesis
      *Lawrence J. Marnett, Michael J. Bienkowski, William R. Pagels, and
      Gregory A. Reed*

153   Direct and Indirect Involvement of Radical Scavengers During Prosta-
      glandin Biosynthesis
      *Robert W. Egan, Paul H. Gale, George C. Beveridge, Lawrence J. Marnett,
      and Frederick A. Kuehl, Jr.*

157   Interaction of Arachidonic Acid and Heme Iron in the Synthesis of
      Prostaglandins
      *D. A. Peterson, J. M. Gerrard, G. H. R. Rao, E. L. Mills, and J. G.
      White*

163   Identification of Prostaglandin D$_2$-Isomerase in Rat Basophilic Leukemia
      and Rat Mast Cells
      B. A. Jakschik, M. M. Steinhoff, and L. H. Lee

Radioimmunoassay

167 New Approach to the RIA of Prostaglandins and Related Compounds Using Iodinated Tracers
F. Dray, K. Gerozissis, B. Kouznetzova, S. Mamas, P. Pradelles, and G. Trugnan

181 Radioimmunologic Determination of 15-Keto-13,14-Dihydro-PGE$_2$: A Method for Its Stable Degradation Product, 11-Deoxy-15-Keto-13,14-Dihydro-11β,16-Cyclo-PGE$_2$
Elisabeth Granström and Hans Kindahl

183 Radioimmunoassay for 13,14-Dihydro-15-Keto, Prostaglandin E$_2$ in Human Plasma: Applications and Artifacts
Stewart A. Metz, Maureen G. Rice, and R. Paul Robertson

187 Radioimmunoassay of Serum Thromboxane B$_2$: A Simple Method of Assessing Pharmacologic Effects on Platelet Function
C. Patrono, G. Ciabattoni, F. Pugliese, E. Pinca, G. Castrucci, A. De Salvo, M. A. Satta, and M. Parachini

193 A Radioimmunoassay for 6-Keto Prostaglandin$_{1\alpha}$
Laurence M. Demers and Dennis D. Derck

201 Radioimmunoassay of Urinary Prostaglandins
M. Korteweg, J. De Boever, D. Vandevivere, and G. Verdonk

207 Biologic and Methodologic Variables Affecting Urinary Prostaglandin Measurement
G. Ciabattoni, F. Pugliese, E. Pinca, G. A. Cinotti, A. De Salvo, M. A. Satta, and C. Patrono

213 Radioimmunoassay of the Main Urinary Metabolite of Prostaglandin F$_{2\alpha}$ in Normal Subjects After Oral Administration of Prostaglandins E$_2$ and F$_{2\alpha}$
Satoshi Kitamura and Yoko Ishihara

Phospholipases

219 Diglyceride Lipase: A Pathway for Arachidonate Release from Human Platelets
R. L. Bell, Nancy Stanford, Donald A. Kennerly, and Philip W. Majerus

225 Release of Arachidonic Acid and its Conversion to Prostaglandins in Various Diploid Cell Types in Culture
Peter Polgar, William H. J. Douglas, Louis Terracio, and Linda Taylor

231 Effects of Divalent Cations on Prostaglandin Biosynthesis and Phospholipase A$_2$ Activation in Rabbit Kidney Medulla Slices
A. Raz and A. Erman

235 Synthesis and Biological Activities of Arachidonic and α- and β-Alkyl
     Substituted Arachidonic Acid Derivatives
     *C. D. Liang, John S. Baran, James E. Miller, D. H. Steinman, and
     R. N. Saunders*

239 Activation of Arachidonic Acid Turnover in Adrenal Phospholipids by
     ACTH, A23187, and Ca^{2+}
     M. P. Schrey and R. P. Rubin

243 Role of Phospholipase in the Regulation of Prostaglandin E_2 Biosynthesis
     by Rabbit Renomedullary Interstitial Cells in Tissue Culture: Effects
     of Angiotensin II, Potassium, Hyperosmolality, Dexamethasone, and
     Protein Synthesis Inhibition
     Randall M. Zusman and C. Alan Brown

249 Role of Extracellular Arachidonate in Regulation of Prostaglandin Bio-
     synthesis in Cultured 3T3 Fibroblasts
     K. A. Chandrabose, R. W. Bonser, and P. Cuatrecasas

255 Time-Synchronized Activation of Lipolysis and Fatty Acids Reacylation
     by Bradykinin and Angiotensin II in the Perfused Rabbit Kidney
     A. Raz and M. Schwartzman

259 Thrombin and Bradykinin Modulate Prostaglandin Synthetase Indepen-
     dently of Phospholipase
     R. W. Bonser, K. A. Chandrabose, and P. Cuatrecasas

263 Glucocorticoids and the Prostaglandin System in Adipose Tissue
     Carmen Vigo, G. P. Lewis, and Priscilla J. Piper

                          Platelets

267 Biosynthesis of Thromboxanes
     Sven Hammarström and Ulf Diczfalusy

275 Effects of Platelet Aggregation and Adenosine 3′:5′-Monophosphate on
     the Synthesis of Thromboxane B_2 in Human Platelets
     *Jan Åke Lindgren, Hans-Erik Claesson, Hans Kindahl, and Sven Hammar-
     ström*

283 Thromboxane A_2 and Prostaglandin H_2 Form Covalently Linked Deriva-
     tives with Human Serum Albumin
     J. Maclouf, H. Kindahl, E. Granström, and B. Samuelsson

287 Heparin Potentiates Synthesis of Thromboxane A_2 in Human Platelets
     W. H. Anderson, S. F. Mohammad, H. Y. K. Chuang, and R. G. Mason

293 *In Vivo* Inhibition of Thromboxane Biosynthesis by Hydralazine
     *James E. Greenwald, Lan K. Wong, Michael Alexander, and Joseph R.
     Bianchine*

297 Thromboxane B₂ Production and Lipid Peroxidation in Human Blood Platelets
L. C. Best, P. B. B. Jones, M. B. McGuire, and R. G. G. Russell

301 PGD₃ is the Mediator of the Antiaggregatory Effects of the Trienoic Endoperoxide PGH₃
M. O. Whitaker, P. Needleman, A. Wyche, F. A. Fitzpatrick, and H. Sprecher

305 Inhibition of Platelet Aggregation by Novel Benzolpyrrole Derivatives
Seizi Kurotumi, Akiro Ohtsu, Kenji Hoshina, Makiko Jimba, Keiji Komoriya, Tatsuyuki Naruchi, Toshio Wakabayashi, Yoshinobu Hashimoto, and Sachio Ishimoto

309 Altered Arachidonic Acid Metabolism in Platelets Inhibited by Onion or Garlic Extracts
Amar N. Makheja, Jack Y. Vanderhoek, Robert W. Bryant, and J. Martyn Bailey

313 Effect of Oral Aspirin Dose on Platelet Aggregation and Arterial Prostacyclin Synthesis: Studies in Humans and Rabbits
E. F. Ellis, P. S. Jones, K. F. Wright, D. W. Richardson, and C. K. Ellis

317 Differential Inhibition of Prostacyclin Production and Platelet Aggregation by Aspirin in Humans
Giulio Masotti, Giorgio Galanti, Loredana Poggesi, Rosanna Abbate, and Gian Gastone Neri Serneri

321 Serine-Esterase (Protease) Inhibitors Block Stimulus-Induced Mobilization of Arachidonate in Platelets
Maurice B. Feinstein, Jack Y. Vanderhoek, and Ronald Walenga

327 Syntheses of New Prostacyclin Analogs
K. Shimoji, Y. Arai, H. Wakatsuka, and M. Hayashi

331 Comparison of the Activities of Prostacyclin and its Stable Analogues on the Platelet Aggregation and Cardiovascular Systems
Akiyoshi Kawasaki, Kenji Ishii, Korekiyo Wakitani, and Masami Tsuboshima

337 Syntheses and Biological Activities of Some Prostacyclin Analogs
S. Ohuchida, S. Hashimoto, H. Wakatsuka, Y. Arai, and M. Hayashi

341 Vasodilator and Antiplatelet Activities of Prostacyclins with Modified ω-Side Chain
B. A. Schölkens, W. Bartmann, G. Beck, U. Lerch, E. Konz, and U. Weithmann

347   Pharmacological Evaluation of ONO 1206, Prostaglandin E_1 Derivative,
      as Antianginal Agent
      Toshimichi Tsuboi, Naonobu Hatano, Katsuyoshi Nakatsuji, Buichi Fuji-
      tani, Kouichi Yoshida, and Masanao Shimizu

                     Structure-Activity Relationship

351   Influence of Sulprostone upon Platelet Function: *In Vitro* and *In Vivo*
      Studies
      R. C. Briel and T. H. Lippert

355   Synthesis and Biological Activity of 9-Deoxo-9-Methylene and Related
      Prostaglandins
      G. L. Bundy, F. A. Kimball, A. Robert, J. W. Aiken, K. M. Maxey,
      O. K. Sebek, N. A. Nelson, J. C. Sih, W. L. Miller, and R. S. P. Hsi

365   Comparative Luteolytic Effects of Prostaglandin $F_{2\alpha}$ and Its 13-Dehydro
      Analogs *In Vivo*
      J. A. McCracken, M. E. Glew, S. S. Hull, Jr., L. Bovaird, L. Underwood,
      and J. Fried

381   Structure-Activity Relationships: A Look at the Structures of PG-Related
      Molecules
      George T. DeTitta, David A. Langs, and Mary G. Erman

385   Evidence for Separate PGD_2 and $PGF_{2\alpha}$ Receptors in the Canine Mesen-
      teric Vascular Bed
      Larry Feigen and Barry Chapnick

389   Evaluation of Prostaglandin and Prostacyclin Antagonism at Platelet
      Receptors by Aggregometry
      Thomas L. Eggerman, Lawrence A. Harker, Niels H. Andersen, and
      Cynthia H. Wilson

395   ^{3}H-PGD_2 Binding by Intact Human Platelets
      A. M. Siegl, J. B. Smith, and M. J. Silver

399   PGI_2 or PGE_2 Selectively Antagonise Responses to Excitatory PGs in
      Human Isolated Myometrium
      G. J. Sanger and A. Bennett

401   Prostaglandin-Specific Binding to Several Microsomal Fractions from
      Bovine Myometrium
      Mary E. Carsten and Jordan D. Miller

407   Prostaglandin Receptor: Induction of Density Changes in Rat Liver
      Plasma Membrane
      Maureen G. Rice, John R. McRae, and R. Paul Robertson

411 Fenalcomine Hydrochloride Inhibits the Action of PG on the Smooth Muscle but Stimulates that of TXA$_2$
Pham Huu Chanh, A. Pham Huu Chanh, and M. Nguyen van Thoai

TX Synthetase Inhibition

417 Biochemical and Pharmacological Evaluation of Thromboxane Synthetase Inhibitors
Robert R. Gorman

427 Synthesis and Biological Properties of Selective Inhibitors of the Prostaglandin Cascade
Josef Fried, J. Barton, S. Kittisopikul, Philip Needleman, and A. Wyche

437 Effect of SQ 80,338 [1-(3-Phenyl-2-Propenyl)-1*H*-Imidazole] on Thromboxane Synthetase Activity and Arachidonic Acid-Induced Platelet Aggregation and Bronchoconstriction
D. N. Harris, R. Greenberg, M. B. Phillips, G. H. Osman, Jr., and M. J. Antonaccio

443 Selective Inhibitor of Thromboxane Synthetase: Pyridine and its Derivatives
Tsumoru Miyamoto, Ken Taniguchi, Tadao Tanouchi, and Fumio Hirata

447 Inhibition of Thromboxane Synthesis and Platelet Aggregation by Pyridine and its Derivatives
Hsin-Hsiung Tai, Nancy Lee, and Chen L. Tai

453 Inhibition of Arachidonate Metabolism by Selected Compounds *In Vitro* with Particular Emphasis on the Thromboxane A$_2$ Synthase Pathway
L. D. Tobias and J. G. Hamilton

457 Inhibition of Dog Platelet Reactivity Following 1-Benzylimidazole Administration
R. H. Harris, T. Fitzpatrick, J. Schmeling, R. Ryan, P. Kot, and P. W. Ramwell

463 Effect of an Inhibitor of TXA$_2$ Synthesis and of PGE$_2$ on the Formation of 12L-Hydroxy-5,8,10 Heptadecatrienoic Acid in Human Platelets
J. E. Vincent, F. J. Zijlstra, and H. van Vliet

TX Antagonists

467 Partial Agonism Shown by Prostaglandin H$_2$ Analogues and 11-Deoxy Prostaglandin F$_{2\alpha}$ on Thromboxane-Sensitive Preparations
R. L. Jones and N. H. Wilson

477 Thromboxane Molecules are not Hairpin Conformers
D. A. Langs, G. T. DeTitta, M. G. Erman, and S. Fortier

481   Synthesis of Thromboxane A_2 Analogs
      K. C. Nicolaou, R. L. Magolda, and D. A. Claremon

485   A Structural Analogue of Thromboxane A_2
      *M. F. Ansell, M. P. L. Caton, M. N. Palfreyman, K. A. J. Stuttle,
      D. Tuffin, and J. L. Walker*

489   Pinane Thromboxane A_2(PTA_2): A TXA_2 Antagonist with Antithrom-
      botic Properties
      *D. Aharony, J. B. Smith, E. F. Smith, A. M. Lefer, R. L. Magolda,
      and K. D. Nicolaou*

493   Stereocontrolled Synthesis of 7-Oxabicyclo[2.2.1]Heptane Prostaglandin
      Analogs as TXA_2 Antagonists
      P. W. Sprague, J. E. Heikes, D. N. Harris, and R. Greenberg

497   Thromboxane A_2 Receptor Antagonism Selectively Reverses Platelet Ag-
      gregation
      G. C. Le Breton and D. L. Venton

505   Vasopressin Stimulates Thromboxane Synthesis in the Toad Urinary
      Bladder: Effects of Thromboxane Synthesis Inhibition
      Ronald M. Burch, Daniel R. Knapp, and Perry V. Halushka

511   Use of Inhibitors of P.G. Synthesis in Patients with Breast Cancer
      T. J. Powles, P. J. Dady, Judith Williams, G. C. Easty, and R. C. Coombes

517   Prostaglandin Enhancement of Skin Tumor Initiation and Promotion
      *Susan M. Fischer, Greta L. Gleason, Jeffrey S. Bohrman, and Thomas
      J. Slaga*

523   Effects of Diazepam on Tumor Growth and Plasma PGE_2 in Rats
      R. A. Karmali, A. Volkman, P. Muse, and T. M. Louis

525   The VX-2 Carcinoma: Humoral Effects and Arachidonic Acid Metabo-
      lism
      W. C. Hubbard, A. Hough, A. R. Brash, R. M. Johnson, and J. A. Oates

529   Increased Prostaglandin Synthesis in Hodgkin's Disease: A Lymphocyte–
      Monocyte Interaction
      P. L. Amlot, A. Chivers, D. Heinzelmann, and L. J. F. Youlten

535   Prostaglandin and Thromboxane Production by Fibroblasts and Vascular
      Endothelial Cells
      A. E. Ali, J. C. Barrett, and T. E. Eling

537   Regeneration of Prostacyclin Synthetase Activity in Cultured Vascular
      Cells Following Aspirin Treatment
      K. F. Salata, J. D. Whiting, and J. M. Bailey

541 Endogenous Prostaglandin E₂ Production Inhibits Proliferation of Polyoma Virus Transformed 3T3 Cells: Correlation with Cellular Levels of Cyclic AMP
Hans-Erik Claesson, Jan Åke Lindgren, and Sven Hammarström

547 Prostacyclin Potently Resorbs Bone *In Vitro*
A. Bennett, D. Edwards, N. N. Ali, D. Auger, and M. Harris

549 Essential Fatty Acid Requirements and Metabolism of Cells in Tissue Culture
J. Martyn Bailey

567 Improved Anticancer Effect by Combining Cytotoxic Drugs with an Inhibitor of Prostaglandin Synthesis
D. A. Berstock, J. Houghton, and A. Bennett

571 Human Breast Carcinomas Release Prostaglandin-Like Material Into the Blood
I. F. Stamford, J. MacIntyre, and A. Bennett

575 Prostaglandin Production and Metabolism in Human Breast Cancer
Pierre H. Rolland, Pierre M. Martin, Jocelyne Jacquemier, Anne M. Rolland, and M. Toga

581 Human Benign Breast Disease: Relationships Between Prostaglandin E₂, Steroid Hormones, and Thermographic Effects of the Inhibitors of PG Biosynthesis
Pierre H. Rolland, Pierre M. Martin, Marielle Bourry, Anne M. Rolland, and Henri Serment

585 Perioperative Behavior of PGE₂ and 13,14-dihydro-15-keto-PGF₂α in Serum of Bronchial Carcinoma Patients
L. Fiedler, H. P. Zahradnik, and G. Schlegel

587 Interactions of Cytotoxic and Anti-Inflammatory Agents on Normal and Neoplastic Tissue
T. J. Powles, G. J. Franks, and J. L. Millar

591 Reduction by Flurbiprofen of Primary Tumor Growth and Local Metastasis Formation in Mice
D. J. Leaper, B. French, and A. Bennett

595 Prostaglandins and Their Relationships to Malignant and Benign Human Breast Tumors
A. Bennett, D. A. Berstock, M. Harris, B. Raja, D. J. F. Rowe, I. F. Stamford, and J. E. Wright

Contents of Volume 7

Heart

601 Role of Prostaglandins in Ventricular Reflexes
Gabor Kaley, Thomas H. Hintze, and Edward J. Messina

609 Significance of Prostaglandins and Thromboxane A_2 for the Mode of Action of Cardiovascular Drugs
W. Förster

619 Cardiovascular Effects of Prostacyclin in Man
S. J. Warrington and J. O'Grady

625 Physiological and Biochemical Parameters of Prostacyclin Action on the Heart and the Coronary Vasculature
K. Schrör, R. Rösen, H. -B. Link, and P. Rösen

631 Effect of Prostacyclin on Coronary Blood Flow and Cardiac Activity in Normotensive and Spontaneously Hypertensive Rats
I. E. Smirnov, P. R. Mentz, and Ch. M. Markov

635 Blockage of Partially Obstructed Coronary Arteries with Platelet Thrombi: Comparison Between Its Prevention with Cyclooxygenase Inhibitors Versus Prostacyclin
James W. Aiken, Ronald J. Shebuski, and Robert R. Gorman

641 Comparison of the Effects of PGI_2 and PGE_1 on Coronary and Systemic Hemodynamics and Coronary Arterial Cyclic Nucleotide Levels in Dogs
T. Ito, K. Ogawa, I. Enomoto, H. Hashimoto, I. Kai, and T. Satake

647 Actions of Prostaglandins I_2 and E_2 on Coronary Occlusion-Induced Arrhythmias in the Rat
T. L. S. Au, G. A. Collins, C. J. Harvie, and M. J. A. Walker

651 Effect of Prostacyclin on Ventricular Arrhythmias After Coronary Artery Occlusion in Cats
Robert K. Dix, Gerald J. Kelliher, Theodore Lawrence, and Nancy Jurkiewicz

655 $PGE_{2\alpha}$ Stimulates Release of PGE_2 and PGI_2 in the Isolated Perfused Rat Heart
E. A. M. de Deckere and F. ten Hoor

659 Augmented PGI_2 Synthesis in Dog Heart–Lung Preparation
Shoichi Imai, Yumi Katano, Norio Shimamoto, Yuko Nishikawa, Kouwa Yamashita, Masataka Ishibashi, and Hiroshi Miyazaki

665 Increase of Coronary Flow and Levels of PGE_1 and $PGF_{2\alpha}$ from Ischemic Area of Experimental Myocardial Infarction
K. Ogawa, T. Ito, I. Enomoto, H. Hashimoto, I. Kai, and T. Satake

671 Myocardial Recovery Following Ischemia: *In Vivo* Effects of PGB_1, A Polymeric Derivative of PGB_1
E. T. Angelakos, R. West, and E. Wudarski

675 Dissimilar Effects of PGE_1 and PGE_2 on Myocardial Infarct Size After Coronary Occlusion in Conscious Dogs
Bodh I. Jugdutt, Grover M. Hutchins, Bernadine H. Bulkley, and Lewis C. Becker

Hemodynamics

679 Modification of the Cardiovascular Actions of Prostaglandins by Thromboxane B_2
Peter A. Kot, John C. Rose, Peter W. Ramwell, Thomas M. Fitzpatrick, Miriam F. Bloom, and Lawrence S. Friedman

683 Interactions Between Different Prostaglandins and Other Relaxing Agents on Isolated Vascular Smooth Muscle
Y. Hatano, J. D. Kohli, L. I. Goldberg, and J. Fried

687 Prostacyclin in Therapy of Peripheral Arterial Disease
A. Szczeklik, R. J. Gryglewski, R. Niżankowski, J. Szczeklik, S. Skawiński, and P. Głuszko

695 Modulation of Peritoneal Transport Rates by Prostaglandins
John F. Maher, Przemyslaw Hirszel, and Mark Lasrich

701 Cardiovascular Research on $PGI_{2\alpha}$, 6-Keto-$PGF_{1\alpha}$, $PGF_{2\alpha}$ and 15-(15) 15-Methyl $PGF_{2\alpha}$
Emilio Marmo, Francesco Rossi, Enrico Lampa, Lucio Giordano, Achille P. Caputi, Ciro Vacca, Bruno Ariello, and Federico Rosatti

711 Prostaglandin Endoperoxide D-Isomerase Activity in Vascular Tissue
Thomas P. Parks and Morton P. Printz

715 Release of Prostacyclin into the Bloodstream in Humans After Local Blood Flow Changes (Ischemia and Venous Stasis)
Gian Gastone Neri Serneri, Giulio Masotti, Loredana Poggesi, and Giorgio Galanti

719   Microcirculatory Responses to PGI_2 and PGE_2 in the Rat Cremaster
      Muscle
      Edward J. Messina and Gabor Kaley

723   Hemodynamic Evaluation of Prostaglandin D_2 in the Conscious Baboon
      J. R. Fletcher and P. W. Ramwell

727   A Comparison of the Vascular Responses to Various Prostanoic Com-
      pounds in the Puppy and Adult Dog
      T. Fitzpatrick, R. Harris, P. Ramwell, and P. Kot

                        Pulmonary Vasculature

731   Differential Actions of the Prostaglandins on the Pulmonary Vascular
      Bed
      *Philip J. Kadowitz, Ernst Wm. Spannhake, James L. Levin, and Albert
      L. Hyman*

745   Pulmonary Hypertension Correlated to Pulmonary Thromboxane Synthe-
      sis
      J. C. Frölich, M. Ogletree, B. A. Peskar, and K. L. Brigham

751   Pulmonary Vascular Responses to Prostaglandins in the Conscious New-
      born Lamb
      James E. Lock, Flavio Coceani, and Peter M. Olley

755   Effects of Prostaglandin E_1, Prostacyclin, and Tolazoline on Elevated
      Pulmonary Vascular Resistance in Neonatal Swine
      M. B. Starling, J. M. Neutze, and R. L. Elliott

759   Effect of Prostaglandins E_1 and E_2 on Rabbit Pulmonary Artery and
      Aorta Strips
      Satoshi Kitamura, Yoko Ishihara, and Konori Kosaka

765   Disparate Actions of Arachidonic Acid on Feline Pulmonary Vascular
      Bed
      Albert L. Hyman, Ernst Wm. Spannhake, and Philip J. Kadowitz

                 Cardiovascular Aspects of Hypertension

769   Hemodynamic Effects of Prostacyclin in Man
      J. Szczeklik, A. Szczeklik, and R. Niżankowski

777   Endogenous Mechanisms Which Regulate Prostacyclin Release
      R. J. Gryglewski, J. Spławinski, and R. Korbut

789   An Antihypertensive Effect of Prostacyclin
      Dorothy M. Sutter and James R. Weeks

791   Prostaglandins A + E Levels in Human Essential Hypertension
      T. Michibayashi

797   Ontogeny of Aortic PGI$_2$ Formation in the Developing Spontaneously
      Hypertensive Rat—Correlation with Elevations in Blood Pressure
      C. R. Pace-Asciak and M. C. Carrara

803   Vascular PG Synthesis in Hypertensive and Normotensive Rats
      Randal A. Skidgel and Morton P. Printz

807   A Prostaglandin Mechanism May Contribute to the Regulation of Blood
      Pressure in Spontaneously Hypertensive Rats During Pregnancy
      B. Zamorano, A. Terragno, J. C. McGiff, and N. A. Terragno

811   *In Vitro* and *In Vivo* Effects of Antihypertensive Drugs on PG Metabolism
      in Different Organs
      *W. Förster, Ch. Taube, H. -U. Block, A. Fahr, K. Pönicke, P. Mentz,
      Ch. Giebier, and B. -L. Bayer*

815   Angiotensin-Induced Prostacyclin Release May Contribute to the Hypo-
      tensive Action of Converting Enzyme Inhibitors
      G. J. Dusting, Elizabeth M. Mullins, and A. E. Doyle

Shock and Trauma

821   Indomethacin Improves Survival After Endotoxin in Baboons
      John R. Fletcher and Peter W. Ramwell

829   Effect of Indomethacin on Blood Pressure, Catecholamine, and Renin
      Response to Acute Hemorrhage
      Giora Feuerstein, Nili Feuerstein, and Zvi Gimmon

835   Beneficial Actions of a New Thromboxane Analog in Traumatic Shock
      *Haruo Araki, Allan M. Lefer, J. Bryan Smith, Kyriacos C. Nicolaou,
      and Ronald L. Magolda*

839   Endotoxin-Induced Hypotension and Blood Levels of 6-Keto-Prostaglan-
      din F$_{1\alpha}$
      H. Bult, J. Beetens, P. Vercrysse, and A. G. Herman

851   Prostaglandins, Lysosomes, and Radiation Injury
      Paul J. Trocha and George N. Catravas

857   Time–Course of Arachidonic Acid, Prostaglandins E$_2$ and F$_{2\alpha}$ Production
      in Human Abdominal Skin, Following Irradiation with Ultraviolet
      Wavelengths (290–320 n.m.)
      *C. N. Hensby, N. A. Plummer, A. K. Black, N. Fincham, and M. W.
      Greaves*

861   Characterization of Chemotactic Factors in Corneal Wound Healing
      B. D. Srinivasan, P. S. Kulkarni, and K. E. Eakins

865   Prostaglandins in Wound Healing: Possible Regulation of Granulation
      *Jonathan T. Lord, Vincent A. Ziboh, William D. Cagle, Sevil Kursunoglu,
      and Gregory Redmond*

                            Neonatology

871   Considerations on the Role of Prostaglandins in the Ductus Arteriosus
      F. Coceani and P. M. Olley

879   Prostaglandin E_1 in the Neonate with Heart Disease
      *Margo M. Schleman, Alfonso Casta, Add Mongkolsmai, and Iain F. S.
      Black*

883   Plasma Indomethacin Levels in Preterm Newborns with Symptomatic
      Patent Ductus Arteriosus: Clinical and Echocardiographic Assess-
      ments of Response
      *Bruce S. Alpert, Michael J. Lewins, Dale W. Rowland, Myles J. Grant,
      Peter M. Olley, Steven J. Soldin, Paul R. Swyer, Flavio Coceani, and
      Richard D. Rowe*

887   Ductus Arteriosus: Developmental Response to Endogenous Prostaglan-
      dins, Oxygen, and Indomethacin
      Ronald Ian Clyman

891   6-Keto-$PGF_{1\alpha}$: Concentrations in Human Umbilical Plasma and Pro-
      duction by Umbilical Vessels
      M. D. Mitchell, D. R. S. Jamieson, Susan M. Sellers, and A. C. Turnbull

897   Placental Transfer and Fetal Effects of $PGF_{1\alpha}$ in the Rat
      T. V. N. Persaud

901   Inhibition of Fetal Bone Growth and Augmentation of PGE_2 Resorptive
      Response by Indomethacin
      J. M. Goodson, S. Offenbacher, F. E. Dewhirst, and R. B. Bloomfield

905   Indications and Pharmacological Effects of Therapy with Prostaglandin
      E_1 in the Newborn
      *Johannes G. Schöber, Maximilian Kellner, Rolf Mocellin, Gebhard Schu-
      macher, and Konrad Bühlmeyer*

913   Clinical Use of Prostaglandins and Prostaglandin Synthetase Inhibitors
      in Cardiac Problems of the Newborn
      P. M. Olley, F. Coceani, R. D. Rowe, and P. R. Swyer

                         Respiratory System

917   Pharmacological Control of Thromboxane A_2 Generation in Lungs
      G. C. Folco, C. Omini, T. Vigano, G. Iantorno, and F. Berti

927 Slow Reacting Substance of Anaphylaxis Enhances the Generation of 12-L-Hydroxy-5,8,10,14-Eicosa Tetraenoic Acid in Isolated Lungs
C. Omini, L. Sautebin, G. Galli, G. C. Folco, and F. Berti

933 Metabolism of ^{3}H-Arachidonic Acid by Male Dog Lung *In Vitro* Using a Perfusion System Designed to Mimic Physiological Conditions
P. Barnes, C. T. Dollery, and C. N. Hensby

937 Dissimilar *In Vivo* Effects of Arachidonic Acid on the Canine Pulmonary Vascular Bed and Airways
Ernst Wm. Spannhake, Albert L. Hyman, and Philip J. Kadowitz

943 Ventilatory and Cardiovascular Effects of Prostacyclin and 6-Oxo-PGF$_{1\alpha}$ by Inhalation
M. Pasarglikian and S. Bianco

953 Effects of Lung Toxins on PGF$_{2\alpha}$ and PGE$_2$ Levels in Plasma and Combined Pleural Effusion and Lung Lavage of Rats
S. N. Giri and M. A. Hollinger

957 Release of Dilator Prostaglandins from Rat Lung During Angiotensin II-Induced Vasoconstriction
N. F. Voelkel, J. G. Gerber, I. F. McMurtry, J. T. Reeves, and A. S. Nies

961 Effects of Captopril on Bradykinin-Induced, Prostaglandin-Mediated Bronchoconstriction in the Guinea Pig
R. Greenberg, G. H. Osman, Jr., E. H. O'Keefe, and M. J. Antonaccio

965 Clinical Evaluation of Main Urinary Metabolite of PGF in Chronic Lung Diseases
Makoto Murao, Kyoichi Uchiyama, Wataru Takahashi, Fumio Hirata, and Toshio Inagawa

969 Prostaglandins and Human Respiratory Tract Smooth Muscle: Structure Activity Relationship
S. M. M. Karim, P. G. Adaikan, and S. R. Kottegoda

981 Thromboxane B$_2$ Inhibits the Pulmonary Metabolism of PGE$_2$ in the Anesthetized Dog
Lawrence S. Friedman, Thomas M. Fitzpatrick, Peter W. Ramwell, and Peter A. Kot

985 Studies on 20-Isopropylidene PGE$_2$ as a New Aerosol Bronchodilator
Makoto Murao, Kyoichi Uchiyama, Akira Shida, Kiyoshi Sakai, Takashi Yusa, and Takeshi Yamaguichi

989 Synthesis and Bronchodilation Activity of 8,10,12-Triazaprostaglandin Analogues
D. R. Adams, A. F. Barnes, J. Bermudez, and F. Cassidy

993 Aspirin, Prostaglandins, and Bronchial Asthma
     *A. Szczeklik, R. J. Gryglewski, G. Czerniawska-Mysik, and E. Nizan-
     kowska*

995 Prostaglandins as Mediators of Tachyphylaxis to Histamine in Canine
     Tracheal Smooth Muscle
     W. H. Anderson, J. J. Krzanowski, J. B. Polson, and A. Szentivanyi

1003 Receptors for E and F Prostaglandins in Airways
     P. J. Gardiner and H. O. J. Collier

1009 Interactions of Vasopressin in Renal Prostaglandins in the Homozygous
     Diabetes Insipidus Rat
     *Michael J. Dunn, Lewis B. Kinter, Reinier Beeuwkes III, David Shier,
     Harold P. Greeley, and Heinz Valtin*

                              ✓ Diuresis

1017 Water Diuresis is a Major Regulator of PGE Excretion in Man
     Z. Kaye, R. Zipser, J. Hahn, P. Zia, and R. Horton

1021 Interaction Between Renal Prostaglandin Metabolism and Salt and Water
     Balance in Healthy Man
     *Herbert J. Kramer, Werner Prior, Bruno Stinnesbeck, Angela Bäcker,
     Jutta Eden, and Rainer Düsing*

1027 Monovalent Cations and Renomedullary Prostaglandin Release
     Howard R. Knapp and John A. Oates

1033 Urinary Prostaglandins in the Newborn: Relationship to Urinary Osmo-
     lality, Urinary Potassium, and Blood Pressure
     Burkhard Scherer and Peter C. Weber

1039 Effects of Meclofenamate on the Renal Actions of Mannitol Infusion
     in Conscious Rabbits. Evidence for Osmotic Control of Renal P. G.
     Synthesis?
     J. Bhattacharya and L. J. Beilin

1047 A Role of Renal Cortical Prostaglandins in the Control of Glomerular
     Filtration Rate in Rat Kidneys
     Jürgen Schnermann and Peter C. Weber

1053 Stimulation of Rabbit Renal PGE_2 Biosynthesis by Dietary Restriction
     of Sodium
     *Rolf A. K. Stahl, Ahmad A. Attallah, Dean L. Bloch, and James B.
     Lee*

1057 Comparison of the Effects of PGE_2 and PGI_2 in Salt-Loaded and Salt-
     Depleted Dogs
     M. L. Watson and R. L. Jones

1061   Effect of Chronic Intrarenal Prostaglandin E_2 Infusion and Angiotensin II Blockade on Arterial Pressure in the Dog
       Gregory M. Hockel and Allen W. Cowley, Jr.

1067   Possible Significance of Renal Prostaglandins for Renin Release and Blood Pressure Control
       Peter C. Weber, Burkhard Scherer, Wolfgang Siess, Eckhard Held, and Jürgen Schnermann

1079   Furosemide-Induced Renal Vasodilation: The Role of the Release of Arachidonic Acid
       John G. Gerber and Alan S. Nies

1083   Restoration of the Diuretic Response to Acetylcholine by Prostaglandin E_2 in Indomethacin-Treated Dogs
       John C. H. Yun, John R. Gill, Jr., Leslie Costello, Harry R. Keiser, and Gerald Kelly

1089   Relationship Between Urinary Prostaglandin (PGE_2 and PGF_2) and Sodium Excretion in Various Stages of Chronic Liver Disease
       H. Wernze, G. Müller, and M. Goerig

1097   Formation of Prostaglandins in Rat and Rabbit Kidney: Effect of Furosemide
       J. E. Vincent and F. J. Zijlstra

1103   Possible Role for Ca^{2+}-Dependent Arachidonate Release and Prostaglandin Synthesis in Expression of the Action of Osmolality on Renal Inner Medullary cGMP
       Patricia A. Craven and Frederick R. De Rubertis

1107   Differential Effects of Deamino-8-D-Arginine Vasopressin on Urinary PGE_2 and $PGF_{2\alpha}$ Excretion
       Larry Walker and J. C. Frölich

1111   The Renal Prostaglandin System in Central Diabetes Insipidus: Effects of Desamino-Arginine Vasopressin
       R. Düsing, R. Herrmann, and H. J. Kramer

1115   Inhibition of Prostaglandins Biosynthesis Lowers Antidiuretic Hormone Excretion in Man
       Philippe Glasson and Michel B. Vallotton

Renal Aspects of Hypertension

1119   Prostaglandins and Plasma Renin Activity in Hypertensive Patients
       A. Hornych, G. London, M. Safar, Y. Weiss, A. Simon, T. T. Guyene, J. Bariéty, and P. Milliez

1123 Prostaglandin-Mediated Renin Release from Renal Cortical Slices
A. R. Whorton, J. D. Lazar, M. D. Smigel, and J. A. Oates

1131 Identification of Thromboxane A_2 in Glycerol-Induced Acute Renal Failure in the Rabbit
Aubrey R. Morrison, Julio E. Benabe, and Michael K. Hoffmann

1135 Prostaglandins Mediate the Macula Densa Stimulated Renin Release
Richard D. Olson, Marcia L. Skoglund, Alan S. Nies, and John G. Gerber

1139 Prostaglandins of Blood Vessels and the Vessel Reactivity in Rats Receiving Sodium Chloride and Indomethacin
A. A. Nekrasova, R. N. Sokolova, Yu. Levitskaya, N. V. Speranskaya, V. P. Kulagina, and N. P. Leghonkaya

1145 Reduction of Renal Prostaglandin E Formation in Essential Hypertension
Peter C. Weber, Burkhard Scherer, Eckhard Held, and Wolfgang Siess

1149 Angiotensin II-Induced Renal Prostacyclin Release Suppresses Platelet Aggregation in the Anesthetized Dog
Ronald J. Shebuski and James W. Aiken

1153 Interrelationship Between Renal Prostaglandin E, Renin, and Renal Vascular Tone in Conscious Dogs
Ben G. Zimmerman, Craig Mommsen, and Edward Kraft

1159 Prostacyclin Release Induced by Bradykinin May Contribute to the Antihypertensive Action of Angiotensin-Converting Enzyme Inhibitors
K. M. Mullane, S. Moncada, and J. R. Vane

Renal Pathology

1163 Role of Prostaglandins in Potassium-Depletion Nephropathy
Frederic C. Bartter

1171 Exaggerated Prostaglandin and Thromboxane Synthesis in the Renal Vein-Constricted Rabbit
Stuart Myers, Robert Zipser, and Philip Needleman

1175 The Role of Prostaglandins and Thromboxane in Modulation of Perfusion Pressure in the Hydronephrotic Rabbit Kidney
Mark Sivakoff, Sandra Holmberg, and Philip Needleman

1177 Prostaglandin Synthesis in Glomeruli from Rats with Unilateral Ureteral Obstruction
Detlef Schlondorff and Vaughn W. Folkert

1181 Prostaglandin Biosynthesis in Normal and Ureteral Obstructed Rabbit Kidney: Formation of a Novel Metabolite
Dina Van Praag and Saul J. Farber

1185 The Principal Metabolites of Arachidonic Acid are Overproduced in Bartter's Syndrome
Hans-George Güllner, J. Bryan Smith, and Frederic C. Bartter

1189 The Effect of Potassium Depletion on Urinary Prostaglandins in Normal Man
R. Düsing, J. R. Gill, Jr., F. C. Bartter, and H. G. Güllner

1193 Contribution of Urine Volume to the Elevated Urinary Prostaglandin E in Bartter's Syndrome and Central and Nephrogenic Diabetes Insipidus
M. Fichman, P. Zia, and R. Zipser

1199 Is the Platelet Defect in Bartter's Syndrome Associated with a Plasma Prostaglandin?
D. E. MacIntyre, M. Smith, L. Levine, J. S. Stoff, M. Stemerman, M. L. Steer, E. W. Salzman, and R. S. Brown

1203 The Clinical Entity of Pseudo-Bartter's Syndrome
Laurence M. Demers, Johannes D. Veldhuis, and Emilio Ramos

Contents of Volume 8

Nervous System

1207 Local Analgesic Effect of Morphine on the Hyperalgesia Induced by cAMP, Ca^{2+}, Isoprenaline, and PGE_2
Sergio H. Ferreira

1217 Formation of Prostaglandins in Rat Brain. Lack of Effect of Enkephalin
J. E. Vincent, F. J. Zijlstra, and M. R. Dzoljic

1221 Metabolism of PGH_2 in the Feline Brain
I. Bishai and F. Coceani

1225 Pressor Action of Centrally Administered Prostaglandin E_1
Nancy J. Kenney and Eve Perara

1231 Effects of Intracerebroventricular Arachidonic Acid and Indomethacin on Angiotensin-Induced Drinking
Steven J. Fluharty and Alan N. Epstein

1235 Factors Affecting Brain Prostaglandin Formation
C. Galli, C. Spagnuolo, and A. Petroni

1241 Sympathetic Nerve Stimulation of the Isolated Rat Heart: Release of a Prostaglandin-like Substance and the Inhibitory Effect of Prostacyclin on the Output of [^{3}H]-Norepinephrine
K. U. Malik

1245 Aspects of Prostaglandin Action on Autonomic Neuroeffector Transmission
Per Hedqvist, Lars Gustafsson, Paul Hjemdahl, and Kerstin Svanborg

1249 Influence of Prostacyclin on Sympathetic Neurotransmission in the Feline Intestinal Vascular Bed
Howard L. Lippton, Barry M. Chapnick, Albert L. Hyman, and Philip J. Kadowitz

1255 Modulatory Role of Prostaglandins on Cholinergic Neurotransmission in the Guinea Pig Ileum
Ondřej Kadlec, Isidor Šeferna, and Karel Mašek

1259 The Plasma Membrane Sodium Pump, PGE_2 Release, and Acidic Phospholipid Turnover in the Guinea Pig Taenia Coli
R. F. Coburn, M. Cunningham, J. Diegel, and J. F. Strauss, III

1263 Production and Effects of Prostaglandins in the Detrusor from Homo, Cat, Rabbit, and Rat
Carin Larsson

1269 Prostacyclin Stimulates Short Circuit Current in the Isolated Toad *(Bufo marinus)* Urinary Bladder
Perry V. Halushka, Alain Levanho, and Miklos Auber

1273 Effects of Indomethacin on Quantal Acetylcholine Release at the Frog Neuromuscular Junction
Kathleen Shaver Madden and William Van der Kloot

1277 Sex and Gonadal Steroid Effects on Arachidonate Uptake into Rat Platelets
E. M. K. Leovey, E. R. Ramey, Y. Maddox, and P. W. Ramwell

Endocrinology

1283 An Imbalance in Arachidonic Acid Metabolism in Diabetes
M. Johnson, A. H. Reece, and H. E. Harrison

1287 Improvement of Defective Insulin Responses to Glucose, Arginine, and β-Adrenergic Stimulation in Diabetics by Sodium Salicylate
John R. McRae, Mei Chen, and R. Paul Robertson

1291 A Role for Prostaglandins as Mediators of α-Adrenergic Inhibition of the Acute Insulin Response to Glucose
Stewart A. Metz, Wilfred Y. Fujimoto, and R. Paul Robertson

1295 Effects of Prostaglandins H_2, D_2, I_2, and Thromboxane on *In Vitro* Secretion of Glucagon and Insulin
S. Pek, W. E. M. Lands, J. Akpan, and M. Hurley

1299 Endogenous Prostaglandins Modulate Glucagon Secretion by Isolated Guinea Pig Islets
A. S. Luyckx and P. J. Lefebvre

1303 Effects of Prostaglandin Inhibitors on Pituitary and Thyroid Responses to Thyrotropin Releasing Hormone in Man: PGs and Pituitary-Thyroid System
E. Pasargiklian, G. De Rosa, L. Troncone, I. Modugno, M. A. Satta, and M. Maussier

1309 Effects of Arachidonic Acid on the Thyroid Gland *In Vitro*
J. M. Boeynaems, J. Van Sande, C. Decoster, and J. E. Dumont

1313 $PGF_{2\alpha}$ Regulation of LH Action on Testicular Testosterone Production
Udon Chantharaksri and Anna-Riitta Fuchs

1317 Lactogenesis Induced by Prostaglandin $F_{2\alpha}$ in Pregnant Rabbits
R. P. Deis, L. M. Houdebine, and C. Delouis

1321 Role of Prostaglandins on Growth Hormone Secretion: PGE_2, A Physiological Stimulator
F. Dray, B. Kouznetzova, D. Harris, and P. Brazeau

1329 Hormone Receptor Control of Prostaglandin $F_{2\alpha}$ Secretion by the Ovine Uterus
John A. McCracken

Reproductive Physiology

1345 Uterine Prostaglandin-Forming Cyclooxygenase: Relationship to Luteolysis and Subcellular Localization
William L. Smith, Richard L. Huslig, Thomas E. Rollins, and R. L. Fogwell

1351 On the Control of Prostaglandin Release During the Bovine Estrous Cycle
Hans Kindahl, Lars-Eric Edqvist, and Jan-Otto Lindell

1357 Characterization of Rat Ovarian Prostaglandin Synthetase
Martin R. Clark, Gagan B. N. Chainy, John M. Marsh, and William J. LeMaire

1361 Arachidonic Acid in Guinea Pig Uterus and Plasma
H. Anne Leaver and Norman L. Poyser

1365 Is Vascular Innervation a Prerequisite for PG-Induced Luteolysis in the Human Corpus Luteum?
L. Hamberger, B. Dennefors, B. Hamberger, P. O. Janson, L. Nilsson, A. Sjögren, and N. Wiqvist

1369 Catechol Oestrogens Stimulate Uterine Prostaglandin Production
Rodney W. Kelly and Margaret H. Abel

1371 Significance of Prostaglandins in the Regulation of Cyclic Events in the Ovary and Uterus
H. R. Lindner, U. Zor, F. Kohen, S. Bauminger, A. Amsterdam, M. Lahav, and Y. Salomon

1391 Prostaglandins and Implantation in the Rat
Christine A. Phillips and N. L. Poyser

1395 Inhibition of PG Biosynthesis as the Maintenance Mechanism of Pregnancy of hCG
Kunio Itoh, Ming-Hung Kuo, Katsuo Omi, Hiroshi Suzuki, Keikichi Kunimoto, and Yoshimaro Hata

1401 Prostaglandin Levels in Cord Venous Plasma at Delivery Related to Labor
I. Z. MacKenzie, Susan Bradley, and M. D. Mitchell

1407 Sequential Prostaglandin Metabolite Values in Pregnant Patients Delivering at Term and Preterm
J. W. C. Johnson, N. H. Dubin, S. Calhoun, R. B. Ghodgaonkar, and J. C. Beck

1409 Plasma Levels of Prostaglandin Metabolites During Spontaneous Delivery
B. Weppelmann, H. O. Hoppen, U. Gethmann, and E. Schuster

1413 Spatial and Temporal Variations in Prostacyclin Production by the Rat Pregnant Uterus
K. I. Williams and K. E. H. El Tahir

1419 Bioconversion of Arachidonic Acid in Human Amnion During Pregnancy and Labor
Katsuyuki Kinoshita, Kazuo Satoh, Takehiko Yasumizu, Shoichi Sakamoto, and Krister Green

1423 Concentrations of Thromboxane B_2 and 6-Oxo-Prostaglandin $F_{1\alpha}$ in Amniotic Fluid, Decidual Tissue, and Placenta in the Later Stages of Pregnancy in the Rat
J. Zamecnik, T. G. Kennedy, and D. T. Armstrong

1431 Arachidonic Acid Content of Decidua, Fetal Membranes, and Amniotic Fluid in Early and Near-Term Pregnancy
Anders Ölund and Nils-Olov Lunell

Obstetrics and Gynecology

1435 The Role of a Long-Acting Vaginal Suppository of 15-ME-PGF$_{2\alpha}$ in First and Second Trimester Abortion
Niels H. Lauersen and Kathleen H. Wilson

1443 Prostaglandin Levels in Menstrual Fluid of Nondysmenorrheic and of Dysmenorrheic Subjects With and Without Oral Contraceptive or Ibuprofen Therapy
W. Y. Chan and M. Yusoff Dawood

1449 Mefenamic Acid Therapy in Dysmenorrhea
Penny W. Budoff

1455 Prostaglandin F_2 and E_2 in Primary Dysmenorrhea
Viveca Lundström and Marc Bygdeman

1459 Management of Uterine Bleeding by PGs or Their Synthesis Inhibitors
M. Toppozada, A. El-Attar, M. A. El-Ayyat, and Y. Khamis

1465 Treatment of Premature Labor with Indomethacin
David A. Blake, Jennifer R. Niebyl, Robert D. White, Karen M. Kumor, Norman H. Dubin, J. Courtland Robinson, and Patricia G. Egner

1469 Systemic Absorption from the Vagina of PGE_2 Administered for the
      Induction of Labor
      M. G. Elder and A. P. Gordon-Wright

1477 Intravaginal PGE_2 Gel Prior to Labor Induction
      I. Z. MacKenzie and M. P. Embrey

1483 The Use of Two-Channel Telemetric Systems in Obstetrics: An Ideal
      Monitoring Method for Oral PGE_2 Induction of Labor
      H. Steiner, D. Robrecht, W. Deichsel, M. Breckwoldt, and H. G. Hille-
      manns

1487 Treatment of Primary Dysmenorrhea and Dysmenorrhea Because of IUP
      with PG-Synthetase Inhibitors
      E. Dreher and B. von Fischer

                          Gastrointestinal

1495 Prostaglandin-Synthesizing System in Rat Liver Changes with Aging
      and Various Stimuli
      Sei-itsu Murota and Ikuo Morita

1507 Comparison of the Effect of Continuous Intravenous Infusion of Prosta-
      glandins E_1, E_2, I, or 6-Keto-$PGF_{1\alpha}$ on Lower Esophageal Sphincter
      Pressure
      D. R. Sinar, J. R. Fletcher, and D. O. Castell

1511 Synthesis and Metabolism of Endogenous Prostaglandins by Human Gas-
      tric Mucosa
      B. M. Peskar, H. W. Seyberth, and B. A. Peskar

1515 Prostaglandin Synthesis by Dog Gastrointestinal Tract
      Louise E. LeDuc and Philip Needleman

1519 Protection Against Topical Damaging Agents and Stimulation of Gastric
      Nonparietal Cell Secretion by 16, 16-Dimethyl PGE_2
      I. H. M. Main and R. Melarange

1521 Gastric Antisecretory and Cardiovascular Actions of a Stable 16-Phenoxy
      Prostacyclin Analog in the Dog
      G. L. Kauffman, Jr., B. J. R. Whittle, D. Aures, and M. I. Grossman

1525 Prevention of Aspirin-Induced Fecal Blood Loss in Men with Prostaglan-
      din E_2
      Max M. Cohen, Gladys Cheung, and Donald M. Lyster

1529 Inhibition of Acid Secretion from the Rat Isolated Gastric Mucosa by
      Arachidonic Acid and Identification of Major Metabolites
      M. H. Frame, C. N. Hensby, and I. H. M. Main

1533 Prostaglandins and Digestive Diseases
      André Robert

1543 Selectivity of Action of Prostaglandins on Acid-Secretion Induced by Histamine, Gastrin, and Nerve Stimulation, *In Vitro*
A. W. Baird, I. H. M. Main, and J. B. Pearce

1547 A Hypothesis Concerning the Protective Action of Paracetamol Against the Erosive Activity of Acetylsalicylic Acid in the Rat Stomach
A. J. M. Seegers, L. P. Jager, and J. van Noordwijk

1553 Effects of Prostaglandins on Gastric Acid and Mucus Secretion
T. Metsä-Ketelä, J. Parantainen, and H. Vapaatalo

1557 Effect of Prostacyclin on Gastric Emptying and Secretion in Rhesus Monkeys
P. T. Shea-Donohue, L. Myers, D. O. Castell, and A. Dubois

1559 Trimethoquinol Selectively Antagonizes Contractions of Rat Gastric Fundus to TXB_2 and Epoxymethano Analogs of PGH_2
G. J. Sanger and A. Bennett

1561 Effect of Prostacyclin on Pancreatic Secretion in Dogs
Stanislaw J. Konturek, Janina Tasler, Jolanta Jaworek, and Marek Cieszkowski

1569 Effects of Various Prostanoids on Gallbladder Muscle
J. R. Wood, S. H. Saverymuttu, A. B. Ashbrooke, and I. F. Stamford

1573 Prostaglandins, Bradykinin, and Rat Ileum
R. Walker and K. A. Wilson

1577 Effects of 16,16-Dimethyl PGE_2 on Bile-Induced Increases in H^+ Permeability of Rabbit Esophagus
John W. Harmon, Lawrence F. Johnson, and Corinne L. Maydonovitch

1581 E Prostaglandins and the Stomach: Pathophysiological Mediators or Therapeutic Agents?
André Dubois

1587 PGE_2 Involvement in the Regulation of Gastric Emptying
D. Nompleggi, L. Myers, P. Ramwell, D. Castell, and A. Dubois

1589 Effects of Prostaglandin E_1, Administered by Gastric Intubation, on Mucus Secretory Patterns in Rat Small Intestine
Marie M. Cassidy and Fred G. Lightfoot

1595 Saturation Kinetics Applied to the Inhibition by PGE_2 of Ion Transport in the Isolated Human Jejunum
J. Rask-Madsen and K. Bukhave

1603 Mechanism of Stimulation of Gastrointestinal Propulsion in Postoperative Ileus Rats by 16,16-Dimethyl PGE_2
M. J. Ruwart, M. S. Klepper, and B. D. Rush

1609   PGF$_{2\alpha}$—A New Therapy for Paralytic Ileus?
       L. Fiedler

1611   Changes in Electromyogram of Isolated Cat Colon Induced by Prosta-
       glandin E$_2$
       N. L. Shearin and K. Kowalewski

1617   Activation of Human Colonic Mucosal Adenylate Cyclase by Prostaglan-
       dins
       Bernd Simon, Horst Kather, and Burkhard Kommerell

1621   Rectal Mucosal Prostaglandin E Release and Electrolyte Transport in
       Ulcerative Colitis
       *D. S. Rampton, G. E. Sladen, K. K. Bhakoo, D. I. Heinzelmann, and
       L. J. F. Youlten*

1627   An Approach to Evaluation of Local Intestinal PG Production and Clini-
       cal Assessment of Its Inhibition by Indomethacin in Chronic Diarrhoea
       K. Bukhave and J. Rask-Madsen

1633   Mechanism of Action of Castor Oil: A Biochemical Link to the Prosta-
       glandins
       *John R. Luderer, Laurence M. Demers, Charles T. Nomides, and Arthur
       H. Hayes, Jr.*

Inflammation

1637   Prostaglandins and Inflammation: Receptor/Cyclase Coupling as an Ex-
       planation of why PGEs and PGI$_2$ Inhibit Functions of Inflammatory
       Cells
       Gerald Weissmann, James E. Smolen, and Helen Korchak

1655   Human and Animal Monocyte Heterogeneity Expressed Through the
       Synthesis of Prostaglandins and Related Lipids
       Marc E. Goldyne, Mike S. Kennedy, and John D. Stobo

1661   Prostaglandin and Thromboxane Production by Rabbit Polymorphonu-
       clear Leukocytes and Rat Macrophages
       *E. M. Davidson, M. V. Doig, A. W. Ford-Hutchinson, and M. J. H.
       Smith*

1665   Metabolism of Arachidonic Acid and Prostaglandin Endoperoxide by
       Assorted Leukocytes
       J. C. McGuire and F. F. Sun

1669   Regulatory Role of Prostaglandins in the Primary and Secondary Immune
       Response to SRBC in Mice. The *In Vivo* and *In Vitro* Effect on Plaque-
       Forming Cell Response of Primed Spleen Cells
       *Y. Hokama, M. Matsuo, M. P. Lam, B. S. Joyo, C. E. Siu, A. H. Morita,
       J. K. Teraoka, N. Oishi, and L. H. Kimura*

1675   Effects of Prostaglandin E_1 on T Cell Function *In Vivo*
     M. J. Parnham, G. A. P. Schoester, and Th. van der Kwast

1679   Dexamethasone Inhibits the Release of Prostaglandins and the Formation of Autophagic Vacuoles from Stimulated Macrophages
     K. Brune, H. Kälin, K. D. Rainsford, and K. Wagner

1685   E-Rosette Formation in Multiple Sclerosis
     Paula Dore-Duffy and Robert B. Zurier

1691   Prostaglandin E_2 and Prostacyclin Elevate Cyclic AMP Levels in Elicited Populations of Mouse Peritoneal Macrophages
     Robert J. Bonney, Sharon Burger, Philip Davies, Fred A. Kuehl, Jr., and John L. Humes

1695   Lysosomal Enzyme Release from Human Granulocytes is Inhibited by Indomethacin, ETYA, and BPB
     James E. Smolen and Gerald Weissmann

1701   Secretion of Inflammatory Mediators from Synovial Fibroblasts: Dissociation of Collagenase and Prostaglandin Release
     Rodger M. McMillan, John V. Fahey, Constance E. Brinckerhoff, and Edward D. Harris, Jr.

1705 PGE_2, $PGF_{2\alpha}$, and TXB_2 Biosynthesis by Human Rheumatoid Synovia
     F. Blotman, J. Chaintreuil, P. Poubelle, O. Flandre, A. Crastes de Paulet, and L. Simon

1709   Stimulation of Prostaglandin Biosynthesis Induced by Mononuclear Cell Factor Added to Cells from Human Gingiva, Cartilage, Synovium, and Endometrium
     D. J. Englis, S. M. D'Souza, J. E. Meats, J. Wright, M. B. McGuire, and R. G. G. Russell

1713   Alteration of Granuloma Formation by PGE_1: Effects of an Adenylate Cyclase Inhibitor and Splenectomy
     M. J. Parnham, M. J. P. Adolfs, and I. L. Bonta

1717 PGE_1 but not PGI_2 Desensitizes the PGI_2 Receptor–Adenylate Cyclase Complex in Human Foreskin Fibroblasts
     Robert R. Gorman and Nancy K. Hopkins

1723   Flurbiprofen and Human Intraocular Inflammation
     Jeffrey S. Hillman, G. J. Frank, and M. B. Kheskani

1727   Differential Inflammatory Effects of Arachidonic Acid on Rabbit Conjunctiva and Iris: A Possible Role of Lipoxygenase in the Conjunctival Response
     P. Bhattacherjee, P. S. Kulkarni, and K. E. Eakins

1733   Changes of Prostaglandin and Thromboxane Levels in Pleural Fluid of
       Rat Carrageenin-Induced Pleurisy
       *M. Katori, Y. Harada, K. Tanaka, H. Miyazaki, M. Ishibashi, and Y.
       Yamashita*

1739   Cyclic AMP and Prostaglandins in Periodontal Disease
       Tawfik M. A. ElAttar and Hsien S. Lin

1741   Mechanisms of Action of Antiinflammatory Drugs
       W. Dawson

1747   Effect of Prostaglandins on Complement Receptors of Human Lympho-
       cytes
       D. Venza-Teti and A. Misefari

1751   Potentiation of Thromboxane B_2 Release from Guinea Pig Lung During
       Anaphylaxis Following Exposure to 100% O_2
       David J. Crutchley, Jeff A. Boyd, and Thomas E. Eling

1755   Enhancement of Antigen-Induced Tracheal Contraction by Cyclooxy-
       genase Inhibition
       J. F. Burka and N..A. M. Paterson

1759   Radioimmunoassay of Thromboxane B_2 in Plasma of Normal and Asth-
       matic Subjects
       *Helen G. Morris, Nancy A. Sherman, Frances T. Shepperdson, and John
       C. Selner*

1765   Prostaglandin-Like Substances in Urine of Asthmatic Patients
       Helen G. Morris and Nancy A. Sherman

Nutrition

1771   Dietary Manipulation of Prostaglandin and Thromboxane Synthesis in
       Heart, Aorta, and Blood Platelets of the Rat
       *F. ten Hoor, E. A. M. de Deckere, E. Haddeman, G. Hornstra, and
       J. F. A. Quadt*

1783   Effect of Fasting and Sex Steroids on Arachidonate Uptake into Rat
       Platelets
       E. M. K. Leovey, E. R. Ramey, Y. Maddox, and P. W. Ramwell

1787   Effects of Diets Varying in Fat and P/S Ratio on Arachidonic Acid
       Metabolism in Human Platelets
       N. W. Schoene, J. T. Judd, M. W. Marshall, V. Reeves, and A. Carvalho

1791   Effects of Dietary Linoleic Acid on the Biosynthesis of PGE_2 and $PGF_{2\alpha}$
       in Kidney Medullae in Spontaneously Hypertensive Rats
       N. W. Schoene, V. B. Reeves, and A. Ferretti

1793 Effect of Different Amounts of Linoleic Acid in the Diet on the Excretion of Urinary Prostaglandin Metabolites in the Rat
D. H. Nugteren, W. C. van Evert, W. J. Soeting, and J. H. Spuy

1797 Essential Fatty Acid Supplementation Inhibits the Effect of Dietary Zinc Deficiency
S. C. Cunnane, G. E. Sella, and D. F. Horrobin

1799 Effects of Dietary Variation in Linoleic Acid Content on the Major Urinary Metabolites of the E Prostaglandins (PGE-M) in Infants
Zvi Friedman, Hannsjorg Seyberth, Jurgen Frölich, and John Oates

1807 Mammary Gland Prostaglandin Synthesis: Effect of Dietary Lipid and Propyl Gallate
D. To, F. L. Smith, and M. P. Carpenter

1813 Influence of Various Lipid Components of Kidneys of Rats Fed Diets Rich or Poor in Linoleic Acid on Prostacyclin Biosynthesis
J. Beitz and W. Förster

1817 Subject Index

Contributors

A

Abbate, Rosanna, 317
Abel, Margaret H., 1369
Adaikan, P. G., 969
Adams, D. R., 989
Adolfs, M. J. P., 1713
Aharony, D., 489
Aiken, James W., 355,635,1149
Alexander, Michael, 293
Ali, A. E., 535
Ali, N. N., 547
Alpert, Bruce S., 883
Amlot, P. L., 529
Amsterdam, A., 1371
Andersen, Niels H., 389
Anderson, W. H., 287,995
Angelakos, E. T., 671
Ansell, M. F., 485
Antonaccio, M. J., 437,961
Arai, Y., 19,327,337
Araki, Haruo, 835
Ariello, Bruno, 701
Armstrong, D. T., 1423
Ashbrooke, A. B., 1569
Attallah, Ahmad A., 1053
Au, T. L. S., 647
Auber, Miklos, 1269
Auger, D., 547
Aures, D., 1521

B

Bäcker, Angelo, 1021
Bailey, J. Martyn, 95,309,537,549
Baird, A. W., 1543
Baran, John S., 235
Barirty, J., 1119
Barnes, A. F., 989
Barnes, P., 933
Barrett, J. C., 535
Bartmann, W., 341
Barton, J., 427

Bartter, Frederic C., 1163,1185,1189
Bauminger, S., 1371
Bayer, B.-L., 811
Beck, G., 341
Beck, J. C., 1407
Becker, Lewis C., 675
Beetens, J., 839
Beeuwkes, R. III, 1009
Beilin, L. J., 1039
Beitz, J., 1813
Bell, R. L., 219
Benabe, Julio E., 1131
Bennett, A., 399,547,567,571,591,
   595,1559
Bermudez, J., 989
Berstock, D. A., 567,595
Berti, F., 917,927
Best, L. C., 297
Beveridge, George C., 153
Bhakoo, K. K., 1621
Bhattacharya, J., 1039
Bhattacherjee, P., 1727
Bianchine, Joseph R., 293
Bianco, S., 943
Bienkowski, Michael J., 149
Bishoi, I., 1221
Black, A. K., 857
Black, Iain F. S., 879
Blake, David A., 1465
Bloch, Dean L., 1053
Block, H.-U., 811
Bloom, Miriam F., 679
Bloomfield, R. B., 901
Blotman, F., 1705
Boeynaems, J. M., 1309
Bohrman, Jeffrey S., 517
Bonney, Robert J., 1691
Bonser, R. W., 249,259
Bonta, I. L., 1713
Borgeat, P., 1
Bourry, Marielle, 581
Bovaird, L., 365

Boyd, Jeff A., 1751
Bradley, Susan, 1401
Brash, A. R., 525
Brazeau, P., 1321
Breckwoldt, M., 1483
Briel, R. C., 351
Brigham, K. L., 745
Brinckerhoff, Constance E., 1701
Brown, C. Alan, 243
Brown, R. S., 1199
Brown, V. R., 111
Brune, K., 1679
Bryant, Robert W., 95,309
Budoff, Penny W., 1449
Bühlmeyer, Konrad, 905
Bukhave, K., 1595,1627
Bulkley, Bernadine H., 675
Bult, H., 839
Burch, Ronald M., 505
Burger, Sharon, 1691
Burka, J. F., 1755
Buytenhek, M., 139
Bygdeman, Marc, 87

C

Cagle, William D., 865
Calhoun, S., 1407
Caputi, Achille, 701
Carpenter, M. P., 1807
Carrara, M. C., 797
Carsten, Mary E., 401
Carvalho, A., 1787
Cassidy, F., 989
Cassidy, Marie M., 1589
Casta, Alfonso, 879
Castell, D. O., 1507,1557,1587
Castrucci, G., 187
Caton, P. L., 485
Catravas, George N., 851
Chaing, Gagan B. N., 1357
Chaintreuil, J., 1705
Chan, W. Y., 1443
Chandrabose, K. A., 249,259
Chanh, Pham Huu, 411
Chanh, Pham Huu A., 411
Chantharaksri, Udon, 1313
Chapnick, Barry, 385,1249
Chen, Mei, 1287

Cheung, Gladys, 1525
Chivers, A., 529
Christ-Hazelhof, E., 129
Chuang, H. Y. K., 287
Ciabattoni, G., 187,207
Cieszkowski, Marek, 1561
Cinotti, G. A., 207
Claesson, Hans-Erik, 275,541
Claremon, D. A., 481
Clark, Martin R., 1357
Clyman, Ronald Ian, 887
Coburn, R. F., 1259
Coceani, Flavio, 751,871,883,913,1221
Cohen, Max M., 1525
Collier, H. O. J., 1003
Collins, G. A., 647
Coombs, R. C., 511
Corey, E. J., 19
Costello, Leslie, 1083
Cowley, Allen W., Jr., 1061
Craven, Patricia A., 1103
Crutchley, David J., 1751
Cuatrecasas, P., 249,259
Cunnane, S. C., 1797
Cunningham, M., 1259
Czerniawska-Mysik, G., 993

D

Dady, P. J., 511
Davidson, E. M., 1661
Davies, Philip, 1691
Dawood, M. Yusoff, 1443
Dawson, W., 1741
De Boever, J., 201
Decoster, C., 1309
de Deckere, E. A. M., 655,1771
Deichsel, W., 1483
Deis, R. P., 1317
Delouis, C., 1317
Demers, Lawrence M., 193,1203,1633
Derck, Dennis D., 193
De Rosa, G., 1303
De Rubertis, Frederick R., 1103
De Salvo, A., 187,207
De Titta, George T., 381,477
Dewhirst, F. E., 901

Diczfslusy, Ulf, 267
Diegel, J., 1259
Dix, Robert K., 651
Doig, M. V., 1661
Dollery, C. T., 933
Dore-Duffy, Paula, 1685
Dougherty, H. W., 77
Douglas, William H. J., 225
Doyle, A. E., 815
Dray, F., 167,1321
Dreher, E., 1487
D'Souza, S. M., 1709
Dubin, Norman H., 1407,1465
Dubois, A., 1557,1581,1587
Dumont, J. E., 1309
Dunn, Michael J., 1009
Düsing, Rainer, 1021,1111,1189
Dusting, G. J., 815
Dutilh, C. E., 101
Dzoljic, M. R., 1217

E

Eakins, K. E., 861,1727
Easty, G. C., 511
Eden, Jutta, 1021
Edqvist, Lars-Eric, 1351
Edwards, D., 547
Egan, Robert W., 77,153
Eggerman, Thomas L., 389
Egner, Patricia G., 1465
El-Attar, A., 1459,1739
El-Ayyat, M. A., 1459
Elder, M. G., 1469
Eling, Thomas E., 535,1751
Elliott, R. L., 755
Ellis, C. K., 313
Ellis, E. F., 313
Embrey, M. P., 1477
Englis, D. J., 1709
Enomoto, I., 641,665
Epstein, Alan N., 1231
Erman, A., 231
Erman, Mary G., 381,477

F

Fahey, John V., 1701
Fahr, A., 811
Falck, J. R., 19

Farber, Saul J., 1181
Feigen, Larry, 385
Feinstein, Maurice B., 321
Ferreira, Sergio H., 1207
Ferretti, A., 1791
Feuerstein, Giora, 829
Feuerstein, Nili, 829
Fichman, M., 1193
Fiedler, L., 585,1609
Fincham, N., 857
Fischer, Susan M., 517
Fitzpatrick, F. A., 301
Fitzpatrick, Thomas M., 457,679,
    727,981
Flandre, O., 1705
Fletcher, John R., 723,821,843,1507
Fluharty, Steven J., 1231
Fogwell, R. L., 1345
Folco, G. C., 917,927
Folkert, Vaughn W., 1177
Ford-Hutchinson, A. W., 1661
Förster, W., 609,811,1813
Fortier, S., 477
Frame, M. H., 1529
Frank, G. J., 587,1723
French, B., 591
Fried, Josef, 365,427,683
Friedman, Lawrence S., 679,981
Friedman, Zvi, 1799
Frölich, Jurgen C., 745,799,1107
Fuchs, Anna-Riitta, 1313
Fujimoto, Wilfred Y., 1291
Fujitani, Buichi, 347

G

Galanti, Giorgio, 317,715
Gale, Paul H., 153
Galli, C., 1235
Galli, G., 927
Gardiner, P. J., 1003
Gerber, John G., 957,1079,1135
Gerkens, John F., 35
Gerozissis, K., 167
Gerrard, J. M., 157
Gethmann, U., 1409
Ghodgaonkar, R. B., 1407
Giebier, Ch., 811
Giel, John R., Jr., 1083,1189

Gimmon, Zvi, 829
Giordano, Lucio, 701
Giri, S. N., 953
Glasson, Philippe, 1115
Gleason, Greta L., 517
Glew, M. E., 365
Głuszko, P., 687
Goerig, M., 1089
Goldberg, L. I., 683
Goldyne, Marc E., 1655
Goodson, J. M., 901
Gordon-Wright, A. P., 1469
Gorman, Robert R., 417,635,1717
Granström, Elisabeth, 69,181,283
Grant, Myles J., 883
Greaves, M. W., 857
Greeley, Harold P., 1009
Gréen, Krister, 1419
Greenberg, R., 437,493,961
Greenwald, James E., 293
Grossman, M. I., 1521
Gryglewski, R. J., 687,777,993
Güllner, Hans-George, 1185,1189
Gustafson, Lars, 1245
Guyene, T. T., 1119

H

Haddeman, E., 101,1771
Hahn, J., 1017
Halushka, Perry V., 505,1269
Ham, E. A., 77
Hamberger, B., 1365
Hamberger, L., 1365
Hames, J. L., 77
Hamilton, J. G., 453
Hammarström, Sven, 1,267,275,541
Harada, Y., 1733
Harker, Lawrence A., 389
Harmon, John W., 1577
Harris, D. N., 437,493,1321
Harris, Edward D., Jr., 1701
Harris, M., 547,595
Harris, R. H., 457,727,843
Harrison, H. E., 1283
Harvie, C. J., 647
Hashimoto, H., 641,665
Hashimoto, S., 337
Hashimoto, Yoshinobu, 305

Hata, Yoshimaro, 1395
Hatano, Naonobu, 347
Hatano, Y., 683
Hayaishi, Osamu, 27
Hayashi, M., 327,337
Hayes, Arthur H., Jr., 1633
Hedqvist, Per, 1245
Heinzelmann, D. I., 1529,1621
Heikes, J. E., 493
Held, Eckhard, 1067,1145
Hensby, C. N., 857,933,1529
Herman, A. G., 839
Herrmann, R., 1111
Hillemanns, H. G., 1483
Hillman, Jeffrey S., 1723
Hintze, Thomas H., 601
Hirata, Fumio, 443,965
Hirzel, Przemyslaw, 695
Hjemdahl, Paul, 1245
Hockel, Gregory M., 1061
Hoffmann, Michael K., 1131
Hokama, Y., 1669
Hollinger, M. A., 953
Holmberg, Sandra, 1175
Hopkins, Nancy K., 1717
Hoppen, H. O., 1409
Hornstra, G., 1771
Hornych, A., 1119
Horrobin, D. F., 1797
Horton, R., 1017
Hoshina, Kenji, 305
Houdebine, L. M., 1317
Hough, A., 525
Houghton, J., 567
Hsi, R. S. P., 355
Hubbard, W. C., 525
Hull, S. S., Jr., 365
Humes, John L., 1691
Hurley, M., 1295
Huslig, Richard L., 1345
Hutchins, Grover M., 675
Hyman, Albert L., 731,765,937,1249

I

Iantorno, G., 917
Imai, Shoichi, 659
Inagawa, Toshio, 965
Ishibashi, Masataka, 659,1733

Ishihara, Yoko, 213,759
Ishii, Kenji, 331
Ishimoto, Sachio, 305
Ito, T., 641,665
Itoh, Kunio, 1395

J

Jacquemier, Jocelyne, 575
Jager, L. P., 1547
Jakschik, B. A., 163
Jamieson, D. R. S., 891
Janson, P. O., 1365
Jaworek, Jolanta, 1561
Jimba, Makiko, 305
Johnson, J. W. C., 1407
Johnson, Lawrence F., 1577
Johnson, M., 1283
Johnson, R. M., 525
Jones, P. B. B., 297
Jones, P. S., 313
Jones, R. L., 107,467,1057
Joyo, B. S., 1669
Judd, J. T., 1787
Jugdutt, Bodh I., 675
Jurkiewicz, Nancy, 651

K

Kadlec, Ondřej, 1255
Kadowitz, Philip J., 731,765,937,1249
Kai, I., 641,665
Kaley, Gabor, 601,719
Kälin, H., 1679
Karim, S. M. M., 969
Karmali, R. A., 523
Katano, Yumi, 659
Kather, Horst, 1617
Katori, M., 1733
Kauffman, G. L., Jr., 1521
Kawasaki, Akiyoshi, 331
Kaye, Z., 1017
Keiser, Harry R., 1083
Kelliher, Gerald J., 651
Kellner, Maximilian, 905
Kelly, Gerald, 1083
Kelly, Rodney W., 1369
Kennedy, Mike S., 1655
Kennedy, T. G., 1423
Kennerly, Donald A., 219

Kenney, Nancy J., 1225
Kerry, P. J., 107
Khamis, Y., 1459
Kheskani, M. B., 1723
Kimball, F. A., 355
Kimura, L. H., 1669
Kindahl, Hans, 181,275,283,1351
Kinoshita, Katsuyuki, 1419
Kinter, Lewis B., 1009
Kitamura, Satoshi, 213,759
Kittisopikul, S., 427
Klepper, M. S., 1603
Knapp, Daniel R., 505
Knapp, Howard R., 1027
Kohen, F., 1371
Kohli, J. D., 683
Kommerell, Burkhard, 1617
Komoriya, Keiji, 305
Konturek, Stanisław J., 1561
Konz, E., 341
Korbut, R., 777
Korteweg, M., 201
Kosaka, Konori, 759
Kot, Peter A., 457,679,727,981
Kottegoda, S. R., 969
Kouznetzova, B., 167,1321
Kowalewski, K., 1611
Kraft, Edward, 1153
Kramer, Herbert J., 1021,1111
Krzanowski, J. J., 995
Kuehl, Frederick A., Jr., 77,153,1691
Kulagina, V. P., 1139
Kulkarni, P. S., 861,1727
Kumor, Karen M., 1465
Kunimoto, Keikichi, 1395
Kuo, Ming-Hung, 1395
Kurozumi, Seizi, 305
Kursunoglu, Sevil, 865

L

Lahav, M., 1371
Lam, M. P., 1669
Lampa, Enrico, 701
Lands, W. E. M., 1295
Langs, David A., 381,477
Larsson, Carin, 1263
Lasrich, Mark, 695
Lauersen, Nills H., 1435

Lawrence, Theodore, 651
Lazar, J. D., 1123
Leaper, D. J., 591
Leaver, H. Anne, 1361
Le Breton, G. C., 497
LeDuc, Louise E., 1515
Lee, James B., 1053
Lee, L. H., 163
Lee, Nancy, 447
Lefer, Allan M., 489,835
Leghonkaya, N. P., 1139
LeMaire, William J., 1357
Leovey, E. M. K., 1277,1783
Lerch, U., 341
Levanho, Alain, 1269
Levin, James L., 731
Levine, L., 1199
Levitskaya, Yu, 1139
Lewins, Michael J., 883
Lewis, G. P., 263
Liang, C. D., 235
Lightfoot, Fred G., 1589
Lin, Hsien S., 1739
Lindell, Jan-Otto, 1351
Lindgren, Jan Åke, 275,541
Lindner, H. R., 1371
Link, H.-B., 625
Lippert, T. H., 351
Lippton, Howard L., 1249
Lipter, Donald M., 1525
Lock, James E., 751
London, G., 1119
Lord, Jonathan T., 865
Louis, T. M., 523
Luderer, John R., 1633
Lunell, Nils-Olov, 1431
Luyckx, A. S., 1299

M

Maas, Richard N., 35
MacIntyre, D. E., 1199
MacIntyre, J., 571
MacKenzie, J. Z., 1401,1477
Maclouf, J., 283
Maddox, Y., 843,1277,1783
Magolda, Ronald L., 481,489,835
Maher, John F., 695
Main, I. H. M., 1519,1529,1543

Majerus, Philip W., 219
Makheja, Amar N., 309
Malik, K. U., 1241
Mamas, S., 167
Marfat, A., 19
Markov, Ch.M., 631,691
Marmo, Emilio, 701
Marnett, Lawrence J., 149,153
Marsh, John M., 1357
Marshall, M. W., 1787
Martin, Pierre M., 575,581
Mašek, Karel, 1255
Mason, R. G., 287
Masotti, Giulio, 317,715
Matsuo, M., 1669
Maussier, M., 1303
Maxey, K. M., 355
Maydonovitch, Corinne L., 1577
McCracken, John A., 365,1329
McGiff, J. C., 807
McGuire, J. C., 111,1665
McGuire, M. B., 297,1709
McMillan, Rodger M., 1701
McMurtry, I. F., 957
McRae, John R., 407,1287
Meats, J. E., 1709
Melarange, R., 1519
Mentz, P. R., 631,811
Messina, Edward J., 601,719
Metsä-Ketelä, T., 1553
Metz, Stewart A., 183,1291
Michibayashi, T., 791
Millar, J. L., 587
Miller, James E., 235
Miller, Jordan D., 401
Miller, W. L., 355
Milliez, P., 1119
Mills, E. L., 157
Mioskowski, C., 19
Misefari, A., 1747
Mitchell, M. D., 891,1401
Miyamoto, Tsumoru, 443
Miyazaki, Hiroshi, 659,1733
Mocellin, Rolf, 905
Modugno, I., 1303
Mohammad, S. F., 287
Mommsen, Craig, 1153
Moncada, S., 43,1159

Mongkolsmai, Add, 879
Morita, A. H., 1669
Morita, Ikuo, 1495
Morris, Helen G., 1759,1765
Morris, H. R., 121
Morrison, Aubrey R., 1131
Mullane, K. M., 1159
Müller, G., 1089
Mullins, Elizabeth M., 815
Murao, Makoto, 965,985
Murota, Sei-Itsu, 1495
Murphy, R. C., 1
Muse, P., 523
Myers, L., 1557,1587
Myers, Stuart, 1171

N

Nakatsuji, Katsuyoshi, 347
Naruchi, Tatsuyuki, 305
Needleman, Philip, 61,301,427,
    1171,1175,1515
Nekrasova, A. A., 1139
Nelson, N. A., 355
Neri Serneri, Gian Gastone, 317,715
Neutze, J. M., 755
Nicolaou, Kyriacos C., 481,489,835
Niebyl, Jennifer R., 1465
Nies, Alan S., 957,1079,1135
Nilsson, L., 1365
Nishikawa, Yuko, 659
Niwa, H., 19
Niżankowska, E., 993
Niżankowski, R., 687,769
Nomides, Charles T., 1633
Nompleggi, D., 1587
Nugteren, D. H., 129,1793

O

Oates, John A., 35,525,1027,1123,1799
O'Brien, Peter J., 145
Offenbacher, S., 901
Ogawa, K., 641,665
Ogino, Nubuchika, 27
Ogletree, M., 745
O'Grady, J., 619
Ohki, Shiro, 27
Ohtsu, Akiro, 305
Ohuchida, S., 337

Oishi, N., 1669
O'Keefe, E. H., 961
Olley, Peter M., 751,871,883,913
Olson, Richard D., 1135
Ölund, Anders, 1431
Omi, Katsuo, 1395
Omini, C., 917,927
Osman, G. H., Jr., 437,961

P

Pace-Asciak, C. R., 797
Pagels, William R., 149
Palfreyman, M. N., 485
Parachini, M., 187
Parantainen, J., 1553
Parks, Thomas P., 711
Parnham, M. J., 1675,1713
Pasargiklian, E., 1303
Pasargiklian, M., 943
Paterson, N. A. M., 1755
Patrono, C., 187,207
Pearce, J. B., 1543
Pek, S., 1295
Perara, Eve, 1225
Persaud, T. V. N., 897
Peskar, B. A., 745,1511
Peterson, D. A., 157
Petroni, 1235
Phillips, Christine A., 1391
Phillips, M. B., 437
Pinca, E., 187,207
Pinelis, V. G., 691
Piper, Priscilla J., 121,263
Plummer, N. A., 857
Poggesi, Loredana, 317,715
Polgar, Peter, 225
Polson, J. B., 995
Pönicke, K., 811
Poubelle, P., 1705
Powles, T. J., 511,587
Poyser, Norman L., 1361,1391
Pradelles, P., 167
Printz, Morton P., 711,803
Prior, Werner, 1021
Pugliese, F., 187,207

Q

Quadt, J. F. A., 1771

R

Rahimtula, Anver D., 145
Rainsford, K. D., 1679
Raja, B., 595
Ramey, E. R., 1277,1783
Ramos, Emilio, 1203
Rampton, D. S., 1621
Ramwell, Peter W., 457,679,723,
727,821,843,981,1277,1587,1783
Rao, G. H. R., 157
Rask-Madsen, J., 1595,1627
Raz, A., 231,255
Redmond, Gregory, 865
Reece, A. H., 1283
Reed, Gregory A., 149
Reeves, J. T., 957
Reeves, V., 1787,1791
Rice, Maureen G., 183,407
Richardson, D. W., 313
Robert, A., 355,1533
Roberts, L. Jackson II, 35
Robertson, R. Paul, 183,407,1287,1291
Robinson, J. Courtland, 1465
Robrecht, D., 1483
Rolland, Anne M., 575,581
Rollins, Thomas E., 1345
Rosatti, Federico, 701
Rose, John C., 679
Rösen, P., 625
Rösen, R., 625
Rossi, Francesco, 701
Rowe, D. J. F., 595
Rowe, Richard D., 883,913
Rowland, Dale W., 883
Rubin, R. P., 239
Rush, B. D., 1603
Russell, R. G. G., 297,1709
Ruwart, M. J., 1603
Ryan, R., 457

S

Safar, M., 1119
Sakai, Kiyoshi, 985
Sakamoto, Shoichi, 1419
Salata, K. F., 537
Salomon, Y., 1371
Salzman, E. W., 1199

Samuelsson, B., 1,283
Sanger, G. J., 399,1559
Satake, T., 641,665
Satoh, Kazuo, 1419
Satta, M. A., 187,207,1303
Saunders, R. N., 235
Sautebin, L., 927
Saverymuttu, S. H., 1569
Scherer, Burkhard, 1033,1067,1145
Schlegel, G., 585
Schleman, Margo, 879
Schlondorff, Detlef, 1177
Schmeling, J., 457
Schnerman, Jürgen, 1047,1067
Schöber, Johannes G., 905
Schoene, N. W., 1787,1791
Schoester, G. A. P., 1675
Schölkens, B. A., 341
Schrey, M. P., 239
Schrör, K., 625
Schumacher, Gebhard, 905
Schuster, E., 1409
Schwartzman, M., 255
Sebek, O. K., 355
Seegers, A. J. M., 1547
Šěferna, Isidor, 1255
Sella, G. E., 1797
Sellers, Susan M., 891
Selner, John C., 1759
Serment, Henri, 581
Seyberth, Hannsjorg W., 1511,1799
Shaver Madden, Kathleen, 1273
Shea-Donohue, P. T., 1557
Shearin, N. L., 1611
Shebuski, Ronald J., 635,1149
Shepperdson, Frances T., 1759
Sherman, Nancy A., 1759,1765
Shida, Akira, 985
Shier, David, 1009
Shimamoto, Norio, 659
Shimizu, Masanao, 347
Shimizu, T., 27
Shimoji, K., 327
Siegl, A. M., 395
Siess, Wolfgang, 1067,1145
Sih, J. C., 355
Silver, M. J., 395
Simon, A., 1119

Simon, Bernd, 1617
Simon, L., 1705
Sinar, D. R., 1507
Sirois, Pierre, 125
Siu, C. E., 1669
Sivakoff, Mark, 1175
Sjögren, A., 1365
Skawiński, S., 687
Skidgel, Randal A., 803
Skoglund, Marcia L., 1135
Sladen, G. E., 1621
Slaga, Thomas J., 517
Smigel, M. D., 1123
Smirnov, I. E., 631
Smith, E. F., 489
Smith, F. L., 1807
Smith, J. B., 395,489,835,1185
Smith, M., 1199
Smith, M. J. H., 1661
Smith, William L., 1345
Smolen, James E., 1695
Soeting, W. J., 1793
Sokolova, R. N., 1139
Soldin, Steven J., 883
Spagnuolo, C., 1235
Spannhake, Ernst Wm., 731,765,937
Speranskaya, N. V., 1139
Spławinski, J., 777
Sprague, P. W., 493
Sprecher, Howard, 61,301
Spuy, J. H., 1793
Srinivasan, B. D., 861
Stahl, Rolf A. K., 1053
Stamford, I. F., 571,595,1569
Stanford, Nancy, 219
Starling, M. B., 755
Steer, M. L., 1199
Steiner, H., 1483
Steinhoff, M. M., 163
Steinman, D. H., 235
Stemerman, M., 1199
Stinnesbeck, Bruno, 1021
Stobo, John D., 1655
Stoff, J. S., 1199
Strauss, J. F. III, 1259
Stuttle, K. A. J., 485
Sun, F. F., 111,1665
Sutter, Dorothy M., 789

Suzuki, Hiroshi, 1395
Svanborg, Kerstin, 1245
Sweetman, Brian J., 35
Swyer, Paul R., 883,913
Szczeklik, A., 687,769,933
Szczeklik, J., 687,769
Szentivanyi, A., 995

T

Taber, Douglass F., 35
Tai, Chen L., 447
Tai, Hsin-Hsiung, 447
Takahashi, Wataru, 965
Tanaka, K., 1733
Taniguchi, Ken, 443
Tanouchi, Tadao, 443
Tasler, Janina, 1561
Taube, Ch., 811
Tawfik, M. A., 1739
Taylor, G. W., 121
Taylor, Linda, 225
ten Hoor, F., 101,655,1771
Teraoka, J. K., 1669
Terracio, Louis, 225
Terragno, N. A., 807
Tippins, J. R., 121
To, D., 1807
Tobias, L. D., 453
Toga, M., 575
Toppozada, M., 1459
Trocha, Paul J., 851
Troncone, L., 1303
Trugnan, G., 167
Tsuboi, Toshimichi, 347
Tsuboshima, Masami, 331
Tuffin, D., 485
Turnbull, A. C., 891

U

Uchiyama, Kyoichi, 965,985
Underwood, L., 365

V

Vacca, Ciro, 701
Vallotton, Michel B., 1115
Valtin, Heinz, 1009
Vanderhoek, Jack Y., 309,321
Van der Kloot, William, 1273

Van der Kwast, Th., 1675
Van der Ouderaa, F. J., 139
Vandevivere, D., 201
Van Dorp, D. A., 139
Vane, J. R., 43, 1159
Van Evert, W. C., 1793
Van Noordwijk, J., 1547
Van Praag, Dina, 1181
Van Sande, J., 1309
Van Thoai, M. Nguyen, 411
Van Vliet, H., 463
Vapaatalo, H., 1553
Veldhuis, Johannes D., 1203
Venton, D. L., 497
Venza-Teti, D., 1747
Vercrysse, P., 839
Verdonk, G., 201
Vigano, T., 917
Vigo, Carmen, 263
Vincent, J. E., 463,1097,1217
Volkman, A., 523
Voelkel, N. F., 957
Von Fischer, B., 1487

W

Wagner, K., 1679
Wakabayashi, Toshio, 305
Wakatsuka, H., 327,337
Wakitani, Korekujo, 331
Walenga, Ronald, 321
Walker, Irene C., 107
Walker, J. L., 115,485
Walker, Larry, 1107
Walker, M. J. A., 647
Walker, R., 1573
Wallach, D. P., 111
Warrington, S. J., 619
Watanabe, Kikuko, 27
Watson, M. L., 1057
Weber, Peter C., 1033,1047,1067,1145
Weeks, James R., 789
Weiss, Y., 1119
Weissmann, Gerlad, 1637,1695
Weithmann, U., 341
Weppelmann, B., 1409
Wernze, H., 1089

West, R., 671
Whitaker, Mark O., 61,301
White, J. G., 157
White, Robert D., 1465
Whiting, J. D., 537
Whittle, B. J. R., 1521
Whorton, A. R., 1123
Williams, Judith, 511
Williams, K. I., 1413
Wilson, Cynthia H., 389
Wilson, Kathleen H., 1435
Wilson, K. A., 1573
Wilson, N. H., 107,467
Wiqvist, N., 1365
Wong, Lan K., 293
Wood, J. R., 1569
Wright, J. E., 595, 1709
Wright, K. F., 313
Wudarski, E., 671
Wyche, Angela, 61,301,427

Y

Yamaguichi, Takeshi, 985
Yamamoto, Shozo, 27
Yamashita, Kouwa, 659
Yamashita, Y., 1733
Yasumizu, Takehiko, 1419
Yoshida, Kouichi, 347
Yoshimoto, T., 27
Youlten, L. J. F., 529,1621
Yun, John C. H., 1083
Yusa, Takashi, 985

Z

Zahradnik, H. P., 585
Zamecnik, J., 1423
Zamorano, B., 807
Zia, P., 1017,1193
Ziboh, Vincent A., 865
Zijlstra, F. J., 463,1097,1217
Zimmerman, Ben G., 1153
Zipser, R., 1017,1171,1193
Zmudka, M., 843
Zor, U., 1371
Zurier, Robert B., 1685
Zusman, Randall M., 243

Advances in Prostaglandin and Thromboxane Research,
Vol. 6, edited by B. Samuelsson, P. W. Ramwell,
and R. Paoletti. Raven Press, New York © 1980.

Leukotrienes: A New Group of Biologically Active Compounds

B. Samuelsson, P. Borgeat, S. Hammarström, and R. C. Murphy

Department of Chemistry, Karolinska Institutet, S-104 01 Stockholm, Sweden

Our knowledge about the oxygenation and further transformation of polyunsaturated fatty acids into biologically active derivatives has increased considerably during recent years. The products consist of prostaglandins (including prostacyclin), thromboxanes, and various hydroxylated fatty acids formed in lipoxygenase catalyzed reactions (1,2). This chapter describes some new developments in our laboratory which have taken place since the third International Conference on Prostaglandins (3).

METABOLISM OF ARACHIDONIC ACID IN POLYMORPHONUCLEAR LEUKOCYTES

The major metabolites of arachidonic acid and 8,11,14-eicosatrienoic acid in rabbit polymorphonuclear leukocytes (PMNL) were recently identified as 5(S)-hydroxy-6,8,11,14-eicosatetraenoic acid and 8(S)-hydroxy-9,11,14-eicosatrienoic acid, respectively (4). Subsequently, several new metabolites have been detected (5,6).

Rabbit peritoneal PMNL were incubated with arachidonic acid. Products were isolated by diethyl ether extraction and purified using silicic acid chromatography and high-pressure liquid chromatography (HPLC). Metabolites were identified by spectrophotometric and gas chromatographic-mass spectrometric techniques. Figure 1 shows a high pressure liquid chromatogram of five polar products in a typical experiment (6). The mass spectra of several derivatives of compounds I, II, and III were practically identical, indicating that the three compounds were isomers, and demonstrated the presence of hydroxyl groups at C-5 and C-12. The ultraviolet spectra of compounds I–V (cf. Fig. 2) showed the characteristic absorption bands of three conjugated double bonds (6,7). Infrared spectometric analysis demonstrated that the conjugated triene in compounds I and II had the *trans* geometry whereas similar analysis indicated the presence of two *trans* and one *cis* ethylenic bonds in the conjugated triene of compound III. Steric analysis of the alcohols indicated that compounds I, II, and III had the (S) configuration at C-5 and that compounds I and III had the (R) configuration at C-12, whereas compound II had the (S) configuration at C-

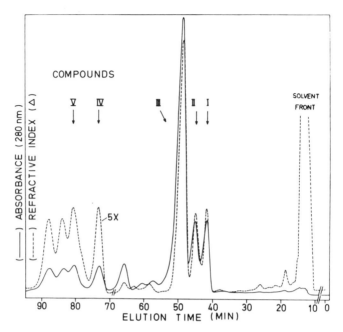

FIG. 1. Dihydroxylated metabolites of arachidonic acid formed by rabbit PMNL. An ether extract was purified by silicic acid column chromatography and the ethyl acetate fraction was subjected to RP-HPLC. The traces show ultraviolet absorbance at 280 nm *(solid line)* and the change in refractive index *(broken line)*. Column: μC_{18} Bondapack; solvent: methanol/water, 70/30, v/v plus 0.01% acetic acid at 0.3 ml/min.

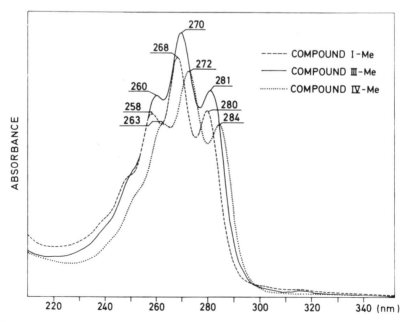

FIG. 2. Ultraviolet spectra of the methyl esters (Me) of some metabolites of arachidonic acid in rabbit PMNL. The spectra of compounds II and V were identical to those of compounds I and III, respectively. Spectra were recorded in methanol.

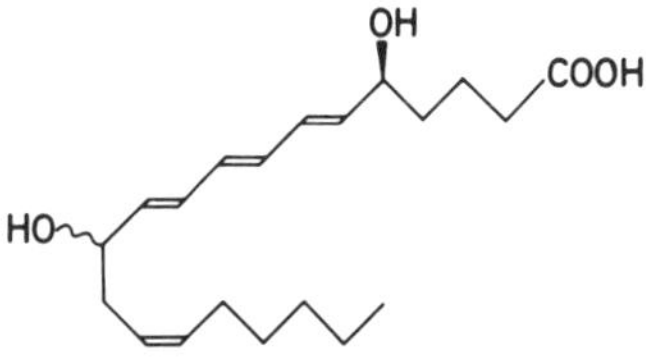

COMPOUND I (12R-HYDROXY-)

COMPOUND II (12S-HYDROXY-)

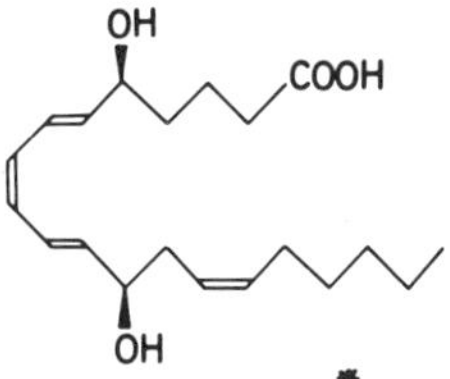

COMPOUND III *

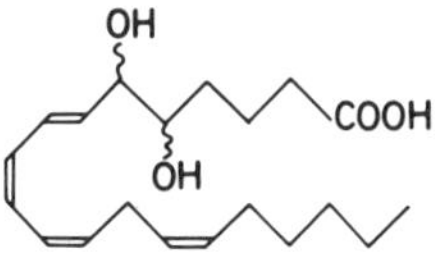

COMPOUNDS IV - V *
(DIASTEREOISOMERS)

FIG. 3. Structures of dihydroxylated metabolites of arachidonic acid in rabbit PMNL. * Indicates an ambiguity in the structure (see text).

12 (Fig. 3). Compounds I, II, and III are thus stereoisomeric 5,12-dihydroxy-6,8,10,14-eicosatetraenoic acids.

Mass spectrometric analyses of compounds IV and V indicated that they were 5,6-dihydroxy derivatives of arachidonic acid (6). The ultraviolet spectra of compounds IV and V were identical (Fig. 2) and showed the presence of three conjugated double bonds in the molecules (6). Infrared spectrometry and steric analyses of the alcohols were not performed because of the limited amount of material available. The gas chromatographic, mass spectrometric, and ultraviolet spectrometric data indicated that compounds IV and V were diastereoisomeric 5,6-dihydroxy-7,9,11,14-eicosatetraenoic acids (6). The proposed mechanism of formation of compound IV and V (see below) requires that the compounds are epimers at C-6 (Fig. 3).

The conversions of arachidonic acid to compounds I-V were 0.12, 0.12, 0.8, 0.035, and 0.035%, respectively. For comparison, the conversion to 5S-hydroxy-6,8,11,14-eicosatetraenoic acid was 5 to 10 times that of compound III (6).

EVIDENCE FOR AN UNSTABLE INTERMEDIATE IN THE FORMATION OF DIHYDROXYEICOSATETRAENOIC ACIDS

$^{18}O_2$ Labeling Experiments

Rabbit PMNL were incubated with arachidonic acid under an atmosphere of $^{18}O_2$ (8). The products, purified by reversed phase (RP)-HPLC, were esterified with diazomethane and subjected to catalytic hydrogenation over PtO_2. The presence and position of ^{18}O in the molecules were determined by mass spectrometry. Compounds I–V each contained a single atom of ^{18}O located at C-5. The 5S-hydroxy-eicosatetraenoic acid was also labeled at C-5. These data show that the hydroxyl groups at C-5 in the metabolites of arachidonic acid in Fig. 3 are derived from molecular oxygen. Incubation of rabbit peritoneal PMNL in $H_2{}^{18}O$-enriched buffer confirmed that the hydroxyl groups at C-12 in compounds I, II, and III originated in water. Based on these observations, it was postulated that an unstable intermediate was generated from arachidonic acid by the leukocytes which would undergo nucleophilic attack by water, alcohols, and other nucleophiles.

Trapping Experiments with Alcohols

Rabbit peritoneal PMNL were incubated for 30 sec with arachidonic acid before addition of 10 volumes of methanol (A), 10 volumes of ethanol (B), or 0.2 volumes of 1 N HCl (C). After extraction and silicic acid column chromatography, the products were analyzed by RP-HPLC. The chromatogram in Fig. 4 shows the pattern of products obtained (polar metabolites only). The material formed upon trapping with methanol (or ethanol) consisted of two compounds present in equal amounts. These compounds were further purified (as methyl esters) by silicic acid HPLC. Their ultraviolet spectra were identical to those of compounds I and II (Fig. 2), indicating the presence of three conjugated double bonds. Infrared spectrometry further indicated that the conjugated double

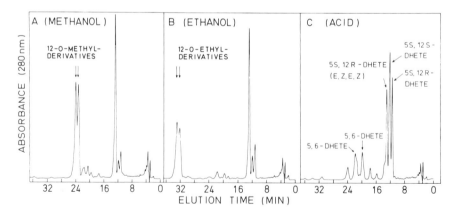

FIG. 4. RP-HPLC chromatograms of the products obtained upon addition of (A) 10 volumes methanol; (B) 10 volumes ethanol; and (C) 0.2 volumes 1N HCl, to suspensions of PMNL incubated for 30 sec with arachidonic acid. The samples were fractionated by silicic acid column chromatography and the ethyl acetate fractions were analyzed by RP-HPLC: (Nucleosil C_{18}); solvent, methanol/H_2O, 75/25, v/v + 0.01% acetic acid at 1 ml/min.

bonds had *trans* geometry. Gas chromatographic-mass spectrometric analyses of several derivatives of the two compounds showed that they were isomeric and carried hydroxyl groups at C-5 and methoxy groups at C-12. Steric analyses showed that the alcohol groups had (S) configuration. Although the configurations at C-12 were not determined, it is clear that the compounds are the C-12 epimers of 5(S)-hydroxy,12-methoxy-6,8,10,14(E,E,E,Z)eicosatetraenoic acid (cf. Fig. 3).

Analogous derivatives were identified when ethanol or ethylene glycol were used for trapping. These data show that a metabolite of arachidonic acid in leukocytes can undergo a facile nucleophilic reaction with alcohols. Interestingly, RP-HPLC analysis of samples obtained from trapping experiments performed under various conditions always indicated inverse relationships between the amount of compounds I and II formed and their 12-*O*-alkyl derivatives (Fig. 5). This suggests that compounds I and II are formed nonenzymatically from the same intermediate that gives rise to the 12-*O*-alkyl derivatives.

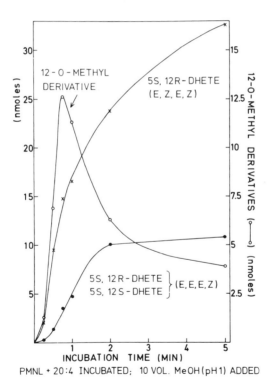

FIG. 5. Time course of the formation of compounds I + II (●——●), of compound III (x——x), and time course of the formation and disappearance of an unstable intermediate, measured as 12-*O*-methyl compounds I + II (○——○) in PMNL incubated with arachidonic acid. Prostaglandin B₂ was added prior to purification as an internal standard.

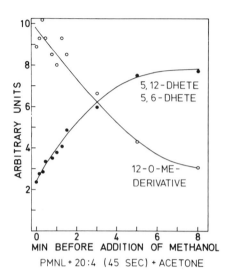

FIG. 6. Time course of the formation of compounds I, II, IV, or V (●——●) and of the disappearance of the unstable intermediate measured as 12-O-methyl compounds I–II (○——○) in a mixture of water/acetone, 1/1, v/v at pH 7.4 and 37°C. Prostaglandin B_2 was added as an internal standard for quantitation by RP-HPLC.

Stability of the Intermediate

Rabbit PMNL were incubated with arachidonic acid for 45 sec before addition of 1 volume of acetone (to stop enzymatic activity). At different time intervals, aliquots of the mixture were transferred to flasks containing 15 volumes of methanol. The relative amounts of metabolites were estimated by RP-HPLC. Figure 6 shows the decay of the intermediate, measured as the 12-O-methyl derivative, at pH 7.4 and 37°C ($t_{1/2}$ = 3–4 min). Simultaneously, the concentrations of compounds I, II, IV, and V (●——●) increased with time. The concentrations of compounds III and 5-hydroxy-6,8,11,14-eicosatetraenoic acid remained constant (not shown). This suggests that compounds I, II, IV, and V are formed nonenzymatically by hydrolysis of a common unstable intermediate, whereas compound III arises by enzymatic hydrolysis of the same intermediate. Similar experiments performed at acid and alkaline pH indicated that the intermediate was acid-labile and somewhat stabilized at alkaline pH.

Structure of the Unstable Intermediate

Based on the experimental data described above, the structure 5(6)-oxido-7,9,11,14-eicosatetraenoic acid (Fig. 7) is proposed for the intermediate. Hydrolysis of epoxides is acid-catalyzed and opening of allylic epoxides is favored at allylic positions (C-6 in this case). This agrees with the retention of ^{18}O at C-5 in compounds IV and V. A mechanism for the formation of compounds I–V from the epoxide intermediate is proposed in Fig. 7. Except for compound III, these are formed by chemical hydrolysis of the epoxide through a mechanism involving a carbonium ion. The latter adds hydroxyl anion preferentially at

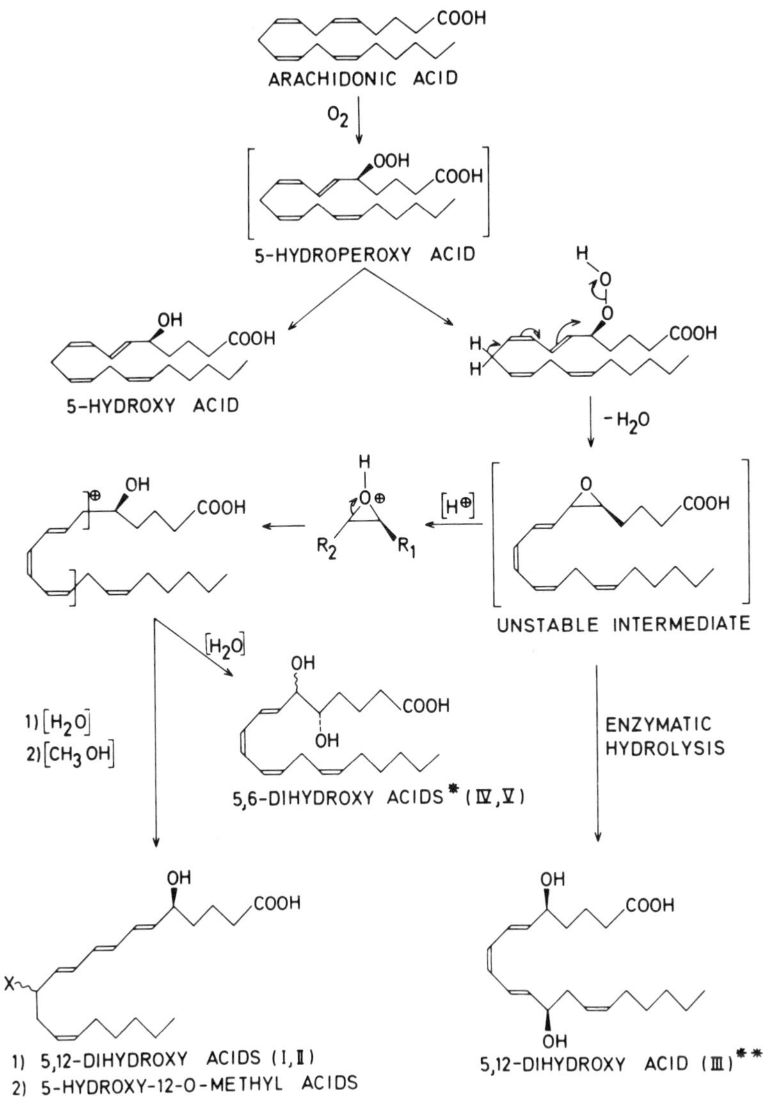

FIG. 7. Scheme of transformations of arachidonic acid in PMNL. Compounds within brackets have not been isolated. (*): The geometry of the double bonds and the configuration of the alcohol groups are unknown. (**): The position of the *cis* double bond in the conjugated triene is unknown.

C-6 and C-12 to yield four isomeric products which contain the stable conjugated triene structure. Compound III is formed enzymatically from the intermediate since it is not racemic at C-12 and because it is only formed by nondenatured cell preparations.

A hypothetical pathway for the formation of the epoxide from arachidonic acid is shown in Fig. 7. It involves initial formation of 5-hydroperoxy-6,8,11,14-eicosatetraenoic acid (5-HPETE) which is the precursor of the 5-hydroxy acid. The epoxide is formed from 5-HPETE by abstraction of a proton at C-10, and elimination of hydroxyl anion from the hydroperoxy group. It should be noted that the geometry of the epoxide ring and of the double bonds as shown in Fig. 7 are uncertain. It is likely that the configuration at C-5 is (S) and that the geometry of the double bonds at Δ^{11} and Δ^{14} is *cis.*

TRANSFORMATION OF ARACHIDONIC ACID IN HUMAN PERIPHERAL BLOOD PMNL

Incubation of human peripheral blood PMNL with arachidonic acid gave the same metabolites as described above for rabbit peritoneal PMNL (9). Interestingly, the percent conversion of substrate to different products varied significantly (more than 10-fold) between cells from separate donors.

Recent experiments have shown that the divalent cation ionophore A23187 stimulates the formation of prostaglandins and thromboxanes in leukocytes (10–12). The effect of the ionophore (2×10^{-5}M) on the biosynthesis of mono- and dihydroxy acids from endogenous and exogenous arachidonic acid in human PMNL is shown in Table 1. The results suggested that in addition to activating a phospholipase (13), the ionophore also stimulated the further transformations of arachidonic acid. These data also pointed out some striking differences in the capacity of leukocytes isolated from different donors to transform arachidonic acid.

CHEMICAL STRUCTURE OF A SLOW-REACTING SUBSTANCE FROM MURINE MASTOCYTOMA CELLS

In 1938, Feldberg and Kellaway (14) described a smooth muscle-contracting factor from perfused guinea pig lungs, after treatment with cobra venom, which

TABLE 1. *Effect of ionophore A23187 on the metabolism of arachidonic acid in human PMNL*

	Compounds formed (nmoles)		
Additions	5-hydroxy acid	15-hydroxy acid	5,12-dihydroxy acid
None	0.6	<0.15	<0.15
A23187	11.2	<0.22	4.2
Arachidonic acid	2.2	4.1	<0.15
A23187 + arachidonic acid	42.8	2.2	7.14

Human PMNL were incubated 4 min at 37°C in the presence or absence of ionophore A23187 and arachidonic acid, as indicated. Incubations were stopped by addition of methanol containing prostaglandin B_2 as internal standard. The amount of compounds formed was measured by RP-HPLC.

they termed "slow-reacting substance" (SRS). Kellaway and Trethewie (15) demonstrated appearance of SRS in effluents from sensitized lungs following challenge with specific antigen. Subsequent work has suggested that SRS plays important roles as a mediator in asthma and other types of immediate hypersensitivity reactions (reviewed in 16 and 17).

A link between the transformations of arachidonic acid in leukocytes described above and SRS formation was suggested by the ionophore stimulation of the pathway and the spectroscopic properties of the products. After having surveyed published procedures (16) for SRS-generation we found a new system (mast cell tumor) which gave a better yield of SRS (18).

The mast cell tumor was propagated in the peritoneal cavity of syngenic mice. SRS was generated by preincubation with [$^3H_8$] arachidonic acid or labeled cysteine, and challenging with the ionophore A23187 in the presence or absence of unlabeled cysteine.

To purify SRS, incubation mixtures were centrifuged, supernatants mixed with ethanol to 80%, filtered, and evaporated to dryness. The residue was hydro-

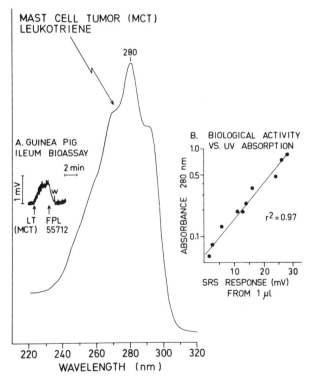

FIG. 8. Ultraviolet spectrum of a slow-reacting substance, SRS (leukotriene C), from mast cell tumor. **Inset A.** Contraction of guinea pig ileum after addition of UV-absorbing material. Note the addition of FPL 55712 at the second arrow. **Inset B.** Correlation between the log absorbance at 280 nm from a purification of the mast cell tumor-leukotriene C and the biological response on isolated guinea pig ileum (least square linear regression).

lyzed with base, purified by Amberlite XAD-8 and silicic acid chromatography followed by two steps of RP-HPLC. This afforded essentially pure SRS.

Purifications were monitored by bioassay on isolated guinea pig ileum in the presence of atropine and pyrilamine maleate. Reversal of contractions by the SRS antagonist FPL 55712 was used as a criterion for biological activity. A preparation of SRS prepared by ionophore challenge of human leukocytes was used to standardize the contractile response.

Purified preparations of mast cell tumor SRS gave a characteristic ultraviolet spectrum (Fig. 8). Inset A of this figure shows the biologic effect of a small aliquot of this fraction. The absorbance at 280 nm and the SRS response of

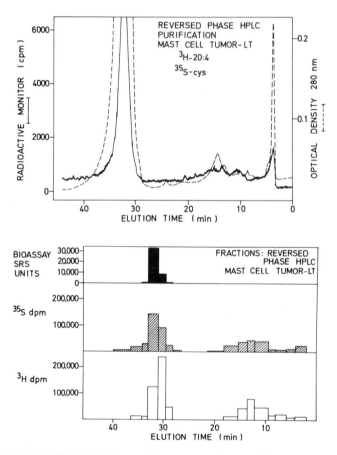

FIG. 9. Upper panel: RP-HPLC (Nucleosil C_{18}, methanol/water, 65/35, v/v + 0.01% acetic acid) of mast cell tumor leukotriene C, purified by silicic acid chromatography and Polygosil C_{18} RP-HPLC. The tumor cells were prelabeled with [$^3H_8$]-arachidonic acid and [^{35}S]-cysteine. A radioactive monitor and an ultraviolet detector (280 nm) were connected in series after the HPLC column. **Lower panel:** Biological activity, ^3H-, and ^{35}S-contents of fractions collected during the RP-HPLC.

TABLE 2. Incorporation of [3H8]arachidonic acid and [3,3H]-, [U-14C]-, and [35S]cysteine into SRS from MCT cells after reversed phase HPLC purification[a]

Component	Retention time[b], min	Exp. A[c] incorporation, dpm		Exp. B[d] incorporation, dpm		Exp. C[e] incorporation, dpm	
		[3H]C20:4	[35S]Cys	[3-3H]Cys	[35S]Cys	[3-3H]Cys	[U-14C]Cys
LTC-1[f]	31.8	1,490,000 (0.027%)	410,000 (0.056%)	97,200 (0.014%)	181,000 (0.020%)	15,700 (0.0020%)	1910 (0.0022%)
LTC-2[g]	35.2	31,000 (0.006%)	13,200 (0.002%)	14,100 (0.002%)	34,400 (0.003%)	12,500 (0.0016%)	1030 (0.0012%)

Numbers in parentheses are calculated percent of added precursor incorporated.

[a] Mobile phase, 65:35 methanol/water. Prior HPLC used 70:30.

[b] Retention time calculated at the maximum of the UV absorbance.

[c] [3H] Arachidonic acid ($C_{20:4}$) (250 μCi) in 2 ml methanol was added dropwise to the cell suspension (9.6 × 10^9 cells) 60 min prior to A23187. [35S]Cysteine (330 μCi) was added 15 min prior to A23187.

[d] [3-3H] Cysteine (300 μCi) and [35S] cysteine (400 μCi) were combined and added to the cell suspension (7.4 × 10^9 cells) 15 min prior to addition of A23187.

[e] [3-3H] Cysteine (355 μCi) and [U-14C] cysteine (39 μCi) were combined and added to the cell suspension (5 × 10^9 cells) 15 min prior to addition of A23187.

[f] UV spectrum with λ_{max} 280 nm, shoulders at 270 and 292 nm.

[g] UV spectrum with λ_{max} 278 nm, shoulders at 268 and 290 nm.

ten fractions collected during a final HPLC purification were highly correlated (inset B, Fig. 8). This suggested that the UV-absorbing material and SRS are identical. The spectrum is similar to the spectra of dihydroxylated arachidonic acid metabolites in rabbit PMNLs (Fig. 2) but shifted 8 to 12 nm bathochromically, indicating that the SRS contained a conjugated triene with an α-auxochrome (vide infra).

Incubations with [^{3}H$_8$]arachidonic acid and [^{35}S]cysteine yielded purified SRS which contained ^{3}H and ^{35}S. Figure 9 shows a high-pressure liquid chromatogram in which high energy β-radiation (^{35}S) and absorbance at 280 nm were monitored continuously (upper panel). Biological activity, ^{35}S and ^{3}H radioactivity were determined in fractions collected during the chromatography (lower panel). The difference in elution profile for ^{35}S and ^{3}H is due to isotope separation during the HPLC.

Dual isotope experiments with [3-^{3}H, ^{35}S]cysteine and [3-^{3}H, U-^{14}C]cysteine and amino group analyses of purified SRS (Table 2) indicated that besides sulfur, the three carbon atoms, the amino group, and hydrogen at C-3 of cysteine were present in the SRS.

Purified SRS from [^{3}H$_8$]arachidonic acid was treated with Raney nickel. The desulfurized product was esterified and purified by silicic acid chromatography. Figure 10 shows a gas-liquid radiochromatogram obtained after trimethylsilylation. The mass spectrum of the major radioactive component was nearly identical to that of similarly derivatized 5-hydroxyarachidic acid (Fig. 11). This suggested that 20 carbon atoms of arachidonic acid occurred in the SRS. Furthermore, the hydroxy group at C-5 as well as the UV spectrum of the molecule indicated

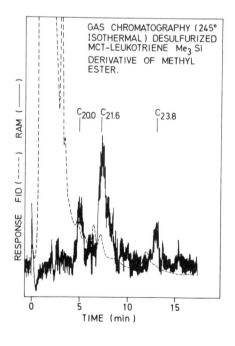

FIG. 10. Gas-liquid radiochromatogram of Raney-nickel desulfurized mast cell tumor leukotriene C (methyl ester, TMS derivative; 1% SE-30; FID, flame ionization detector; RAM, radioactivity monitor).

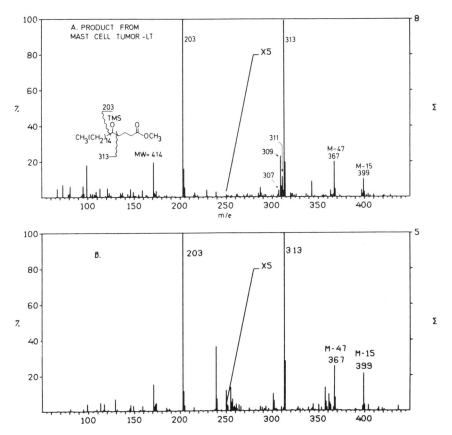

FIG. 11. (A) Mass spectrum of the radioactive product with an equivalent carbon number of 21.6 (Fig. 10). (B) Mass spectrum of the methyl ester, TMS derivative of 5-hydroxyarachidic acid.

that the SRS is structurally related to the dihydroxylated arachidonic acid metabolites in rabbit PMNLs described above.

The purified SRS from [³H₈]arachidonic acid was further degraded by reductive ozonolysis. This yielded an ether extractable radioactive product which cochromatographed with carrier 1-hexanol on RP-HPLC and gas-liquid radiochromatography (alcohol or trimethylsilylether) (Fig. 12). The results showed that the Δ^{14} double bond of arachidonic acid remained in the SRS.

An experiment with soybean lipoxygenase was essential for the final structure elucidation of the mast cell tumor SRS. The lipoxygenase requires a methylene-interrupted *cis,cis*-1,4-pentadiene to introduce a molecule of oxygen at the methylene group. Simultaneously, the ω-6 double bond is isomerized to ω-7 (19). Figure 13 shows the spectral changes observed after 5-min and 1-hr incubations of purified SRS with the lipoxygenase. The 30-nm bathochromic shift showed that the conjugated triene was extended to a conjugated tetraene. Since the Δ^{14} double bond was most likely isomerized to Δ^{13}, the experiment indicated

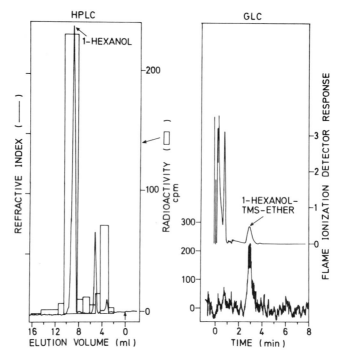

FIG. 12. Reductive ozonolysis of mast cell tumor leukotriene C from [³H₈]-arachidonic acid: *Left:* HPLC of ether extractable products. 1-Hexanol was added as internal reference (μ C₁₈ bondapak; 50% aqueous methanol/water, 1/1, + 0.01% acetic acid at 1 ml/min). Radioactivity was determined after addition of Instagel to HPLC fractions. *Right:* Gas-liquid radio chromatogram of ether extractable products (TMS derivative). 1-Hexanol was added prior to derivative formation (1.6% OV-1 at 52°C).

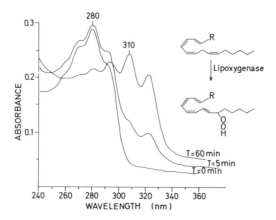

FIG. 13. Alteration of the ultraviolet spectrum of mast cell tumor leukotriene C during an incubation with soybean lipoxygenase.

that the SRS had additional double bonds at $\Delta^{7,9,11}$. Therefore, the SRS was a cysteine-containing derivative of 5-hydroxy-7,9,11,14-eicosatetraenoic acid.

This amino acid was attached at C-6 of the eicosatetraenoic acid for the following reasons: *(a)* Oxidative and reductive ozonolysis yielded 1,5-pentane-dioic acid and 1-hexanol, respectively, excluding substitution at C-1 through C-5 and C-15 through C-20; *(b)* C-7 through C-12 were excluded based on the ultraviolet spectrum since a substituent on the triene chromophore should give a higher λ_{max} than that observed (20); *(c)* For the same reason, substitution at C-13 or C-14 would give a higher λ_{max} than that observed for lipoxygenase-treated SRS. Furthermore, attachment of an amino acid at these sites would most likely prevent conversion by soybean lipoxygenase.

A sulfur substituent at C-6 is in agreement with the ultraviolet spectrum of SRS since a thioether bond α to a conjugated triene gives a bathochromic shift of approximately 10 nm (21).

Figure 14 shows the structure of the mouse mast cell tumor SRS and summa-rizes the experimental evidence for it. It should be noted that the stereochemistry at C-5 and C-6 is unknown as well as the geometry of the double bonds at Δ^7 and Δ^9. The lipoxygenase experiment requires that the other double bonds are *cis*. Also, although the experiments with labeled cysteines indicated that all carbon atoms of the amino acid are incorporated into LTC, the data do not rule out that the substituent at C-6 is a derivative of cysteine.

The structure of the SRS suggests that it may be formed from the 5,6-oxido-7,9,11,14-eicosatetraenoic acid, described above as an intermediate in the biosyn-thesis of 5(S),12(R)-dihydroxy-6,8,10,14-(e,z,e,z)-eicosatetraenoic acid (Fig. 15). This confers considerable importance to the lipoxygenase which leads to the formation of these products. The term *leukotriene* has been introduced (22)

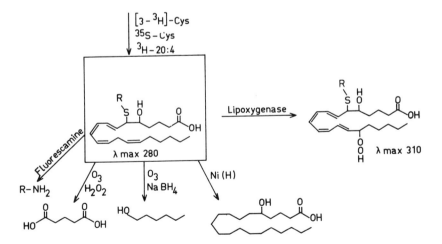

FIG. 14. Precursor experiments and chemical and enzymological transformations of mouse mast cell tumor leukotriene C (SRS).

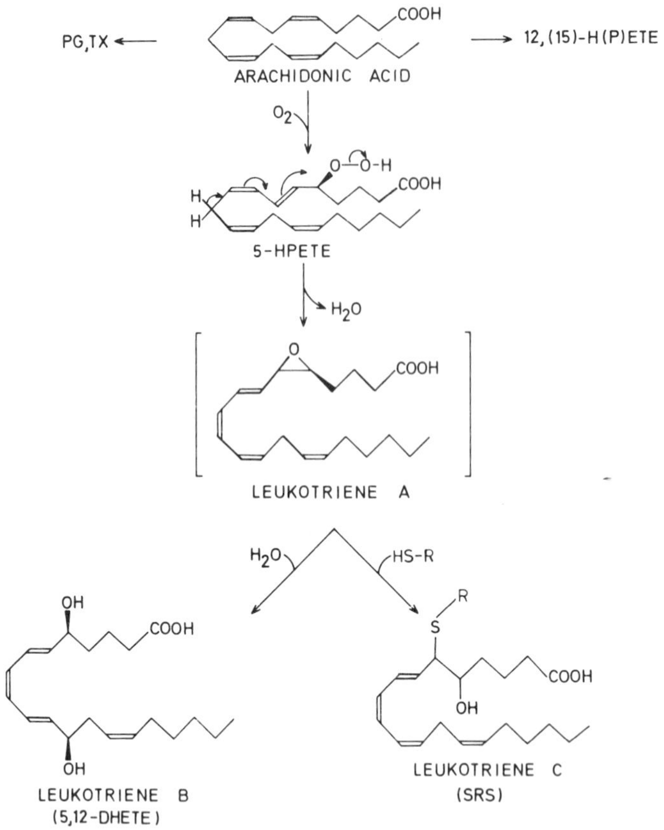

FIG. 15. Proposed scheme of transformations of arachidonic acid leading to 5,6(oxido)-7,9, 11,14-eicosatetraenoic acid (leukotriene A) and 5(S),12(R)-dihydroxy-6,8,11,14-(e,z,e,z)-eicosatetraenoic acid (leukotriene B) in leukocytes and to a 6-cysteinyl derivative of 5-hydroxy-7,9,11,14-eicosatetraenoic acid (leukotriene C) (SRS) in murine mastocytoma cells.

for compounds of this pathway which contain a conjugated triene. Leukotriene A, LTA is the 5,6-oxido-intermediate, LTB the 5,12-dihydroxy compound, and LTC the slow-reacting substance from mouse mast cell tumor. Additional studies indicate the presence of a structurally related leukotriene in rat basophilic leukemia cells. This suggests that there is a family of leukotrienes and preliminary studies indicate that their occurrence is not restricted to leukocytes and mast cells.

The leukotriene pathway, which is initiated by oxygenation at C-5, constitutes a system parallel to that of the prostaglandins and thromboxanes (Fig. 16). The formation of the latter group of compounds does also involve a lipoxygenase type reaction; however, in this case oxygen is initially introduced at C-11. The formation of leukotrienes should therefore be amenable to pharmacologic control without affecting prostaglandin synthesis. It is thus conceivable that new types

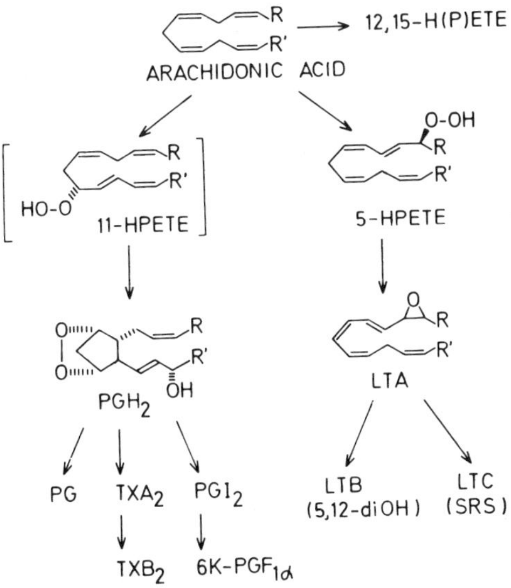

FIG. 16. General principles in the oxygenation and further transformations of arachidonic acid.

of drugs intervening with the formation and action of leukotrienes could be developed for use in asthma and other immediate hypersensitivity reactions.

ACKNOWLEDGMENT

This project was supported by a grant from the Swedish Medical Research Council (project 03X-217).

REFERENCES

1. Samuelsson, B., Granström, E., Gréen, K., Hamberg, M., and Hammarström, S. (1975): *Annu. Rev. Biochem.,* 44:669–695.
2. Samuelsson, B., Goldyne, M., Granström, E., Hamberg, M., Hammarström, S., and Malmsten, C. (1978): *Annu. Rev. Biochem.,* 47:997–1029.
3. Samuelsson, B. (1976): In: *Advances in Prostaglandin and Thromboxane Research,* edited by B. Samuelsson and R. Paoletti, Vol. 1, pp. 1–6. Raven Press, New York.
4. Borgeat, P., and Samuelsson, B. (1976): *J. Biol. Chem.,* 251:7816–7820. See also correction: (1977) *J. Biol. Chem.,* 252:8772.
5. Borgeat, P., and Samuelsson, B. (1979): *J. Biol. Chem.,* 254:2643–2646.
6. Borgeat, P., and Samuelsson, B. (1979): *J. Biol. Chem. (in press).*
7. Crombie, L., and Jacklin, A. G. (1957): *J. Chem. Soc.,* 1632–1646.
8. Borgeat, P., and Samuelsson, B. (1979): *Proc. Natl. Acad. Sci. USA (in press).*
9. Borgeat, P., and Samuelsson, B. (1979): *Proc. Natl. Acad. Sci. USA,* 76:2148–2152.
10. Knapp, H. R., Oelz, O. O., Roberts, J., Sweetman, B. J., Oates, J. A., and Reed, P. W. (1977): *Proc. Natl. Acad. Sci. USA,* 74:4251–4255.
11. Weidemann, M. J., Peskar, B. A., Wrogemann, K., Rietschel, E. T., Staudinger, H., and Fischer, H. (1978): *FEBS Lett.,* 89:136–140.
12. Wentzell, B., and Epand, R. M. (1978): *FEBS Lett.,* 86:255–258.
13. Pickett, W., Jesse, R. L., and Cohen, P. (1977): *Biochim. Biophys. Acta,* 486:209–213.

14. Feldberg, W., and Kellaway, C. H. (1938): *J. Physiol.*, 94:187–226.
15. Kellaway, C. H., and Trethewie (1940): *J. Exp. Physiol.*, 30:121–145.
16. Austen, K. (1978): *J. Immunol.*, 121:793–805.
17. Orange, R. P., and Austen, K. F. (1969): *Adv. Immunol.*, 10:105–144.
18. Murphy, R. C., Hammarström, S., and Samuelsson, B. (1979): *Proc. Natl. Acad. Sci. USA (in press).*
19. Hamberg, M., and Samuelsson, B. (1967): *J. Biol. Chem.*, 242:5329–5335.
20. Williams, D. H., and Fleming, I. (1966): In: *Spectroscopic Methods in Organic Chemistry*, pp. 6–39. McGraw-Hill, New York.
21. Koch, H. P. (1949): *J. Chem. Soc.*, 387:394.
22. Samuelsson, B., Borgeat, P., Hammarström, S., and Murphy, R. C. (1979): *Prostaglandins*, 17:785–787.

Advances in Prostaglandin and Thromboxane Research,
Vol. 6, edited by B. Samuelsson, P. W. Ramwell,
and R. Paoletti. Raven Press, New York © 1980.

Recent Studies on the Chemical Synthesis of Eicosanoids

E. J. Corey, H. Niwa, J. R. Falck, C. Mioskowski, Y. Arai, and
A. Marfat

Department of Chemistry, Harvard University, Cambridge, Massachusetts 02138

The chemical synthesis of stable prostanoids—including such naturally occurring prostaglandins as $PGF_{2\alpha}$, PGE_2, PGI_2, and a multitude of structural analogs—is now at a highly developed stage, with the result that these substances can be satisfactorily produced synthetically (for review, see ref. 5). However, challenging synthetic problems still abound, partly as a result of recent discoveries of new and, in some cases, quite unstable biologically active substances originating from polyunsaturated C_{20} fatty acids. It is convenient to use the term "eicosanoids" to describe the broad group of compounds derived from C_{20} fatty acids. The eicosanoid family thus includes prostaglandins, thromboxanes, Samuelsson's HETE (12,13), lipoxygenase-derived hydroperoxides or alcohols (4,12,13,16,18), slow-reacting substance of anaphylaxis (2,15), etc. In order to achieve a meaningful capability of producing by chemical synthesis novel, or unstable, members of the eicosanoid family, new synthetic methodology is needed. Potentially, the most useful chemistry in this regard would be reactions which effect *highly selective chemical oxidation* of polyunsaturated fatty acids such as arachidonic acid. This paper is concerned with these matters and, specifically, with new synthetic methods for selective oxidation and specific synthesis of certain biologically interesting, non-PG eicosanoids.

The eicosanoid *(S)*-12-hydroxy-5,8,14-*cis,* 10-*trans*-eicosatetraenoic acid (Samuelsson's HETE), formed biochemically from arachidonic acid presumably via the corresponding hydroperoxide in a lipoxygenase-type reaction, is of considerable interest but is available in only submilligram amounts from natural sources. A chemical synthesis of this substance **1** (Fig. 1) has been developed which leads *directly* to the natural antipode without the need for resolution. Starting from the 2-methoxypropyl ether of *S*-(-)-malic acid ethyl ester, the synthesis proceeds via the intermediates shown in Fig. 1, the crucial step being the coupling of the aldehydo ester **15** with the β-oxido ylide **16** (10). This synthesis lends itself to the production of gram amounts of HETE. It has not thus far been extended to the synthesis of the corresponding 12-hydroperoxide, which is currently unknown, but which is an extremely interesting candidate for biological studies (see, for example, ref. 14).

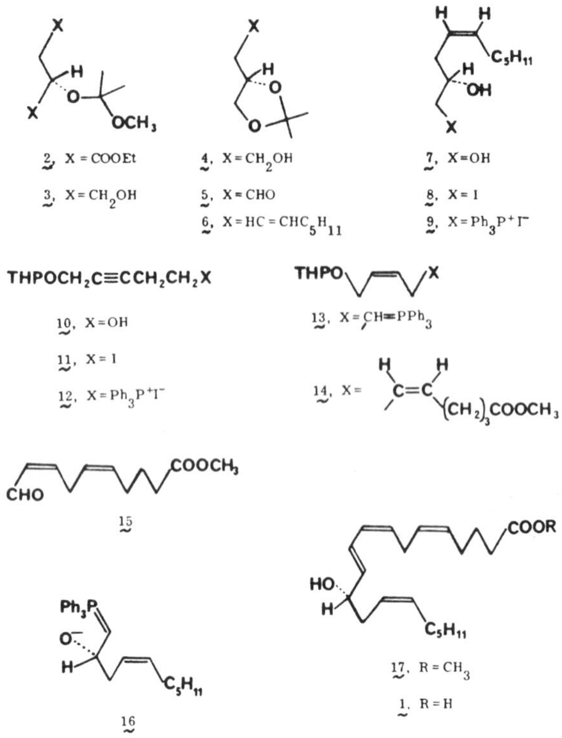

FIG. 1. Total synthesis of HETE.

Along with studies on the synthesis of HETE by multistep approaches such as outlined in Fig. 1, we investigated the transformation of the natural precursor arachidonic acid to HETE by selective chemical oxidation. The long-known free-radical-initiated autoxidation of polyunsaturated fatty acids is obviously completely unsuited for this purpose, since it produces hopelessly complex mixtures. From a purely logical point of view, it seemed attractive to consider the possibility of some kind of internally directed oxidation process which depends on the carboxylic function of arachidonic acid as a controller group. Although there are a number of reasonable reaction sequences utilizing this principle which might be workable for the synthesis of lipoxygenase-type products from arachidonic acid, we chose for our initial studies the scheme which is depicted in general form in Fig. 2. The successful realization of such a scheme would depend on the ability to perform three chemical steps: (a) utilization of the carboxyl function to epoxidize selectively only *one* of the *cis* bonds, (b) the application of the known base-catalyzed epoxide to allylic alcohol rearrangement (17,19,20), and finally, (c) the conversion of an allylic alcohol to corresponding allylic hydroperoxide. Both the first and final steps involve new chemistry. As might be expected, the *bimolecular* epoxidation of polyunsaturated fatty

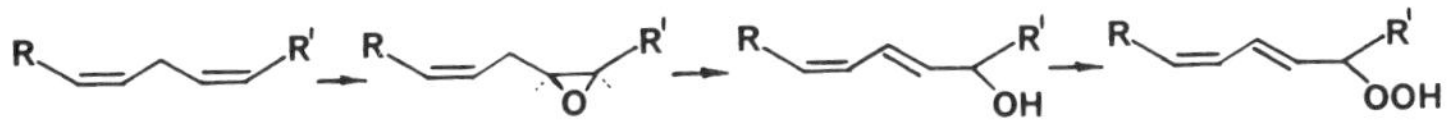

FIG. 2. Strategy for the selective conversion of a *cis,cis*-1,4-diene unit to a lipoxygenase-type unit.

acids by peroxy acid reagents is essentially nonselective and all double bonds are attacked to some degree (7), so that this is not a viable approach.

The strategy which was adopted, and which proved remarkably successful, involved the conversion of arachidonic acid (**1** in Fig. 4) to the corresponding peroxy acid (**2**) which was then allowed to react *internally* in dilute solution (ca. 0.01 M). It was anticipated that internal epoxidation from peroxyarachidonic acid would not lead to oxygen transfer to either the Δ^5- or Δ^8-double bonds, since the bicyclic structures corresponding to the normal transition site for the peroxy acid olefin reaction (Fig. 3) in these cases would be quite strained (judging, for example, from examination of CPK space-filling models). Thus there seemed a reasonable chance for considerable chemical selectivity, although it was not possible to decide *a priori* whether internal attack would favor Δ^{11}- or Δ^{14}-epoxidation.

No peroxy-polyunsaturated fatty acids had been made prior to this investigation, and it was not a complete surprise when it was discovered that the standard methods of synthesis failed. However, a new process for the conversion of carboxylic acids to peroxycarboxylic acids under mild, nonacidic conditions was devised (9) which was extremely effective. A solution of arachidonic acid (purity > 99%) in dry methylene chloride was allowed to react with an equivalent of carboxyldiimidazole at 25°C for 20 min to form arachidonylimidazole and this solution was treated with excess, cold anhydrous hydrogen peroxide in ether in the presence of a catalytic amount of lithium imidazolide. After stirring with powdered sodium bisulfate (to remove the imidazole), drying and dilution with methylene chloride a 0.01 M solution of peroxyarachidonic acid was obtained, which on storage at 20°C for 6 hr and isolation afforded a *single product,* the 14,15-epoxide **3** in 98% isolated yield (Fig. 4). The structure of **3** was confirmed by physical methods, as well as chemical degradation. Hydrogenation of the methyl ester **4** followed by exposure to periodic acid water–tetrahydrofuran produced the known ester aldehyde **5**. In addition, oxidation of **4** by periodate–permanganate followed by esterification with CH_2N_2 gave the epoxy ester **6** (9).

In a similar way, *cis*-8,11,14-eicosa-trienoic acid was converted into the corresponding peroxy acid derivative, which at 0°C for 70 hr in ether–methylene

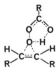

FIG. 3. Transition state for the reaction of a *cis*-olefin with a peroxycarboxylic acid.

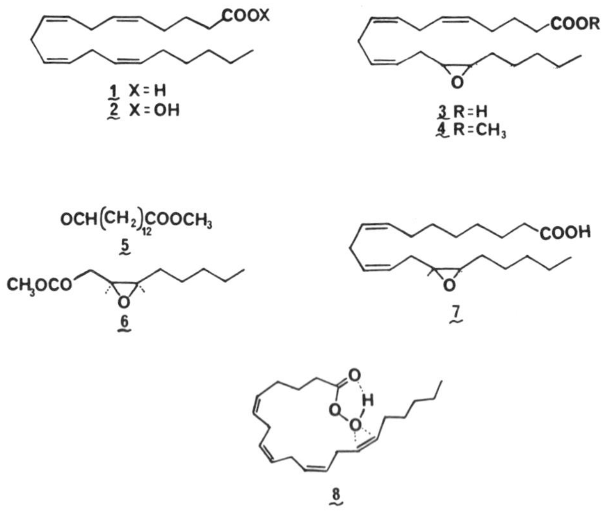

FIG. 4. Internal epoxidation of arachidonic and *cis*-8,11,14-eicosatrienoic acids.

chloride transferred oxygen preferentially to the Δ^{14}-double bond to give a $\Delta^{14,15}$-epoxide **7** in 92% isolated yield.

The large preference for transfer of oxygen to the Δ^{14}-double bond of arachidonic acid (and the somewhat smaller, but still impressive, tendency for *cis*-8,11,14-eicosa-trienoic acid) may be due in large measure to a favoring of that transition state geometry for oxygen transfer in which the center of the $C=C$ pi electron cloud is back side to and colinear with the O—O bond being broken (see formula **8** in Fig. 4). In essence, this S_N2-like arrangement allows optimal transfer of the pi electrons into the O—O antibonding molecular orbital. The colinear geometry is readily attained for transfer to the Δ^{14}-double bond but not the Δ^{11}-double bond. The internal epoxidation is probably also favored by the relatively favorable energy of a J-like shape for arachidonic acid.

Conversion of $\Delta^{14,15}$-epoxyarachidonic acid to the corresponding peroxy acid and subsequent internal oxygen transfer as described above produced in a mixture of two diastereomeric $\Delta^{11,12},\Delta^{14,15}$-bis-epoxides excellent yield (Fig. 5, **1**). Methylation of this product with diazomethane forms the methyl ester, which on treatment with lithium diisopropylamide at $-90°C$ gives the rearranged epoxy alcohol **2** reaction, which with potassium selenocyanate in methanol at 65°C effects deoxygenation (3) to produce ±-HETE methyl ester (**3**). This synthesis provides one indication of the utility of internal, carboxyl-directed oxidation in the synthesis of eicosanoids from polyunsaturated fatty acids. The further conversion of **3** to the corresponding hydroperoxide is now under study.

Figure 6 summarizes the results of experiments on internal epoxidation by intramolecular oxidation transfer for a number of other polyunsaturated fatty acids. An investigation (still under way) of the internal oxidation of arachidonic

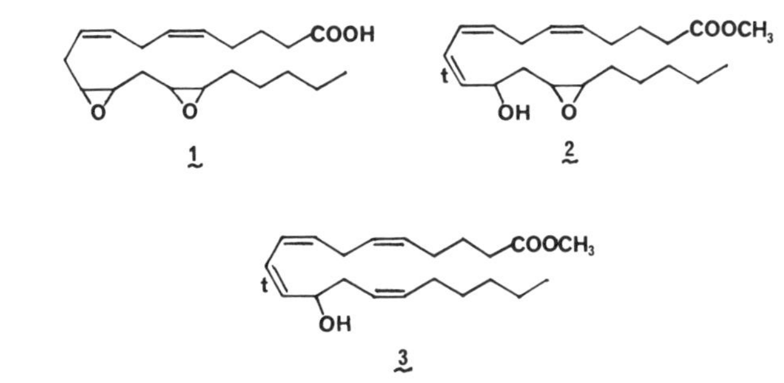

FIG. 5. Conversion of arachidonic acid to HETE.

acid derivatives in which the carboxyl function is displaced by the use of a "spacer group" has yielded interesting results, as illustrated by cases 1 and 2 in Fig. 6. The numbers shown refer to the percent yield of isolated epoxide obtained from the corresponding peroxy acid. It seems possible that by the use of appropriate spacer groups, the selective oxidation of any particular double bond in, for example, arachidonic acid, may be attainable. Example 3 shows that internal oxygen transfer to the $\Delta^{17,18}$-double bond in eicosapentaenoic acid is competitive with reaction at the $\Delta^{14,15}$-double bond. In the case of 5,8,11,14, 17,20-cis-docosahexaenoic acid, oxidation at the three double bonds at the omega end of the chain was preferred.

Recently, the formation of a new eicosanoid from arachidonic acid by rabbit polymorphonuclear leukocytes has been observed by Borgeat and Samuelsson (6; personal communication). The results of this elegant study allowed the assignment of structure 1 (Fig. 7) to this new metabolite with the exception of the exact configuration at each of the double bonds in the conjugated triene part of the diol which was not determined. It seemed to us that the most reasonable biogenetic pathway to 1 was from the epoxide intermediate 2, which could in

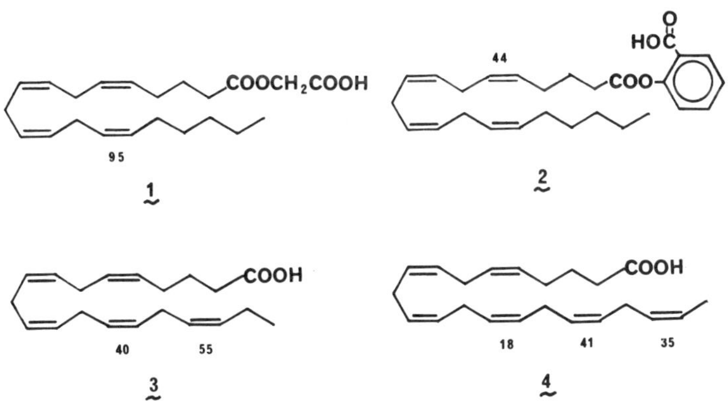

FIG. 6. Internal epoxidation of some polyunsaturated fatty acid derivatives.

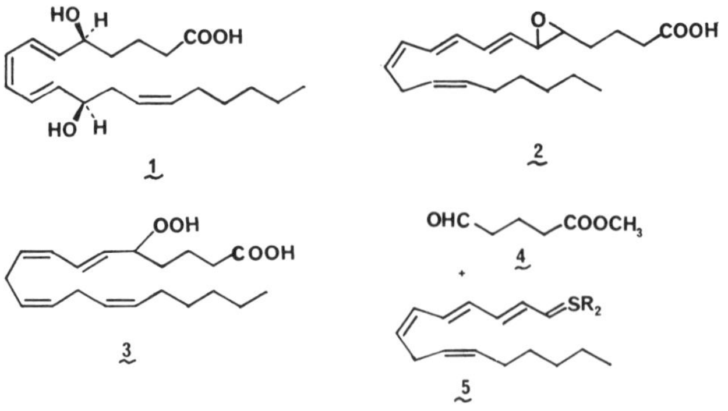

FIG. 7. Eicosanoids from rabbit polymorphonuclear leukocytes.

turn be formed from the lipoxygenase-like intermediate **3** (1). We therefore embarked on a synthesis of these substances to verify this hypothesis.

A successful synthesis of **2**, as well as the isomer about the oxirane ring, has now been completed, and biological studies with the synthetic material are now underway in the laboratories of Professor Samuelsson. The pathway of synthesis involves as the key step the reaction of the aldehyde **4** with a sulfur ylide **5**, methodology developed several years ago in our laboratory (8).

The 5,6-epoxide of arachidonic acid has been obtained via the 5,6-iodo lactone in good yield (9). The conversion of this intermediate to the hydroperoxide **3** via the corresponding alcohol is now under study.

ACKNOWLEDGMENT

The authors are grateful to the National Science Foundation (U.S.) for a grant in support of this research.

REFERENCES

1. Agata, I., Corey, E. J., Hortman, A. G., Klein, J., Proskow, S., and Ursprung, J. J. (1965): *J. Org. Chem.*, 30:1698–1710.
2. Bach, M. K., Brashler, J. R., and German, R. R. (1977): *Prostaglandins*, 14:21–38.
3. Behan, J. M., Johnstone, R. A. W., and Wright, M. J. (1975): *J. Chem. Soc. [Perkin I.]*, 1216–1217.
4. Bild, G. S., Ramacloss, C. S., Lim, S., and Axelrod, B. (1977): *Biochem. Biophys. Res. Commun.*, 74:949–954.
5. Bindra, J. S., and Bindra, R. (1977): *Prostaglandin Synthesis*. Academic Press, New York.
6. Borgeat, P., and Samuelsson, B. (1979): *J. Biol. Chem.*, 254:2643–2646.
7. Chung, S. K., and Scott, A. I. (1974): *Tet. Lett.*, 3023–3026.
8. Corey, E. J., and Chaykovsky, M. (1965): *J. Am. Chem. Soc.*, 87:1353–1364.
9. Corey, E. J., Niwa, H., and Falck, J. R. (1979): *J. Am. Chem. Soc.*, 101:1586–1587.
10. Corey, E. J., Niwa, H., and Knolle, J. (1978): *J. Am. Chem. Soc.*, 100:1942–1943.
11. Corey, E. J., and Oppolzer, W. (1964): *J. Am. Chem. Soc.*, 86:1899–1900.
12. Hamberg, M., and Samuelsson, B. (1974): *Proc. Natl. Acad. Sci. USA*, 71:3400–3404.
13. Hamberg, M., Svensson, J., and Samuelsson, B. (1974): *Proc. Natl. Acad. Sci. USA*, 71:3824.

14. Hammerström, S., Hamberg, M., Samuelsson, B., Duell, E. A., Stawiski, M., and Voorhees, J. J. (1975): *Proc. Natl. Acad. Sci. USA,* 72:5130–5134.
15. Jakschik, B. A., Falkenheim, S., and Parker, C. W. (1977): *Proc. Natl. Acad. Sci. USA,* 74:4577–4586.
16. Jones, R. L., Kerry, P. J., Poyser, N. L., Walker, I. C., and Wilson, N. H. (1978): *Prostaglandins,* 16:583–589.
17. Kissel, C. L., and Rickborn, B. (1972): *J. Org. Chem.,* 37:2060–2063.
18. Samuelsson, B., and Hamberg, M. (1967): *J. Biol. Chem.,* 242:5336–5343.
19. Thummel, R. P., and Rickborn, B. (1970): *J. Am. Chem. Soc.,* 92:2064–2067.
20. Yasuda, A., Tanaka, S., Oshima, K., Yamamoto, H., and Nozaki, H. (1974): *J. Am. Chem. Soc.,* 96:6513–6514.

Advances in Prostaglandin and Thromboxane Research,
Vol. 6, edited by B. Samuelsson, P. W. Ramwell,
and R. Paoletti. Raven Press, New York © 1980.

Enzymes Involved in the Formation and Further Transformations of Prostaglandin Endoperoxides

Shozo Yamamoto,[1] Shiro Ohki,[2] Nubuchika Ogino,[3] Takao
Shimizu, Tanihiro Yoshimoto,[1] Kikuko Watanabe,
and Osamu Hayaishi

*Department of Medical Chemistry, Kyoto University Faculty of Medicine, Sakyo-ku,
Kyoto, Japan*

Studies on prostaglandin (PG) biosynthesis started shortly after the isolation and structure determination of PGE and PGF, and it was soon elucidated that the precursors of PGEs were eicosapolyenoic acids. The enzyme preparation used earlier was a homogenate or a microsomal fraction of vesicular gland, which catalyzed an overall conversion of the eicosapolyenoic acids to PGE (1,2,17,18). A hypothetical mechanism was proposed to explain how PG biosynthesis proceeded in a series of reactions. A characteristic and important feature of this hypothesis was the involvement of an endoperoxide intermediate (5,9). However, it was not known at that time whether such an endoperoxide was an enzyme-bound intermediate or an isolable product.

MICROSOMAL PG SYNTHETASE SYSTEM

Based on these previous findings and hypothesis, we started our enzymological studies on the PG synthetase system. The starting material was a microsomal fraction of bovine vesicular gland. When the microsomes were incubated with ^{14}C-labeled 8,11,14-eicosatrienoic acid and the etherial extract from the reaction mixture was examined by silica gel thin-layer chromatography, a major reaction product comigrated with PGE_1 (Fig.1).

In the above reaction mixture, three compounds were included as activators. A variety of compounds had been found to stimulate the overall PGE synthesis. These compounds were different in structure from one another, and as a result of our further investigation, they were divided into three categories: hemoglobin (20), tryptophan (8), and glutathione (9).

On the other hand, the microsomes were treated with a nonionic detergent

Present addresses: [1] Department of Biochemistry, Tokushima University School of Medicine, Kuramoto-cho, Tokushima, Japan; [2] Ono Central Research Institute, Shimamoto-cho, Mishima-gun, Osaka, Japan; [3] Department of Ophthalmology, Kyoto University Faculty of Medicine, Sakyo-ku, Kyoto, Japan.

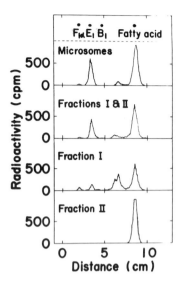

FIG. 1. Reactions of [^{14}C] 8, 11, 14-eicosatrienoic acid with fraction I or fraction II or both.

to solubilize the enzyme, and the supernatant solution obtained by high-speed centrifugation was subjected to DEAE-cellulose column chromatography. The enzyme was resolved into two fractions I and II by increasing buffer concentration.

Reactions were carried out with these two enzyme fractions and the three activators in various combinations. When all these components were present, eicosatrienoic acid was converted to PGE$_1$, as in the microsomal incubation (Fig. 1). Fraction II was inactive with eicosatrienoic acid, while fraction I produced a compound migrating faster than PGE$_1$. The compound was not converted to PGE$_1$ on further incubation with fraction II. The result indicated that the compound produced by fraction I was not an intermediate between eicosatrienoic acid and PGE$_1$.

Shortly after this finding, the actual isolation and identification of two PG endoperoxides were reported by Nugteren and Hazelhof (10) and Hamberg et al. (6). These reports described PG endoperoxides as unstable at room temperature and suggested that the reaction product of fraction I be isolated cautiously, particularly at subzero temperatures. The results obtained under refined experimental conditions demonstrated a series of reactions from eicosatrienoic acid to PGE$_1$, namely, the reaction of eicosatrienoic acid with fraction I produced PGG$_1$ as a major product. Heme was required for this reaction. Another enzyme also contained in fraction I transformed PGG$_1$ to PGH$_1$ in the presence of heme and tryptophan. The conversion of PGH$_1$ to PGE$_1$ was catalyzed by fraction II. Glutathione was required for this reaction (7).

PG ENDOPEROXIDE SYNTHETASE

As a peculiar nature of the enzyme, both the production of PGG$_1$ and its conversion to PGH$_1$ were catalyzed by the same enzyme fraction I. Purification of enzyme was necessary to conclude whether the two types of reaction were catalyzed by a single enzyme or two separate enzymes. Fortunately, the enzyme was highly purified by isoelectrofocusing to a specific activity of approximately 2 μmoles/min/mg of protein. Disc gel electrophoresis of the purified enzyme gave an essentially single band of protein. On isoelectrofocusing, the two enzyme activities were associated and detected around pH 7.0 (7,14). On heat treatment, both enzyme activities were lost in parallel as the temperature was raised (14).

Since both reactions required hemoglobin, the specificity of the heme requirement was investigated with various heme compounds and other metalloporphyrins. The heme was active either as hematin or as a protein-bound form such as hemoglobin and myoglobin. Horseradish peroxidase and cytochrome c were ineffective. The characteristic heme requirement was essentially identical in both reactions (7,14). Among other metalloprotoporphyrins tested (Mn, Co, Zn), only manganese protoporphyrin was as active as hematin. However, the addition of manganese protoporphyrin resulted in the production of PGG_1 not only in the absence of tryptophan, but also in its presence. This was in sharp contrast to the effect of iron protoporphyrin. Thus the two enzyme activities could be discriminated by the use of manganese protoporphyrin instead of hematin (12).

In addition to tryptophan, a variety of compounds have been reported by many investigators to stimulate PG synthesis (Fig. 2). Most of these compounds were described first as activators for the overall synthesis of PGE, but are now known to be required for the step from PGG to PGH. It was reported earlier that the cytosol of vesicular gland contained certain activators (15). Our further investigation on this active principle has recently led to the isolation of a new activator, which was identified as uric acid. Among the other purine derivatives tested, only 2,8-dihydroxyadenine was as active as uric acid (13).

We investigated extensively the role of these compounds. The results were complicated, but could be discussed in terms of three categories. First, some

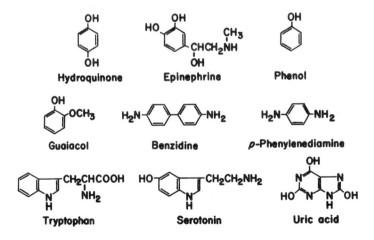

FIG. 2. Compounds which stimulate the PG hydroperoxidase reaction.

of these compounds (for example, epinephrine and guaiacol) were shown by spectrophotometric studies to be dehydrogenated in a stoichiometric quantity along with the conversion of PGG_1 to PGH_1. This is a typical peroxidase reaction, with epinephrine or guaiacol as a hydrogen donor and PGG_1 as a hydrogen acceptor. With tryptophan, however, such a stoichiometric transformation was not detected (14). Second, these compounds increased the affinity of the enzyme for the heme (14). Third, all the compounds tested were stabilizers of the enzyme and protected the enzyme from the inactivation caused by its interaction with the heme (12). All these findings are still phenomenological, and to the best of the present knowledge, it is difficult to explain the function of these activators by a simple principle.

CYCLOOXYGENASE AND HYDROPEROXIDASE

In view of a peroxidatic reduction of PGG_1 with epinephrine or guaiacol, hydroperoxide specificity was investigated with various hydroperoxides. As presented in Fig. 3, the enzyme showed higher activity and affinity for those with PG-like structures, as examined with guaiacol (14).

As illustrated in Fig. 4, the purified enzyme, tentatively referred to as PG endoperoxide synthetase, can produce either PGG or PGH depending on the choice of the activators. Available experimental findings indicate that both the production of PGG and its conversion to PGH are catalyzed either by a single enzyme or by two tightly associated enzymes. The first step is an oxygenative cyclization of eicosapolyenoic acid, to which a term of fatty acid cyclooxygenase is applicable, as proposed by Samuelsson and others (6). The second step is the conversion of the 15-hydroperoxide of PGG to a hydroxyl group of PGH. Although a precise mechanism for this reaction is still unclarified, we refer to

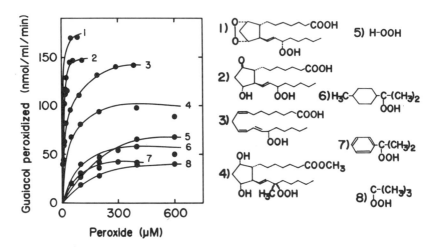

FIG. 3. Hydroperoxide specificity of the PG hydroperoxidase reaction.

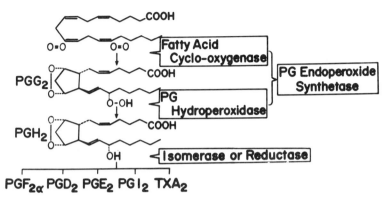

FIG. 4. Enzymes involved in the formation and further transformations of PG endoperoxides.

this enzyme as PG hydroperoxidase merely in the sense that the enzyme attacks hydroperoxides, preferentially those with PG-like structures. Thus PG endoperoxide synthetase has both the cyclooxygenase and hydroperoxidase activities.

Several investigators have implicated a possible involvement of glutathione peroxidase in the step from PGG to PGH. The glutathione peroxidase prepared from bovine red blood cells did catalyze a glutathione-dependent conversion of PGG_1 to PGH_1 (Table 1). In contrast, PG endoperoxide synthetase peroxidized glutathione only in a negligible amount either with cumene hydroperoxide or with PGG_1, as compared with the tryptophan-dependent conversion of PGG_1 to PGH_1 (14). The possibility cannot be ruled out that the PG hydroperoxidase is merely an adventitious activity of the cyclooxygenase, and under physiological conditions, glutathione peroxidase is actually involved in the step from PGG_1 to PGH_1.

PG ENDOPEROXIDE ISOMERASES

The endoperoxide moiety of PGH is cleaved and rearranged in various ways to produce other PG and thromboxanes (TX). Each type of rearrangement is catalyzed by a specific isomerase. We recently purified PGD synthetase from

TABLE 1. *Glutathione peroxidase and PG hydroperoxidase*

Enzyme	Hydrogen donor	Hydrogen acceptor	Enzyme activity (μmole/min/mg protein)
Glutathione peroxidase	Glutathione	Cumene hydroperoxide	1.24
		PGG_1	0.37
PG hydroperoxidase	Glutathione	Cumene hydroperoxide	0.00
		PGG_1	0.03
	(Tryptophan)	PGG_1	1.16

the rat brain cytosol (16) and solubilized PGE synthetase from the bovine vesicular gland cytosol (11), PGI synthetase from the rabbit aorta microsomes (19), and TXA synthetase from the bovine platelet microsomal fraction (22).

Among these isomerases, only PGE synthetase required glutathione (11), whereas the other isomerases were active without glutathione (16,19,22). In contrast to PGD synthetase of rat brain cytosol, glutathione was required for the enzyme of rat spleen cytosol purified by Christ-Hazelhof and Nugteren (3). Glutathione is known as an oxidoreduction coenzyme. Along with the isomerization of PGH_1 to PGE_1, there was no stoichiometric oxidation of glutathione (11). The result suggests a role of glutathione other than as an oxidoreduction coenzyme.

When PGH_1 was utilized as substrate, PGE_1 and PGD_1 were produced by the corresponding isomerases (11,16), but PGI synthetase and TXA synthetase did not produce PG and TX as major products. As shown in Fig. 5, on the reaction of PGI synthetase with PGH_1, the product comigrated with 12-L-hydroxy-8,10-heptadecadienoic acid (HHD), which was produced by the reaction of PGH_1 and ferrous chloride. The reactions with PGH_2 and PGH_1 occurred at almost the same rate, and both reactions were inhibited by 15-hydroperoxyarachidonic acid. Both enzyme activities were lost in parallel as the temperature

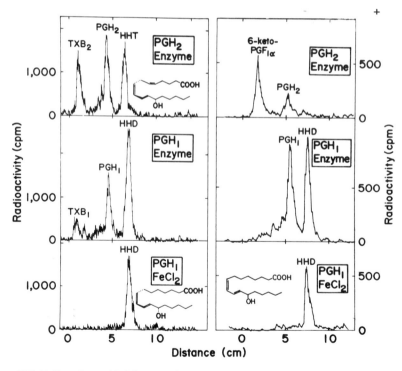

FIG. 5. Reactions with PGH_2 or PGH_1 with TXA synthetase and PGI synthetase.

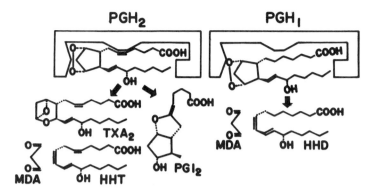

FIG. 6. Side reactions of TXA synthetase and PGI synthetase with PGH$_1$ as substrate analog.

was raised (19). A similar result was obtained with TXA synthetase. As reported by Diczfalusy et al. (4), on incubation with PGH$_1$ the enzyme produced TXB$_1$ only in a small amount, and a major product was HHD. Reactions with both PGH$_2$ and PGH$_1$ occurred at nearly the same rate and were inhibited in a parallel fashion by 1-carboxyheptylimidazole, a potent selective inhibitor of the enzyme (21).

As illustrated in Fig. 6, PGH$_2$ fits the active site of TXA synthetase or PGI synthetase, and the endoperoxide moiety is so rearranged as to produce TXA$_2$ or PGI$_2$, respectively. When PGH$_1$ is bound to the active site, the substrate analog may misfit the active site to some extent. Thus the endoperoxide may be subjected to a distorted reaction, and the whole molecule may be split into HHD and malondialdehyde. If under physiological conditions these enzymes react with PGH$_1$ in this way, it may cause a waste of PG endoperoxide. Therefore, a certain physiological mechanism may operate to avoid wasting PG endoperoxide in this way, for example, at the step of the release of eicosatrienoic acid from phospholipid.

ACKNOWLEDGMENTS

This work was supported in part by a grant-in-aid for scientific research from the Ministry of Education, Science and Culture of Japan; by a research grant from the Intractable Diseases Division, Public Health Bureau, Ministry of Health and Welfare of Japan; and by grants from the Japanese Foundation on Metabolism and Diseases, the Kanae Foundation of the New Medicine Research Association, and the Research Foundation for Cancer and Cardiovascular Diseases.

REFERENCES

1. Bergström, S., Danielsson, H., Klenberg, D., and Samuelsson, B. (1964): *J. Biol. Chem.,* 239:PC4006–4008.

2. Bergström, S., Danielsson, H., and Samuelsson, B. (1964): *Biochim. Biophys. Acta,* 90:207–210.
3. Christ-Hazelhof, E., and Nugteren, D. H. (1979): *Biochim. Biophys. Acta,* 572:43–51.
4. Diczfalusy, D., Falardeau, P., and Hammarström, S. (1977): *FEBS Lett.,* 84:271–274.
5. Hamberg, M., and Samuelsson, B. (1967): *J. Biol. Chem.,* 242:5336–5343.
6. Hamberg, M., Svensson, J., Wakabayashi, T., and Samuelsson, B. (1974): *Proc. Natl. Acad. Sci. USA,* 71:345–349.
7. Miyamoto, T., Ogino, N., Yamamoto, S., and Hayaishi, O. (1976): *J. Biol. Chem.,* 251:2629–2636.
8. Miyamoto, T., Yamamoto, S., and Hayaishi, O. (1974): *Proc. Natl. Acad. Sci. USA,* 71:3645–3648.
9. Nugteren, D. H., Beerthuis, R. K., and van Dorp, D. A. (1966) *Rec. Trav. Chim.,* 85:405–419.
10. Nugteren, D. H., and Hazelhof, E. (1973): *Biochim. Biophys. Acta,* 326:448–461.
11. Ogino, N., Miyamoto, T., Yamamoto, S., and Hayaishi, O. (1977): *J. Biol. Chem.,* 252:890–895.
12. Ogino, N., Ohki, S., Yamamoto, S., and Hayaishi, O. (1978): *J. Biol. Chem.,* 253:5061–5068.
13. Ogino, N., Yamamoto, S., Hayaishi, O., and Tokuyama, T. (1979): *Biochem. Biophys. Res. Commun.,* 87:184–191.
14. Ohki, S., Ogino, N., Yamamoto, S., and Hayaishi, O. (1979): *J. Biol. Chem.,* 254:829–836.
15. Samuelsson, B. (1969): *Prog. Biochem. Pharmacol.,* 5:109–128.
16. Shimizu, T., Yamamoto, S., and Hayaishi, O. (1979): *J. Biol. Chem.,* 254:5222–5228.
17. van Dorp, D. A., Beerthuis, R. K., Nugteren, D. H., and Vonkeman, H. (1964): *Biochim. Biophys. Acta,* 90:204–207.
18. van Dorp, D. A., Beerthuis, R. K., Nugteren, D. H., and Vonkeman, H. (1964): *Nature,* 203:839–841.
19. Watanabe, K., Yamamoto, S., and Hayaishi, O. (1979): *Biochem. Biophys. Res. Commun.,* 87:192–199.
20. Yoshimoto, A., Ito, H., and Tomita, K. (1970): *J. Biochem.,* 68:487–499.
21. Yoshimoto, T., Yamamoto, S., and Hayaishi, O. (1978): *Prostaglandins,* 16:529–540.
22. Yoshimoto, T., Yamamoto, S., Okuma, M., and Hayaishi, O. (1977): *J. Biol. Chem.,* 252:5871–5874.

Advances in Prostaglandin and Thromboxane Research,
Vol. 6, edited by B. Samuelsson, P. W. Ramwell,
and R. Paoletti. Raven Press, New York © 1980.

Metabolism of the Prostaglandins and Thromboxanes

John A. Oates, L. Jackson Roberts II, Brian J. Sweetman,
Richard L. Maas, John F. Gerkens, and Douglass F. Taber

*Departments of Pharmacology and Medicine, Vanderbilt University, School of Medicine,
Nashville, Tennessee 37232*

The metabolism of a prostaglandin (PG) by the lung determines the extent to which its actions are limited to its site of origin as opposed to exerting systemic effects. The pulmonary vascular bed efficiently removes most of PGE_2 and $PGF_{2\alpha}$ from the circulation (4); approximately 96% of PGE_2 is extracted by the lung. PGE_2 also is removed by the liver and kidney, which function as secondary organs of disposition. In contrast, a substantial fraction of PGI_2 escapes removal by the lung, thus yielding to the kidney and particularly to the liver primary roles in the removal of this PG from the circulation (6). As it is not inactivated by the lung, PGI_2 can enter the systemic circulation to function as a hormone.

Present evidence suggests that the failure of the lung to extract PGI_2 is not due to lack of number or affinity of metabolizing enzymes. Hawkins and his colleagues (10) demonstrated that PGI_2 was not removed by the perfused rat lung, but was readily metabolized by rat lung homogenates. These findings led to the conclusion that a transport system to enable passage of PGs from the blood to lung parenchyma was rate limiting in determining its disposition by the lung and that such a transport system for PGI_2 was lacking.

The initial insights into the chemical mechanisms of biotransformation derived from the studies of Änggård and Samuelsson (1) demonstrating that PGs of the E and F series undergo rapid dehydrogenation of the 15-hydroxyl group by the lung, followed by reduction of the 13,14-double bond to yield 15-keto-13,14-dihydro-PGs. Further studies (5,9) demonstrated that *in vivo* β- and ω-oxidation take place in the liver and other organs to further metabolize the 15-keto-13,14-dihydro-PGs, yielding a number of metabolites. The major urinary metabolite of PGE_2 in man is the 16-carbon dicarboxylic acid, 7α-hydroxy-5,11-diketo-tetranorprostane dioic acid. $PGF_{2\alpha}$ undergoes similar biotransformation to a 16-carbon dicarboxylic acid metabolite.

The 15-keto-13,14-dihydro-PGs are not as rapidly removed from the circulation as the primary PGs and persist in the circulation with half-lives of about

8 min (17). Thus these circulating metabolites can accumulate in blood and provide indicators of rapid changes in PG production.

The urinary metabolites of PGs may be measured as an index of PG production by the body. Methods for measuring the urinary metabolites of PGE_2 and $PGF_{2\alpha}$ were devised by Hamberg (7,8), employing gas chromatography–mass spectrometry to measure the ratio of metabolite to a deuterium-labeled analog of the metabolite which serves as a standard. Isotope ratios are quantified by continuous monitoring of selected ions as they emerge from the gas chromatograph (selected ion monitoring). Utilizing these methods for measuring the urinary metabolites of PGE_2 or $PGF_{2\alpha}$, it has been possible to demonstrate the inhibition of the synthesis of these PGs in man by nonsteroidal antiinflammatory drugs (7) and to demonstrate that the dose–response curve for this biochemical effect closely correlates with the doses employed in antiinflammatory therapy (12).

Analysis of the urinary metabolite of PGE_2 has also been useful in elucidating the participation of cyclooxygenase metabolites in disease states. For example, after the demonstration by Tashian et al. (22) that PGs mediated the hypercalcemia associated with a fibrosarcoma of the mouse, Hannsjorg Seyberth and I examined the possibility that the hypercalcemias associated with human solid tumors might be mediated by PGs. Levels of the urinary PGE metabolite (PGE-M) were found to be elevated, sometimes to a marked degree, in many patients who had hypercalcemia produced by solid tumors (20). However, not all patients with tumor-associated hypercalcemia had increased excretion of PGE-M, suggesting that there might be different etiologies for the hypercalcemias associated with solid tumors. That hypercalcemia itself was not a cause for increased PGE-M excretion was apparent from the normal levels of PGE-M found both in patients with hyperparathyroidism and those with hematological neoplasms such as multiple myeloma. Studies with the cyclooxygenase inhibitors, aspirin and indomethacin, were conducted to ascertain whether the increased production of PGE_2 was indeed a reflection of an etiological role of cyclooxygenase metabolites in the hypercalcemias. Tumors that were not associated with clinical evidence for metastases to bone were considered most representative of "endocrine hypercalcemia." In patients whose tumor-induced hypercalcemia was not associated with evidence for bone metastases, an elevated urinary excretion of PGE-M always predicted that the serum calcium could be lowered to normal levels with the cyclooxygenase inhibitors (19). In patients with evident bone metastases, elevated levels of PGE-M predicted statistically significant reductions in serum calcium, but these reductions were not into the normal range and were of little clinical consequence. In contrast, when there was no elevation of PGE-M, tumor-induced hypercalcemia was not suppressed by aspirin or indomethacin at all. These findings led to the conclusion that the hypercalcemia produced by one subset of solid tumors is PG dependent and that a separate and distinct group of tumors produces hypercalcemia by some other humoral substance that is independent of the PG system.

The overproduction of PGE_2 coupled with improvement of the hypercalcemia by indomethacin treatment cannot be taken as proof that PGE_2 is the mediator of the hypercalcemia. These data simply reflect that the hypercalcemia is due to an excess of some cyclooxygenase product; PGE_2 could be either the mediator or simply a byproduct of the excessive metabolism of polyunsaturated fatty acids by the cyclooxygenase pathway in these tumors.

In clinical conditions where PG production is more sporadic, the measurement of the circulating metabolite may be a more accurate indicator. An example is a patient with metastatic medullary carcinoma of the thyroid who had both diarrhea and episodic attacks of flushing (13). This patient was found to have normal excretion of PGE-M. However, during diagnostic studies it was found that calcium infusion predictably evoked a flushing episode, and this maneuver was employed to study possible PG release during the flushing attacks. During episodes of vasodilatation evoked by infusion of calcium, it was found that the concentration of 15-keto-13,14-dihydro-$PGF_{2\alpha}$ increased markedly and reproducibly concurrently with the clinical flush. With the more severe flushing episodes, an increase in 15-keto-13,14-dihydro-PGE_2 also could be detected, though these increases were always smaller than those of 15-keto-13,14-dihydro-$PGF_{2\alpha}$. These findings led us to evaluate the effects of inhibiting PG synthesis on the clinical problems of flushing and diarrhea. In a controlled study it was demonstrated that both the flushing and diarrhea improved on aspirin. These studies therefore implicate a cyclooxygenase metabolite in the clinical syndrome. Whether a cyclooxygenase metabolite exerts effects within the tumor and causes release of other hormones such as calcitonin or whether it acts as a primary mediator of the flushing episodes is yet to be elucidated. The studies in this patient illustrate the utility of measuring the circulating metabolites of these and other PGs in assessing PG release that is limited to a brief period of time.

To provide a basis for assessing the metabolism of PGD_2 *in vivo*, its metabolic fate was examined in the monkey (3). A major pathway for biotransformation of PGD_2 was through reduction at the 11-keto-position, yielding a series of metabolites with a PGF type of ring structure. The most abundant metabolite of PGD_2 was dinor-$PGF_{2\alpha}$. In addition, there were metabolites retaining the PGD ring structure, the most abundant of which was 9,20-dihydroxy-11,15-dioxo-2,3-dinorprost-5-enoic acid. Knowledge of these D-ring metabolites affords an opportunity to assess whether PGD_2 is formed to an appreciable extent *in vivo*. The metabolism of PGD_2 into metabolites with the F-ring obviously influences interpretation of any quantitative changes in levels of $PGF_{2\alpha}$ and its metabolites *in vivo*.

As thromboxane A_2 is a highly labile and potent compound, assessment of its metabolic fate is more complex. Thromboxane A_2 is known to undergo relatively rapid nonenzymatic degradation to thromboxane B_2 in aqueous solutions. Thus assessment of the metabolic fate of thromboxane B_2 would provide information on the further biotransformation of that fraction of thromboxane A_2 which was transformed to thromboxane B_2. In addition, it is conceivable that thromboxane A_2 itself undergoes enzymatic transformation in some tissues.

Furthermore, the binding of thromboxane A_2 to proteins provides yet an additional pathway for its disposition.

As an initial approach to assessing the fate of thromboxane A_2, we have investigated the metabolism of thromboxane B_2 in the monkey and man. This approach is based in part on the fact that neither thromboxane A_2 nor thromboxane B_2 is metabolized within the platelet, enabling it to secrete these two molecules unmetabolized, whereas any tissues containing metabolizing enzymes could initiate biotransformation before thromboxane A_2 or thromboxane B_2 reaches the circulation. Thus it seemed that the metabolic fate of thromboxane B_2 was more likely to be relevant to assessing thromboxane A_2 production in the platelet than in any tissues which might contain thromboxane A_2-metabolizing enzymes.

The metabolism of thromboxane B_2 was initially assessed in the monkey following the infusion of ^{3}H-thromboxane B_2 (14,15). These studies revealed that a novel and major pathway of thromboxane B_2 metabolism was via dehydrogenation of the 11-hydroxyl group, leading to the formation of 11-dehydrothromboxane B_2, a δ-lactone. A number of metabolites containing this ring structure were identified. The mass spectrum of the methyl ester-trimethyl silylether derivative of the lactone or tetrahydropyran ring form of putative 11-dehydro thromboxane B_2 was identical to synthetic 11-dehydro thromboxane B_2 (provided courtesy of Dr. Norman Nelson). Further evidence for the lactone structure was derived by reaction with sodium methoxide in methanol, yielding the dicarboxylic acid methylester. The lactone structure was further confirmed by reaction with methoxyamine to yield the acyclic amide. In addition to 11-dehydro-thromboxane B_2, other metabolites with this ring structure were also identified (Fig. 1). The major urinary metabolite of thromboxane B_2 was 2,3-dinor thromboxane B_2 (accounting for approximately 15% of the radioactivity excreted in the urine).

To facilitate the nomenclature of the various metabolites of thromboxane B_2, several of the groups working in the area have proposed a system of nomenclature for the thromboxanes based on the tetrahydropyran ring form (18). The 20-carbon parent structures for the nomenclature are thrombane and thrombanoic acid (Fig. 2). In the β-oxidized products, the original carbon numbers are retained by designation of the deleted methylene groups. For example, the product of a single β-oxidation of 11-dehydro-thromboxane B_2 would be 9,15-dihydroxy-11-oxo-2,3-dinor-thromba-5,13-dienoic acid.

The metabolism of tritium-labeled thromboxane B_2 also was investigated in man following its slow infusion over several hours (14–16). 2,3-Dinor-thromboxane B_2 was the major metabolite, representing 23% of the recovered radioactivity. Twenty-one metabolites were identified, and 11-dehydrogenation was a major pathway. The sum of the various metabolites containing the 11-oxo-ring structure accounted for approximately 48% of total recovered metabolites; these included 11-dehydro-thromboxane B_2 itself, as well as compounds with this ring structure that had undergone 15-dehydrogenation, 13,14-reduction, and varying degrees

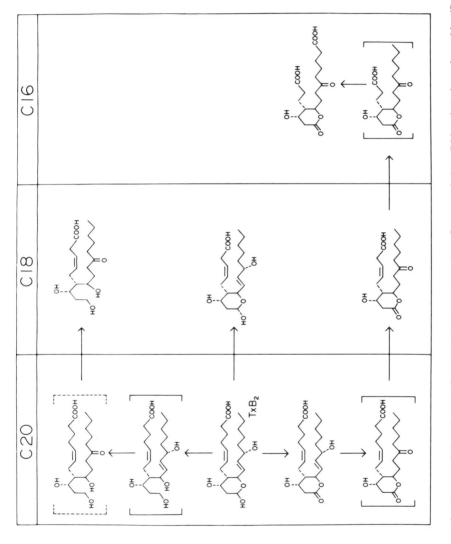

FIG. 1. Proposed pathways of thromboxane B₂ metabolism in the monkey. Compounds in solid brackets have been identified. The compound in dashed brackets has been identified from the *in vitro* incubation of thromboxane B₂ with 100,000 × *g* supernatant of guinea pig liver (but not in the urine of monkeys).

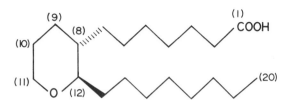

FIG. 2. Schematic of the thrombanoic acid molecule.

of β- and ω-oxidation. Of particular note was the failure to find any 15-oxo-metabolite that retained the original thromboxane B_2 ring structure with the 11-hydroxyl group.

In further investigation of the dehydrogenation, the metabolism of thromboxane B_2 in the $100,000 \times g$ supernatant of the guinea pig liver was examined. When nicotinamide adenine dinucleotide was present, thromboxane B_2 was converted to 11-dehydro-thromboxane B_2, as well as to the 15-oxo-13,14-dihydro metabolite of 11-dehydro-thromboxane B_2. Even though PGE_2 readily undergoes 15-dehydrogenation in this system, no 15-oxo-metabolite was found with the original thromboxane B_2 ring structure.

When studying the metabolic fate of arachidonic acid in the guinea pig lung following anaphylaxis, Dawson et al. (2) found that in association with the intrapulmonary formation of thromboxane A_2, 15-oxo-13,14-dihydro-thromboxane B_2 was released from the lung. This metabolite was found in substantial amounts only in sensitized lungs. The sum of the *in vitro* and *in vivo* evidence to date raises the possibility that the 15-oxo-13,14-dihydro-thromboxane B_2 metabolite may result from direct dehydrogenation of thromboxane A_2 itself by the sensitized lung. This pathway clearly requires further study.

With the observation that dinor-thromboxane B_2 is the major metabolite of thromboxane B_2 in man, we have devised a method for its measurement in urine as one means of assessing thromboxane B_2 production in man. 2,3-Dinor-thromboxane B_2 is analyzed by gas chromatography—mass spectroscopy in the selected ion monitoring mode, utilizing a chemically synthesized standard with three deuteriums on ω-carbon. Normal humans have been found to excrete only a few hundred picograms of 2,3-dinor-thromboxane B_2 per milligram of creatine. In one patient with thrombocytosis, urinary excretion of 2,3-dinor-thromboxane B_2 was several times normal values.

The metabolic fate of PGI_2 and its degradation product, 6-keto-$PGF_{1\alpha}$, have been investigated in the rat and monkey (11,21; M. D. Smigel and A. R. Wharton, *unpublished observations*). The composite of the findings in these two species suggests that PGI_2 hydrolyzes to 6-keto-$PGF_{1\alpha}$ to some extent *in vivo*, probably by a nonenzymatic mechanism. PGI_2 is a better substrate for the 15-dehydrogenase enzyme, but 6-keto-$PGF_{1\alpha}$ can be converted to the 15-keto metabolite *in vivo*. Thus 6,15-diketo-13,14-dihydro $PGF_{1\alpha}$ is formed by two pathways. From this metabolite β-oxidation to 18-carbon compounds occurs, as well as varying degrees of ω-oxidation.

Determination of the metabolic fate of PGI_2 in man should enable better evaluation of the yin/yang of the thromboxane A_2/PGI_2 systems in humans as they are perturbed by drugs and disease.

ACKNOWLEDGMENTS

The authors are indebted to Dr. J. Throck Watson for his advice and support in mass spectrometry. These investigations have been supported by National Institutes of Health Grants GM 15431 and HL 14192. Dr. Oates is the Joe and Morris Werthan Professor of Investigative Medicine.

REFERENCES

1. Änggård, E., and Samuelsson, B. (1964): *J. Biol. Chem.,* 239:4097–4102.
2. Dawson, W., Boot, J. R., Cockerill, A. F., Mallen, D. N. B., and Osborne, D. J. (1976): *Nature,* 262:699–702.
3. Ellis, C. K., Sweetman, B. J., Smigel, M. D., and Oates, J. A. (1979): *J. Biol. Chem.,* 254:4152–4163.
4. Ferreira, S. H., and Vane, J. R. (1967): *Nature,* 216:868–873.
5. Ganström, E., and Samuelsson, B. (1971): *J. Biol. Chem.,* 246:5254–5263.
6. Gerkens, J. F., Friesinger, G. C., Branch, R. A., Shand, D. G., and Gerber, J. G. (1978): *Life Sci.,* 22:1837–1842.
7. Hamberg, M. (1972): *Biochem. Biophys. Res. Commun.,* 49:720–726.
8. Hamberg, M. (1973): *Anal. Biochem.,* 55:368–378.
9. Hamberg, M., and Samuelsson, B. (1971): *J. Biol. Chem.,* 246:6713–6721.
10. Hawkins, H. J., Smith, J. B., Nicolau, K. C., and Eling, T. E. (1978): *Prostaglandins,* 16:871–884.
11. Pace-Asciak, C. R., Carrara, M. C., and Domazet, Z. (1977): *Biochem. Biophys. Res. Commun.,* 78:115–121.
12. Rane, A., Oelz, O., Frolich, J. C., Seyberth, H. W., Sweetman, B. J., Watson, J. T., and Oates, J. A. (1978): *Clin. Pharmacol. Ther.,* 23:658–668.
13. Roberts, L. J. II, McKenna, T. J., Hubbard, W. C., Bloomgarden, Z. T., Bertagna, Z. Y., McLean, G. W., Rabinowitz, D., and Oates, J. A. (1979): *Clin. Res.,* 27:506A.
14. Roberts, L. J. II, Sweetman, B. J., and Oates, J. A. (1978): *Clin. Res.,* 26:294A.
15. Roberts, L. J. II, Sweetman, B. J., and Oates, J. A. (1978): *J. Biol. Chem.,* 253:5305–5318.
16. Roberts, L. J. II, Sweetman, B. J., Payne, N. A., and Oates, J. A. (1977): *J. Biol. Chem.,* 252:7415–7417.
17. Samuelsson, B. (1973): In: *Advances in Biosciences, Vol. 9, International Conference on Prostaglandins,* edited by S. Bergstrom, pp. 7–14. Pergamon Press, Oxford.
18. Samuelsson, B., Hamberg, M., Roberts, L. J. II, Oates, J. A., and Nelson, N. A. (1978): *Prostaglandins,* 16:875–860.
19. Seyberth, H. W., Segre, G. V., Hamet, P., Sweetman, B. J., Potts, J. T., Jr., and Oates, J. A. (1976): *Trans. Assoc. Am. Physicians,* 89:92–104.
20. Seyberth, H. W., Segre, G. V., Morgan, J. L., Sweetman, B. J., Potts, J. T., Jr., and Oates, J. A. (1975): *N. Engl. J. Med.,* 293:1278–1283.
21. Sun, F. F., and Taylor, B. M. (1978): *Biochemistry,* 17:4096–4101.
22. Tashian, A. H., Jr., Voelkel, E. F., Levine, L., and Goldhaber, P. (1973): *J. Exp. Med.,* 136:1329–1343.

Advances in Prostaglandin and Thromboxane Research,
Vol. 6, edited by B. Samuelsson, P. W. Ramwell,
and R. Paoletti. Raven Press, New York © 1980.

Prostacyclin in the Cardiovascular System

S. Moncada and J. R. Vane

Department of Prostaglandin Research, The Wellcome Research Laboratories,
Beckenham, Kent BR3 3BS, United Kingdom

Prostacyclin was originally found as a product of the transformation of prostaglandin (PG) endoperoxides by a microsomal fraction of pig aorta (105). This compound, originally called PGX (18,56,106), was later chemically identified as an intermediate in the formation of 6-oxo-$PGF_{1\alpha}$, a compound already known (33,129). PGX was then given the name of prostacyclin, with the abbreviation of PGI_2 (83).

Prostacyclin is formed by vascular tissues of all species so far tested, including rabbit, ox, and human (18,39,108), and is the main metabolic product of arachidonic acid in isolated vascular tissue (83,143). Prostacyclin is the most potent endogenous inhibitor of platelet aggregation yet discovered. It is 30 to 40 times more potent than PGE_1 (111) and more than 1,000 times more active than adenosine (14). *In vivo,* applied locally in low concentrations, prostacyclin inhibits thrombus formation due to adenosine diphosphate (ADP) in the microcirculation of the hamster cheek pouch (70); and given systemically to the rabbit, it prevents electrically induced thrombus formation in the carotid artery and increases bleeding time (158). The duration of these effects *in vivo* is short, disappearing within 30 min of administration. Prostacyclin disaggregates platelets *in vitro* (106,158) and in extracorporeal circuits where platelet clumps have formed on collagen strips (57,58), and in the circulation of man (154).

Prostacyclin is unstable and its activity disappears within 15 sec on boiling or within 10 min at 22°C at neutral pH. In blood at 37°C, prostacyclin has a half-life of 2 to 3 min (37,40). Alkaline pH increases the stability of prostacyclin (83), so that at pH 10.5 at 25°C, it has a half-life of 100 hr.

In the anesthetized dog, prostacyclin is hypotensive in doses ranging from 50 to 1,000 ng/kg/min (5). In anesthetized rabbit or rat, intravenous prostacyclin causes a fall in blood pressure and is 4 to 8 times more potent than PGE_2. Prostacyclin is at least 100 times more active than its degradation product, 6-oxo-$PGF_{1\alpha}$ (5). Since it is not inactivated by the pulmonary circulation, prostacyclin is equipotent as a vasodilator when given either intra-arterially or intravenously in the rat, rabbit, or dog (6,37,40). This is an important difference from PGE_1 or PGE_2, which, because of strong metabolism in the pulmonary circulation, are much less active when given intravenously (45). Many authors have suggested a vasodilator role for locally generated PGE_2 in the vascular wall, and others have suggested that PGE_1 is released. There is little evidence that PGE_1 is a naturally occurring PG in the cardiovascular system of mammals, and prostacyclin is the main product of vascular tissue.

In the heart, local injections of arachidonic acid into the coronary circulation of the dog cause vasodilatation, and because this effect was abolished by indomethacin (75), it was assumed that PGE_2 was the likely mediator. However, there were some major difficulties with this proposal. In isolated Langendorff-perfused hearts of the rabbit, arachidonic acid dilated the coronary vasculature, but PGE_2 was inactive (12,115). Isolated strips of bovine, canine, and human coronary artery were relaxed by arachidonic acid, but PGE_2 contracted them (88). Arachidonate-induced relaxation of these strips was abolished by indomethacin, and it was therefore suggested that the metabolite responsible must be the endoperoxide intermediate PGH_2 (88).

It was later shown that bovine coronary arteries were relaxed by prostacyclin and PGH_2 (39,134) (which sometimes induced an initial transient contraction), but after treatment with 15-hydroperoxyarachidonic acid (15-HPAA) an inhibitor of prostacyclin synthetase, the relaxation induced by arachidonic acid was abolished, whereas that induced by PGH_2 was reversed to a contraction (39). Thus arachidonic acid-induced relaxation of coronary arteries is due to intramural metabolism to prostacyclin. This study further confirmed that the intrinsic activity of PGH_2 on isolated blood vessels is contractile (39).

In isolated Langendorff-perfused hearts of the guinea pig and rabbit, prostacyclin is not only a potent vasodilator, but is also the predominant metabolite of arachidonic acid (144). Similarly, using chromatographic procedures, others have identified 6-oxo-$PGF_{1\alpha}$, the degradation product of prostacyclin, as the major product from rat and rabbit hearts perfused with arachidonic acid (34). We, and others, have investigated the coronary actions of prostacyclin in the intact heart of open chest dogs (5,36). Local injection of prostacyclin (50–500 ng) into the coronary circulation increased coronary blood flow without systemic effects, and it was a more potent coronary dilator than PGE_2. Furthermore, profound and prolonged coronary vasodilatation was rapidly elicited by prostacyclin (20–100 µg) absorbed through the myocardium after dripping a solution onto the ventricular surface of the left ventricle (36). Interestingly, when endogenous synthesis is inhibited by indomethacin or meclofenamate, the coronary circulation is sensitized to the vasodilator effects of exogenous prostacyclin but not to PGE_2 (36,75). These inhibitors of cyclooxygenase decrease resting coronary blood flow in anesthetized, open-chest dogs. Although this is not seen in conscious dogs without acute surgery (128), it does indicate that the generation of a vasodilator metabolite of arachidonic acid increases or maintains coronary blood flow during mildly traumatic conditions. It is clear that this metabolite is prostacyclin.

Bradycardia accompanying the hypotension induced by prostacyclin has been observed in anesthetized dogs (5,36,76), and only transient weak tachycardia accompanied prostacyclin infusion in anesthetized cats (92). In contrast, the hypotension induced by PGE$_2$ always causes tachycardia, which is presumably mediated by baroreceptors (98). Although there is no clear difference in the overall systemic vasodilator effects of these two PGs as assessed by total peripheral resistance, PGE$_2$ has a more pronounced effect on cardiac output and myocardial contractility (as indicated by maximum acceleration of aortic blood flow). These observations indicate that in equihypotensive doses, prostacyclin reduces cardiac work more than PGE$_2$.

The bradycardia induced by prostacyclin is a reflex response mediated at least partially by vagal pathways, since it is reduced or abolished by atropine (24,25). However, the afferent arc is also subserved by vagal fibers, for vagotomy (but not atropine treatment) reduces the hypotensive effects of prostacyclin. Therefore, the hypotension induced by prostacyclin has at least two components: a direct relaxant effect on vascular smooth muscle, and reflex, noncholinergic vasodilatation. Similar results have been obtained by Hintze et al. (76).

Prostacyclin, infused intravenously in the renal circulation of the dog, reduces vascular resistance and increases renal blood flow and urinary excretion of sodium, potassium, and chloride ions at doses below those needed for a systemic effect (13,73). There is now good evidence that prostacyclin mediates the release of renin from the renal cortex. Arachidonic acid, PG endoperoxides, and prostacyclin all stimulate renin release from slices of rabbit renal cortex, but PGE$_2$ has no such effect (161,164). Furthermore, indomethacin reduces renin release in animals and man (31,46,91). Prostacyclin-like activity and 6-oxo-PGF$_{1\alpha}$ have been identified in incubates of PGG$_2$ or PGH$_2$ with renal cortical microsomes (137,165), and prostacyclin may be the obligatory endogenous mediator of renin secretion by the kidney. Indeed, Gerber et al. (49) have demonstrated that prostacyclin induces renin release when infused intrarenally into dogs, and Hill et al. (74) have demonstrated increased concentrations of angiotensin II in arterial blood during intrarenal infusions of prostacyclin. 6-Oxo-PGF$_{1\alpha}$ is also formed by collecting tubule cells isolated from rabbit papillae (54).

Prostacyclin is also a strong vasodilator in the mesenteric and hind limb circulations of the dog (where thromboxane A$_2$ (TXA$_2$) is a vasoconstrictor) (41) and on arterioles of the microcirculation of the hamster cheek pouch (72), where it also reverses epinephrine-induced vasoconstriction. Interestingly, in this preparation 6-oxo-PGF$_{1a}$ had 1/20th the vasodilator activity of prostacyclin and was more potent then PGE$_2$. Prostacyclin also induces vasodilatation and hypotension in man when given either intravenously or by inhalation (60,127, 153). This is accompanied by tachycardia.

Prostacyclin relaxes most vascular strips *in vitro,* including rabbit celiac and mesenteric arteries (18), bovine coronary arteries (39,116), human and baboon cerebral arteries (15), and lamb ductus arteriosus (27). Exceptions to this include the porcine coronary arteries (38), some strips of rat venous tissue, and isolated human saphenous vein (93), which are contracted by prostacyclin. Whether these same effects are induced in the corresponding circulations in the intact animal or man has not been studied. In the human umbilical arterial strip, prostacyclin induces a dose-dependent relaxation at low concentrations ($<10^{-6}$ M) and a dose-dependent contraction at higher concentrations ($>10^{-5}$ M) (132). As already mentioned, prostacyclin, and not PGE$_2$, is the main metabolite of arachidonic acid in isolated vascular tissue, and this has led to an intense study to reassess the effects of arachidonic acid and its metabolites on vascular tissue and the cardiovascular system. Arachidonic acid infused intravenously into dogs is converted mainly into a substance with prostacyclin-like activity as measured by bioassay (114).

PROSTACYCLIN RELEASE AND ROLE IN VASCULAR HOMEOSTASIS

Vessel microsomes in the absence of cofactors utilize PG endoperoxides, but not arachidonic acid, to synthesize prostacyclin (105). Fresh vascular tissue can utilize both precursors, although it is far more effective in utilizing endoperoxides (18). Moreover, vessel microsomes, fresh vascular rings, or endothelial cells treated with indomethacin can, when incubated with platelets, generate a prostacyclin-like antiaggregating activity (18,20,56). The release of this substance is inhibited by 15-hydroperoxy arachidonic acid (15-HPAA), a selective inhibitor of prostacyclin formation (56,106). From all these results it was concluded that the vessel wall can synthesize prostacyclin not only from its own endogenous precursors, but can also utilize PG endoperoxides released by the platelets, thus suggesting a biochemical cooperation between platelets and vessel wall (112,113).

This hypothesis has proved to be controversial. Needleman and associates demonstrated that although arachidonic acid was rapidly converted to prostacyclin by perfused rabbit hearts and kidneys, PGH$_2$ was not readily used. The authors concluded that some degree of vascular damage is necessary for the endoperoxide to be utilized by prostacyclin synthetase (116). On the other hand, incubation of platelet-rich plasma with fresh indomethacin-treated arterial tissue leads to an increase in platelet cyclic adenosine monophosphate (AMP), which parallels the inhibition of the aggregation (10) and which can be abolished by previous treatment of the vascular tissue with tranylcypromine, a less active inhibitor of prostacyclin formation (56). Additionally, Tansik et al. (156) showed that lysed aortic smooth muscle cells could be fed PG endoperoxides by lysed human platelets, and Nordoy et al. (122) have demonstrated that endothelial cells can be fed with endoperoxides released from platelets during collagen-induced aggregation. Further, undisturbed endothelial cell monolayers readily utilize PGH$_2$ to transform it into prostacyclin (101).

In contrast, recent work by Needleman et al (120) and Hornstra et al. (79), using vessel microsomes and fresh vascular tissue, suggests that the feeding of endoperoxides from platelets does not take place under their experimental circumstances. However, Needleman et al. (120) made the interesting observation that when platelets were treated with a TXA$_2$ synthetase inhibitor, platelet endoperoxides were utilized by the vessel wall. This supports our suggestion that TXA_2 synthetase inhibitors might have a superior antithrombotic effect to simple cyclooxygenase inhibitors (111,112). It is important to realize, however, that all these observations have been made *in vitro* and that *in vivo* experiments are necessary in order to clarify further the nature of the interaction between platelets and normal or damaged vessel wall.

In the vasculature, the enzyme system which generates prostacyclin is most highly concentrated in the intimal surface and progressively decreases in activity towards the adventitial surface (107). Production of prostacyclin by cultured cells from vessel walls also shows that endothelial cells are active producers of prostacyclin (61,95,163); moreover, this production persists after numerous subcultures *in vitro* (26).

Generation of prostacyclin could be the main mechanism by which the vessel wall is protected from deposition of platelet aggregates, thus providing a comprehensive explanation of the long-recognized fact that contact with healthy vascular endothelium is not a stimulus for platelet clumping. An imbalance between formation of prostacyclin and TXA_2 could be of dramatic consequence.

Vascular damage leads to platelet adhesion but not necessarily to thrombus formation. When the injury is minor, platelet thrombi are formed that break away from the vessel wall and are washed into the circulation. The degree of injury is an important determinant, and there is general agreement that for the development of a thrombus, severe damage or physical detachment of the endothelium must occur. All these observations are in accord with the distribution of prostacyclin synthetase, being abundant in the intima and progressively decreasing in concentration from the intima to the adventitia. Moreover, the proaggregating elements increase from the subendothelium to the adventitia. These two opposing tendencies render the endothelial lining antiaggregatory and the outer layers of the vessel wall thrombogenic (107).

The ability of the vascular wall actively to prevent aggregation has been postulated before (142). For instance, the presence of an ADP-ase in the vessel wall has led to the suggestion that this enzyme, by breaking down ADP, limits platelet aggregation (67,94). We have confirmed the presence of an ADP-ase in the vascular wall. However, the antiaggregating activity of the vascular wall is mainly related to the release of prostacyclin, for 15-HPAA or 13-hydroperoxy linoleic acid, two inhibitors of prostacyclin formation which have no activity on the ADP-ase system, abolish most if not all of the antiaggregatory activity of vascular endothelial cells (20). Similar results have been obtained using an antiserum which cross-reacts with and neutralizes prostacyclin *in vitro* (19). Endothelial cells pretreated with this antiserum lose the ability to inhibit ADP-induced aggregation (26). It is not yet clear whether or not prostacyclin is responsible for all the thromboresistant properties of the vascular endothelium. However, recent work by Czervionke et al. (30) with endothelial cell cultures has demonstrated that platelet adherence in the presence of thrombin increases from 4 to 44% after 1 mM aspirin treatment. This increase was parallel to a decrease in 6-oxo-PGF$_{1\alpha}$ formation from 107 to <3 nM and could be reversed by addition of 25 nM of exogenous prostacyclin. This work suggests that prostacyclin, although probably not responsible for all the thromboresistant properties of vascular endothelium, plays a very important role in the control of platelet aggregability.

The fact that prostacyclin inhibits platelet aggregation (platelet–platelet interaction) at much lower concentrations than those needed to inhibit adhesion (platelet–collagen interaction) (68) suggests that prostacyclin, indeed, allows platelets to stick to vascular tissue and to interact with it, while at the same time preventing or limiting thrombus formation. Certainly, platelets adhering to a site where prostacyclin synthetase is present could feed the enzyme with endoperoxide, thereby producing prostacyclin and preventing other platelets from clumping onto the adhering platelets, limiting the cells to a monolayer. It is also possible that formed elements of blood such as the white cells, which produce endoperoxides and TXA$_2$ (32,51,69), interact with the vessel wall to allow formation of prostacyclin, as do the platelets. This suggestion, coupled with the fact that prostacyclin may modulate white cell behavior (71,162), could well mean that prostacyclin plays a role in the control of white cell migration during the inflammatory response (see below).

Unlike other prostaglandins such as PGE$_1$ and PGF$_{2\alpha}$, prostacyclin is not inactivated on a passage through the pulmonary circulation (40), and this is probably due to the fact that prostacyclin, although a good substrate for lung dehydrogenase, is not a substrate for the uptake mechanism responsible for transport from the circulation to the intracellular enzyme (66). Indeed, the lung constantly releases small amounts of prostacyclin into the circulation (57,110). The concentrations of prostacyclin are higher in arterial than in venous blood due to overall inactivation of about 50% in one circulation through peripheral tissues (40). Thus platelet aggregability *in vivo* is modulated by circulating prostacyclin, which will reinforce the actions of locally produced prostacyclin throughout the vasculature.

MECHANISM OF ACTION

Prostacyclin inhibits platelet aggregation by stimulating adenylate cyclase, leading to an increase in cyclic AMP levels in the platelets (53,157). In this respect prostacyclin is much more potent than either PGE$_1$ or PGD$_2$ (157). 6-Oxo-PGF$_{1\alpha}$ has very weak antiaggregating activity and is almost devoid of activity on platelet cyclic AMP (157).

Prostacyclin is not only more potent than PGE$_1$ in elevating cyclic AMP, but the elevation persists longer. The elevation induced by PGE$_1$ starts falling after 30 sec, whereas prostacyclin stimulation is not maximal until after 30 sec and is maintained for 2 min, after which it gradually declines over 30 min (53). Prostacyclin is also a strong direct stimulator of adenylate cyclase in isolated membrane preparations (53).

Prostacyclin, as well as the less active PGE_1 and PGD_2, seems to increase adenylate cyclase activity by acting on specific receptors on the platelet membrane (103,166). However, PGE_1 and prostacyclin act on a receptor separate from that for PGD_2, since N0164, a PG antagonist (43), selectively reverses the inhibition of platelet aggregation induced by PGD_2, but not that induced by prostacyclin or PGE_1 (166). Moreover, studies of agonist-specific sensitization of cyclic AMP accumulation in platelets show that PGE_1 or PGE_2 can desensitize for subsequent PGE_1 or prostacyclin activation and that subthreshold concentrations of prostacyclin desensitize PGE_1 stimulation. PGD_2, however, desensitizes to a further dose of PGD_2 but not to PGE_1 or prostacyclin (103). These results suggest (103,166) that the previously recognized PGE_1 receptor in platelets (104) might in fact be a prostacyclin receptor.

There have not been many detailed studies on the mechanism of action of prostacyclin. In contrast to TXA_2, it enhances Ca^{2+} sequestration (84). Moreover, an inhibitory effect on platelet phospholipase (90,104) and platelet cyclooxygenase have been described (99). All these effects are related to its ability to increase cyclic AMP in platelets. Moreover, prostacyclin inhibits PG endoperoxide-induced aggregation, suggesting additional sites of action, still undefined, but dependent on the cyclic AMP effect (104). These observations have extended and given important biological significance to the original observation of Vargaftig and Chignard (159), who demonstrated that substances that increase cyclic AMP in platelets such as PGE_1 inhibit the release of TXA_2 [measured as Rabbit Aorta Contracting Substance (RCS)] in platelets (159). Prostacyclin, by inhibiting several steps in the activation of the arachidonic acid metabolic cascade, exerts an overall control of platelet aggregability *in vivo*.

The fact that prostacyclin increases cyclic AMP levels in cells other than platelets (78), and the possibility that in those cells an interaction with the TX system could lead to a similar control of cell behavior to that observed in platelets, suggests that the PGI_2–TXA_2 system has wider biological significance in regulation of other cell functions.

PROSTACYCLIN AND TXA_2: THROMBOSIS AND HEMOSTASIS

It is now clear that PG endoperoxides are at the crossroads of arachidonic acid metabolism, for they are precursors of substances with opposing biological properties. On the one hand, TXA_2 produced by the platelets is a strong constrictor of large blood vessels and induces platelet aggregation. On the other hand, prostacyclin produced by the vessel wall is a strong vasodilator and the most potent inhibitor of platelet aggregation known. Each substance has the opposite effect on cyclic AMP concentrations, thereby giving a balanced control mechanism which will therefore affect thrombus and hemostatic plug formation. Selective inhibition of the formation of TXA_2 should lead to an increased bleeding time and inhibition of thrombus formation, whereas inhibition of prostacyclin formation should be propitious for a "prothrombotic state." The amount of control exerted by this system can be tested, for selective inhibitors of each pathway have been described (112,121).

The utilization of aspirin as a pharmacological tool to investigate the interaction between these two substances has been fruitful. Aspirin is highly active against platelet cyclooxygenase *in vivo* and *in vitro*. Whereas the analgesic and anti-inflammatory dose in humans is about 1.5 g a day, a single tablet of aspirin (325 mg) inhibits the cyclooxygenase of platelets by about 90% (22). Moreover, this effect is long lasting, because aspirin acetylates the active site of the enzyme, leading to irreversible inhibition (140,141). Platelets are unable to synthesize new protein (100) and cannot replace inactivated cyclooxygenase. Therefore, the inhibition will only be overcome by new platelets coming into the circulation after the block of cyclooxygenase in megakaryocytes has worn off (22). Interestingly, the cyclooxygenase of vessel walls is much less sensitive to aspirin than that of platelets (8). It has also been suggested that endothelial cells *in vitro* and *in vivo* recover from aspirin inhibition by regeneration of cyclooxygenase (29,85). This has been reinforced by the observation that the recovery of the endothelial cell synthetase in cell cultures can be prevented by treatment with the protein synthesis inhibitor, cycloheximide (30).

Studies in rabbits (3,87) suggest that low doses of aspirin reduce TXA_2 formation to a greater extent than prostacyclin formation. These experiments also showed that inhibition of TXA_2 formation is longer lasting than that of prostacyclin. Indeed, it has been recently shown that infusions of arachidonic acid into rabbits and cats lead to an antithrombotic effect and to an increase in bleeding time, which can be potentiated by low doses of aspirin and blocked by larger doses (which would inhibit prostacyclin and TXA_2 formation) (3,87).

Any antithrombotic activity of dipyridamole can also be linked with the prostacyclin system, for this substance is an inhibitor of phosphodiesterase and thus amplifies the effects of the increase in cyclic AMP induced by circulating prostacyclin (109). Dipyridamole is most effective when there is a favorable PGI_2/TXA_2 ratio, after a small dose of aspirin, or more than 24 hr after a high dose. These experiments have provided the explanation for the well-recognized synergism of small doses of aspirin and dipyridamole in experimental models or in clinical experience (62,77). A selective inhibitor of TX formation and a phosphodiesterase inhibitor should now be tested for antithrombotic efficacy, since this theoretically provides an advantage over aspirin in leaving endoperoxides from platelets available for the vessel walls or other cells to synthesize prostacyclin. These results also suggest that aspirin used in small daily dose or a large dose at weekly intervals alone or in combination with a phosphodiesterase inhibitor such as dipyridamole, would be a useful therapeutic combination. Clearly, it is important not to use too high a dose of aspirin, for that will neutralize the whole system, including prostacyclin formation.

Until the discovery of prostacyclin, the use of aspirin as an antithrombotic, based on its effect on platelet function, looked very clear (97). However, the situation now needs further clarification, especially with respect to the optimal dose of aspirin. Aspirin in high doses (200 mg/kg) increases thrombus formation in a model of venous thrombosis in the rabbit (85), and *in vitro* treatment of endothelial cells with aspirin enhances thrombin-induced platelet adherence to them (29). In addition, there is an inverse correlation between platelet adhesion and aggregation and the amount of prostacyclin produced by the tissue; moreover, aspirin treatment of arterial tissue increases its thrombogenicity (H. Baumgartner, *personal communication*).

In humans, O'Grady and Moncada have demonstrated that a single low dose of aspirin (0.3 g) increases bleeding time 2 hr after ingestion, whereas a high dose (3.9 g) has no effect (126). These results have been confirmed by others (133). Moreover, platelet aggregation and TXA$_2$ formation are blocked 2 hr after a single high dose of aspirin (3.9 g) and slowly recover towards pretreatment levels over a period of 168 hr. The bleeding time remains unchanged for the first 2 hr; but 24 and 72 hr after aspirin, it is increased and slowly recovers toward pretreatment levels over a period of 168 hr, in a manner which is a mirror image of the recovery of TXA$_2$ formation and platelet aggregability (2). All these results clearly demonstrate that the balance between TXA$_2$ and PGI$_2$ is an important mechanism of control of platelet aggregability *in vivo*. Recently (139), it has been demonstrated that tranylcypromine, an inhibitor of prostacyclin formation, enhances platelet aggregation in an experimental model of thrombosis in the microcirculation of the brain of the mouse. Clearly, manipulation of this control mechanism might lead to pro- or antithrombotic states of clinical relevance. In this context, it is interesting to note that recently, it has been shown that hydrocortisone treatment of normal or thrombocytopenic rats blocks prostacyclin formation in the vessel wall and decreases the bleeding time (11), a result which would be expected from the above-mentioned aspirin studies. It is also relevant to observe that the authors mention that for years it has been the clinical impression that steroids decrease the bleeding time in thrombocytopenic patients without increasing the platelet count. Whether other drugs exert their antithrombotic effect by acting on this mechanism is not yet known, but studies using sulfinpyrazone in cultured endothelial cells (52) and ticlopidine given orally to rats (7) suggest that these compounds have little or no effect on prostacyclin formation at concentrations at which they affect platelet behavior. A compound which might stimulate prostacyclin formation in humans after oral ingestion has also been described (160).

Selective inhibition of prostacyclin formation by lipid peroxides could also lead to a condition in which platelet aggregation is increased, and this could play a role in the development of atherosclerosis. Indeed, lipid peroxidation takes place in plasma as a nonenzymic reaction (64), and it is known to occur in certain pathological conditions (148). Hence lipid peroxides present in these conditions could be shifting the balance of the system in favor of TXA$_2$ and predispose to thrombus formation. In this context it is interesting that Dembinska-Kiec and associates (35) have found that there is a strong reduction in prostacyclin formation by hearts or vessel walls of rabbits made atherosclerotic.

Similarly, it has been reported that human atherosclerotic tissue does not produce prostacyclin, whereas tissue obtained from a nearby normal vessel does (4).

The role of lipid peroxides in the development of atherosclerosis has been debated for the last 25 years since Glavind et al. (50) described the presence of lipid peroxides in human atherosclerotic aortae. They found the peroxide content in diseased arteries to be directly proportional to the severity of the atherosclerosis. Subsequent investigations by Woodford et al. (169) suggested the artifactual nature of Glavind's findings, ascribing the presence of lipid peroxides to their formation during the preparative procedure (169). Despite this, the presence of conjugated diene hydroperoxides in lipids of human atheroma has again been reported (47,48), and lipid peroxides have been found in atherosclerotic rabbit aortae (80) subjected to an extraction procedure which avoids lipid peroxidation *in vitro.* Some authors (17,63) favor the suggestion that lipid peroxides are present in atherosclerotic plaques, whether or not these peroxides act by inhibiting prostacyclin formation, and as a consequence reduce the wall's defense mechanism. This theory is of interest, especially since other substances related to atherosclerosis such as the cholesterol carriers, low-density lipoproteins, have also been shown to inhibit prostacyclin formation in endothelial cell cultures (124).

THERAPEUTIC POTENTIAL OF PROSTACYCLIN

Prostacyclin or chemical analogs may find a use as a "hormone replacement" therapy in conditions such as acute myocardial infarction or "crescendo angina" and other states in which excessive platelet aggregation takes place in the circulation. Moreover, we have suggested its use in extracorporeal circulation systems such as cardiopulmonary bypass and renal dialysis (113). In these systems the main problems are platelet loss with the formation of microaggregates which, when returning to the patient, are responsible for the cerebral and renal impairment observed after bypass (1,16). In addition, there are side effects associated with the chronic use of heparin, especially the development of osteoporosis (55).

Several antiplatelet drugs have been suggested to deal with these two problems and some have been used with moderate success. PGE_1 has been reported to be beneficial during cardiopulmonary bypass (9). However, PGs of the E type induce diarrhea (96), an effect not shared by prostacyclin (158). Therefore, prostacyclin is not only more potent but more specific in achieving platelet protection. Prostacyclin has now been beneficially used in several systems of extracorporeal circulation in experimental animals, including renal dialysis, cardiopulmonary bypass, and charcoal hemoperfusion (21,28,170). In one of these systems (renal dialysis), prostacyclin can replace heparin altogether (170). In charcoal hemoperfusion, heparin is also necessary, since charcoal particles seem to activate directly the clotting cascade (21).

Following reports that PGE_1 has been used successfully in the treatment of peripheral vascular disease (23), prostacyclin has been shown to have a similar effect, producing a long-lasting increase in muscle blood flow, disappearance of ischemic pain, and healing of ulcers after an intra-arterial infusion to the affected limb (155).

UNSTABLE DERIVATIVES OF OTHER FATTY ACIDS

Endoperoxides derived from dihomo-γ-linolenic acid and eicosapentaenoic acid have been described and some of their biological activities studied. Needleman et al. (118) showed the formation of PGG_1, PGH_1, PGG_3, and PGH_3 when sheep seminal vesicles were incubated with the appropriate precursor. Moreover, they showed that when PGH_3 was incubated with indomethacin-treated platelet microsomes (TX synthetase), TXA_3 was formed. However, they could not detect the formation of TXA_1 when PGG_1 or H_1 were incubated with the same enzyme preparation. The existence of TXA_1 has been demonstrated by Falardeau et al. (44), although the conversion rate of the endoperoxide precursor is low.

PGH_1 contracts the rabbit aortic strip (about one-fifth as active as PGH_2), the pig coronary artery strip (equiactive to PGH_2), and the bovine coronary artery, a preparation on which PGH_2 is relaxant or has a biphasic effect (117). PGH_3 also relaxes the bovine coronary artery but is less potent than PGH_2 (117). It contracts the rabbit aortic strip, where it is one-fifth as potent as PGH_2. TXA_3 also contracts the three bioassay tissues and is approximately one-fifth as active as TXA_2.

In Platelets

In contrast to arachidonic acid, dihomo-γ-linolenic acid and eicosapentaenoic acid do not induce aggregation but prevent the second phase of ADP-induced aggregation (146). Originally, Willis et al. showed that PGG_1 and PGH_1 do not aggregate human platelets, nor do they inhibit the aggregation induced by PGH_2 (168). On the other hand, PGH_3 or TXB_3 have little or no proaggregating effect (135).

The study of the unstable intermediates of dihomo-γ-linolenic and eicosapentaenoic acid has gained momentum as a result of the theories on the use of these fatty acids as dietary components with "antithrombotic" properties. Before the discovery of prostacyclin, it was suggested that the use of dietary dihomo-γ-linolenic acid, the precursor of the E_1 series of PGs, could be an approach to the prevention of thrombosis, for PGG_1 was not proaggregating (167). Furthermore, if the platelet made PGE_1, it might inhibit aggregation. Some reports tended to agree with this proposal (147), but there is some doubt, for in the rabbit, feeding with dihomo-γ-linolenic acid leads to an increase in the tissue content of this acid without change in platelet responsiveness, at least to ADP (125). Most of the positive studies were made *in vitro* in situations in which platelets have no contact with vessel walls (86).

The use of dihomo-γ-linolenic acid in an attempt to direct the synthetic machinery of the platelets is not the most rational approach for prevention of thrombosis, because the endoperoxides PGG_1 and PGH_1 are not substrates for prostacyclin synthesis and an accumulation of these substances or their precursor might adversely affect the prostacyclin protective mechanism. Indeed, it has recently been shown that in endothelial cell cultures (123), the addition of dihomo-γ-linolenic acid to the culture medium reduces the release of prostacy-clin-like material.

Eicosapentaenoic acid, the precursor of the PG_3 series, can, however, act as a precursor for an antiaggregating agent, probably Δ^{17}-prostacyclin (140,169). This compound has been synthesized chemically and has similar properties and potency to prostacyclin (82). TXA_3 is synthesized by platelet microsomes and is less proaggregatory than TXA_2 (59,119,135,149). Originally, Needleman and colleagues reported that TXA_3 and PGH_3 directly stimulate platelet adenylate cyclase and inhibit aggregation (119). However, it is now clear that in this work the formation of PGD_3 and PGE_3 from PGH_3 and their possible interaction was underestimated. Since these compounds strongly counteract the proaggrega-tory effect of PGH_3 and TXA_3 (59), the net effect of the transformation of eicosapentaenoic acid in the platelets, unlike that of arachidonic acid, is not a proaggregatory effect. Thus the ingestion of this fatty acid could afford a dietary protection against thrombosis (42). Indeed, we and others (42) have suggested that the low incidence of myocardial infarction in Eskimos and their increased tendency to bleed could be due to the high eicosapentaenoic acid and low arachi-donate content of their diet and consequently of their tissue lipids.

METABOLISM OF PROSTACYCLIN

Prostacyclin or 6-oxo-PGF$_{1\alpha}$ metabolism has been studied in whole animals and *in vitro* in tissue slices or homogenates. *In vitro* in the rat, 6-oxo-PGF$_{1\alpha}$ is partially excreted intact and partially as dinor-6-oxo-PGF$_{1\alpha}$ and dinor-ω-1-hydroxy-6-keto PGF$_{1\alpha}$ (130). Sun and Taylor (151) have identifed seven metabo-lites of prostacyclin in urine after intravenous administration. It was found that 77% of the administered dose is excreted within 3 days (33% in urine and 44% in feces). Most of the metabolism was by 15-hydroxy-PG dehydrogenase, giving 15-oxo-PGI$_2$ as the first degradation step. However, some compounds formed suggested that some of the compound had first been converted nonenzy-mically to 6-oxo-PGF$_{1\alpha}$ and then metabolized. This study demonstrates that *in vivo*, 6-oxo-PGF$_{1\alpha}$ is not a major metabolite of prostacyclin, and that 6-oxo-PGF$_{1\alpha}$ should be considered mainly as a chemical degradation product.

In vitro studies have demonstrated that in lung (102) and blood vessel (150), prostacyclin is rapidly oxidized by the 15-hydroxy-PG dehydrogenase to the corresponding 15-oxo compound. However, under the same conditions, 6-oxo-$PGF_{1\alpha}$ was a poor substrate for this enzyme (102,150).

PROSTACYCLIN IN PATHOLOGICAL STATES

Increased production of PG endoperoxides or TXA_2 *in vitro* by platelets has been found in patients with arterial thrombosis, deep venous thrombosis, or recurrent venous thrombosis. These conditions are associated with a shortened platelet survival time (89). In addition, increased sensitivity to aggregating agents and increased release of "rabbit aorta contracting substance" has been described in rabbits made atherosclerotic by diet (145) and in patients who have survived myocardial infarction (152). Moreover, platelets from rats made diabetic release more TXA_2 (65,81). Diseases associated with changes in prostacyclin production have been described. An increased production has been suggested in uremic patients to explain their hemostatic defect (136). On the other hand, a lack of prostacyclin production has been suggested in patients with idiopathic thrombocytopenic purpura (138). Both diseases are linked by the accumulation during uremia or the lack of production during idiopathic thrombocytopenia purpura of an ill-defined "plasma factor" which stimulates prostacyclin synthesis (95).

More recently, a decreased production of prostacyclin by the blood vessels of rats made diabetic has also been described (65,81); this decreased production can be corrected by chronic treatment with insulin (65). Finally, increased prostacyclin production has been described in blood vessels of spontaneously hypertensive rats (131).

As yet, a clear relationship between different diseases and the prostacyclin–TXA_2 balance is not established. However, it seems that conditions which favor the development of thrombosis are associated with an increase in TXA_2 and a decrease in prostacyclin formation, whereas an increased prostacyclin formation plus decreased TXA_2 is present in some conditions associated with an increased bleeding tendency. Much of the cited work, however, needs confirmation before it is possible to make more definite conclusions.

REFERENCES

1. Abel, R. M., Buckley, M. J., Austen, W. G., Barnett, G. O., Beck, C. H., and Fischer, J. E. (1976): *J. Thorac. Surg.,* 71:323–333.
2. Amezcua, J-L., O'Grady, J., Salmon, J. A., and Moncada, S. (1979): *Thromb. Res.,* 16:69–79.
3. Amezcua, J-L., Parsons, M., and Moncada, S. (1978): *Thromb. Res.,* 13:477–488.
4. Angelo, V. D., Villa, S., Myskiewiec, M., Donati, M. B., and de Gaetano, G. (1978): *Thromb. Haematol.,* 39:535–536.
5. Armstrong, J. M., Chapple, D. J., Dusting, G. J., Hughes, R., Moncada, S., and Vane, J. R. (1977): *Br. J. Pharmacol.,* 61:136P.
6. Armstrong, J. M., Lattimer, N., Moncada, S., and Vane, J. R. (1978): *J. Pharmacol.,* 62:125–130.
7. Ashida, S-I., and Abiko, Y. (1978): *Thromb. Res.,* 13:901–908.
8. Baenziger, N. L., Dillender, M. J., and Majerus, P. W. (1977): *Biochem. Biophys. Res. Commun.,* 78:294–301.

9. Balanowski, P. J. P., Bauer, J., Machiedo, G., and Neville, W. E. (1977): *J. Thorac. Cardiovasc. Surg.*, 73:221–224.

10. Best, L. C., Martin, T. J., Russell, R. G. G., and Preston, F. E. (1977): *Nature*, 267:850–851.

11. Blajchman, M. A., Senyi, A. F., Hirsh, J., Surya, Y., Buchanan, M., and Mustard, J. F. (1979): *J. Clin. Invest.*, 63:1026–1035.

12. Block, A. J., Feinberg, H., Herbaczynska-Cedro, K., and Vane, J.R. (1975): *Circ. Res.*, 36:34–42.

13. Bolger, P. M., Eisner, G. M., Ramwell, P. W., and Slotkoff, L. M. (1978): *Nature*, 271:457–469.

14. Born, G. V. R. (1962): *Nature*, 194:927–929.

15. Boullin, D. J., Bunting, S., Blaso, W. P., Hunt, T. M., and Moncada, S. (1979): *Br. J. Clin. Pharmacol.*, 7:139–147.

16. Branthwaite, M. A. (1972): *Thorax*, 27:748–753.

17. Brooks, C. J. W., Steel, G., Gilbert, J. D., and Harland, W. A. (1971): *Atherosclerosis*, 13:223–237.

18. Bunting, S., Gryglewski, R., Moncada, S., and Vane, J. R. (1976): *Prostaglandins*, 12:897–913.

19. Bunting, S., Moncada, S., Reed, P., Salmon, J. A., and Vane, J. R. (1978): *Prostaglandins*, 15:565–574.

20. Bunting, S., Moncada, S., and Vane, J. R. (1977): *Lancet*, 2:1075–1076.

21. Bunting, S., Moncada, S., Vane, J. R., Woods, H. F., and Weston, M. J. (1979): In: *Prostacyclin*, edited by J. R. Vane and S. Bergstrom, pp. 361–369. Raven Press, New York.

22. Burch, J. W., Stanford, N., and Majerus, P. W. (1978): *J. Clin. Invest.*, 61:314–319.

23. Carlson, L. A., and Olsson, A. G. (1976): *Lancet*, 2:810p.

24. Chapple, D. J., Dusting, G. J., Hughes, R., and Vane, J. R. (1978): *J. Physiol.*, 281:43–44P.

25. Chapple, D. J., Dusting, G. J., Hughes, R., and Vane, J. R. (1979): *Br. J. Pharmacol. (in press).*

26. Christofinis, G. J., Moncada, S., MacCormick, C., Bunting, S., and Vane, J. R. (1979): In: *Prostacyclin*, edited by J. R. Vane and S. Bergstrom, pp. 77–84. Raven Press, New York.

27. Coceani, F., Bishai, I., White, E., Bodach, E., and Olley, P. M. (1978): *Am. J. Physiol.*, 234:H117–H122.

28. Coppe, D., Wonders, T., Snider, M., and Salzman, E. W. (1979): In: *Prostacyclin*, edited by J. R. Vane and S. Bergstrom, pp. 371–383. Raven Press, New York.

29. Czervionke, R. L., Hoak, J. C., and Fry, G. L. (1978): *J. Clin. Invest.*, 62:847–856.

30. Czervionke, R. L., Smith, J. B., Fry, G. L., and Hoak, J. C. (1979): *J. Clin. Invest.*, 63:1089–1092.

31. Data, J. L., Crump, W. J., Hollifield, J. W., Frolich, J. C., and Nies, A. S. (1976): *Clin. Res.*, 24:397A.

32. Davison, E. M., Ford-Hutchinson, A. W., Smith, M. J. H., and Walker, J. R. (1978): *Br. J. Pharmacol.*, 63:407P.

33. Dawson, W., Boot, J. R., Cockerill, A. F., Mallen, D. N. B., and Osborne, D. J. (1976): *Nature*, 262:699–702.

34. De Dekere, E. A. M., Nugteren, D. H., and Ten Hoor, F. (1977): *Nature*, 268:160–163.

35. Dembinska-Kiec, A., Gryglewska, T., Zmuda, A., and Gryglewski, R. J. (1977): *Prostaglandins*, 14:1025–1034.

36. Dusting, G. J., Chapple, D. J., Hughes, R., Moncada, S., and Vane, J. R. (1978): *Cardiovasc. Res.*, 12:720–730.

37. Dusting, G. J., Moncada, S., and Vane, J. R. (1977): *Br. J. Pharmacol.*, 62:414–415P.

38. Dusting, G. J., Moncada, S., and Vane, J. R. (1977): *Eur. J. Pharmacol.*, 45:301–304.

39. Dusting, G. J., Moncada, S., and Vane, J. R. (1977): *Prostaglandins*, 13:3–15.

40. Dusting, G. J., Moncada, S., and Vane, J. R. (1978): *Br. J. Pharmacol.*, 64:315–320.

41. Dusting, G. J., Moncada, S., and Vane, J. R. (1978): *Eur. J. Pharmacol.*, 49:65–72.

42. Dyerberg, J., Bang, H. O., Stoffersen, E., Moncada, S., and Vane, J. R. (1978): *Lancet*, 2:117–119.

43. Eakins, K. E., Raja dhyaksha, V., and Schroer, R. (1976): *Br. J. Pharmacol.*, 58:333–339.

44. Falardeau, P., Hamberg, M., and Samuelsson, B. (1976): *Biochim. Biophys. Acta*, 441:193–200.

45. Ferreira, S. H., and Vane, J. R. (1967): *Nature*, 216:868–873.

46. Frolich, J. C., Hollifield, J. W., Dormois, J. C., Frolich, B. L., Seyberth, H., Michelakis, A. M., and Oates, J. A. (1976): *Circ. Res.,* 39:447–452.
47. Fukazumi, K. (1965): *Yukagaku,* 14:119–122.
48. Fukazumi, K., and Iwata, Y. (1963): *Yukagaku,* 12:93–97.
49. Gerber, J. G., Branch, R. A., Nies, A. S., Gerkens, J. F., Shand, D. G., Hollifield, J., and Oates, J. A. (1978): *Prostaglandins,* 15:81–88.
50. Glavind, J., Hartmann, S., Clemmesen, J., Jessen, K. E., and Dam, H. (1952): *Acta. Pathol. Microbiol. Scand.,* 30:1.
51. Goldstein, I. M., Malmsten, C. L., Kaplan, H. B., Kindahl, H., Samuelsson, B., and Weissman, G. (1977): *Clin. Res.,* 25:518A.
52. Gordon, J. L., and Pearson, J. D. (1978): *Br. J. Pharmacol.,* 64:481–483.
53. Gorman, R. R., Bunting, S., and Miller, O. V. (1977): *Prostaglandins,* 13:377–388.
54. Grenier, F. C., and Smith, W. L. (1978): *Prostaglandins,* 16:759–772.
55. Griffith, G. C., Nichols, G., Asher, J. D., and Flanagan, B. (1965): *J. Am. Med. Assoc.,* 193:91–94.
56. Gryglewski, R. J., Bunting, S., Moncada, S., Flower, R. J., and Vane, J. R. (1976): *Prostaglandins,* 12:685–714.
57. Gryglewski, R. J., Korbut, R., and Ocetkiewicz, A. C. (1978): *Nature,* 273:765–767.
58. Gryglewski, R. J., Korbut, R., and Ocetkiewicz, A. C. (1978): *Prostaglandins,* 15:637–644.
59. Gryglewski, R. J., Salmon, J. A., Ubatuba, F. B., Weatherly, B. C., Moncada, S., and Vane, J. R. (1979): *Prostaglandins,* 18:453–478.
60. Gryglewski, R. J., Szczeklik, A., and Nizankowski, R. (1978): *Thromb. Res.,* 13:153–163.
61. Harker, L. A., Joy, N., Wall, R. T., Quadracci, L., and Striker, G. (1977): *Thromb. Haematol.,* 38:137 (abstract).
62. Harker, L. A., and Slichter, S. J. (1972): *N. Engl. J. Med.,* 287:999–1005.
63. Harland, W. A., Gilbert, J. D., Steel, G., and Brooks, C. J. W. (1971): *Atherosclerosis,* 13:239–246.
64. Harman, D., and Piette, L. H. (1966): *J. Gerontol.,* 21:560–565.
65. Harrison, H. E., Reece, A. H., and Johnson, M. (1978): *Life Sci.,* 23:351–356.
66. Hawkins, H. J., Smith, B. J., Nicolaou, K. C., and Eling, T. E. (1978): *Prostaglandins,* 16:871–884.
67. Heyns, A. du P., van den Berg, D. J., Potgieter, G. M., and Retief, F. P. (1974): *Thromb. Diath. Haemorrh.,* 32:417–431.
68. Higgs, E. A., Moncada, S., Vane, J. R., Caen, J. P., Michel, H., and Tobelem, G. (1978): *Prostaglandins,* 16:17–22.
69. Higgs, G. A., Bunting, S., Moncada, S., and Vane, J. R. (1976): *Prostaglandins,* 12:749–757.
70. Higgs, G. A., Moncada, S., and Vane, J. R. (1977): *Br. J. Pharmacol.,* 61:137P.
71. Higgs, G. A., Moncada, S., and Vane, J. R. (1978): *J. Physiol.,* 280:55–56P.
72. Higgs, G. A., Moncada, S., and Vane, J. R. (1979): *Microvasc. Res.,* 18:245–254.
73. Hill, T. W. K., and Moncada, S. (1979): *Prostaglandins,* 17:87–98.
74. Hill, T. W. K., Moncada, S., and Vane, J. R. (1978): *Abstract for 7th International Congress of Pharmacology,* Paris.
75. Hintze, T. H., and Kaley, G. (1977): *Circ. Res.,* 40:313–320.
76. Hintze, T. H., Kaley, G., Martin, E. G., and Messina, E. J. (1978): *Prostaglandins,* 15:712.
77. Honour, A. J., Hockaday, T. D. R., and Mann, J. I. (1977): *Br. J. Exp. Pathol.,* 58:268–272.
78. Hopkins, N. K., Sun, F. F., and Gorman, R. R. (1978): *Biochem. Biophys. Res. Commun.,* 85:827–836.
79. Hornstra, G., Haddeman, E., and Don, J. A. (1979): *Nature,* 279:66–68.
80. Iwakami, M. (1965): *Nagoya J. Med. Sci.,* 28:50–66.
81. Johnson, M., Reece, A. H., and Harrison, H. E. (1979): *Adv. Pharmacol. Ther.* 4:865.
82. Johnson, R. A., Lincoln, F. H., Nidy, E. G., Schneider, W. D., Thompson, J. L., and Axen, U. (1978): *J. Am. Chem. Soc.,* 100:7690–7705.
83. Johnson, R. A., Morton, D. R., Kinner, J. H., Gorman, R. R., McGuire, J. C., Sun, F. F., Whittaker, N., Bunting, S., Salmon, J., Moncada, S., and Vane, J. R. (1976): *Prostaglandins,* 12:915–928.
84. Kazer-Glanzman, R., Jakabova, M., George, J., and Luscher, E. (1977): *Biochim. Biophys. Acta,* 466:429–440.

85. Kelton, J. G., Hirsch, J., Carter, C. J., and Buchanan, M. R. (1978): *J. Clin. Invest.*, 62:892–895.
86. Kernoff, P. B. A., Willis, A. L., Stone, K. J., Davies, J. A., and McNicol, G. P. (1977): *Br. Med. J.*, 2:1441–1444.
87. Korbut, R., and Moncada, S. (1978): *Thromb. Res.*, 13:489–500.
88. Kulkarni, P. S., Roberts, R., and Needleman, P. (1976): *Prostaglandins*, 123:337–353.
89. Lagarde, M., and Dechavanne, M. (1977): *Lancet*, 1:88.
90. Lapetina, E. G., Schmitges, C. J., Chandrabose, K., and Cuatrecasas, P. (1977): *Biochem. Biophys. Res. Commun.*, 76:828–835.
91. Larsson, C., Weber, P., and Anggard, E. (1974): *Eur. J. Pharmacol.*, 28:391–394.
92. Lefer, A. M., Ogletree, M. L., Smith, J. B., Silver, M. J., Nicolaou, K. C., Barnette, W. E., and Gasic, G. P. (1978): *Science*, 200:52–54.
93. Levy, S. V. (1978): *Prostaglandins*, 16:93–97.
94. Lieberman, G. E., Lewis, G. P., and Peters, T. J. (1977): *Lancet*, 2:330–332.
95. MacIntyre, D. E., Pearson, J. D., and Gordon, J. L. (1978): *Nature*, 271:549–551.
96. Main, I. H. M., and Whittle, B. J. R. (1975): *Br. J. Pharmacol.*, 54:309–317.
97. Majerus, P. W. (1976): *Circulation*, 54:357–359.
98. Malik, K. U., and McGiff, J. C. (1976): In: *Prostaglandins: Physiological, Pharmacological and Pathological Aspects*, edited by S. M. Karim, M. T. P. Press, Ltd., Lancaster, pp. 103–200.
99. Malmsten, C., Granström, E., and Samuelsson, B. (1976): *Biochem. Biophys. Res. Commun.*, 68:569–576.
100. Marcus, A. J. (1978): *J. Lipid Res.*, 19:793–826.
101. Marcus, A. J., Weksler, B. B., and Jaffe, E. A. (1978): *J. Biol. Chem.*, 253:7138–7141.
102. McGuire, J. C., and Sun, F. F. (1978): *Arch. Biochem. Biophys.*, 189:92–96.
103. Miller, O. V., and Gorman, R. R. (1976): *J. Cyclic Nucleotide Res.*, 2:79–87.
104. Minkes, M., Stanford, M., Chi, M., Roth, G., Raz, A., Needleman, P., and Majerus, P. (1977): *J. Clin. Invest.*, 59:449–454.
105. Moncada, S., Gryglewski, R. J., Bunting, S., and Vane, J. R. (1976): *Nature*, 263:663–665.
106. Moncada, S., Gryglewski, R. J., Bunting, S., and Vane, J. R. (1976): *Prostaglandins*, 12:715–733.
107. Moncada, S., Herman, A. G., Higgs, E. A., and Vane, J. R. (1977): *Thromb. Res.*, 11:323–344.
108. Moncada, S., Higgs, E. A., and Vane, J. R. (1977): *Lancet*, 1:18–21.
109. Moncada, S., and Korbut, R. (1978): *Lancet*, 1:1286–1289.
110. Moncada, S., Korbut, R., Bunting, S., and Vane, J. R. (1978): *Nature*, 273:767–768.
111. Moncada, S., and Vane, J. R. (1977): In: *Biochemical Aspects of Prostaglandins and Thromboxanes*, edited by N. Kharasch and J. Fried, Academic Press, New York, pp. 155–177.
112. Moncada, S., and Vane, J. R. (1978): *Br. Med. Bull.*, 34:129–135.
113. Moncada, S., and Vane, J. R. (1979): *N. Engl. J. Med.*, 300:1142–1147.
114. Mullane, K. M., Dusting, G. J., Salmon, J. A., Moncada, S., and Vane, J. R. (1979): *Eur. J. Pharmacol.*, 54:217–228.
115. Needleman, P. (1976): *Fed. Proc.*, 35:2376–2381.
116. Needleman, P., Bronson, S. D., Wyche, A., Sivakoff, M., and Nicolaou, K. C. (1978): *J. Clin. Invest.*, 61:839–849.
117. Needleman, P., Kulkarni, P. S., and Raz, A. (1977): *Science*, 195:409–412.
118. Needleman, P., Minkes, M., and Raz, A. (1976): *Science*, 193:163–165.
119. Needleman, P., Raz, A., Minkes, M. S., Ferrendelli, J. A., and Sprecher, H. (1979): *Proc. Natl. Acad. Sci. USA*, 76:944–948.
120. Needleman, P., Wyche, A., and Raz, A. (1979): *J. Clin. Invest.*, 63:345–349.
121. Nijkamp, F. P., Moncada, S., White, H. L., and Vane, J. R. (1977): *Eur. J. Pharmacol.*, 44:179–187.
122. Nordoy, A., Svensson, B., and Hoak, J. C. (1978): *Thromb. Res.*, 12:597–608.
123. Nordoy, A., Svensson, B., and Hoak, J. C. (1979): *Eur. J. Clin. Invest.*, 9:5–10.
124. Nordoy, A., Svensson, B., Wiebe, D., and Hoak, J. C. (1978): *Circ. Res.*, 43:527–534.
125. Oelz, O., Seyberth, H. W., Knapp, H. R., Sweetman, B. J., and Oates, J. A. (1976): *Biochim. Biophys. Acta*, 431:268–277.
126. O'Grady, J., and Moncada, S. (1978): *Lancet*, 2:780.
127. O'Grady, J., Warrington, S., Moti, M. J., Bunting, S., Flower, R. J., Fowle, A. S. E., Higgs,

E. A., and Moncada, S. (1979): In: *Prostacyclin,* edited by J. R. Vane and S. Bergstrom, pp. 409–417. Raven Press, New York.

128. Owen, T. L., Ehrhart, I. C., Weidner, W. J., Scott, J. B., and Haddy, F. J. (1975): *Proc. Soc. Exp. Biol. Med.,* 149:871–876.
129. Pace-Asciak, C. (1976): *J. Am. Chem. Soc.,* 98:2348–2349.
130. Pace-Asciak, C. R., Carrara, M. C., and Domazer, Z. (1977): *Biochem. Biophys. Res. Commun.,* 78:115–121.
131. Pace-Asciak, C. R., Carrara, M. C., Rangaraj, G., and Nicolaou, K. G. (1978): *Prostaglandins,* 15:1005–1012.
132. Pomerantz, K., Sintetos, A., and Ramwell, P. (1978): *Prostaglandins,* 15:1035–1044.
133. Rajah, S. M., Penny, S., and Kester, R. (1978): *Lancet,* 2:1104.
134. Raz, A., Isakson, P. C., Minkes, M. S., and Needleman, P. (1977): *J. Biol. Chem.,* 252:1123–1126.
135. Raz, A., Minkes, M. S., and Needleman, P. (1977): *Biochim. Biophys. Acta,* 488:305–311.
136. Remuzzi, G., Cavenaghi, A. E., Mecca, G., Donati, M. B., and de Gaetano, G. (1977): *Thromb. Res.,* 11:919–920.
137. Remuzzi, G., Cavenaghi, A. E., Mecca, G., Donati, M. B., and de Gaetano, G. (1978): *Thromb. Res.,* 12:363–366.
138. Remuzzi, G., Misiani, R., Marchesi, D., Livio, M., Mecca, G., de Gaetano, G., and Donati, M. B. (1978): *Lancet,* 2:871–872.
139. Rosenblum, W. I., and El-Sabban, F. (1978): *Circ. Res.,* 43:238–241.
140. Roth, G. J., and Majerus, P. W., (1975): *J. Clin. Invest.,* 56:624–632.
141. Roth, G. J., and Siok, C. J. (1978): *J. Biol. Chem.,* 253:3782–3784.
142. Saba, S. R., and Mason, R. G. (1974): *Thromb. Res.,* 5:747–757.
143. Salmon, J. A., Smith, D. R., Flower, R. J., Moncada, S., and Vane, J. R. (1978): *Biochim. Biophys. Acta,* 523:250–262.
144. Schror, K., Moncada, S., Ubatuba, F. B., and Vane, J. R. (1978): *Eur. J. Pharmacol.,* 47:103–114.
145. Shimamoto, T., Kobayashi, M., Takahashi, T., Takashima, Y., Sakamoto, M., and Morooka, S. (1978): *Jpn. Heart J.,* 19:748–753.
146. Silver, M. J., Smith, J. B., Ingerman, C., and Kocsis, J. J. (1973): *Prostaglandins,* 4:863–875.
147. Sim, D. K., and McCraw, A. P. (1977): *Thromb. Res.,* 10:385–397.
148. Slater, T. F. (1972): *Free Radical Mechanisms in Tissue Injury.* Pion Ltd., London.
149. Smith, D. R., Weatherly, B. C., Salmon, J. A., Ubatuba, F. B., Gryglewski, R. J., and Moncada, S. (1979): *Prostaglandins,* 18:423–438.
150. Sun, F. F., McGiff, J. C., and Wong, P. Y. K. (1978): *Fed. Proc.,* 37:916.
151. Sun, F. F., and Taylor, B. M. (1978): *Biochemistry,* 17:4096–4101.
152. Szczeklik, A., Gryglewski, R. J., Musial, J., Grodzinska, L., Serwonska, M., and Marcinkiewicz, E. (1978): *Thromb. Haematol.,* 40:66–74.
153. Szczeklik, A., Gryglewski, R. J., Nizankowska, E., Nizankowski, R., and Musial, J. (1978): *Prostaglandins,* 16:654–660.
154. Szczeklik, A., Gryglewski, R. J., Nizankowski, R., Musial, J., Pieton, R., and Mruk, J. (1978): *Pharmacol. Res. Commun.,* 10:545–556.
155. Szczeklik, A., Nizankowski, R., Skawinski, S., Szczeklik, J., Gluszko, P., and Gryglewski, R. J. (1979): *Lancet,* 1:1111–1114.
156. Tansik, R. L., Namm, D. H., and White, H. L. (1978): *Prostaglandins,* 15:399–408.
157. Tateson, J. E., Moncada, S., and Vane, J. R. (1977): *Prostaglandins,* 13:389–399.
158. Ubatuba, F. B., Moncada, S., and Vane, J. R. (1979): *Thromb. Haematol.,* 41:425–434.
159. Vargaftig, B. B., and Chignard, M. (1975): *Agents Actions,* 5:137–144.
160. Vermylen, J., Chamone, D. A. F., and Verstraete, M. (1979): *Lancet,* 1:518–520.
161. Weber, P. C., Larsson, C., Anggard, E., Hamberg, M., Corey, E. J., Nicolaou, K. C., and Samuelsson, B. (1976): *Circ. Res.,* 39:868–874.
162. Weksler, B. B., Knapp, J. M., and Jaffe, E. A. (1977): *Blood (Suppl. 1),* 50:287.
163. Weksler, B. B., Marcus, A. J., and Jaffe, E. A. (1977): *Proc. Natl. Acad. Sci. USA,* 74:3922–3926.
164. Wharton, A. R., Misono, K., Hollifield, J., Frolich, J. C., Inagami, T., and Oates, J. A. (1977): *Prostaglandins,* 14:1095–1104.

165. Wharton, A. R., Smigel, M., Oates, J. A., and Frolich, J. C. (1977): *Prostaglandins,* 13:1021.
166. Whittle, B. J. R., Moncada, S., and Vane, J. R. (1978): *Prostaglandins,* 16:373–388.
167. Willis, A. L., Comai, K., Kuhn, D. C., and Paulsrud, J. (1974): *Prostaglandins,* 8:509–519.
168. Willis, A. L., Vane, F. M., Kuhn, D. C., Scott, C. G., and Petrin, M. (1974): *Prostaglandins,* 8:453–507.
169. Woodford, F. P., Bottcher, C. J. F., Oette, K., and Ahrens, E. H., Jr. (1965): *J. Atheroscler. Res.,* 5:311–316.
170. Woods, H. F., Ash, G., Weston, M. J., Bunting, S., Moncada, S., and Vane, J. R. (1978): *Lancet,* 2:1075–1077.

Advances in Prostaglandin and Thromboxane Research,
Vol. 6, edited by B. Samuelsson, P. W. Ramwell,
and R. Paoletti. Raven Press, New York © 1980.

Mechanism Underlying the Inhibition of Platelet Aggregation by Eicosapentaenoic Acid and Its Metabolites

Philip Needleman, *Howard Sprecher, Mark O. Whitaker, and
Angela Wyche

*Department of Pharmacology, Washington University Medical School, St. Louis, Missouri
63110; and *Department of Physiological Chemistry, Ohio State University,
Columbus, Ohio 43210*

The fatty acid 5,8,11,14,17-eicosapentaenoic acid (EPA) was enzymatically converted by ram cyclooxygenase into the prostaglandin (PG)-endoperoxide PGH_3 (8,9). The purified PGH_3 was converted by the appropriate enzyme source into thromboxane A_3 or Δ^{17}-prostacyclin (PGI_3) (7,9). Surprisingly, the 3-series fatty acid (EPA), endoperoxide (PGH_3), or thromboxane A_3 did not induce aggregation in human platelet-rich plasma (PRP) (8); furthermore, preincubation of human PRP with exogenous PGH_3 or thromboxane A_3 inhibited aggregation with conventional stimuli (e.g., PGH_2, arachidonate, adenosine diphosphate, thrombin) by elevating platelet cyclic adenosine monophosphate (AMP) levels (9). Dyerberg et al. (1) found that Greenland Eskimos have a bleeding tendency and have elevated EPA and depressed arachidonic acid (AA) levels in their blood lipid fraction. These authors proposed that the bleeding disorder resulted from the vascular synthesis of PGI_3. In the current study, we attempted to investigate the mechanisms by which EPA or its metabolites could alter platelet function.

MATERIALS AND METHODS

Materials

5,8,11,14,17-[1-^{14}C]-Eicosapentaenoic acid (20:5), 7.2 Ci/mole, was prepared by total organic synthesis (13). [^{14}C]PGH$_3$ and [^{14}C]PGH$_2$ were enzymatically synthesized and purified with acetone–pentane powder of sheep seminal vesicles as previously described (2,8).

PG standards, PGE_2, D_2, A_2, prostacyclin (PGI_2), 6-keto-$PGF_{1\alpha}$, PGE_3, and thromboxane B_2 were kindly supplied by the Upjohn Company, Kalamazoo, Michigan. The 2',5'-dideoxyadenosine was purchased from P. L. Biochemicals Inc., Milwaukee, Wisconsin.

Platelet Experiments

Citrated human PRP or washed human platelet suspensions were prepared as previously described (6). Platelet cyclic AMP levels (at 60 sec) were determined by radioimmunoassay as previously described (14).

Blood Vessel–Fatty Acid Incubations

Rabbit thoracic aorta was dissected into fine rings (120 mg) and incubated with the ^{14}C-labeled fatty acid (AA or EPA) (10^6 cpm) in 10 ml 100 mM PO_4 buffer, pH 7.8, at 37°C for 1 hr. The media was acidified, extracted, and chromatographed in organic phase of the A9 solvent system (ethyl acetate:acetic acid:2,2,4-trimethylpentane:H_2O,110:20:50:100).

RESULTS AND DISCUSSION

Potency of 3-Series PGs as Contractile Agents

We previously demonstrated that the 3-series endoperoxide and thromboxane were less potent contractile agents on rabbit thoracic aorta strips than the corresponding 2-series compounds [i.e., PGH_2 and thromboxane A_2 (8)]. Similarly, PGI_3 relaxes isolated coronary arterial strips but is less potent than PGI_2 (9). A similar comparison of vascular and nonvascular smooth muscle contractile efficacy showed that PGE_3 was 6 to 20 times less potent than either PGE_2 or PGE_1 (Table 1).

Differential Aggregation and Cyclic AMP Responses of Human or Rabbit PRP to PGH_3

In order to test the hypothesis that platelet aggregation could be depressed by EPA and its metabolites, we planned to initiate feeding experiments substitut-

TABLE 1. *Comparative contractile potency of PGEs on vascular and nonvascular smooth muscle[a]*

Assay tissue	ED$_{50}$		
	PGE$_2$	PGE$_3$	PGE$_1$
Bovine coronary artery contraction (4)	140 ± 20 ng	2200 ± 300 ng	—
Porcine coronary artery contraction (4)	1.02 ± 0.3 μg	24 ± 3 μg	—
Rat stomach strip (5)	8 ± 2 ng	45 ± 6 ng	13 ± 3 ng
Chick rectum (4)	15 ± 3 ng	80 ± 5 ng	15 ± 5 ng
Rabbit aorta (4)	1.0 ± 0.4 μg	14 ± 2 μg	—

[a]The values represent the means $\pm$ SE, and the number of animals are indicated in the parentheses. ED$_{50}$ designates the dose of PGE needed to elicit a 50% maximal contractile in the tissue, and the values are obtained from the parallel dose–response curves.

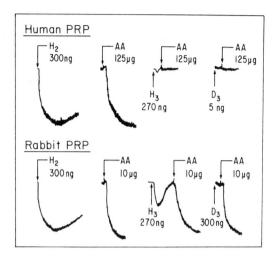

FIG. 1. Response of human and rabbit PRP to various treatments. H_2, PGH_2, AA, arachidonic acid, H_3, PGH_3, D_3-, PGD_3. The PGH_3 or PGD_3 was preincubated with the PRP for 1 min prior to the addition of the stimulating AA dose.

ing 9,12,15-linolenic acid (EPA precursor) for 9, 12-linoleic acid (AA precursor) in the diet of laboratory animals. During control experiments, we discovered that exogenous PGH_3 did not inhibit aggregation in rat or rabbit PRP. This observation was reminiscent of the finding that PGD_2 inhibits aggregation only in human platelets (12). In Fig. 1 it can be seen that human PRP is aggregated by exogenous PGH_2 or AA and that both PGH_3 and PGD_3 preincubation readily inhibit the response to subsequently added agonist. Furthermore, PGD_3 is much more potent than PGH_3; thus the concentration of PGD_3 needed to cause a 50% inhibition of human PRP aggregation is 2.1 ± 0.5 ng ($n = 5$), whereas the IC_{50} for PGH_3 is 26 ± 6 ng (Fig. 2). At their 50% inhibitory doses, PGD_3 and PGH_3 both caused (at 1 min) a 40% increase in platelet cyclic AMP levels and at their IC_{100} caused a 400 to 500% increase. On the other hand, neither PGD_3, PGH_3 nor PGD_2 elevated rabbit PRP cyclic AMP levels or inhibited aggregation at doses up to 1 $\mu g/ml$ (Fig. 1).

We initially rejected the possibility that the inhibition of platelet aggregation by PGH_3 (or thromboxane A_3) could be mediated by PGD_3 because the 3-series endoperoxide, thromboxane, and prostacyclin were all less active on vascular smooth muscle than their 2-series counterparts (7–9). Furthermore, we also observed that PGE_3 was 6 to 20 times less active than PGE_2 as a contractile agent on nonvascular and vascular smooth muscle (Table 1). It is therefore quite surprising that PGE_3 is so active on human platelets and that the PGH_3 breakdown to PGD_3 is much more rapid than anticipated. We showed that the PGD_3 ($\sim 7\%$) spontaneously generated ($t_{1/2}$ 90 sec) during the 1-min preincubation of PGH_3 (IC_{50}, 26 ng) with human PRP is adequate to quantitatively

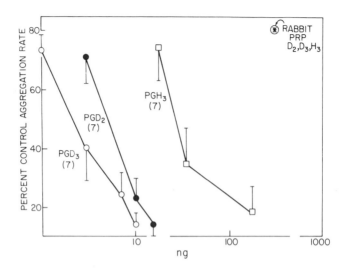

FIG. 2. Dose-dependent inhibition of human PRP aggregation by PGD_3, PGD_2, and PGH_3. All the antagonists are preincubated with the PRP for 1 min prior to (AA) agonist addition. The values are means $\pm$ SE, with the number of human donors shown in parentheses. No dose of PGD_2, PDG_3, or PGH_3 inhibited rabbit PRP, whereas PGI_2 and PGE_1 were still effective inhibitors.

account for the elevation of platelet cyclic AMP and inhibition of aggregation by the endoperoxide (see Whitaker et al., *this volume*). This observation was confirmed with the PGH antisera, which abolished the PGD_3 and PGH_3 inhibition of aggregation (15). These experiments seem to preclude the possible intrinsic platelet role of PGH_3, thromboxane A_3, or PGD_3 as an inhibitor of aggregation. However, it is apparent that exogenous PGD_3 has considerable potential as a therapeutic agent, since it is a potent inhibitor of platelet aggregation. In addition, PGD proves to be a very poor substrate for pulmonary PG-dehydrogenase, with a K_m that is two orders of magnitude higher than PGE_2 and a very low V_{max} (11), which suggests that exogenous PGD_3 or an appropriate analog would be expected to act as a circulating antithrombotic agent. Furthermore, if the biological data obtained with the other 3-series products is a useful indication, then PGD_3 probably has a minimal effect on vascular and nonvascular smooth muscle at antithrombotic doses. Thus PGD_3 could possibly avoid the profound vasodilator side effects of PGI_2 (3), as well as the diarrhea and gastrointestinal side effects induced by the conventional PGs (5).

Effects of Endoperoxides After Inhibition of Platelet Adenylate Cyclase

Haslam et al. (4) have demonstrated that 2',5'-dideoxyadenosine (DDA) inhibits the elevation of platelet cyclic AMP by PGE_1 and that DDA does not alter AA-induced aggregation. Preincubation of human PRP with DDA blocks

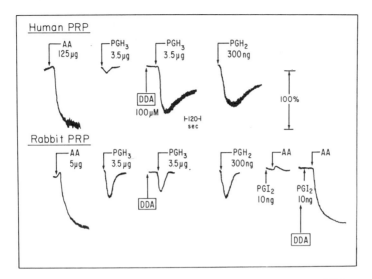

FIG. 3. Effect of the adenylate cyclase inhibitor DDA on human or rabbit PRP aggregation. The DDA was preincubated in the PRP for 2 min before subsequent treatment.

the elevation of platelet cyclic AMP and the inhibition of aggregation produced by PGH_3 (Fig. 3), as well as by PGI_2, PGD_3, and PGD_2 (not shown). DDA has no effect on basal (13.5 fmoles/μl PRP) cyclic AMP levels, but abolishes the increase produced by 3 ng of prostacyclin (89 fmoles/μl PRP) or 20 ng PGD_3 (81.6 fmoles/μl PRP) (Fig. 4). The abolition of the stimulation of platelet adenylate cyclase by DDA did, in fact, unmask a direct but moderate and reversible aggregatory effect of PGH_3 (Fig. 3), as well as abolish the ability of this endoperoxide to inhibit platelet aggregation. Higher doses of PGH_3 did

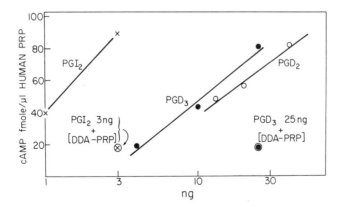

FIG. 4. Dose-dependent stimulation of human PRP cyclic AMP levels by PGI_2, PGD_3, and PGD_2 and the reversal by the adenylate cyclase antagonist (DDA, 100 μM for 2 min).

not produce complete, irreversible aggregation. We also observed that the inhibition of platelet aggregation by PGE_1 and PGD_2 was abolished by DDA (not shown). Furthermore, in rabbit PRP neither PGH_3 nor PGD_3 elevate platelet cyclic AMP or inhibit aggregation, and exogenous addition of PGH_3 (3.5 μg) causes a reversible aggregation not influenced by DDA (Figs. 3 and 4).

Eicosapentoenate Tissue Incorporation, Metabolism, and Effects on Platelet Aggregation

PGD formation by platelet would only be expected to occur on addition of an exogenous source of PG-endoperoxide, since endogenously formed endoperoxide is avidly converted to thromboxane before any significant breakdown to D and E can occur (10). Thus the possible mechanisms whereby high intrinsic eicosapentaenoate could interfere with platelet aggregation require either the demonstraton of adequate levels of PGI_3 production by the vasculature or documentation that eicosapentaenoate is readily incorporated and released from tissue lipids and that this fatty acid competes with AA. We can readily demonstrate that both ^{14}C-EPA and ^{14}C-AA are incorporated into the vascular phospholipid pool (15). However, under incubation conditions that result in a 10 to 20% conversion of AA by blood vessel cyclooxygenase, there was no detectable conversion of ^{14}C-EPA (Fig. 5). Similarily, exogenous ^{14}C-EPA proved to be a poor substrate for heart and kidney cyclooxygenase, although it is readily incorporated into the tissue lipids (not shown). On the other hand, we found that EPA is readily released from tissue lipids from either perfused kidney (15) or platelets (9) by the same conditions that activate the release of AA.

The above data suggest that neither platelet formation of 3-series PGs nor vascular synthesis of PGI_3 is a likely mechanism whereby EPA could interfere with aggregation. What mechanism can explain the potential of EPA to act as an intrinsic antithrombotic substance? An additional possiblility is the competition of EPA with AA for platelet metabolism. We have previously demonstrated that a 1:1 or 2.5:1 ratio of EPA:^{14}C-AA causes a 50% inhibition in the production of ^{14}C-metabolites by platelet cyclooxygenase and lipoxygenase (9). Furthermore, we observed that the simultaneous exposure of human PRP (or rabbit PRP) to EPA and AA in a 1:1 ratio inhibits the AA-induced aggregation. Exogenously added EPA was also capable of inhibiting PRP aggregation induced by exogenous ADP or collagen or by thrombin in washed platelet suspensions. However, these experiments do not preclude that possibility that EPA could be inhibiting platelet aggregation by some other mechanism.

Since EPA acts as a competitive antagonist for platelet AA metabolism, the simultaneous release of EPA could suppress AA conversion to its aggregatory metabolites. The simultaneous lowering of endogenous AA and increase in EPA which must result from a diet of the type that the Greenland Eskimos ingest would be anticipated to markedly reduce the generation of PGH_2 and throm-

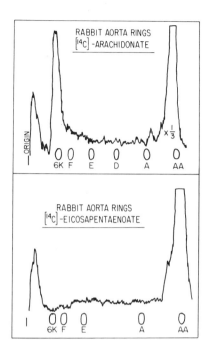

FIG. 5. Metabolism of [^{14}C] arachidonic acid or [^{14}C] eicosapentaenoic acid by rabbit thoracic aorta rings. The incubation media was acidified, extracted, concentrated, and run with unlabeled PG standards on silica gel thin-layer plates. The standards are indicated at the bottom of the chromatogram. 6K,6-keto-PGF$_{1\alpha}$; F, PGF$_{2\alpha}$; E, PGE$_2$; D, PGD$_2$; A, PGA$_2$; AA, arachidonic acid. These silica gel plates cannot distinguish compounds by their degree of unsaturation; therefore, EPA and AA migrate to the same place.

boxane A$_2$. If these suggested mechanisms in fact explain the Eskimo bleeding tendency, then it should be expected that there is little, if any, vascular PGI$_2$ or any other PG production (i.e., a PG deficiency). Obviously, it would be valuable to ascertain the total urinary PG production in this population. Indeed, these subjects would be studied usefully in those situations believed to be mediated by intrinsic PG synthesis (e.g., inflammation, ulcers, renal disease, etc.).

ACKNOWLEDGMENTS

This work was supported by International Rotary Fellowship (M.O.W.) and N.I.H. Grants HL-20787, SCOR-HL-17646, and Contract HV-72945. The authors acknowledge the excellent technical assistance provided by Karin Watters, Sandra Holmberg, and Susan Bronson.

REFERENCES

1. Dyerberg, J., Bang, H. O., Stoffersen, E., Moncada, S., and Vane, J. R. (1978): *Lancet,* 2:117–119.
2. Gorman, R. R., Sun, F. F., Miller, O. V., and Johnson, R. A. (1977): *Prostaglandins,* 13:1043–1056.
3. Gryglewski, R. J., Szczeklik, A., and Nizankowski, R. (1978): *Thromb. Res.,* 13:153–163.
4. Haslam, R. J., Davidson, M. M. L., Fox, J. E. B., and Lynham, J. A. (1978): *Throm. Haemostas.,* 40:232–240.

5. Horton, E. W., Main, I. H. M., Thompson, C. J., and Wright, P. M. (1968): *Gut,* 9:655–665.
6. Minkes, M., Stanford, N., Chi, M., Roth, G. J., Raz, A., Needleman, P., and Majerus, P. W. (1977): *J. Clin. Invest.,* 59:449–454.
7. Needleman, P., Kulkarni, P. S., and Raz, A. (1977): *Science* 195:409–412.
8. Needleman, P., Minkes, M., and Raz, A. (1976): *Science,* 193:163–165.
9. Needleman, P., Raz, A., Minkes, M. S., Ferrendelli, J. A., and Sprecher, H. (1979): *Proc. Natl. Acad. Sci. USA,* 76:944–948.
10. Needleman, P., Wyche, A., and Raz, A. (1979): *J. Clin. Invest.,* 63:345–349.
11. Ohno, H., Morikawa, Y., and Hirara, F. (1978): *J. Biochem.,* 84:1485–1494.
12. Smith, J. B., Silver, M. J., Ingerman, C. M., and Kocsis, J. J. (1974): *Thromb. Res.,* 5:291–299.
13. Sprecher, H. (1971): *Lipids,* 6:889–894.
14. Steiner, A. L., Parker, C. W., and Kipnis, D. M. (1972): *J. Biol. Chem.,* 247:1106–1113.
15. Whitaker, M. O., Wyche, A., Fitzpatrick, F., Sprecher, H., Ferrendelli, J. A., and Needleman, P. (1979): *Proc. Natl. Acad. Sci. USA (in press).*

Advances in Prostaglandin and Thromboxane Research,
Vol. 6, edited by B. Samuelsson, P. W. Ramwell,
and R. Paoletti. Raven Press, New York © 1980.

Assay Methods for Prostaglandins and Thromboxanes

Elisabeth Granström

Department of Chemistry, Karolinska Institute, S-104 01 Stockholm 60, Sweden

Ever since the structures of the first few prostaglandins (PGs) were elucidated around 20 years ago, the PG family has been steadily growing, with new pathways and metabolites being discovered continuously. Finding assay methods sufficiently sensitive and specific for the detection and quantitation of all these compounds constitutes a great problem in PG research.

From the earliest years of research in this field, such methods have often been based on the strong biological activities of these compounds. Later, chemical and physical methods also appeared, such as ultraviolet spectrometry, gas-liquid chromatography with flame ionization detection, and an enzymatic method based on the activities of the metabolizing enzyme 15-hydroxyprostanoate dehydrogenase. These methods were, however, either too insensitive or too nonspecific for use in many biological experiments, and they have more recently been replaced by improved techniques such as gas-liquid chromatography with electron capture detection, quantitative mass spectrometry with deuterium-labeled carriers and multiple ion detection, cascade superfusion techniques in bioassay, radioimmunoassay, and a number of other methods (for reviews, see refs. 49,50). Today, three different types of assay methods have gained particularly widespread use: bioassay, gas chromatography with mass spectrometry, and radioimmunoassay.

Bioassay is based on the fact that the members of the prostaglandin family display both quantitative and qualitative differences in their effects on smooth muscle from different organs, as well as in many other biological systems. The earliest type of bioassay, the organ bath type, is now largely replaced by the superfusion technique, which has further been developed into the cascade technique: in this method several different assay organs are superfused in turn by the same sample (58). A quite specific assay system can be obtained if a combination is made of suitable organs with different reactions to the various compounds (cf. 36,61), and if the organs are pretreated with specific antagonists against other biologically active substances than those of the PG family—e.g., histamine, bradykinin, catecholamines, and serotonin (36).

During the last few years the effects of PGs and thromboxanes on platelet aggregation have also been used for quantitative estimations of these compounds. There are also a number of *in vivo* bioassays, based on PG effects on blood pressure, estrous cycle length, body temperature, development of various inflammatory symptoms, etc.

Gas chromatography–mass spectrometry is an entirely different and very specific type of method. It is based on the addition to the sample of a comparatively large amount of the deuterium-labeled compound to be measured (see refs. 20,49,50). This acts as a carrier during the chromatographic purification steps and as an internal standard during the final mass spectrometry. The small amount of the natural, protium form of the compound can be accurately calculated from the known amount of the added deuterium form and the measured proportion between the protium and the deuterium forms in the final mass spectrometry of the purified compound.

Some of the employed deuterium carriers have several deuterium atoms close to the carboxyl group, as in the 3,3,4,4-tetradeutero compounds used for the common prostaglandins and their plasma metabolites. Others, such as thromboxane B_2 (TXB_2) and 12-hydroxy-5,8,10,14-eicosatetraenoic acid (HETE), are commonly prepared from octadeutero-arachidonic acid. For some highly degraded urinary metabolites, the deuterium label is sometimes introduced at a later stage, during the preparation of derivatives such as deuterium-labeled methyl oximes (see ref. 20).

Radioimmunoassay is today the most commonly employed assay method in this field (for reviews, see refs. 13,14,49,50). The method is based on the competition between radiolabeled and unlabeled molecules of the compound for the binding sites of an antibody directed against this compound. The more cold molecules present in the incubation, the more radioactive ones will be displaced from the antibody binding sites, with the radioactivity increasing in the free fraction. Absolute amounts of the compound are obtained by comparison with a set of standards with known amounts.

All these assay methods have their specific advantages and shortcomings, but since these are well known, they will not be the topic of the present discussion. However, there are also several problems with the assay of compounds in this field that are common to all the methods and are related to the chemical and metabolic fates of the measured compounds (cf. 18,49,50). Some of these problems are less well recognized and will therefore be discussed in somewhat more detail here.

It has now widely been accepted that measurement of the primary PGs such as E_2 or $F_{2\alpha}$ in the peripheral circulation or in urine does not give a true picture of the total body synthesis of these compounds. In the blood the actual, endogenous levels may be totally "buried" in the large artifactual amounts formed during the sample collection. In urine, levels of primary PGs only reflect the renal synthesis of these compounds or, in men, even the contamination from the seminal fluid, instead of reflecting the production in other organs (12,62). In order to avoid drawing erroneous conclusions from PG measurements, it is thus necessary to monitor the proper compound in each study. In the case of blood measurements, this means the stable, circulating 15-keto-13,14-dihydro compounds, and for urine, the relevant tetranor metabolites (49,50).

Since this necessity became well known and accepted, a great number of studies have been successfully carried out on the roles of $PGF_{2\alpha}$ in the body by using 15-keto-13,14-dihydro-$PGF_{2\alpha}$ as a target for measurements in the peripheral circulation. However, this has not been the case with the corresponding PGE_2 metabolite, 15-keto-13,14-dihydro-PGE_2. Very few assays for it exist, and very few data have been published on its occurrence in biological fluids (19,26,29,35,43,48,56). The reason for this is likely to be pronounced chemical instability in aqueous media. The compound seems to be dehydrated easily to form the corresponding PGA_2 metabolite, which subsequently cyclizes by an attack by C-16 at C-11 to form 11-deoxy-15-keto-13,14-dihydro-11β,16-cyclo-PGE_2 (see refs. 4,30). Like other PGE compounds, it can also undergo isomerization at C-8. Furthermore, in protein-containing samples such as plasma, a large fraction of the metabolite is trapped by proteins, mainly albumin, to form covalent derivatives. All these reactions occur spontaneously and rapidly.

Published data for this metabolite may thus be uncertain, particularly when obtained by radioimmunoassay. With the exception of the protein binding, the same degradations also occur in the radioimmunoassay reagents, i.e., the tracer and the standards. In assays for 15-keto-13,14-dihydro-PGE_2, reagents and samples of different ages have been incubated, thus constituting unknown and variable mixtures of all the degradation products. In addition, it is uncertain what compound the antibody was actually directed against. This depends on the age of the hapten used for coupling, the coupling conditions, the time for the dialysis of the conjugate, etc. Furthermore, incubation in the assay has been carried out under conditions which lead to further degradation.

A possible solution to the problem is to develop an assay for the stable bicyclic degradation product instead, and to induce this degradation to completion in all the samples prior to assay. This can be done efficiently if proteins are first removed by extraction (15).

Measurements of TX have been carried out using a variety of methods. The first ones were aimed at TXA_2 itself and were bioassays, utilizing its high potency for induction of platelet aggregation or its strong contracting effects on various vessels, with rabbit aorta as the most commonly used preparation (25,44,54, 55,59).

Methods other than bioassay had to be aimed at a stable degradation product, such as TXB_2, formed by spontaneous hydrolysis of TXA_2. Several such methods have been developed, starting with a double-isotope method for exogenous TX formation (25) and followed by several radioimmunoassays, mass spectrometric methods, and electron capture methods for endogenous thromboxane formation (2,10,11,16,24,51).

When TXB_2 was measured during platelet aggregation *in vitro,* a rapid rise was seen coinciding with the aggregation, and the TXB_2 amounts then remained at high, constant levels (10,16,17). When it was desirable to study the kinetics of the formation and disappearance of TXA_2, this method was not sufficient, and a different approach was used. TXA_2 was converted by excess methanol into mono-*O*-methyl-TXB_2 (25), and this latter derivative was measured instead. Its levels reflect the amount of TXA_2 present in the sample at the very moment the methanol was added (17).

When this method was applied to studies on platelet aggregation, it was indeed found that TXA_2 is formed only during the earliest phase. Furthermore, when the platelets were rapidly removed by filtration, so as to exclude any possibility of a later formation of TXA_2, the disappearance of the compound could be selectively studied (17). It was found to disappear with a half-life of 32 sec in a buffer of pH 7.4, which was exactly what had been reported for TXA_2 using other methods (25). Thus it seems that under these circumstances, mono-*O*-methyl-TXB_2 is a reliable indicator of TXA_2 formation.

The further development of this area should, of course, preferably include the measurement of the TX production *in vivo*. However, this seems to be very difficult. TXB_2 cannot be monitored in plasma for the same reason as primary PGs; the endogenous levels become completely overshadowed by the large amounts formed as artifacts during collection and handling of the sample. In fact, as the TX pathway is the major one in platelets (24), the problem can be expected to be even greater here than for the primary PGs.

A possible solution to this problem would be either to find a relatively stable, circulating metabolite which is not formed during sampling or to measure the excretion into urine of a suitable urinary metabolite. Unfortunately, when the further fates of TXB_2 were investigated in several species, no conversion into 15-keto-13,14-dihydro-TXB_2 was seen (28,45,46). This compound was hoped to be a major circulating metabolite in analogy with the classical PGs.

The main urinary metabolite of TXB_2 is dinor-TXB_2 in several species (28, 45,46,53). A mass spectrometric method was recently developed for this compound and used to quantitate TXB_2 production *in vivo* in the guinea pig (53). The basal TXB_2 production was low, only around 500 ng/day. When the guinea pigs were sensitized and anaphylaxis later induced by challenge with the immunogen, no increase was seen at all in the excretion of dinor-TXB_2 (53). This was surprising, as sensitized guinea pig lungs are known to produce large amounts of TX during challenge (44,23). A likely explanation was that TXA_2 had been degraded by a different pathway *in vivo* and thus escaped detection when only dinor-TXB_2 was measured.

This hypothesis was corroborated by the identification of the long-sought metabolite 15-keto-13,14-dihydro-TXB_2 in perfusion experiments with anaphylactic guinea pig lungs (7,33). In nonsensitized lungs it was a rather minor product but dominated the picture after sensitization; interestingly, its relative importance increased with repeated challenges (5).

Thus it seems that although TXB_2 is not a substrate for the enzyme 15-hydroxy-prostanoate dehydrogenase, TXA_2 itself may be, and may become converted into first, e.g., 15-keto-13,14-dihydro-TXA$_2$, which is then spontaneously hydrolyzed into 15-keto-13,14-dihydro-TXB$_2$. A radioimmunoassay was recently developed for the latter metabolite, and the findings of large amounts of this compound from anaphylactic guinea pig lungs *in vitro* were confirmed (3).

To turn back to the earlier *in vitro* experiments, measurement of the TX production by platelets under these circumstances still seemed a fairly simple matter: assay of the stable end product, TXB$_2$, when the total TX synthesis was studied, and assay of mono-*O*-methyl-TXB$_2$ in a methanol-treated sample when it was necessary to know the exact amounts of TXA$_2$ in a particular instant.

However, the situation is more complicated that this, even in this relatively simple biological system. In studies on PGH$_2$-induced aggregation in platelet-rich plasma, a peculiar phenomenon was noticed (9,31,32). Different results were obtained when the removed aliquots were treated in different ways. If acetone was used to quench the reaction, the normal increase of TXB$_2$ to a high, constant level was found. However, if the aliquots were quenched by addition of acid, a rapid burst in TXB$_2$ production was seen, followed by an apparent disappearance as reflected by a decrease in detected TXB$_2$ levels. As TXB$_2$ itself is stable under these conditions, the compound that disappeared must be its precursor, TXA$_2$. It turned out that TXA$_2$ was quickly trapped by proteins, mainly albumin, to form covalently bound derivatives (31,32). The same phenomenon was seen when arachidonic acid was used as a substrate (32).

Thus if TXB$_2$ is monitored in any sample that contains albumin, such as plasma, it is possible that it only reflects a minor portion of the TXA$_2$ actually released. The major portion has become protein bound and thus escapes detection. The true amounts of formed TXA$_2$ can only be detected during the first few seconds after the release, and then only if the pH is quickly lowered, because at a low pH the hydrolysis into TXB$_2$ is much more rapid than the reaction with proteins.

To summarize the assay problems for TX, this area has become very complicated. A few years ago, TXB$_2$ was almost automatically believed to be the end-product of the TX pathway and a reliable indicator of TXA$_2$ formation. Now it seems that under many circumstances TXB$_2$ is a very minor and insignificant product. TXA$_2$ seems to be metabolized to a great extent via different pathways into protein-bound derivatives or 15-keto-13,14-dihydro metabolites and thus escapes detection when only TXB$_2$ or its breakdown products are monitored.

Measurement of the PGI$_2$ (prostacyclin) production is still a relatively new problem. Most measurements are carried out by bioassay, either utilizing the effects of PGI$_2$ on various smooth muscle preparations or its antiaggregatory effects, which is perhaps the most commonly used assay for this compound (6,8,37,61). Generally this is done *in vitro*, and changes in the light transmission of a platelet preparation are measured. Recently, advantage has been taken of the reverse effects of PGI_2 on collagen-induced platelet aggregation on a strip of tendon, which results in changes in the weight of this strip that can be recorded (22).

As PGI_2 is a very unstable compound, methods other than bioassay must be aimed at a stable degradation product instead. For assay of the amount of PGI_2 in a sample, the spontaneously formed hydrolysis product, 6-keto-$PGF_{1\alpha}$, is probably the best choice (27,40). A few radioimmunoassays, gas chromatographic, and mass spectrometric methods for this compound already exist (1, 34,41,47,57). For the measurement of the PGI_2 production and release *in vivo*, however, 6-keto-$PGF_{1\alpha}$ may not be the best indicator. It has been demonstrated that PGI_2 survives passage through the lung, and this suggests that the compound should be a circulating hormone (8,21,38,60,64); but several other studies indicate that its actions are of very short duration *in vivo*, and furthermore, that it is efficiently extracted and metabolized by other organs and tissues (39,63,65). In contrast to 6-keto-$PGF_{1\alpha}$ (42), PGI_2 is a very good substrate for the enzyme 15-hydroxyprostanoate dehydrogenase, and for studies on plasma levels reflecting the prostacyclin pathway, 6,15-diketo-13,14-dihydro-$PGF_{1\alpha}$ may prove to be the best indicator; the situation is thus analogous to the TX area. For urinary measurements, relevant dinor metabolites seem to be the most suitable compounds to assay, at least in the few species studied so far (52,63).

ACKNOWLEDGMENTS

This study was supported by grants from the World Health Organization and the Swedish Medical Research Council.

REFERENCES

1. Abdel-Halim, M. S., Ekstedt, J., and Änggård, E. (1979): *Prostaglandins,* 17:405–409.
2. Anhut, H., Bernauer, W., and Peskar, B. A. (1977): *Eur. J. Pharmacol.,* 44:85–88.
3. Anhut, H., Peskar, B. A., and Bernauer, W. (1978): *Naunyn Schmiedebergs Arch. Pharmacol.,* 305:247–252.
4. Beal, R. F., Babcock, J. C., and Lincoln, F. H. (1967): In: *Prostaglandins. Nobel Symposium 2,* edited by S. Bergström and B. Samuelsson, pp. 219–230. Almqvist and Wiksell, Uppsala, Sweden.
5. Boot, J. R., Cockerill, A. F., Dawson, W., Mallen, D. N. B., and Osborne, D. J. (1978): *Int. Arch. Allergy Appl. Immunol.,* 57:159–164.
6. Bunting, S., Gryglewski, R., Moncada, S., and Vane, J. R. (1976): *Prostaglandins,* 12:897–913.
7. Dawson, W., Boot, J. R., Cockerill, A. F., Mallen, D. N. B., and Osborne, D. J. (1976): *Nature,* 262:699–702.
8. Dusting, G. J., Moncada, S., and Vane, J. R. (1978): *Br. J. Pharmacol.,* 64:315–320.
9. Fitzpatrick, F. A., and Gorman, R. R. (1977): *Prostaglandins,* 14:881–889.
10. Fitzpatrick, F. A., Gorman, R. R., McGuire, J. C., Kelly, R. C., Wynalda, M. A., and Sun, F. F. (1977): *Anal. Biochem.,* 82:1–7.
11. Fitzpatrick, F. A., Gorman, R. R., and Wynalda, M. A. (1977): *Prostaglandins,* 13:201–208.
12. Frölich, J. C., Wilson, T. W., Sweetman, B. J., Smigel, M., Nies, A. S., Carr, K., Watson, J. T., and Oates, J. A. (1975): *J. Clin. Invest.,* 55:763–770.
13. Granström, E. (1978): *Prostaglandins,* 15:3–17.

14. Granström, E., and Kindahl, H. (1978): In: *Advances in Prostaglandin and Thromboxane Research, Vol. 5,* edited by J. C. Frölich, Raven Press, New York, pp. 119–210.
15. Granström, E., and Kindahl, H. (1980): *this volume.*
16. Granström, E., Kindahl, H., and Samuelsson, B. (1976): *Anal. Lett.,* 9:611–627.
17. Granström, E., Kindahl, H., and Samuelsson, B. (1976): *Prostaglandins,* 12:929–941.
18. Granström, E., and Samuelsson, B. (1978): In: *Advances in Prostaglandin and Thromboxane Research, Vol. 5,* edited by J. C. Frölich, pp. 1–13. Raven Press, New York.
19. Gréen, K., and Granström, E. (1973): In: *Prostaglandins in Fertility Control, Vol. 3,* edited by S. Bergström, pp. 55–61. Karolinska Institutet, Stockholm, Sweden.
20. Gréen, K., Hamberg, M., Samuelsson, B., Smigel, M., and Frölich, J. C. (1978): In: *Advances in Prostaglandin and Thromboxane Research, Vol. 5.,* edited by J. C. Frölich, pp. 39–94. Raven Press, New York.
21. Gryglewski, R. J., Korbut, R., and Ocetkiewicz, A. (1978): *Nature,* 273:765–767.
22. Gryglewski, R. J., Korbut, R., Ocetkiewicz, A., and Stachwa, T. (1978): *Naunyn Schmiedebergs Arch. Pharmacol.,* 302:25–30.
23. Hamberg, M., Svensson, J., Hedqvist, P., Strandberg, K., and Samuelsson, B. (1976): In: *Advances in Prostaglandin and Thromboxane Research, Vol. 1,* edited by B. Samuelsson and R. Paoletti, pp. 495–501. Raven Press, New York.
24. Hamberg, M., Svensson, J., and Samuelsson, B. (1974): *Proc. Natl. Acad. Sci. USA,* 71:3824–3828.
25. Hamberg, M., Svensson, J., and Samuelsson, B. (1975): *Proc. Natl. Acad. Sci. USA,* 72:2994–2998.
26. Hubbard, W. C., and Watson, J. T. (1976): *Prostaglandins,* 12:21–35.
27. Johnson, R. A., Morton, D. R., Kinner, J. H., Gorman, R. R., McGuire, J. C., Sun, F. F., Whittaker, N., Bunting, S., Salmon, J., Moncada, S., and Vane, J. R. (1976): *Prostaglandins,* 12:915–928.
28. Kindahl, H. (1977): *Prostaglandins,* 13:619–629.
29. Levine, L. (1977): *Prostaglandins,* 14:1125–1139.
30. Lincoln, F. H., Schneider, W. P., and Pike, J. E. (1973): *J. Org. Chem.,* 38:951–956.
31. Maclouf, J., Kindahl, H., Granström, E., and Samuelsson, B. (1979): Fourth International Prostaglandin Conference, Washington, D.C., May 1979, Abstract.
32. Maclouf, J., Kindahl, H., Granström, E., and Samuelsson, B. (1979): *submitted for publication.*
33. Mallen, D. N. B., Osborne, D. J., Cockerill, A. F., Boot, J. R., and Dawson, W. (1978): *Biomed. Mass Spectr.,* 5:449–452.
34. Mitchell, M. D. (1978): *Prostaglandins Med.,* 1:13–21.
35. Mitchell, M. D., Sors, H., and Flint, A. P. F. (1977): *Lancet,* 2(8037):558.
36. Moncada, S., Ferreira, S. H., and Vane, J. (1978): In: *Advances in Prostaglandin and Thromboxane Research, Vol. 5,* edited by J. C. Frölich, pp. 211–236. Raven Press, New York.
37. Moncada, S., Gryglewski, R. J., Bunting, S., and Vane, J. R. (1976): *Prostaglandins,* 12:715–739.
38. Moncada, S., Korbut, R., Bunting, S., and Vane, J. R. (1978): *Nature,* 273:767–768.
39. Needleman, P., Bronson, S. D., Wycke, A., Sivakoff, M., and Nicholaou, K. C. (1978): *J. Clin. Invest.,* 61:839–849.
40. Pace-Asciak, C. (1976): *Experientia,* 32:291–292.
41. Pace-Asciak, C. R. (1977): *Anal. Biochem.,* 81:251–255.
42. Pace-Asciak, C. R., Carrara, M. C., and Domazet, Z. (1977): *Biochem. Biophys. Res. Commun.,* 78:115–121.
43. Peskar, B. A., Holland, A., and Peskar, B. M. (1974): *FEBS Lett.,* 43:45–48.
44. Piper, P., and Vane, J. R. (1969): *Nature,* 223:29–35.
45. Roberts, L. J., II, Sweetman, B. J., and Oates, J. A. (1978): *J. Biol. Chem.,* 253:5305–5318.
46. Roberts, L. J., II, Sweetman, B. J., Payne, N. A., and Oates, J. A. (1977): *J. Biol. Chem.,* 252:7415–7417.
47. Salmon, J. A. (1978): *Prostaglandins,* 15:383–397.
48. Samuelsson, B., and Gréen, K. (1974): *Biochem. Med.,* 11:298–303.
49. Samuelsson, B., Granström, E., Gréen, K., Hamberg, M., and Hammarström, S. (1975): *Ann. Rev. Biochem.,* 44:669–695.
50. Samuelsson, B., Goldyne, M., Granström, E., Hamberg, M., Hammarström, S., and Malmsten, C. (1978): *Annu. Rev. Biochem.,* 47:997–1029.

51. Sors, H., Pradelles, P., Dray, F., Rigaud, M., Maclouf, J., and Bernard, P. (1978): *Prostaglandins,* 16:277–290.
52. Sun, F. F., and Taylor, B. M. (1978): *Biochemistry,* 17:4096–4101.
53. Svensson, J. (1979): *Prostaglandins,* 17:351–365.
54. Svensson, J., Hamberg, M., and Samuelsson, B. (1974): *Acta Physiol. Scand.,* 94:222–228.
55. Svensson, J., Hamberg, M., and Samuelsson, B. (1976): *Acta Physiol. Scand,* 98:285–294.
56. Tashjian, A. H. Jr., Voelkel, E. F., and Levine, L. (1977): *Prostaglandins,* 14:309–317.
57. Ubatuba, F. B. (1978): *J. Chromatogr.,* 161:165–177.
58. Vane, J. R. (1969): *Br. J. Pharmacol.,* 35:209–242.
59. Vargaftig, B., and Zirinis, P. (1973): *Nature [New Biol.],* 244:114–116.
60. Waldman, H. M., Alter, I., Kot, P. A., Rose, J. C., and Ramwell, P. W. (1978): *J. Pharmacol. Exp. Ther.,* 204:289–293.
61. Whittle, B., Mugridge, K., and Moncada, S. (1979): *Eur. J. Pharmacol.,* 53:167–172.
62. Williams, W. M., Frölich, J. C., Nies, A. S., and Oates, J. A. (1977): *Kidney Int.,* 11:256–260.
63. Wong, P. Y.-K., McGiff, J. C., Cagen, L., Malik, K. U., and Sun, F. F. (1979): *J. Biol. Chem.,* 254:12–14.
64. Wong, P. Y.-K., McGiff, J. C., Sun, F. F., and Malik, K. U. (1978): *Biochem. Biophys. Res. Commun.,* 83:731–738.
65. Wong, P. Y.-K., Sun, F. F., and McGiff, J. C. (1978): *J. Biol. Chem.,* 253:5555–5557.

Advances in Prostaglandin and Thromboxane Research,
Vol. 6, edited by B. Samuelsson, P. W. Ramwell,
and R. Paoletti. Raven Press, New York © 1980.

Inflammation: The Role of Peroxidase-Derived Products

F. A. Kuehl, Jr., J. L. Humes, E. A. Ham, R. W. Egan, and H. W. Dougherty

Merck Institute for Therapeutic Research, Rahway, New Jersey 07065

The initial enzymes in the prostaglandin (PG) biosynthetic pathway, cyclooxygenase and PG hydroperoxidase, are common to a single protein (17). Although it has not yet been established whether these activities are expressed by a bifunctional catalytic site or by two distinct sites associated with a single protein, it is clear that the enzymatic activities are quite independent of each other. Thus nonsteroidal anti-inflammatory agents such as indomethacin block the cyclooxygenase with no effect on the peroxidase (3). There is also a requirement for oxidizable cofactors for full peroxidase and cyclooxygenase activity (17), and the substitution of the hematin by a manganese porphyrin complex has no effect on the cyclooxygenase reaction but significantly reduces the peroxidase activity (16). In examining the scheme in Fig. 1, it is evident that the prime function of the peroxidase is to effect the conversion of PGG_2 to PGH_2, and there is a large body of evidence to support this view. However, with the isolation of hydroperoxy PGEs, it is evident that the peroxidase is relatively nonspecific with respect to substrate, a fact that will be discussed in detail later.

The peroxidase reaction leads to all biologically active compounds of the PG cascade (Fig. 1). Since these are formed subsequent to the cyclooxygenase step and are thus subject to control by NSAIDs, all must be considered as potential mediators of inflammation until proven otherwise. In addition to these organic reaction products, an oxidizing equivalent that has been heretofore ignored is also produced during the peroxidatic conversion of PGG_2 to PGH_2. The reason for this lack of attention probably derives from the fact that peroxidases have been generally considered to be enzymatic mechanisms for the conversion of oxidants to a lower and less lethal oxidizing state. The action of glutathione peroxidase is the classic example of the phenomenon wherein hydroperoxides are reduced in the presence of a specific obligatory reductant, glutathione. In contradistinction to glutathione peroxidase, PG-hydroperoxidase is quite nonspecific with respect to the nature of reducing agents and thus must be considered as a multisubstrate peroxidase. Futhermore, unlike glutathione peroxidase, in the absence of added reducing species, PG-hydroperoxidase

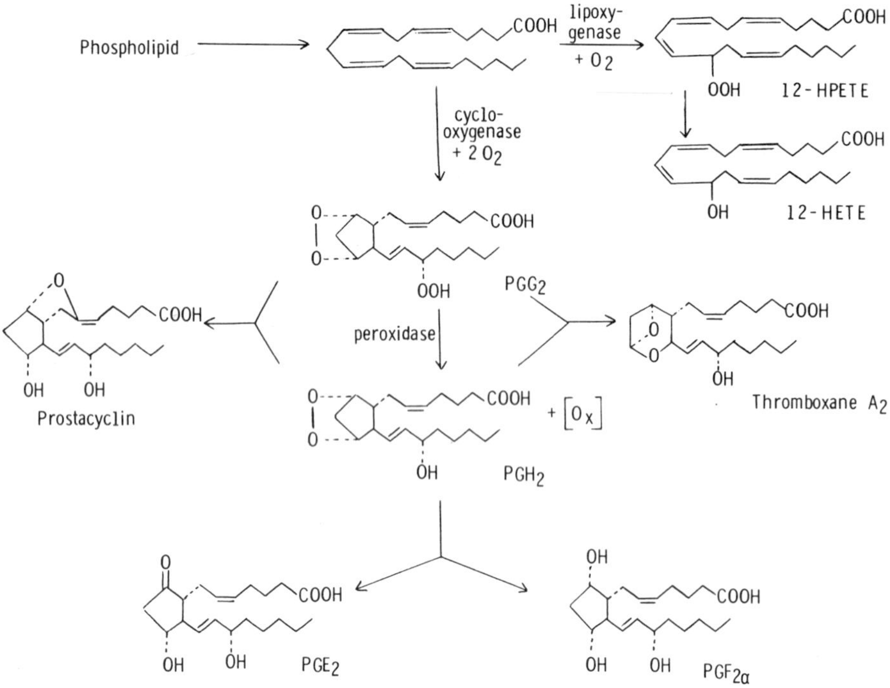

FIG. 1. Scheme showing arachidonic acid cascade.

proceeds normally to yield hydroxy acids, and the oxidant produced attacks available sensitive compounds, including the peroxidase itself (5). Available data imply that this oxidant, $[O_x]$, a byproduct of the PG biosynthetic pathway, is a uniquely potent one, with an oxidizing capacity equivalent to hydroxyl radical. Thus under appropriate conditions, it may be predicted to have pathological significance.

SUBSTRATES FOR PG HYDROPEROXIDASE

Having established that PGG_2 is capable of releasing an oxidizing species $[O_x]$ on reaction with the peroxidase component of PG synthetase, it was of interest to examine the enzyme for substrate specifity (5). The parameters studied were conversion of hydroperoxy to hydroxy acid, release of $[O_x]$ as measured by an electron paramagnetic (EPR) signal, and deactivation of enzymes. PGG_1, the precursor of the PGE_1 series, like PGG_2, is an excellent substrate. 15-Hydroperoxyeicosa-5,8,11,13-tetraenoic acid (15-HPETE), the principle product of the reaction of arachidonic acid with soybean lipoxygenase, is also an excellent substrate. 12-HPETE, a product of the reaction of arachidonic acid with a lipoxygenase present in platelets is next on the list (see Fig. 1). 15-Hydroperoxy PGE_1 (15-HPE_1) is a somewhat poorer substrate. The finding that hydrogen peroxide is also a substrate, although a poorer one, demonstrates that the peroxidase associated with PG synthetase is quite nonspecific and thus capable of generating $[O_x]$ from a number of hydroperoxy compounds. This pathway also offers an alternate catabolic route for H_2O_2 that differs from the catalase route in that a more potent oxidant, $[O_x]$, is generated in place of a less potent one (O_2).

EVIDENCE THAT $[O_x]$ IS AN INFLAMMATORY MEDIATOR

The first evidence for the involvement of an oxidizing radical species in the PG biosynthetic pathway derived from studies with an experimental drug, an active anti-inflammatory agent, in animal models of inflammation. This compound, MK-447 (2-aminomethyl-4-t-butyl-6-iodophenol), was found to be ineffective in inhibiting the synthesis of prostaglandins *in vitro* as do indomethacin, aspirin, and other nonsteroidal anti-inflammatory agents (10). When a comparison was made of the separated products following the enzymatic oxygenation of arachidonic acid, the effect of MK-447 was to increase the utilization of substrate arachidonic acid, a reflection of enhanced cyclooxygenase activity, and to facilitate even more markedly the conversion of PGG_2 to PGH_2, a reflection of increased peroxidase activity resulting in an overall increase in PG synthesis (10). A number of radical scavengers including phenol, methional, and aminopyrine had an effect similar to MK-447, suggesting their action to be a common one, that of preventing deactivation of the cyclooxygenase and peroxidase components of PG synthetase by an oxidizing moiety generated during the enzymatic sequence. The pinpointing of the site of oxidant release at the peroxidase was accomplished by measuring the direct conversion of PGG_2 to PGH_2 with attendant destruction of the enzyme, an action partially reversed by scavengers (5). Evidence that the peroxidatic reduction is a free-radical-related event was established by EPR studies (3). In this experiment the reaction was quenched by freezing to $-196°C$ to give an EPR signal, an effect observable only in the presence of PGG_2 and active enzyme, and blocked by phenol but not by indomethacin (3). The peak was centered at a g-value of about 2.0 and had a peak-to-peak line width of about 25 G with no discernible hyperfine structure. Because of the absence of distinguishing characteristics, this technique did not provide information regarding the nature of the oxidant or whether this EPR signal represents the initial oxidant or is a product of radical-chain-induced events. It is clear, however, that the deactivation of the cyclooxygenase and peroxidase are dependent on the peroxidatic release of an activated oxygen $[O_x]$ from PGG_2.

With evidence that $[O_x]$ is destructive to enzymes, it was of interest to determine what amino acids are particularly susceptible to oxidation. This property was determined by measuring the ability of the compounds to stimulate the conversion of PGG_2 to PGH_2 and to depress the EPR signal associated with the peroxidase (5). Interestingly, tryptophan is by far the most sensitive to the action of $[O_x]$, a finding consistent with its established role as an efficient cofactor of the peroxidase reaction. The relatively lower potency of histidine and cysteine attests to the unique properties of this oxidant. There have been several published reports on the fatty acid-dependent co-oxygenation of a wide variety of organic compounds by the PG-synthetase reaction (11,15,21). It seems most probable that such co-oxygenation is attributable to $[O_x]$ released in the peroxidatic conversion of PGG_2 to PGH_2. All of these data are consistent with the character of $[O_x]$ as a short-lived, extremely potent oxidizing agent.

NATURE OF $[O_x]$

Both methional and aminopyrine are free radical scavengers and have been suggested to have specificity for hydroxyl radical (OH·). $[O_x]$ does oxidize these substrates and releases ethylene from the former. However, there is little evidence to support this alleged specificity; in fact, the use of methional to identify OH· has been the subject of critical studies in a recent report (19). As an alternative to measuring oxidants by traditional scavengers, our objective was to try to incorporate the oxygen function into an organic compound which by its nature might give some hint of the identity of $[O_x]$ and also be amenable to quantitative measurements. Furthermore, a compound that might bind to the enzyme or associated cyclooxygenase by virtue of its locus might be expected to react with the initial oxidant in an efficient manner.

The sulfoxide sulindac (20) is a prodrug which when administered is converted metabolically to its sulfide, 5-fluoro-2-methyl-1-[p-(methylthio)benzylidene]indene-3-acetic acid, a potent cyclooxygenase inhibitor (2). When similarly administered, this sulfide metabolite, in turn, is significantly converted to the sulfoxide (2), suggesting that this *in vivo* oxidation could stem from an interaction with a peroxidase. On examination, sulindac sulfide was found to be a scavenger of $[O_x]$ and to be exclusively and efficiently reconverted to the parent sulfoxide, sulindac, by the peroxidase reaction (5). Using ^{3}H-sulindac sulfide, it was possible to quantitatively measure the reduction of the hydroperoxide and simultaneous oxidation of the sulfide (5). As shown in Table 1, the reduction of 15-HPE$_1$ and simultaneous oxidation of sulindac sulfide varies depending on enzyme and sulfide levels. However, in the last column, it is apparent that when 132 nmoles of 15-HPE$_1$ are reduced, 125 nmoles of sulindac sulfide are oxidized. Since evidence indicated that the hydroperoxide reduction occurs in the absence of oxygen (3), these data with sulindac sulfide implied that both oxygens of the hydroperoxide are accounted for in the reaction products, one in the remaining hydroxyl and the other in the sulfoxide.

The stoichiometry of this peroxidase reaction and the apparent lack of a requirement for external oxygen posed the possibility of scission between the two oxygen atoms of the hydroperoxy acid. This mechanism was conclusively

TABLE 1. *Quantitative comparison of 15-HPE$_1$ reduction and sulindac sulfide oxidation*[a]

15-HPE$_1$ (nmoles)	Sulindac sulfide (nmoles)	Enzyme	15-HPE$_1$ reduced (nmoles)	Sulindac sulfide oxidized (nmoles)
150	100	−	0	0
150	−	+	25	−
150	50	+	56	29
150	100	+	97	77
150	150	+	132	125

[a] Sheep seminal vesicle microsomes were used as an enzyme source, 0.56 mg protein each incubate. For details, see ref. 5.

confirmed by using hydroperoxy PGE$_2$, containing ^{18}O in the hydroperoxy group at C$_{15}$. Separation of the products of the reaction with PG-hydroperoxidase showed quantitative recovery of the ^{18}O in the oxygenation product of sulindac sulfide, sulindac, and full retention of ^{18}O in the PGE$_2$ formed. Thus in the initial phase of the peroxidatic reaction, a scission occurs between the two oxygens of the hydroperoxide. Homolytic cleavage is possible, which, of course, would result in the formation of hydroxyl radical. However, the oxidation of reduced sulindac involving a quantitative transfer of ^{18}O is more satisfactorily explained as an interaction with an oxygen–enzyme–iron complex such as perferryl iron $(FeO)^{3+}$. In similar ^{18}O experiments involving the reaction of 15-hydroperoxy arachidonic acid with PG-hydroperoxidase, Marnett et al. have recently shown that the cooxygenation of diphenylisobenzofuran, in contrast to our findings with sulindac sulfide, effects a transfer of atmospheric oxygen to the scavenger (12). The transfer of ^{18}O to sulindac sulfide, combined with the results of Marnett et al., suggests that the reaction of hydroperoxides with PG-hydroperoxidase involves the formation of an initial oxidant, which can be followed by a reaction with atmospheric oxygen to yield a second oxidizing species. The fact that the oxidation of diphenylisobenzofuran greatly exceeds the reduction of hydroperoxide compared to sulindac sulfide, which is the equivalent, is consistent with this interpretation.

With the finding that [O$_x$] can lead to other oxidizing species, it seems very likely that most co-oxygenations by the peroxidase are products of the secondary reactions. Despite uncertainty with respect to the ultimate oxidant for other reductants, we conclude that for sulindac sulfide, [O$_x$] is the oxidizing species. It is likely that the second oxidizing species is the hydroxyl radical, since the hydroxyl radical (but not O$_2^-$ or H$_2$O$_2$) is also capable of oxidizing sulindac sulfide. Accordingly, [O$_x$] must be a precursor, possibly perferryl ion as noted. Thus in considering the actions of [O$_x$], it is important to bear in mind that the ultimate oxidizing species may be the product of a secondary action, that with atmospheric oxygen.

PATHOLOGICAL ASPECTS OF [O_x]

In considering pathological aspects of [O_x], the relationship to inflammation stemmed from the anti-inflammatory action of MK-447 in animal models of inflammation as noted. These findings have now been extended to a variety of structures, including phenol, lipoic acid, iodide ion, etc., whose only common feature was the ability to scavenge [O_x] (4). When examined in the mouse ear challenged with the inflammatory agent phorbol myristate acetate, all of these showed significant antiedema properties when applied topically. As an alternative to this indirect approach relating [O_x] to inflammation, studies were undertaken to establish whether [O_x] generated *in situ* would trigger an inflammatory response in this same model. The classical studies of Ferreira and Vane (6) have shown that administered PGEs alone do not cause a significant edematous response. However, in combination with bradykinin or histamine (6), PGEs elicit a full edematous response. We now know that bradykinin has the capacity to effect the release of arachidonic acid from phospholipid pools and thus trigger the PG biosynthetic response. Since [O_x] is one of the products of this response, our goal was to examine whether [O_x] in combination with PGE_2 would trigger a full inflammatory reaction.

Linoleic acid was shown by Hamberg and Samuelsson (9) to react with PG synthetase to give hydroperoxy acids; however, it cannot be converted directly to PGs because of the absence of the 8–9 double bond necessary for endoperoxide formation. Thus it offers a potential for generating [O_x] but not other PG products *in situ*. As shown in Fig. 2, application of arachidonic acid (AA) caused a significantly greater edematous response than PGE_2 alone in the mouse ear inflammatory model (Fig. 3), a finding consistent with the modulator role applied to PGEs by Ferreira and Vane (i.e., both PGE_2 and [O_x] would be formed by AA). In contrast, linoleic acid alone is seen to have no significant effect on

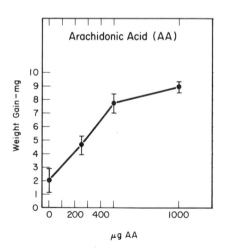

FIG. 2. Effect of topically administered arachidonic acid on ear weight in the mouse. This is a modification of the mouse ear model of inflammation described by Van Arman (22).

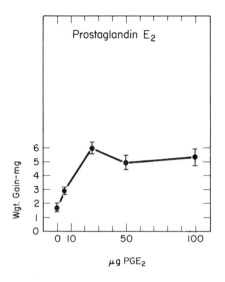

FIG. 3. Effect of topically administered PGE₂ on ear weight in the mouse.

ear weight (Fig. 4). However, in combination with a level of PGE₂ that minimally effects the ear edema, linoleic acid is seen to generate a large inflammatory response. As might be predicted, indomethacin, which prevents the conversion of linoleic acid to hydroperoxy acids and ultimately $[O_x]$, blunts this response, and MK-447, a scavenger for $[O_x]$, has a similar effect.

In considering targets of $[O_x]$ among enzymes of the PG biosynthetic pathway which may have pathological significance, a destructive action on either the cyclooxygenase or peroxidase would have a net effect equivalent to the action of indomethacin, i.e., suppress all subsequent products (Fig. 1). Thus it is not possible to assign a pathological role to these actions. On the other hand, recent reports that the balance between thromboxane A_2 (TXA₂) and PGI₂ may be

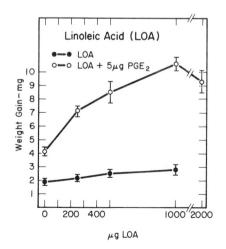

FIG. 4. Comparative effects of linoleic acid alone and linoleic acid combined with PGE₂ on weight in the mouse ear.

important in atherosclerosis and hypertension made it clear that selective sensitivity of PGI_2 synthetase, but not TXA_2 synthetase, to $[O_x]$ could be an important
pathological aspect of these diseases (14). Such a possibility presented itself
by the data showing that 15-HPETE is capable of producing $[O_x]$ on reaction
with peroxidase and by the suggestion by Moncada and Vane (13) that 15-
HPETE inhibits the synthesis of PGI_2 but not TXA_2 *in vitro*. Recently, we
have shown that on co-incubation, 15-HPETE does not suppress the synthesis
of PGI_2 and thus is not an inhibitor of the enzyme (8). However, in experiments
detailed elsewhere (8), we have demonstrated that 15-HPETE suppresses the
formation of PGI_2 as a consequence of the peroxidatic reduction of this hydroperoxy acid and release of $[O_x]$, which is highly destructive to the PGI_2 synthetase.
PGG_2 or PGG_1 and 12-HPETE had similar effects. In sharp contrast, TX
synthetase was completely resistant to deactivation by $[O_x]$. Thus it is evident
that the peroxidatic reduction of hydroperoxy acids to yield $[O_x]$ could have
the potential for altering the PGI_2/TXA_2 ratio in favor of the latter. The suggestion has been made that hydroperoxy acids may be responsible for triggering
diseases associated with high lipoperoxidation (hypertension, atherosclerosis,
etc.) (18). Apparently such effects have been considered to be direct, involving
the prosthetic hydroperoxy groups. The data presented here permit the alternate
suggestion that the oxidant released during the conversion of the hydroperoxy
to a hydroxyl group by the peroxidase associated with PG synthetase, and
perhaps other peroxidases, may be responsible for triggering the pathological
effects alluded to here. Since scavengers of $[O_x]$ prevent deactivation of PGI_2
synthetase, the potential for such compounds as therapeutic agents in diseases
related to lipoperoxidation is an attractive possibility.

OTHER SOURCES OF $[O_x]$

We have shown that H_2O_2 is a substrate for the peroxidase reaction indigenous
to PG synthetase, yielding the same oxidizing species as PGG_2 and 15-HPETE.
Ordinarily, H_2O_2 is disposed of metabolically by catalase, which converts it to
molecular oxygen and water. The obvious question was whether other peroxidases in which H_2O_2 is the preferred substrate resemble that associated with
PG system. To explore this possibility we turned to the polymorphonuclear
leukocytes (PMNs), which after inflammatory challenge, respond with a burst
of oxygen consumption leading to superoxide formation. Dismutation of superoxide (O_2^-) by superoxide dismutase (SOD) produces H_2O_2. The latter is believed
to react nonenzymatically in the presence of iron with another mole of O_2^-,
resulting in the formation of hydroxyl radical (the Haber-Weiss reaction), the
ultimate lethal oxidant produced by the PMN (7). Since $[O_x]$ is produced by
reaction of H_2O_2 with prostaglandin hydroperoxidase, it seemed possible that
the ultimate lethal product of the PMN might also be $[O_x]$ formed by reaction
of H_2O_2 with a membrane-bound peroxidase rather than by the Haber-Weiss
reaction. Accordingly, human PMNs were challenged with opsonized zymosan

in the presence of reduced sulindac, the scavenger for $[O_x]$. From the data in Table 2, it is evident that the stimulated cell caused a significant oxidation of this scavenger. Since the oxidation of reduced sulindac was not depressed by the presence of indomethacin, it was evident that oxidation is not dependent on the PG biosynthetic pathway. The action of catalase to prevent oxidation of reduced sulindac shows the requirement for H_2O_2. On the other hand, the lack of a similar action of SOD implies that O_2^- is not a direct factor in the oxidation of sulindac. Keeping in mind the fact that neither O_2^- nor H_2O_2 alone significantly oxidizes reduced sulindac, two conclusions can be drawn from these studies: The potent oxidizing agent produced by the PMN bears a strong resemblance to that produced by PG hydroperoxidase, and the H_2O_2-dependent oxidant is not formed by the Haber-Weiss reaction. Rather it would appear to be a product of the reaction of H_2O_2 with a peroxidase indigenous to the PMNs, possibly myeloperoxidase. It seems likely that the "hydroxyl radical" produced by phagocytosing PMNs may be identical to that produced by PG hydroperoxidase and thus sensitive to the same scavengers.

To summarize our data, we have shown that an oxidant released during the peroxidatic reduction of PGG_2 to PGH_2 is capable of oxidizing tissue enzymes, as well as organic compounds of a wide variety of structures. Studies using isotopic oxygen have shown this peroxidase reaction to involve a cleavage between the two oxygen atoms of the hydroperoxide. This fact is consistent with identity of the initial oxidant either as a hydroxyl radical in the free state or in a precursor form as a compound I-type oxygen–iron–enzyme complex. Scavengers of this oxidant have shown anti-inflammatory activity in animal models of inflammation. However, the precise targets of $[O_x]$ remain to be established.

Finally, evidence that hydrogen peroxide, rather than being metabolically reduced to a less potent oxidizing species, can be converted to $[O_x]$ by PG hydroperoxidase suggested that peroxidases specific for H_2O_2 may also yield $[O_x]$. Studies with human PMNs, a cell type essential for inflammatory symptoms, revealed the existence of such a peroxidase. It is attractive to suggest that this destructive oxidizing species $[O_x]$ derived from the reaction of H_2O_2

TABLE 2. *Oxidation of sulindac sulfide by activated PMNs[a]*

	Sulfoxide produced (nmoles)	
	Exp. I	Exp. II
PMNs (5×10^6 cells)	0.7 ± 0.1	0.7 ± 0.1
PMNs + zymosan (Z)	4.5 ± 0.0	8.4 ± 0.3
PMNs + (Z) + SOD (50 μg/ml)	4.6 ± 0.02	7.7 ± 0.7
PMNs + (Z) + catalase (3000 U/ml)	0.7 ± 0.4	0.8 ± 0.2
PMNs + (Z) + catalase + SOD	0.5 ± 0.3	0.7 ± 0.1

[a] Human granulocytes purified by the method of Böyum (1) were employed in these studies.

with the peroxidase(s) indigenous to the PMN plays a major role in inflammatory processes and is an important target of scavengers that display anti-inflammatory activity.

REFERENCES

1. Böyum, A. (1967): *Scand. J. Clin. Invest.,* 21:77–89.
2. Duggan, D. E., Hare, L. E., Ditzler, C. A., Lei, B. W., and Kwan, K. C. (1977): *Clin. Pharmacol. Ther.,* 21:326–335.
3. Egan, R. W., Paxton, J., and Kuehl, F. A. Jr. (1976): *J. Biol. Chem.,* 251:7329–7335.
4. Egan, R. W., Gale, P. H., Beveridge, G. C., Phillips, G. B., and Marnett, L. J. (1978): *Prostaglandins,* 16:861–869.
5. Egan, R. W., Gale, P. H., and Kuehl, F. A. Jr. (1979): *J. Biol. Chem.,* 254:3295–3302.
6. Ferreira, S. H., and Vane, J. R. (1974): *Annu. Rev. Pharmacol.,* 14:57–73.
7. Halliwell, B. (1978): *FEBS Lett.,* 92:321–326.
8. Ham, E. A., Egan, R. W., Soderman, D. D., Gale, P. H., and Kuehl, F. A., Jr. (1979): *J. Biol. Chem.,* 254:2191–2194.
9. Hamberg, M., and Samuelsson, B. (1967): *J. Biol. Chem.,* 242:5344–5354.
10. Kuehl, F. A. Jr., Humes, J. L., Egan, R. W., Ham, E. A., Beveridge, G. C., and Van Arman, C. G. (1977): *Nature,* 265:170–173.
11. Marnett, L. J., Wlodawer, P., and Samuelsson, B. (1975): *J. Biol. Chem.,* 250:8510–8517.
12. Marnett, L. J., Bienkowski, M. J., and Pagels, W. R. (1979): *J. Biol. Chem.,* 254:5077–5082.
13. Moncada, S., and Vane, J. R. (1977): In: *Biochemical Aspects of Prostaglandins and Thromboxanes,* edited by N. Kharasch and J. Fried, pp. 155–177. Academic Press, New York.
14. Moncada, S., Korbut, R., Bunting, S., and Vane, J. R. (1978): *Nature,* 273:767–768.
15. Nugteren, D. H., Beerthuis, R. K., and van Dorp, D. A. (1967): In: *Prostaglandins, Proceedings of the Second Nobel Symposium,* edited by S. Bergström and B. Samuelsson, pp. 45–50. Interscience, New York.
16. Ogino, N., Ohki, S., Yamamoto, S., and Hayaishi, O. (1978): *J. Biol. Chem.,* 253:5061–5068.
17. Ohki, S., Ogino, N., Yamamoto, S., and Hayaishi, O. (1979): *J. Biol. Chem.,* 254:829–836.
18. Pace-Asciak, C. R. (1977): *Prostaglandins,* 13:811–817.
19. Prior, W. A., and Tong, R. H. (1978): *Biochem. Biophys. Res. Commun.,* 81:498–503.
20. Shen, T. Y., Witzel, B. E., Jones, H., Linn, B. O., McPherson, J., Greenwald, R., Fordice, M., and Jacobs, A. (1972): *Fed. Proc.,* 31:577.
21. Takeguchi, C., and Sih, C. J. (1972): *Prostaglandins,* 2:169–184.
22. Van Arman, C. G. (1974): *Clin. Pharmacol. Ther.,* 16:900–904.

Advances in Prostaglandin and Thromboxane Research,
Vol. 6, edited by B. Samuelsson, P. W. Ramwell,
and R. Paoletti. Raven Press, New York © 1980.

Clinical Applications

Marc Bygdeman

Department of Obstetrics and Gynecology, Karolinska Hospital, Stockholm, Sweden

The prostaglandins (PGs) are biologically highly active compounds with widespread normal occurrence in the human body. Their biological function may be characterized as modulators involved in the regulation of, for instance, vascular tonus, blood pressure, platelet aggregation, lipolysis, gastric secretion, bronchial tonus, nerve transmission, ovulation, life-span of the corpus luteum, tubal contractility, and nonpregnant and pregnant uterine contractility.

It is not surprising, considering all these possible physiological functions of different PGs, that a variety of clinical applications have been suggested. So far, however, PGs are used routinely only on indications related to the stimulatory effect on human myometrium (11).

The approved indications for routine clinical use so far are termination of pregnancy, treatment of abnormal pregnancy, and induction of labor. Other indications on which PGs are used in clinical trials are, for instance, to facilitate arteriography, to improve circulation in patients with ischemic peripheral vascular diseases, to dilate ductus arteriosus in neonates with certain malformations where a widely patent ductus arteriosus is essential for survival, to prevent bleeding from the gastrointestinal tract induced by prostaglandin biosynthesis inhibitors like aspirin or indomethacin, for menstrual induction, to dilate the cervix prior to vacuum aspiration in late first trimester pregnancy, and to ripen the cervix at or near term.

To cover all possible and approved clinical applications of PGs is naturally not possible here. Many of the presentations in this volume are, however, clinically oriented and discuss many of these areas in detail. My intention is only to discuss briefly a few clearly foreseen possible future indications for clinical use of PGs. I will also try to summarize at least some of the experience gained during recent years from routine clinical use of PGs and the possible future development within these areas. I will, however, not discuss the clinical use of PG biosynthesis inhibitor and will consider only to a very limited extent prostacyclin and thromboxane, since many aspects of these compounds are brilliantly presented by Vane and Needleman in this volume. (13,18).

CARDIOVASCULAR SYSTEM

Circulation

Different PGs can, in different ways, influence the regulation of blood pressure and thrombus formation, two physiological functions of great importance for the pathogenesis of vascular diseases. Therapeutic roles for different PGs from prevention of vascular diseases to treatment of an acute vascular catastrophe may be possible in the future.

An example of a specific PG treatment for vascular diseases is the effect of administration of PGE_1 on patients suffering from advanced arteriosclerosis of the legs with chronic ischemic ulcers and resting pain. Intermittent intra-arterial infusion, intravenous infusion for 72 hr or repeated intravenous injections of PGE_1 resulted in nearly immediate complete or almost complete relief of resting pain in the leg. In many of the patients a healing of the ischemic ulcers was also observed (4).

PGE_1 has several biological effects which are theoretically beneficial. It is a potent vasodilator and an inhibitor of platelet aggregation. Administration of PGE_1 may result in better oxygen delivery and more efficient utilization of delivered oxygen and may also influence the oxidative metabolism in an oxygen-saving direction. There is also evidence that PGE_1 stimulates epidermal growth.

Another example of specific PG treatment on vascular tonus is the effect of PGE_1 on ductus arteriosus of the neonate. Current evidence suggests that ductus arteriosus remains widely patent during fetal life because of a continuous pro-duction of PGE_2. At birth when the arterial oxygen tension rises and ductal sensitivity to the PGs of the E type become markedly reduced, the ductus will close. In certain neonates, however, an open ductus is necessary for survival. To this group belongs, for instance, patients who have severe pulmonary stenosis or pulmonary atresia. PGE_1 could be given to these patients as an arterial infusion during 1 to 2 days to dilate the ductus in order to improve their preopera-tive condition. Inversely, the use of synthesis inhibitors are being studied to investigate if the closure of a patent ductus can be affected without surgery. The dilatation of the ductus will be reflected by a rise in arterial oxygen tension, improved tissue oxygenation, and, as a consequence, a reduced metabolic acido-sis. The results published so far suggest that PG treatment has a significant impact on the frequency of intraoperative deaths and possibly also on the overall mortality of these patients in the neonatal period (14).

Vascular Thrombosis

An exciting possible future application of PG therapy is to prevent or treat vascular thrombosis. The endoperoxides PGG_2 and PGH_2 and thromboxane A_2 strongly stimulate platelet aggregation, while prostacyclin has the opposite effect. It is likely that an important factor in platelet aggregation is the enzymatic formation of thromboxane A_2 in platelet microsomes, while microsomes in the vascular endothelium produce prostacyclin. A balance between thromboxane A_2 formed in the platelets and prostacyclin formed by vascular endothelium may therefore be critical for the formation of thrombosis and possibly be influenced therapeutically by PG administration (13,18).

Hypertension and Cardiac Function

One of the first biological effects of PGs described already by von Euler is the blood pressure lowering effect. An important factor in hypertension is the salt metabolism of the kidney. Different PGs are vasodilators, and some may also inhibit sodium reabsorption in the kidneys. Experimental data from animals also indicate that PGs are deeply involved in the regulation of cardiac function. Unraveling the physiological function of different PGs in more detail will certainly be of importance for future therapy in these clinical situations.

GASTROINTESTINAL TRACT

The PGs have well-known effects on the secretion and motility of the gastrointestinal tract (15). PGE_2 itself in the doses used does not inhibit gastric secretion in humans, whereas the 15-methyl or the 16,16-dimethyl analogs of PGE_2 are very strong inhibitors when given orally and also have a long duration of action. Experiments in animals have shown that PGs also stimulate mucus and nonparietal cell secretion and that experimental ulcerations induced by, for example, PG biosynthesis inhibitors may be prevented by oral PGE_2 therapy. Recently, a protective effect has also been demonstrated in man (5,10).

During conventional oral therapy with aspirin or indomethacine in male volunteers or in male patients with rheumatic diseases, the fecal blood loss increased from around 1 ml/day to 4 to 8 ml/day. Oral administration of PGE_2 in a dose as low as 0.33 mg three times daily or 40 μg 15-methyl PGE_2 three times daily was found to reduce the blood loss to control values. The protective effect of both PGE_2 and 15-methyl PGE_2 in these cases was not due to an inhibition of gastric acid secretion, as the doses were lower than the threshold for these effects.

Both the inhibition of gastric secretion and the protective effect on gastric mucosa are characteristics which certainly support the possibility that some PGs may be used in the future for treatment of gastric ulcer in man.

UTERINE CONTRACTILITY

The clinical use of PGs in the area of obstetrics and gynecology depends on the unique property of these compounds to stimulate uterine contractility during all stages of pregnancy. The classical PGs, E_2 and $F_{2\alpha}$, and different PG analogs are used for menstrual regulation, dilatation of the cervix prior to vacuum aspiration, second-trimester abortions, ripening of the cervix, labor induction, and treatment of abnormal pregnancy.

Termination of Second-Trimester Pregnancy

Intrauterine administration of $PGF_{2\alpha}$ and PGE_2 for termination of second-trimester pregnancy has been used on a routine basis for 6 years. However, randomized comparative studies are few. Those available compare intra-amniotic administration of hypertonic saline with $PGF_{2\alpha}$ given by the same route (9,19).

These studies show that intra-amniotic administration of $PGF_{2\alpha}$ is more effective, with a higher success rate and a shorter induction–abortion interval. It is also likely that PG therapy is associated with a lower risk for serious complications. The frequency of gastrointestinal side effects is higher following $PGF_{2\alpha}$ therapy; possible side effects also include cervical laceration or cervical vaginal fistula. The increased bleeding following abortion which has been reported by some investigators seems more likely to be due to inadequate PG treatment or inadequate management of the third stage than to be specifically related to the compounds (2,9).

More important, however, is the recent development of PG analogs suitable for pregnancy termination. Some of these analogs are more potent and have a longer duration than the classical PGs. In particular, the analogs belonging to the E series generally have a significantly lower frequency of gastrointestinal side effects. The most prospective advantage of PG analogs is, however, that they may be administered by noninvasive routes, e.g., intramuscularly, vaginally, or orally. Noninvasive administration not only has the advantage of simplicity, i.e., complications due to an inadvertent injection might be avoided, but also increases the possibility of using PGs during other periods of gestation.

Promising results on termination of pregnancy have been reported, for instance, following intramuscular injections of 15-methyl $PGF_{2\alpha}$ and 16-phenoxytetranor PGE_2-methylsulfonylamide and vaginal administration of 15-methyl $PGF_{2\alpha}$-methyl ester and 9-deoxo-16,16-dimethyl-9-methylene PGE_2 (3,8,11,12). The latter compound is also active following oral administration, and preliminary results show that effective uterine contractility could be induced, resulting in an abortion in nearly all patients (3). In contrast to all other PG analogs tested orally, 9-deoxo-16,16-dimethyl-9-methylene PGE_2 gives a predictable effect with an acceptable frequency of side effects (Fig. 1).

Dilatation of Cervix Prior to Vacuum Aspiration

It is generally agreed that the frequency of complications with vacuum aspiration increases with increasing gestational age. Some of these complications, e.g., cervical laceration and uterine perforation, are directly related to the mechanical dilatation necessary for the procedure, especially during the last week of the first trimester. Other complications may partly be due to an insufficient or difficult dilatation, e.g., hemorrhage and incomplete evacuation of the conceptus. The increasing concern of a potential cervical injury or long-term effect on reproduc-

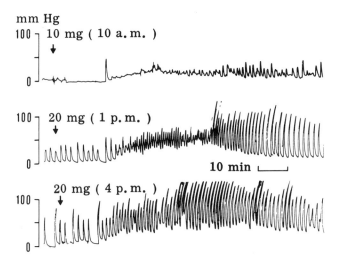

FIG. 1. Uterine contractility following repeated oral administration of 9-deoxo-16,16-dimethyl-9-methylene PGE_2. The initial dose was 10 mg, followed by 20 mg every third hour.

tive behavior has also focused clinicians' interest on more physiological methods of producing cervical dilatation. Several studies have shown that pretreatment mainly with PG analogs by noninvasive routes is therapeutically effective in achieving such a result. Not only is the cervix gradually dilated, but the frequency of immediate complications is also significantly reduced. Also of great importance are the results indicating that the frequency of late sequelae may be related to forceful mechanical dilatation of the cervix.

Menstrual Regulation

While PG therapy has a recognized position in termination of second-trimester pregnancies, the use of PG for menstrual regulation is still in an explorative phase. The ultimate goal is to develop a self-administered, nonsurgical procedure which could compete with vacuum aspiration. The initial trails using classical PGs were mainly discouraging. The only effective route was intrauterine administration, and premedication was necessary to reduce the frequency of side effects. The situation has changed, at least partly, with the availability of PG analogs. Intrauterine administration of different analogs has been shown to be highly effective in terminating early pregnancy.

Encouraging progress has also been reported following vaginal administration of PG analogs (8). Repeated or single vaginal administration of 15-methyl-$PGF_{2\alpha}$-methyl ester has been shown to be highly effective, but even more promising seems use of some new PGE analogs with increased stability in suppository form. To this group belong 16,16-dimethyl-*trans*-Δ^2PGE_1-methyl ester and 9-

deoxo-16,16-dimethyl-9-methylene PGE_2. At present it may be concluded that PG therapy is as effective as vacuum aspiration in terminating very early pregnancy. Both methods are used on an outpatient basis. Vacuum aspiration still has advantages in terms of hospital time, duration of bleeding, and frequency of gastrointestinal side effects. It is likely, however, that in the future the simplicity of vaginal and oral treatment and its potential for self-administration will make PGs competitive alternatives to vacuum aspiration.

Induction of Labor

Intravenous administration of $PGF_{2\alpha}$ and PGE_2 has a recognized therapeutic role for induction of labor. The superiority (at most very slight) of either of these compounds over the other or over intravenous infusion of oxytocin remains a matter of controversy. The advantages and disadvantages of the three compounds were recently summarized by Thiery (16) in the following way. All three compounds are equally effective in patients with favorable prognoses for induction. PG is probably slightly superior for difficult inductions and in pregnancy complicated by fetal death or anencephaly. The margin of effective dose is somewhat narrower for prostaglandin, and occasional gastrointestinal upsets and venous erythema are associated with PG therapy.

PGE_2 may also be given as oral tablets, a therapy which seems most useful in patients with good inducibility, particularly if combined with early amniotomy (16). The design of dose schedules in the past was dependent on clinical results. It has recently been shown by gas chromatography—mass spectrometry that the E metabolite reaches a peak in plasma concentration 1 hr after administration, indicating that hourly administration is preferable (Fig. 2) (1).

Ripening of the Cervix

The possibility of ripening the cervix at or near term is an important new therapeutic possibility for prostaglandins. An unripe cervix in late pregnancy is a bad prognostic sign, especially in the primigravida. If labor has to be induced, it may be protracted and difficult. Although the cervix ripens if given time, few, if any, obstetrical indications for delivery diminish with the passage of time. The normal mechanism by which the cervix ripens before effacement and dilatation during labor is still unknown. Experimental data suggest that PGs, possibly together with placental hormones, have a physiological role (7).

Prostaglandins, mainly PGE_2, have been administered orally, vaginally, into the cervical canal, or into the extra-amniotic space in clinical trials. Data indicate that extra-amniotic administration of 0.5 mg PGE_2 in gel form is advantageous with regard to efficacy in comparison with other routes of administration. If cervical ripening is obtained, reduced fetal and maternal complication rates will result (6,17). The disadvantages of the therapy at present is the risk involved with the introduction of an extra-amniotic catheter and lack of stable PG preparations.

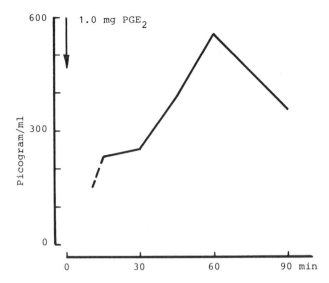

FIG. 2. Mean plasma levels of 15-keto-13,14-dihydro PGE_2 following oral administration of 1.0 mg PGE_2 in tablet form ($n = 4$).

Abnormal Pregnancy

The termination of abnormal pregnancy, hydatidiform mole, and missed abortion have long been gynecological problems. Surgical emptying of the uterus is sometimes associated with serious complications. Oxytocin administration is often insufficient to induce an effective uterine contractility. Intra-amniotic PG administration is not suitable; while intravenous infusion or extra-amniotic administration of classical PG may be used, it is by no means an optimal therapy. Noninvasive administration is preferable, and PGE_2 vaginal suppositories are available for this purpose in a few countries. Clinical trials have shown that intramuscular injections of 16-phenoxy-tetranor-PGE_2-methylsulfonylamide, vaginal administration of 15-methyl-$PGF_{2\alpha}$-methyl ester, or single extra-amniotic injection of dihomo-15-methyl-$PGF_{2\alpha}$-methyl ester are even better alternatives (11).

CONCLUSIONS

Prostaglandins E_2 and $F_{2\alpha}$ have well-established clinical indications when stimulation of uterine contractility is wanted. Clinical trials indicate that the development of stable PG analogs useful for noninvasive administration will not only result in a complete change in abortion technology, but also reduce many of the risks presently associated with induction of labor. In other therapeutic areas, PGs are, as yet, only used clinically to a limited extent. It seems certain, however, that in the near future PGs or their analogs will find an important clinical role, mainly in the cardiovascular and gastroenterological fields.

REFERENCES

1. Bremme, K., Kindahl, H., and Svanborg, K. (1979): to be published.
2. Bygdeman, M. (1978): *Obstet. Gynecol.,* 52:424–429.
3. Bygdeman, M., Gréen, K., Bergström, S., Bundy, G., and Kimball, F. (1979): *Lancet,* 1:1136.
4. Carlsson, L. A., and Olsson, A. G. (1979): In: *Advances in Prostaglandin Research. Practical Application of Prostaglandins and Their Synthetase Inhibitors,* edited by S. M. M. Karim. MTP Press, Lancaster, England.
5. Cohen, M. M. (1978): *Lancet,* 2:1253–1254.
6. Editorial (1979): *Lancet,* 1:17.
7. Ellwood, D. A., Mitchell, M. D., Anderson, A., and Turnball, A. C. (1979): *Lancet,* 1:376–377.
8. Gréen, K., Bygdeman, M., and Bremme, K. (1979): *Contraception,* 18:551–560.
9. Grimes, D. A., Schulz, K. F., Cates, W., and Tyler, C. W. (1977): *Obstet. Gynecol.,* 49:612–616.
10. Johansson, C., Kollberg, B., Nordemar, R., and Bergström, S. (1979): *Lancet,* 1:317.
11. Karim, S. M. M., Choo, H. T., Lim, A. L., Yeo, K. C., and Ratnam, S. S. (1978): *Prostaglandins,* 15:1063.
12. Karim, S. M. M., and Ratnam, S. S. (1977): In *Biochemical Aspects of Prostaglandins and Thromboxanes,* edited by N. Kharasch and J. Fried, p. 115. Academic Press, New York.
13. Needleman, P. (1980): *this volume.*
14. Olley, P. M., Coceani, F., and Rowe, R. D. (1978): In: *Advances in Prostaglandin and Thromboxane Research, Vol. 4,* edited by F. Coceani and P. M. Olley, pp. 345–353. Raven Press, New York.
15. Robert, A. (1980): *this volume.*
16. Thiery, M., and Amy, J. J. (1977): *Obstet. Gynecol. Annu.,* 6:127–171.
17. Ulmsten, U., and Wingerup, L. (1979): *Acta Obstet. Gynecol. Scand., [Suppl.],* 84.
18. Vane, J., (1980): *this volume.*
19. WHO Prostaglandin Task Force (1976): *Br. Med. J.,* 1:1373–1376.

Advances in Prostaglandin and Thromboxane Research,
Vol. 6, edited by B. Samuelsson, P. W. Ramwell,
and R. Paoletti. Raven Press, New York © 1980.

Isolation of Glucose-Sensitive Platelet Lipoxygenase Products from Arachidonic Acid

Robert W. Bryant and J. Martyn Bailey

George Washington University School of Medicine, Washington, D.C. 20037

Platelets have been shown to have two routes for oxidative metabolism of arachidonic acid (AA)—the cyclooxygenase pathway and the lipoxygenase pathway (7). This chapter deals with the identification of novel products of the latter pathway and their formation from 12-hydroperoxy-5,8,10,14-eicosatetraenoic acid (12-HPETE), the initial platelet lipoxygenase product.

Washed human platelets were incubated with $(1\text{-}^{14}C)$-AA and the products were separated by thin-layer chromatography (TLC) and detected by autoradiography as previously described (3). Incubations with high concentrations of AA (80 μg/ml) showed a more complex pattern of metabolites (Fig. 1B) than incubations at lower concentrations of AA (20 μg/ml), where only HETE, 12-hydroxyheptadecatrienoic acid (HHT), thromboxane (TX) B_2 were detected (Fig. 1A). These additional metabolites (i.e., THETE, III, IV, and V) were members of the lipoxygenase pathway, since they were not blocked by aspirin (Fig. 1C) but were inhibited by 5,8,11,14-eicosatetraynoic acid (Fig. 1D).

These novel lipoxygenase metabolites were isolated by preparative TLC in solvent system I (described in Fig. 1) and were analyzed by gas chromatography–mass spectroscopy (GC-MS) after conversion to methyl ester trimethylsilyl ether derivatives. The two bands running just above TXB$_2$ were each identified as a mixture of the positional isomers 8,9,12- and 8,11,12-trihydroxy-eicosatrienoic acids (1,2,8), collectively termed THETE. The two bands appeared to represent diastereomeric pairs of each positional isomer. Hydrogenation (platinum oxide catalyst) of THETE produced a mixture of 8,9,12- and 8,11,12-trihydroxy-eicosanoic acids. Their mass spectral cleavage patterns were analagous to those for a model trihydroxy fatty acid, 8,9,13-trihydroxy-docosonoic acid.

Metabolite V, which co-chromatographed with HHT, was tentatively identified as 10-hydroxy-11,12-epoxy-5,8,14-eicosatrienoic acid. The methyl ester (ME) trimethylsilyl ether (TMS) of this metabolite (C22.1 on 3% SP 2100) gave prominent mass spectral ions (m/e) of 407(M-15); 391(M-31); 332(M-90); 311, loss of CH_3—$(CH_2)_4$—$CH{=}CH$—CH_2; 282, loss of CH_3—$(CH_2)_4$—$CH{=}CH$—CH_2—CHO; and 269, loss of $CH_3(CH_2)_4$—$CH{=}CH$—CH_2—$\underset{\diagdown O \diagup}{CH{-}CH}$.

These fragmentations were supported by spectra obtained with D$_3$-ME, and

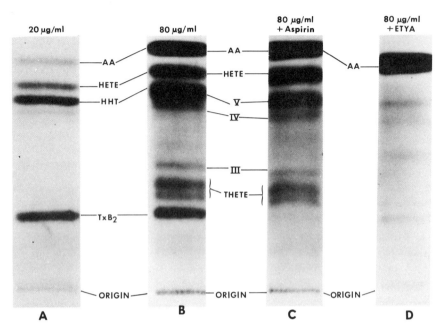

FIG. 1. Stimulation of novel lipoxygenase metabolites by elevated arachidonate concentration. Washed platelets were incubated with ¹⁴C-AA (1.5 μCi/μmole) at 20 μg/ml **(A)** or 80 μg/ml **(B–D)** with addition of aspirin **(C)** or 5,8,11,14-eicosatetraenoic acid **(D)**. Metabolites were separated on silicic acid in the solvent system I, with the composition isooctane:ethyl acetate: acetic acid:water, 5:11:2:10 *(upper phase)*. Radioactive bands were detected by autoradiography.

D_9-TMS derivatives. The structure of this 10-hydroxy-11,12-epoxy-arachidonate (10,11,12-HEPA) was also supported by comparison of its mass spectrum with that of an authentic sample of 11-hydroxy-12,13-epoxy-9-octadecenoic acid, an intramolecular rearrangement product of 13-hydroperoxy-9, 11-octadecadienoic acid (6). The structure of THETE and HEPA and their lipoxygenase origin suggest that they are intramolecular rearrangement products of 12-hydroperoxy-5,8,10,14-eicosatetraenoic acid (12-HPETE).

Platelet conversion of arachidonate to THETE and 10,11,12-HEPA was influenced by a number of factors in addition to arachidonate concentration. For instance, their synthesis was blocked by the presence of glucose (1 mM), as shown in Fig. 2. Similar concentration of galactose or lactate did not show this striking effect. Reduced glutathione (3 mM) also inhibited THETE and 10,11,12-HEPA formation.

These results suggest that these novel lipoxygenase products form in glucose-free incubations at high AA concentrations because the platelet glutathione peroxidase system is incapable of completely reducing 12-HPETE to 12-HETE and thus allowing some 12-HPETE to form THETE and 10,11,12-HEPA. One

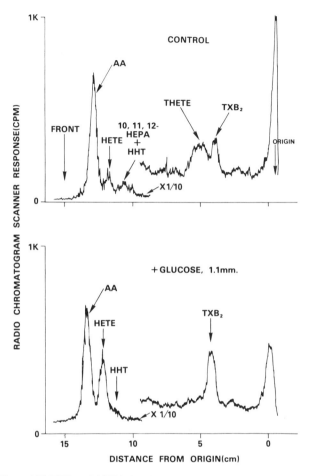

FIG. 2. Inhibition of THETE and HEPA by glucose. Washed platelets were incubated with ^{14}C-arachidonic acid (80 μg/ml) in the absence **(top)** or presence **(bottom)** of 1.1 mM glucose. The chromatogram was developed in system I, and the radioactive bands were detected with a radiochromatogram scanner.

possible mechanism for this conversion is shown in Fig. 3. It involves a free radical epoxide intermediate, similar to those proposed by Gardner (5), which could give rise to both a 10-hydroxy-11,12-epoxide (10,11,12-HEPA) and an 8-hydroxy-11,12-epoxide (8,11,12-HEPA). An analogous version of the latter hydroxy-epoxide was suggested by Falardeau et al. (4) as the precursor of the 8,9,12- and 8,11,12-trihydroxy-eicosadienoic acids formed in platelet incubations with 8,11,14-eicosatrienoic acid. The role of glucose in maintaining platelet-reduced glutathione levels for 12-HPETE reduction and the involvement of a platelet glutathione peroxidase enzyme in determining the distribution of the platelet lipoxygenase products, as suggested in Fig. 3, is under investigation.

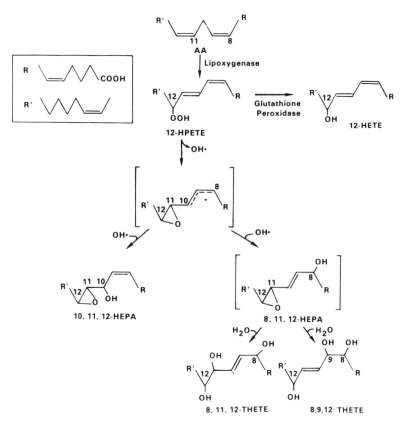

FIG. 3. Possible mechanism for the rearrangement of 12-HPETE to 10,11,12-HEPA and 8,9,12- and 8,11,12-THETE. This scheme also suggests the importance of the glutathione peroxidase system in determining the product distribution of the platelet lipoxygenase pathway.

ACKNOWLEDGMENTS

8,9,13-Trihydroxy-docosanoic acid and 11-hydroxy-12,13-epoxy-9-octadecenoic acid were kindly provided by Robley J. Light, Florida State University, Tallahassee, Florida, and Harold W. Gardner, U. S. Department of Agriculture, Peoria, Illinois, respectively. This work was supported in part by N.I.H. Grants 5S07RR539–17, HL 05062, and CA 15356 and N.S.F. Grant PCM 07147.

REFERENCES

1. Bryant, R. W., and Bailey, J. M. (1978): *Fed. Proc.,* 37:1317.
2. Bryant, R. W., and Bailey, J. M. (1979): *Prostaglandins,* 17:9–18.
3. Bryant, R. W., Feinmark, S. J., Makheja, A. N., and Bailey, J. M. (1978): *J. Biol. Chem.,* 253:8134–8142.
4. Falardeau, P., Hamberg, M., and Samuelsson, B. (1976): *Biochem. Biophys. Acta,* 441:193–200.

5. Gardner, H. W. (1975): *J. Agric. Food Chem.,* 23:129–134.
6. Hamberg, M., and Gotthammar, B. (1973): *Lipids,* 8:737–744.
7. Hamberg, M., and Samuelsson, B. (1974): *Proc. Natl. Acad. Sci. USA,* 71:3400–3404.
8. Jones, R. L., Kerry, P. J. Poyser, N. L., Walker, I. C., and Wilson, N. H. (1978): *Prostaglandins* 16:583–589.

Advances in Prostaglandin and Thromboxane Research,
Vol. 6, edited by B. Samuelsson, P. W. Ramwell,
and R. Paoletti. Raven Press, New York © 1980.

Role of the Arachidonate Lipoxygenase Pathway in Blood Platelet Aggregation

C. E. Dutilh, E. Haddeman, and F. ten Hoor

Unilever Research Vlaardingen, 3130 AC Vlaardingen, The Netherlands

The relationship between the formation of thromboxane A_2 (TXA$_2$) and blood platelet aggregation has been studied extensively, and it is well established that TXA$_2$, formed from prostaglandin endoperoxides, is directly involved in the aggregation process (6,7). However, very little is known about the role of the lipoxygenase pathway (9) and its products 12-hydroperoxyeicosatetraenoic acid (HPETE) and 12-hydroxyeicosatetraenoic acid (HETE). We investigated the relative contributions to the aggregation process of both pathways, using a low concentration of eicosatetraynoic acid (ETYA) to preferentially inhibit lipoxygenase (8), aspirin to inhibit endoperoxide synthase (6), and a high concentration of ETYA to inhibit both. From the results obtained we evaluated the possible contribution of the lipoxygenase pathway to blood platelet aggregation.

METHODS

The various *fatty acids* used, including ETYA, were from our own laboratory stocks; (1-^{14}C)-arachidonic acid (AA) was from Amersham, adenosine diphosphate (ADP) from Boehringer. Fatty acids were dissolved in phosphate-buffered salt solution or platelet poor plasma (PPP).

Human citrated blood from volunteers (aspirin free for at least 2 weeks) was used to prepare platelet-rich plasma (PRP; centrifugation at 120 × g for 10 min), PPP (centrifugation at 1500 × g for 10 min) or platelet suspensions. The latter were prepared by adding 0.1 vol ethylenediaminetetraacetic acid (EDTA) solution (EDTA, 77 mM; NaCl, 0.12 mM) to PRP in siliconized glass tubes and centrifugation at 600 × g for 10 min, after which the supernatant was removed and the platelet pellet resuspended in a phosphate-buffered salt solution (pH 7.4) with 12 mM glucose. For some experiments, PRP was prepared from blood of volunteers 1 hr after ingestion of 500 mg acetylsalicylic acid (ASA). This ASA-PRP neither aggregated nor formed TX degradation products after incubation with arachidonic acid, but did produce HETE.

Platelet aggregation was studied using a Born aggregometer. To 0.8 ml platelet suspension (about 0.3 × 10^9 platelets) with 20 μl CaCl$_2$ (0.1 M), 100 μl of the test substance was added after a 3-min stabilization period. At the same time or after 30 sec, platelet aggregation was induced with 100 μl of a solution containing either ADP (final concentration 1 μM) or ^{14}C-AA (final concentration 2 to 10 μM, depending on individual platelet sensitivity). When product analysis of the contents of the cuvette had to be performed, 0.2 ml citric acid (2.3 M) was added 4 min after the induction of aggregation.

Product analysis was carried out as follows. Radioactive products were extracted from the incubates with diethyl ether, dried, and separated by silica thin-layer chromatography using chloroform : methanol : acetic acid : water (90 : 6 : 1 : 0.75) as the solvent. Identification of HETE and of 12-hydroxyheptade-catrienoic acid (HHT) and TXB$_2$, the end-products of the endoperoxide synthase pathway, was done by co-chromatography of inactive standards of HETE, HHT, and TXB$_2$ (Rf: AA, 0.68; HETE, 0.51; HHT, 0.43; TXB$_2$, 0.12). The radioactive zones were scraped off and quantitated by liquid scintillation counting. To detect any lysis of blood platelets, lactate dehydrogenase was measured with a Boehringer test kit.

The following *experiments* were performed:

(a) The effect of 0.7 and 7.0 μM ETYA on ^{14}C-AA–induced aggregation of blood platelet suspensions was investigated and the formation of HETE, HHT, and TXB$_2$ determined as described,

(b) The effect of various concentrations of AA on ADP-induced aggregation of ASA-PRP was studied; and

(c) The effect of a variety of fatty acids (oleic acid, linoleic acid, dihomo-γ-linolenic acid, Mead acid, ETYA, (5Z,8Z,11Z,14E)-5,8,11,14-eicosatetraenoic acid) on ADP-induced aggregation of ASA-PRP was studied.

RESULTS

At the fatty acid concentrations used, no platelet lysis occurred (lactate dehydrogenase < 150 U/liter). The effect of ETYA on AA-induced aggregation of blood platelet suspensions is shown in Fig. 1. A 0.7 μM concentration of ETYA converts an irreversible AA-induced aggregation into a reversible one, a 7 μM concentration of ETYA completely prevents AA-induced aggregation. Table 1 shows the HETE and HHT + TXB$_2$ production in this experiment. The 0.7 μM ETYA concentration only inhibits HETE formation, while the 7 μM concentration inhibits the formation of both HETE and HHT + TXB$_2$. Figure 2A and B shows the effect of various concentrations of AA on the ADP-induced aggregation of ASA-PRP. The reversible type of ADP-induced aggregation which is obtained in this PRP is converted into an irreversible one by AA, depending on the AA concentration used. Figure 2B shows that dihomo-γ-linolenic acid may have the same, but much less pronounced, effect (curve e). Figure 2C clearly shows that all other fatty acids used have no influence on ADP-induced aggregation of ASA-PRP.

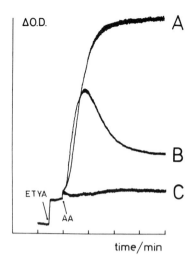

FIG. 1. Influence of ETYA on AA-induced platelet aggregation. Different amounts of ETYA were added to human platelet suspensions and 1 μg ¹⁴C-AA was added to initiate aggregation after 30 sec. ETYA concentrations (μM): A,0; B,0.7; C,7. The optical density (O.D.) is given in arbitrary units. For product analysis, see Table 1.

DISCUSSION

Blood platelet aggregation can be reversible or irreversible. In man reversible aggregation can be induced by moderate amounts of ADP and by prostaglandin endoperoxides or TXA_2 (1,2). In this type of aggregation platelets are entangled with each other through the formation of pseudopodia but do not stick together (11). It is not known which processes are involved in the irreversible type of aggregation.

The results of our experiments show that while a 0.7 μM ETYA solution only inhibits HETE formation (Table 1) and leaves HHT + TXB_2 formation intact, it nevertheless converts an irreversible type of aggregation into a reversible one (Fig. 1). Recently, we have demonstrated that this reduced HETE production is correlated with a decreased serotonin release (4). On the other hand, in blood platelets in which endoperoxide synthase is completely blocked by ASA (as

TABLE 1. *Conversion of ¹⁴C-AA used to induce platelet aggregation at different ETYA concentrations*[a]

Recording	ETYA (μM)	Radioactivity (%)		
		HHT + TXB_2	HETE	AA
A	0	22	30	48
B	0.7	40	6	54
C	7	5	1	94

[a] Amount of ¹⁴C-AA, 1 μg. A–C recordings refer to Fig. 1. For experimental details, see text and legend to Fig. 1.

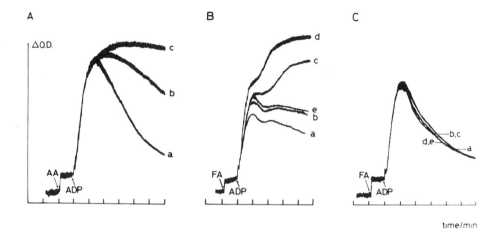

time/min

FIG. 2. Influence of various fatty acids on ADP-induced platelet aggregation. Human PRP was prepared 1 hr after the ingestion of 500 mg ASA. **A** and **C** represent the results obtained with blood from one volunteer, and **B** shows those obtained with blood from another volunteer. Fatty acids (FA) were added dissolved in PPP and ADP (0.5 μg; final concentration 1 μM) was added after 30 sec to initiate the aggregation. **A:** AA at concentration (mM): a, 0; b, 0.16; c, 0.32. **B:** AA at concentrations (mM): a, 0; b, 0.81; c, 1.6; d, 2.4; and e, dihomo-γ-linolenic acid at of 1.6 mM. **C:** Various fatty acids at a concentration of 0.33 mM: a, linoleic acid; b, Mead acid; c, (5Z, 8Z, 11Z, 14E)-5-,8,11,14-eicosatetraenoic acid; d, oleic acid; e, ETYA. The optical density (O.D.) is given in arbitrary units.

shown by the observation that no aggregation occurs or TX derivatives are formed on incubation with AA), an ADP-induced reversible type of aggregation is converted into an irreversible one after addition of AA (Figs. 2A and B).

These data are suggestive of a role of HETE *formation* in irreversible platelet aggregation. This suggestion is supported by the observation that a variety of other fatty acids do not influence the ADP-induced reversible aggregation of ASA-PRP (Fig. 2C). However, HETE *as such* is not responsible for the irreversibility of the aggregation, as it was observed that HETE (as with other fatty acids) inhibits AA-induced platelet aggregation (not shown) (3). We therefore suggest that HETE *formation* during the initially reversible aggregation process can, under certain circumstances, lead to the formation of a HETE gradient around the aggregating platelets, which via a process of chemotaxis similar to that seen in leukocytes (5,10) makes the platelets stick together and thus leads to irreversibility of the process.

The observations that dihomo-γ-linolenic acid has an effect similar to AA, be it less pronounced, and that Mead acid, being a very good substrate for lipoxygenase (4,9), has not, suggest that the proposed mechanism is very specific and only holds for those fatty acids which are a substrate for both lipoxygenase and endoperoxide synthase.

ACKNOWLEDGMENTS

We thank J. A. Don for excellent technical assistance and Mrs. E. L. Zaal, C. Gardien, and P. R. van der Heiden for preparing the manuscript.

REFERENCES

1. Charo, I. F., Feinman, R. D., and Detwiler, T. C. (1977): *J. Clin. Invest.,* 60:866–873.
2. Charo, I. F., Feinman, R. D., Detwiler, T. C., Smith, J. B., Ingerman, C. M., and Smith, M. J. (1977): *Nature,* 269:66–69.
3. Dutilh, C. E., Haddeman, E., Don, J. A., and ten Hoor, F. (1980): *Prostaglandins.*
4. Dutilh, C. E., Haddeman, E., Jouvenaz, G. H., ten Hoor, F., and Nugteren, D. H. (1979): *Lipids,* 14:241–246.
5. Goetzl, E. J., Woods, J. M., and Gorman R. R. (1977): *J. Clin. Invest.,* 59:179–183.
6. Hamberg, M., and Samuelsson, B. (1974): *Proc. Natl. Acad. Sci. USA,* 71:3400–3404.
7. Hamberg, M., Svensson, J., and Samuelsson, B. (1975): *Proc. Natl. Acad. Sci. USA,* 72:2994–2998.
8. Hammarström, S. (1977): *Biochim. Biophys. Acta,* 487:517–519.
9. Nugteren, D. H. (1975): *Biochim. Biophys. Acta,* 380:299–307.
10. Turner, S. R., Tainer, J. A., and Lynn, W. S. (1975): *Nature,* 257:680–681.
11. White, J. G. (1970): *Scand. J. Haematol.,* 7:145–151.

Advances in Prostaglandin and Thromboxane Research,
Vol. 6, edited by B. Samuelsson, P. W. Ramwell,
and R. Paoletti. Raven Press, New York © 1980.

An Epoxy–Hydroxy Product from Arachidonate

Irene C. Walker, R. L. Jones, P. J. Kerry, and N. H. Wilson

Department of Pharmacology, University of Edinburgh, Edinburgh EH8 9JZ, Scotland

Rapid metabolism of arachidonic acid occurs in human platelets by two main pathways. Fatty acid cyclooxygenase generates PGG_2 and PGH_2, which are then enzymatically isomerized to thromboxane A_2, a very potent stimulant of platelet aggregation (3). Lipoxygenase action also produces 12-hydroperoxyeicosa-5,8,10,14-tetraenoic acid (HPETE), which is subsequently transformed to 12-hydroxyeicosa-5,8,10,14-tetraenoic acid (HETE) (2). Our recent studies with washed platelets have resulted in the identification of two trihydroxy acids: 8,11,12-trihydroxyeicosa-5,9,14-trienoic acid and 8,9,12-trihydroxyeicosa-5, 10,14-trienoic acid (THETA)(5). A possible mechanism suggested for the formation of these trihydroxy acids was the conversion of HPETE to 8-hydroxy-11,12-epoxyeicosa-5,9,14-trienoic acid and subsequent hydration of this epoxide. During attempts to detect this epoxy–hydroxy intermediate an analogous compound was detected (6). Gas chromatographic–mass spectrometric (GC-MS) analysis of various derivatives indicated the structure of this novel metabolite as 10-hydroxy-11,12-epoxyeicosa-5,8,14-trienoic acid (EPHETA). The structural assignment and the biological testing of this compound are discussed.

METHODS AND RESULTS

Platelet-rich plasma and washed platelets from citrated human, horse, cat, dog, and rabbit blood were prepared according to Hamberg et al. (4). Washed platelets (at a concentration of 5×10^8 to 5×10^9 ml^{-1}) were incubated with arachidonic acid (1.65×10^{-4} M) (with 1-^{14}C-arachidonic acid as tracer) at 37°C for 30 min. After acidification, the products were extracted with diethyl ether and the ether evaporated. The nonpolar lipids were removed by partition of the material between 67% ethanol and petroleum ether, and after evaporation of the alcoholic phase, the extract was subjected to liquid gel partition chromatography (6). Scintillation counting of the column eluate revealed a more polar shoulder on the HETE peak, which was investigated.

The methyl ester–trimethylsilyl ether (Me/TMS) derivative showed a single GC peak (carbon value 22.05 on a 3% OVI column). The mass spectrum indicated a compound with a molecular weight of 422 as ions were observed at m$^+$/e 422, 407 (—CH$_3$), and 391 (—OCH$_3$). This was consistent with a C_{20}

fatty acid methyl ester having three double bonds, one TMS group, and one keto or epoxy oxygen. Additional significant ions were observed at m^+/e 332 (—TMSOH), 311, 282/281, and 269 (base peak) (Fig. 1). The material did not form an oxime, indicating the absence of a keto group. The ethyl ester–TMS spectrum was consistent with the assignments in Fig. 1.

Following hydrogenation (platinum oxide/methanol) and Me/TMS derivatization, the material showed two marginally separated GC peaks (carbon values 22.80, 22.85). Mass spectra taken at these carbon values were very similar and indicated the presence of three double bonds in the original material. Most noteworthy were large ions at m^+/e 273 and 257, which indicated the TMS group was in the 10 position, as these ions correspond to cleavage on either side of a TMS group in this position. The two marginally resolved GC peaks were present in the single ion chromatograms of the major ions, indicating stereoisomers of the molecule were probably present.

Evidence for the epoxide was provided by treatment of the methyl ester of the material with lithium aluminium hydride (LiAlH$_4$) (this reagent reduces an epoxide to a mono-alcohol, usually forming two positional isomers; an ester is also converted to an alcohol). GC-MS of both the TMS derivative and the *n*-butyl boronate/TMS derivative of the product of the LiAlH$_4$ reaction gave spectra consistent with the expected products. The formation of the boronate derivative provided strong evidence that the hydroxyl group was adjacent to the epoxide in the original molecule, since only 1,2- and 1,3-diols readily form boronates.

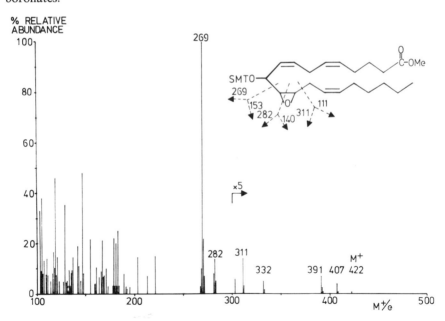

FIG. 1. Mass spectrum of EPHETA (in Me-TMS).

High pressure liquid chromatography (HPLC) of the material gave two partially resolved peaks, which were shown to have identical carbon values on GC as their Me/TMS derivatives and very similar mass spectra. This provided further evidence for the existence of stereoisomers of this molecule (most probably hydroxyl isomers).

The formation of EPHETA was not inhibited by indomethacin (10^{-5} M), but was blocked by eicosa-5,8,11,14-tetraynoic acid (10^{-5} M). A possible mechanism suggested is the transformation of HPETE; analogous conversions of C_{18} fatty acid hydroperoxides have been reported (1).

The EPHETA zone from the liquid–gel chromatography showed no activity on platelets, either pro- or antiaggregatory (10 μg/ml), or on guinea pig ileum (1 μg). However, pronounced chemotactic activity for rabbit peritoneal leukocytes was observed at concentrations of 1 and 5 μg/ml using a modified Boyden chamber. Preliminary data on the HPLC-purified material (two experiments) indicate that the majority of the chemotactic activity is associated with the more polar EPHETA isomer.

ACKNOWLEDGMENT

These studies were supported from an M. R. C. program grant to Professor E. W. Horton.

REFERENCES

1. Hamberg, M. (1975): *Lipids,* 10(2):87–92.
2. Hamberg, M., and Samuelsson, B. (1974): *Proc. Natl. Acad. Sci. USA,* 71:3400–3404.
3. Hamberg, M., Svensson, J., and Samuelsson, B. (1975): *Proc. Natl. Acad. Sci. USA,* 72:2994–2998.
4. Hamberg, M., Svensson, J., Wakabayashi, T., and Samuelsson, B. (1974): *Proc. Natl. Acad. Sci. USA,* 71:345–349.
5. Jones, R. L., Kerry, P. J., Poyser, N. L., Walker, I. C., and Wilson, N. H. (1978): *Prostaglandins,* 16:583–588.
6. Jones, R. L., Kerry, P. J., Poyser, N. L., Walker, I. C., and Wilson, N. H. (1979): In: *Chemistry, Biochemistry and Pharmacological Activity of Prostanoids,* edited by S. M. Roberts and F. Scheinmann, pp. 138–148. Pergamon Press, New York.

Advances in Prostaglandin and Thromboxane Research,
Vol. 6, edited by B. Samuelsson, P. W. Ramwell,
and R. Paoletti. Raven Press, New York © 1980.

Study on the Property and Inhibition of Human Platelet Arachidonic Acid 12-Lipoxygenase

F. F. Sun, J. C. McGuire, D. P. Wallach, and V. R. Brown

*Experimental Biology Research, The Upjohn Company,
Kalamazoo, Michigan 49001*

12-Lipoxygenase is one of the two major oxygenation pathways for arachidonic acid in platelets. The products, 12-hydroperoxy-5,8,10,14-eicosatetraenoic acid and 12-hydroxy-5,8,10,14-eicosatetraenoic acid (HETE), possess interesting biological activities (4). The soluble cytoplasmic fraction of platelet homogenate (9) contains the lipoxygenase, although Ho et al. (7) also found a membrane-bound lipoxygenase. Recent experiments demonstrated additional products generated from polyunsaturated fatty acids by lipoxygenase. The discovery of the dihydroxy acids (3) and trihydroxy acids (2,8) suggest that the animal lipoxygenase may be an entry point into a multienzyme complex which produces an array of hydroxylated polyunsaturated lipids. The increasing interest in this enzyme intensifies the search for potent and specific inhibitors. This report describes our finding that a common organic chemical, acetone phenylhydrazone, blocks the 12-lipoxygenase in human platelets.

A washed human platelet suspension (5) or platelet high-speed supernatant (9) containing various amounts of the inhibitor were incubated with ^{14}C-arachidonic acid. The products were quantitatively extracted with ether after deproteination with acetone and determined by radiometric thin-layer chromatography. The identities of the metabolites were confirmed by gas chromatography–mass spectrometry (10).

Incubation of ^{14}C-arachidonic acid with platelet supernatant generated two metabolites. The fast running peak was identified as HETE and the peak at the origin as 8,11,12-trihydroxy-5,9,14-eicosatrienoic acid (THETA) by their respective mass spectra (5). Indomethacin (10^{-4} M) did not inhibit THETA or HETE formation, while 10^{-4} M eicosatetraynoic acid (ETYA) completely abolished their formation. The HETE formation increased linearly for the first 15 min and then gently leveled off. The ratio of HETE to THETA varied from preparation to preparation but generally remained between $10:1$ and $3:1$.

Preincubation of platelet supernatant with acetone phenylhydrazone (APH) over the concentration range of 10^{-4} to 10^{-7} M resulted in a dose-dependent inhibition of the lipoxygenase activity. APH inhibited THETA and HETE equally, suggesting that THETA originates from the lipoxygenase pathway. The

ED_{50} was 2.3 μM for HETE. Two similar compounds, phenylhydrazine and formaldehyde phenylhydrazone were poor inhibitors. They had an ID_{50} greater than 100 μM.

APH is also a cyclooxygenase inhibitor. When tested against the sheep seminal vesicle cyclooxygenase system, the compound had a ED_{50} of 3.0 $\times$ 10^{-5} M. Formaldehyde phenylhydrazone blocks the cyclooxygenase with approximately equal potency (ED_{50}, 4.5 $\times$ 10^{-5} M).

Since our data showed that APH is more effective against 12-lipoxygenase than cyclooxygenase, this compound was tested in washed human platelets, which contain both enzymes. Under our routine assay conditions, washed platelets produced HETE, 12-hydroxyheptadecatrienoic acid (HHT), and thromboxane (TX) B_2 in the ratio of 3:1:1. Addition of 10^{-4} M of indomethacin completely prevented the formation of HHT and thromboxane B_2, while the yield of HETE increased nearly twofold. ETYA blocked the formation of all three compounds with equal effectiveness. However, APH apparently has greater potency against the lipoxygenase than cyclooxygenase. The ID_{50} (Table 1) was 1.6 μM for lipoxygenase and an average of 15 μM for cyclooxygenase (TXB_2 and HHT). Therefore, APH can be considered a "selective" inhibitor for the lipoxygenase. In comparison with the previously reported selective inhibitor, 5,8,11-eicosatriynoic acid (6), APH is 10 times more potent but slightly less "selective."

Blackwell and Flower (1) reported that 1-phenyl-3-pyrazolidone (phenidone) inhibited both the lipoxygenase and cyclooxygenase pathways in platelets. The compound bears some structural resemblance to APH, but is much less potent (ED_{50} 3.1 $\times$ 10^{-4} M for platelet lipoxygenase). It is possible that the two compounds may act via the same mechanism.

The lack of specific inhibitors for animal lipoxygenase has greatly hampered the investigation of its physiological significance. The identification of this unique chemical structure should lead to the discovery of a better or more specific

TABLE 1. ED_{50} of platelet 12-lipoxygenase inhibitors

Inhibitors	Enzyme source	ID_{50} (μM)		
		HETE	HHT	TXB_2
ETYA	Platelet cytoplasmic fraction	0.03	—	—
ETYA	Washed platelet	2.9	4.5	2.6
EA[a]	Platelet cytoplasmic fraction	4.3	—	—
EA[b]	Washed platelet	24.0	340.0	340.0
Phenidone[c]	Platelet homogenate	308.6	388.8	388.8
APH	Platelet cytoplasmic fraction	2.3	—	—
APH	Washed platelet	1.6	13.0	17.0

[a] EA, 5,8,11-eicosatriynoic acid
[b] From ref. 6.
[c] From ref. 1.

inhibitor. APH can be readily synthesized by mixing acetone with phenylhydrazine reagent, a procedure described in elementary organic chemistry laboratory manuals. By carefully choosing the right dose, one may obtain the maximal utilization of its "selectivity" in biological testings.

REFERENCES

1. Blackwell, G. J., and Flower, R. J. (1978): *Prostaglandins,* 16:417–425.
2. Bryant, R. W., and Bailey, J. M. (1979): *Prostaglandins,* 17:9–18.
3. Falardeau, P., Hamberg, M., and Samuelsson, B. (1976): *Biochim. Biophys. Acta,* 441:193–200.
4. Goetzl, E. J., Wood, J. M., and Gorman, R. R. (1977): *J. Clin. Invest.,* 59:179–183.
5. Hamberg, M., Svensson, J., Wakabayashi, T., and Samuelsson, B. (1974): *Proc. Natl. Acad. Sci. USA,* 71:345–349.
6. Hammarstron, S. (1977) *Biochim. Biophys. Acta,* 487:517–519.
7. Ho, P. P. K., Walters, P., and Sullivan, H. R. (1977) *Biochim. Biophys. Res. Commun.,* 79:398–405.
8. Jones, R. L., Kerry, P. J., Poyser, N. L., Walker, I. C., and Wilson, N. H. (1978): *Prostaglandins,* 16:583–589.
9. Nugteren, H. (1975): *Biochim. Biophys. Acta,* 380:299–307.
10. Sun, F. F. (1977): *Biochem. Biophys. Res. Commun.,* 74:1432–1440.

Advances in Prostaglandin and Thromboxane Research,
Vol. 6, edited by B. Samuelsson, P. W. Ramwell,
and R. Paoletti. Raven Press, New York © 1980.

Interrelationships of SRS-A Production and Arachidonic Acid Metabolism in Human Lung Tissue

J. L. Walker

May & Baker Ltd., Dagenham, Essex RM10 7XS, England

Arachidonic acid (AA) is metabolized by both cyclooxygenase and lipoxygenase, and it has previously been shown (7) that inhibition of cyclooxygenase by indomethacin potentiates the release of slow-reacting substance of anaphylaxis (SRS-A). Hamberg (2) subsequently showed that inhibition of cyclooxygenase increased the formation of lipoxygenase products and found that lipoxygenase activity is high in lung tissue. These findings focused attention on the possible interrelationship between AA metabolism and SRS-A production. In addition, clinical interest was aroused in a possible connection between increased production of the potent bronchoconstrictor substance, SRS-A, induced by indomethacin and the syndrome of aspirin sensitivity. To further investigate these interrelationships, the effects of several nonsteroidal antiinflammatory drugs (NSAI) and of lipoxygenase inhibition, induced by nordihydroguaiaretic acid (NGA) and phenidone, on SRS-A release from human lung were studied.

METHODS

Specimens of macroscopically normal human lung were sensitized in reaginic serum from house-dust sensitive patients as previously described (4). Drug effects on release of SRS-A and histamine were determined by an incubation method (5) using three replicates per treatment. Sensitized lung tissue, washed free of serum, was incubated with NSAI (sodium salt) at room temperature for 1 hr before being divided into aliquots, transferred to a water bath at 37°C, and challenged with antigen (extract of *Dermatophagoides pteronyssinus,* 1 µg/ml final concentration) still in the presence of NSAI. NGA and phenidone were added to the lung incubates immediately before challenge. In both cases the incubation was continued at 37°C for 20 min before removal of the supernatant fluid for fluorimetric assay of histamine and biological assay of SRS-A on the mepyraminized guinea pig ileum. All supernatants were bracket assayed in arbitrary units against the same sample of crude guinea pig SRS-A. SRS-A was characterized by loss of biological activity on incubation with aryl sulfatase and inhibition of spasmogenic activity on the guinea pig ileum by FPL 55712 (0.01 μg/ml). Student's t-test was used to assess the significance of the difference between treatments.

RESULTS

Antigen challenge caused the release of SRS-A and histamine. The effects of NGA, indomethacin, and phenidone on the release of SRS-A and histamine from three specimens of passively sensitized human lung are shown in Table 1. NGA (15 μg/ml) strongly inhibited the release of SRS-A, whereas indomethacin (1 to 3 μg/ml) potentiated the release by approximately 50%. When added to lung incubates treated with indomethacin, NGA reversed the effect of indomethacin and reduced SRS-A release to below that of challenged controls. These drug effects were statistically significant ($p < 0.05$). The effects of NGA and

TABLE 1. *Effect of NGA, phenidone, and indomethacin on the release of SRS-A and histamine from passively sensitized human lung tissue*

Lung specimen	Treatment (drug conc., μg/ml)	SRS-A released[a] (U/ml)	Change in SRS-A released by antigen (%)	Histamine released[a] (% total tissue histamine)	Change in histamine released by antigen (%)
1	Challenged	1311 ± 78	—	40.0 ± 1.89	—
	Unchallenged	0	—	4.6 ± 0.47	—
	NGA (15)	0	−100[c]	31.0 ± 1.30	−25.5[c]
	Indomethacin (1)	1808	+49[c]	22.8	−48.6[c]
	NGA (15) +[b] Indomethacin (1)	0	−100[c]	28.1 ± 1.63	−36.5[c]
2	Challenged	683 ± 88	—	25.7 ± 1.69	—
	Unchallenged	0	—	2.9 ± 0.13	—
	NGA (15)	93 ± 60	−86.5[c]	21.3 ± 1.43	−17.7
	Indomethacin (1)	1048 ± 97	+52.1[c]	28.2 ± 1.14	+11.4
	Indomethacin (3)	986 ± 31	+44.3[c]	25.9 ± 1.47	+1.3
	NGA (15) +[b] Indomethacin (1)	338 ± 71	−50.9[c]	20.5 ± 0.54	−22.5[c]
	NGA (15) +[b] Indomethacin (3)	325 ± 50	−52.7[c]	20.6 ± 1.49	−22.1
3[b]	Challenged	1603	—	33.9	—
	Unchallenged	0	—	5.7	—
	Phenidone (1)	1042	−35	36.8	+10.3
	Phenidone (3)	492	−69	31.5	−8.5
	Phenidone (10)	326	−79	30.7	−11.3
	Phenidone (30)	327	−79	28.9	−17.7

[a] Mean (±SE) of three replicates except for data for indomethacin for specimen 1, mean of two replicates.
[b] Supernatants from three separate replicates pooled before assay; no statistical analysis possible.
[c] Significant effect, $p < 0.05$.

indomethacin on histamine release were inconsistent, varying between no effect and a modest, but significant, reduction. Phenidone (1 to 30 μg/ml) inhibited SRS-A release in a dose-dependent manner but had no marked effect on histamine release. Although statistical analyses of the phenidone results were not possible, percentage changes in mediator release > 25% are usually significant at the 5% level with this technique.

The effects of NSAI on SRS-A release are shown in Fig. 1. The magnitude of the drug effects varied in different lung specimens, but whereas indomethacin, aspirin, and ketoprofen had fairly consistent effects, those of ibuprofen, tolmetin, and fenoprofen were more variable (SEM > ±35%). Indomethacin, ibuprofen, tolmetin, and aspirin potentiated SRS-A release; fenoprofen had little effect at the doses tested, but ketoprofen inhibited SRS-A release. In the majority of experiments, NSAI inhibited histamine release (not shown), but the degree of inhibition was variable and often not significant at the 5% level ($p > 0.05$). None of the drugs tested caused a nonspecific release of SRS-A or histamine, and none interfered with the assays of histamine or SRS-A in the doses used.

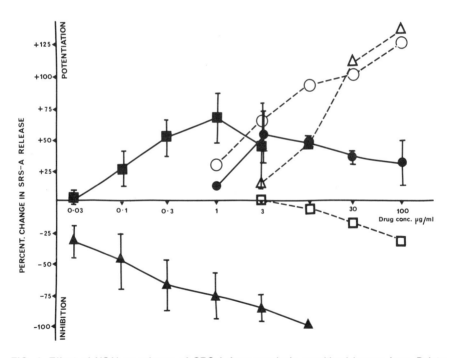

FIG. 1. Effect of NSAI on release of SRS-A from passively sensitized human lung. Points are mean percent changes in SRS-A in three or five (indomethacin) specimens of lung tissue. Bars represent SEM, but for clarity are omitted for ibuprofen, tolmetin, and fenoprofen, where SEM were > ±35%. Symbols used: ■, indomethacin; ▲, ketoprofen; ●, aspirin; □, fenoprofen; △, tolmetin; ○, ibuprofen.

DISCUSSION

AA Metabolism and SRS-A Release

This study confirmed the potentiating effect of indomethacin on SRS-A release. Three explanations for the potentiation of SRS-A release by indomethacin have been suggested: A cyclooxygenase product inhibits SRS-A release *or* a lipoxygenase product enhances it *or* SRS-A is itself formed from AA, possibly via lipoxygenase. If enhancement of SRS-A release by indomethacin occurs because a cyclooxygenase product inhibits SRS-A release, then all cyclooxygenase inhibitors should potentiate SRS-A production, and the additional inhibition of lipoxygenase should not affect this potentiation. This hypothesis must be rejected because (a) ketoprofen, which is approximately equiactive with indomethacin in inhibiting cyclooxygenase in human lung (M. T. Withnall, *personal communication*), did not potentiate SRS-A release; (b) NGA, which inhibits lipoxygenase (2) but does not affect prostaglandin (PG) synthesis (3), reversed the potentiating effect of indomethacin; and (c) phenidone, which inhibits both cyclooxygenase and lipoxygenase (1) reduced the amount of SRS-A released. The concentrations of indomethacin (7; and Withnall, *personal communication*), NGA (2), and phenidone (1) used are known to inhibit the relevant enzymes almost completely. These studies therefore support the concept that SRS-A production is associated with the lipoxygenase pathway, i.e., SRS-A may be formed directly from AA or its synthesis could be closely connected with a lipoxygenase product.

Aspirin Sensitivity

The ability of certain NSAI to cause bronchospasm in "aspirin-sensitive" patients has been correlated with their potency in inhibiting PG synthesis (6), and it has been suggested (7) that increased production of SRS-A might be the cause of the bronchoconstrictor effects of NSAI. Ketoprofen did not potentiate SRS-A production, but in common with the other NSAI tested, does cause bronchospasm in aspirin-sensitive patients. Hence increased SRS-A production cannot be the prime cause of bronchospasm following ingestion of NSAI.

ACKNOWLEDGMENTS

I thank Mrs. M. Ford, Miss J. Lang, and Miss S. Miller for skilled technical assistance; Mr. G. Flavell, F.R.C.S., F.R.C.P., and Mr. E. J. M. Weaver, F.R.C.S., L.R.C.P., for specimens of human lung tissue; and Professor J. Pepys, F.R.C.P., F.R.C.P.E., F.C.Path., for human serum.

REFERENCES

1. Blackwell, G. J., and Flower, R. J. (1978): *Prostaglandins,* 16(3):417–425.
2. Hamberg, M. (1976): *Biochim. Biophys. Acta,* 431:651–654.

3. Morris, H. R., Piper, Priscilla, J., Taylor, G. W., and Tippins, J. R. (1979): *Br. J. Pharmacol.,* 66:452P.
4. Piper, P. J., and Walker, J. L. (1973): *Br. J. Pharmacol.,* 47:291–305.
5. Sheard, P., Killingback, P. G., and Blair, A.M.J.N. (1967): *Nature,* 216:283–284.
6. Szczeklik, A., Gryglewski, R. J., and Czerniawska-Mysik, G. (1975): *Br. Med. J.,* 1:67–69.
7. Walker, J. L. (1973): *Adv. Biosci.,* 9:235–240.

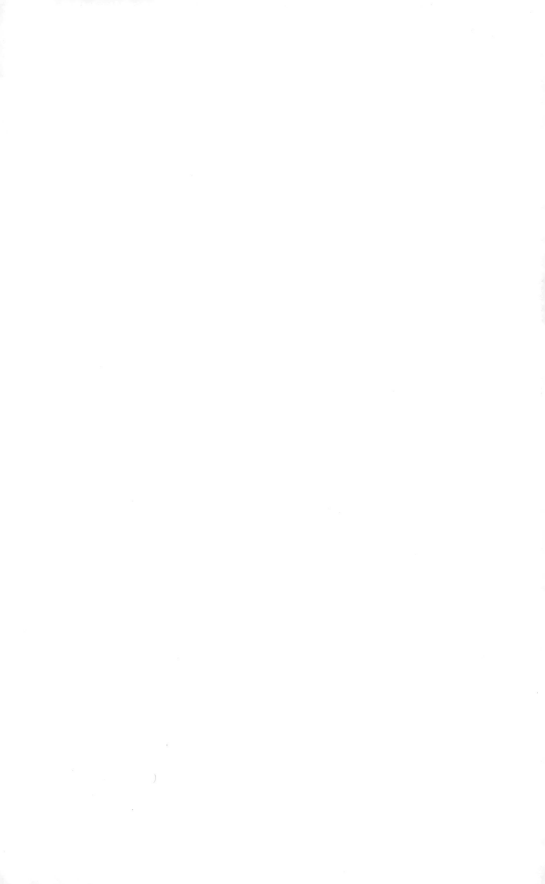

Advances in Prostaglandin and Thromboxane Research,
Vol. 6, edited by B. Samuelsson, P. W. Ramwell,
and R. Paoletti. Raven Press, New York © 1980.

Potentiation of SRS-A Release from Guinea Pig Chopped Lung by Substrates for Arachidonate Lipoxygenase

Priscilla J. Piper, J. R. Tippins, *H. R. Morris, and *G. W. Taylor

*Department of Pharmacology, Royal College of Surgeons of England, London WC2A 3PN, and *Department of Biochemistry, Imperial College of Science and Technology, London S.W.3, England*

Various groups have suggested that slow-reacting substance of anaphylaxis (SRS-A) is formed from arachidonic acid (AA) by the action of lipoxygenase (4). In guinea pig lung the output of SRS-A is potentiated by cyclooxygenase inhibitors (2) which may increase the action of arachidonate lipoxygenase (3). To clarify the mechanism of synthesis and release of SRS-A, the effects of substrates for arachidonate lipoxygenase, including ^{14}C-AA, were investigated.

METHODS

Chopped lung tissue from sensitized guinea pigs was prepared as previously described (6). The actions of the fatty acids shown in Table 1 and indomethacin on SRS-A release were investigated. Prostaglandin (PG) $F_{2\alpha}$ release was measured by radioimmunoassay and histamine by fluorimetric assay (2). The effects of nordihydroguaiaretic acid (NDGA, 1 to 50 μg/ml), eicosatetraynoic acid (ETA, 10 μg/ml), and diethylcarbamazine (DEC, 1 mg/ml) on SRS-A release were studied.

SRS-A was prepared by challenge of lung tissue treated with indomethacin and ^{14}C-AA (7), and combined with SRS-A prepared from perfused lung (2) and purified by an extension of the method of Morris et al (7). The biological activity, ultraviolet (UV) absorbance, and radioactivity of fractions (0.5 ml) eluted from the high pressure liquid chromatography (HPLC) were measured.

RESULTS

Potentiation of SRS-A

Low levels of SRS-A (<0.05 u/ml) were detected when unsensitized lung tissue was incubated with AA (1 μg/ml). Concentrations of SRS-A released

TABLE 1. *Actions of fatty acids and indomethacin on SRS-A release*

Fatty acid (10 μg/ml)	Fatty acid + indomethacin (1 μg/ml)	Increase in SRS-A release (%)
Arachidonic	—	141.0 ± 20.2
—	Arachidonic	198.6 ± 17.1
5,8,11,14,17-Eicosapentaenoic	—	99.7 ± 19.9
—	Eicosapentaenoic	128.5 ± 15.5
4,7,10,13,16,19-Docosahexaenoic	—	22.0 ± 2.3
6,8,12-Octadecatrienoic	—	20.5 ± 5.2
5,8,11-Eicosatrienoic	—	0
Dihomo-γ-linolenic	—	0
11,14-Eicosadienoic	—	0
11,14,17-Eicosatrienoic	—	0
9,12,15-Octadecatrienoic	—	0
Oleic		
	Indomethacin (1 μg/ml)	81.1 ± 9.7

by challenge were increased by indomethacin, AA, 5,8,11,14,17-eicosapentaenoic acid, 4,7,10,13,16,19-docosahexaenoic, and 6,9,12-octadecatrienoic acids (Table 1). The fatty acid-stimulated release of SRS-A was further increased by indomethacin. The other fatty acids shown in Table 1 did not affect SRS-A release. The release of histamine was not potentiated by these acids. In all cases biological activity of SRS-A was antagonized by FPL 55712 (0.1 to 1 μg/ml).

Distribution of Radioactivity

Following reverse-phase HPLC in methanol:water, the peak of the biological activity appeared towards the end of the gradient with the major part of the radioactivity eluting slightly later. At this stage the biological activity and the radiolabeled material were not clearly separated. The samples containing the biologically active material were then subjected to further reverse-phase HPLC in a propanol:acetic acid:water system. The biologically active and UV-active material co-eluted, but were well separated from the peak of radioactivity, which eluted much later.

Inhibition of SRS-A Release

Eicosatetraynoic acid and NDGA inhibited the control release of SRS-A and that stimulated by indomethacin or AA. NDGA (10 μg/ml) converted the indomethacin-induced 81% potentiation of SRS-A release to a 40% reduction compared with control values. NDGA did not inhibit release of $PGF_{2\alpha}$ during antigen challenge. Diethylcarbamazine inhibited control and indomethacin-stimulated release of SRS-A.

DISCUSSION

Incubation of lung tissue with indomethacin and/or exogenous AA or eicosapentaenoic acid increased the amount of SRS-A released. In contrast to results with guinea pig perfused lung (2), histamine release from chopped lung was not potentiated by AA or indomethacin. After extensive purification of SRS-A, the biological activity and UV absorbance became clearly separated from the radioactivity. This shows that although SRS-A may be synthesized from endogenous AA, exogenous ^{14}C-AA did not become incorporated into SRS-A, a finding which agrees with that for SRS-A from rat peritoneum (1), but differs from that in rat basophil leukemia cells (4). The purification system was modified from that originally described (7) because in these experiments the biological activity eluted much earlier than before and was contaminated with at least one other AA-related compound.

The release of SRS-A was potentiated by indomethacin and substrates for arachidonate lipoxygenase with three or more double bonds, although 5,8,11-eicosatrienoic and dihomo-γ-linolenic acids did not increase SRS-A output. Acids which did not have double bonds at n9 and 12 (8) did not potentiate SRS-A release. Indomethacin further increased the effect of the fatty acids. The control and potentiated release of SRS-A was inhibited by inhibitors of lipoxygenase—ETA, NDGA, and DEC. These results ,strongly suggest that the release of SRS-A is stimulated by some aspect of arachidonic acid metabolism by lipoxygenase and that DEC inhibits SRS-A release (9) by inhibition of this enzyme. The fact that ^{14}C-AA was not incorporated into SRS-A is explained by the finding of Jose and Seale (5) that exogenous ^{14}C-AA incorporated into lung phospholipids is not metabolized during antigen challenge. However, this does not discount the possibility that SRS-A may be formed from endogenous AA and that the exogenous fatty acids may act by displacing endogenous AA. Alternatively, SRS-A may be formed by a yet undescribed enzyme for which 5,8,11-eicosatrienoic and dihomo-γ-linolenic acids are not substrates.

ACKNOWLEDGMENTS

We thank the Medical Research Council and the Asthma Research Council for grants.

REFERENCES

1. Bach, M. K., Brashler, J. R., Brooks, C. D., and Neerken, A. J. (1979): *J. Immunol.,* 122:160–165.
2. Engineer, D. M., Niederhauser, U., Piper, P. J. and Sirois, P. (1978): *Br. J. Pharmacol.,* 62:61–66.
3. Hamberg, M. (1976): *Biochim. Biophys. Acta,* 431:651–654.
4. Jakschik, B. A., Falkenhein, S., and Parker, C. W. (1977): *Proc. Natl. Acad. Sci. USA,* 74:4577–4581.
5. Jose, P. J., and Seale, J. P. (1979): *Br. J. Pharmacol. (in press).*

6. Morris, H. R., Piper, P. J., Taylor, G. W., and Tippins, J. R. (1979): *Br. J. Pharmacol.*, 67:179–184.
7. Morris, H. R., Taylor, G. W., Piper, P. J., and Tippins, J. R. (1978): *FEBS. Lett.*, 87:203–206.
8. Nugteren, D. H. (1975): *Biochim. Biophys. Acta*, 380:299–307.
9. Orange, R. P., Valentine, M. D., and Austen, K. F. (1968): *Proc. Soc. Exp. Biol. Med.*, 127:127–132.

Advances in Prostaglandin and Thromboxane Research,
Vol. 6, edited by B. Samuelsson, P. W. Ramwell,
and R. Paoletti. Raven Press, New York © 1980.

Further Studies on the Inactivation of Slow-Reacting Substance of Anaphylaxis by Lipoxidase

Pierre Sirois

Pulmonary Research Unit, Faculty of Medicine, University Hospital Center, University of Sherbrooke, Sherbrooke, Quebec J1H 5N4, Canada

Following the discovery by Kellaway and Trethewie (6) of slow-reacting substance of anaphylaxis (SRS-A) in 1940, the research to unravel the chemical structure of this mediator of hypersensitivity reactions (type 1) has been hampered by so many technical difficulties that until recently, we were completely ignorant of the chemical composition of this entity. Fortunately, during the last five years, three main lines of research produced evidence concerning this important molecule. The first series of evidence was presented by Orange and his co-workers (8) who showed that SRS-A was inactivated by arylsulfatase and suggested the presence of a sulfate ester group. This finding was supported by the abundance of sulfur on spark source mass spectrometric analysis. However, technical limitations prevented this group from obtaining more structural information, despite attempts of conventional derivatization and the use of spark source, electron impact, or chemical ionization mass spectrometry.

The next evidence was presented by Bach et al. (1) and Jakschik et al. (5) in 1977. Both groups have obtained limited amounts of radiolabeled SRS-A following incubation of either rat mononuclear cells or rat basophilic leukemia cells with tritiated arachidonic acid and stimulation by the ionophore A23187, and they concluded that arachidonic acid has a precursor role in the biosynthesis of SRS-A. This finding was further confirmed in Orange's laboratory (12). Recently, a third line of evidence emerging from our laboratories (3,10,11) showed that lipoxidase could inactivate SRS-A, and we postulated the close relationship between SRS-A and fatty acids like arachidonic acid, linoleic acid, or linolenic acid. The purpose of the following investigation was to confirm and further characterize the inactivation of SRS-A by lipoxidase.

METHODS

SRS-A was obtained from rat peritoneal cavity following passive sensitization with rat antiovalbumine (9). Crude dried extracts were stored at $-20°C$. The guinea pig ileum in the presence of hyoscine and mepyramine was used in the bioassay.

Incubations with lipoxidase were performed in Tyrode buffer at 37°C for 1 hr, as described by Sirois (10). SRS-A was used at a final concentration of 50 U/ml.

RESULTS AND DISCUSSION

In previous experiments (10), our results have shown that the inactivation of SRS-A by lipoxidase was dependent on temperature, concentration, and time. In order to further characterize this reaction, the present series of experiments show the effect of various concentrations of arachidonic acid added to the solution of enzyme (5 μg/ml) prior to the addition of SRS-A and incubated for 60 min. As shown in Fig. 1, a high concentration (50 μg/ml) of the lipoxidase natural substrate completely inhibits the inactivation of SRS-A. When lower concentrations of arachidonic acid (0.1, 1.0, and 10 μg/ml) were used, the inhibition decreased, and 22.1 ± 4.1, 20.6 ± 4.0, and 36.5 ± 6.0 U/ml of SRS-A, respectively, were recovered from the total of 50 U added. This inhibition could be due to the large excess of arachidonic acid molecules for the binding sites of the enzyme as compared to the number of SRS-A molecules. Similar results were obtained when 1-phenyl-3-pyrazolidone (phenidone) was added to the enzyme prior to adding SRS-A (Fig. 2). This substance possesses good inhibitory properties against both the lipoxidase and the cyclooxygenase (2). At the highest doses used (100, 1,000, and 10,000 ng/ml), phenidone produced full inhibition of lipoxidase (5 μg/ml) under our experimental conditions. At the lowest doses used (1.0 and 10 ng/ml), 21.9 ± 3.2 and 26.0 ± 3.9 U/ml of SRS-A, respectively, were recovered as compared with 13.2 ± 2.5 U/ml in the absence of the chemical.

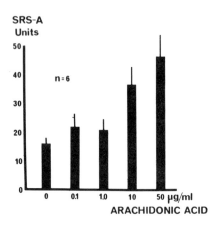

FIG. 1. Effect of arachidonic acid on the inactivation of rat SRS-A (50 U/ml) by lipoxidase (5 μg/ml; E.C.1.13.1.13, type I). Incubations were conducted in Eppendorf tubes (1.5 ml) at 37°C for 1 hr in a final volume of 0.5 ml of Tyrode solution, terminated by boiling for 5 min, and centrifuged. The supernatants were kept for the bioassay. Results are means ± SEM.

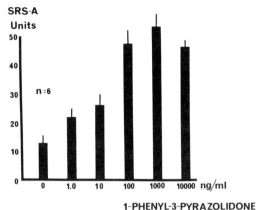

FIG. 2. Effect of phenidone on the inactivation of rat SRS-A (50 U/ml) by lipoxidase (5 μg/ml). Experimental conditions were identical to those described in Fig. 1.

Indomethacin (0.02 to 20 μg/ml) was also used to further characterize this reaction. As shown on the table, the nonsteroid antinflammatory drug did not affect the inactivation of SRS-A by lipoxidase.

These results support previous observations on the inactivation of SRS-A by lipoxidase. A similar mechanism in animals would also appear to be a possible process for the disposition of SRS-A following immediate hypersensitivity reactions. Because of the very strict specificity of this enzyme (4), our results suggest that the structure of SRS-A is very close to arachidonic acid and contains a *cis,cis*-1,4-pentadiene group ($-CH=CH-CH_2-CH=CH-$). In support to this finding, Morris et al. (7) have recently shown that the only fatty acids (20:4, 20:3, 20:5, and 22:6) which potentiated SRS-A release from guinea pig lungs have double bonds at C-9 and C-12 (Fig. 3). If one couples this part of information to other evidence (1,5,12) suggesting that SRS-A could be a metabolite of arachi-

TABLE 1. *Effect of indomethacin on the inactivation of SRS-A by lipoxidase[a]*

Indomethacin (μg/ml)	SRS-A recovered (U/ml)
0	11.9 ± 2.1
0.02	12.0 ± 0.2
0.2	10.4 ± 0.9
2.0	12.4 ± 1.7
20	10.4 ± 1.2

[a] The experimental conditions were identical to the previous series of experiments. $n = 4$.

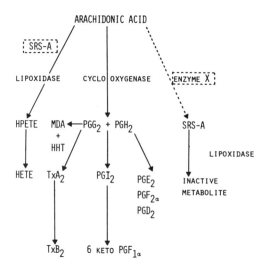

FIG. 3. Hypothetical pathways of metabolism of arachidonic acid. Two pathways in solid lines are well documented and lead to the formation of prostaglandins and thromboxanes through the action of the cyclooxygenase and to the formation of HETE through the lipoxidase. On the *right,* the *dotted line* represents the suggested pathway leading to the formation of SRS-A catalized by an unknown enzyme X. On the basis of the present state of knowledge, one cannot exclude the possibility that SRS-A could be an intermediary product in the formation of 12-hydroperoxy-5,8,10,14-eicosatetraenoic acid (HPETE) and HETE.

donic acid, one has to suppose that SRS-A is an intermediary metabolite in the formation of 12-hydroxy-5,8,10,14-eicosatetraenoic acid (HETE) or that SRS-A is the product of a completely different pathway of metabolism of arachidonic acid.

ACKNOWLEDGMENTS

This work was supported by MRC Grant MA-7143. Rat SRS-A was produced in the laboratory of the late Dr. R. P. Orange (MRC Grant MT-4605).

REFERENCES

1. Bach, M. K., Brashler, J. R., and Gorman, R. R. (1977): *Prostaglandins,* 14:21–31.
2. Blackwell, G. J., and Flower, R. J. (1978): *Prostaglandins,* 16:417–425.
3. Engineer, D. M., Morris, H. R., Piper, P. J., and Sirois, P. (1978): *Br. J. Pharmacol.,* 64:211–218.
4. Holman, R. T., Egwin, P. O., and Christie, W. W. (1969): *J. Biol. Chem.,* 244:1149–1151.
5. Jakschik, B. A., Falkenhein, S., and Parker, C. W. (1977): *Proc. Natl. Acad. Sci. USA,* 74:4577–4581.
6. Kellaway, C. H., and Trethewie, E. R. (1940): *Q. J. Exp. Physiol.,* 30:121–145.
7. Morris, H. R., Piper, P. J., Taylor, G. W., and Tippins, J. R. (1979): *Br. J. Pharmacol.,* 66:452P.
8. Orange, R. P., Murphy, R. C., and Austen, K. F. (1974): *J. Immunol.,* 113:316–322.
9. Orange, R. P., Murphy, R. C., Karnowsky, M. L., and Austen, K. F. (1973): *J. Immunol.,* 110:760–770.
10. Sirois, P. (1979): *Prostaglandins,* 17:395–404.
11. Sirois, P., Engineer, D. M., Piper, P. J., and Moore, E. G. (1979): *Experientia,* 35:361–363.
12. Sirois, P., Moore, E. G., and Orange, R. P. (1979): *Agents and Actions,* 9(4).

Advances in Prostaglandin and Thromboxane Research,
Vol. 6, edited by B. Samuelsson, P. W. Ramwell,
and R. Paoletti. Raven Press, New York © 1980.

Chemical and Enzymic Conversions of the Prostaglandin Endoperoxide PGH$_2$

D. H. Nugteren and E. Christ-Hazelhof

Unilever Research Vlaardingen, 3130 AC Vlaardingen, The Netherlands

At our Vlaardingen laboratory we have always been very interested in nutritional studies on edible oils and fats. The role of the dietary essential fatty acid (EFA) linoleic acid and its conversion products, such as arachidonic acid, has especially received our attention. In 1964, Van Dorp and co-workers combined two separate fields of study by demonstrating that the EFAs could be converted in the body into prostaglandins (PG) (for a review, see ref. 22). Much of our work has been aimed at a better understanding of the structural and dynamic functions of the EFAs and their oxygenation products in the body.

An unstable intermediate of PG biosynthesis, the endoperoxide PGH$_2$, was isolated in 1973 (6,14). Now we know that five different enzymes exist which convert this endoperoxide into five different, biologically active products. Four of these conversions are isomerizations; only in the case of PGF$_{2\alpha}$ formation does a reduction take place and is a reducing agent required. Of these five products, PGF$_{2\alpha}$ is fairly stable; it remains unchanged in aqueous solutions for a long period of time. Two of the other products, PGE$_2$ and PGD$_2$, can be kept under physiological conditions—in water at pH 7.4 and 37°C—for a few hours only. These prostaglandins dehydrate easily. PGE$_2$ then gives PGA$_2$. The recently discovered thromboxane A$_2$ (TXA$_2$) and prostacyclin are both hydrolyzed extremely rapidly in buffer at pH 7.4 and 37°C, with half-lives of approximately 0.5 and 3 min, respectively (7,12).

We want to note, however, that all these products are much more stable in aprotic organic solvents, which is why these compounds can be studied to a certain extent by physicochemical methods. As a matter of fact, total organic syntheses of PGH$_2$ and prostacyclin (but not yet of TXA$_2$) have been described (18,24). From our own experience we know that PGH$_2$, prostacyclin, and even TXA$_2$ can be kept for several days at room temperature in dry diethyl ether, ethyl acetate, or acetone. Solutions of these compounds can be stored for very long periods at −80°C without appreciable decomposition. However, under physiological conditions, water is, of course, always present, and through the years we have made many studies on the chemical and enzymic reactions of the PG endoperoxides in neutral aqueous solution. In nearly every animal system, arachidonic acid is the most abundant and readily convertible substrate during

PG biosynthesis, and we will therefore limit our discussion to the conversions of PGH$_2$.

CHEMICAL REACTIONS OF PGH$_2$ IN AQUEOUS SOLUTIONS

Formation of PGE$_2$ and PGD$_2$

When PGH$_2$ is dissolved in water, it decomposes almost exclusively into a mixture of PGE$_2$ and PGD$_2$ with a constant E/D ratio of 2.4; less than 10% of other products—PGF$_{2\alpha}$ and 12-hydroxy-heptadecatrienoic acid (HHT) + malonaldehyde—are formed (Table 1). This first-order reaction takes place with a half-life of 5 min at 37°C (8) or about 10 min at 20°C (3) in buffer at pH 7 to 8. The pH value has some influence. Below pH 4 and above pH 8 the decomposition is strongly accelerated (14). It is also possible to influence the PGE$_2$/PGD$_2$ ratio. A striking increase in the amount of PGD$_2$ was observed after addition of certain serum albumins, especially from cow, sheep, and pig (3). It is remarkable that not every animal serum albumin gives much PGD$_2$; rabbit and rat albumin are much less active. It appeared that bovine albumin not only altered the E/D ratio, but also simultaneously increased the velocity of the isomerization of the endoperoxide, as shown in Fig. 1.

We found that another group of binding proteins, the ligandins or glutathione S-transferases, could also change the E/D ratio. Again the sheep transferases (isolated from lung or liver) produced more PGD$_2$, while those of the rat yielded larger quantities of PGE$_2$ (see Table 1 and ref. 3). Serum albumins and ligandins have some properties in common. This is apparently also reflected in the species differences with regard to their action on prostaglandin endoperoxide; sheep proteins produce much more PGD$_2$ than those of the rat.

It has been reported that decomposition of the endoperoxide when absorbed

TABLE 1. *Changes in the PGE$_2$/PGD$_2$ ratio during decomposition of PGH$_2$ in the presence of some binding proteins or silica gel[a]*

Addition	Radioactivity (%) after TLC			
	PGE$_2$	PGD$_2$	PGF$_{2\alpha}$	Others
None	66	28	2	4
1.2 mg GSH	65	27	4	4
2 mg sheep serum albumin	22	72	2	4
2 mg rat serum albumin	47	45	2	6
20 µg sheep ligandin[b] + 1.2 mg GSH	11	38	47	4
20 µg rat ligandin[b] + 1.2 mg GSH	56	11	30	3
Adsorbed at SiO$_2$	47	44	5	4

[a] Conditions: 2 to 3 µg (1-^{14}C)-PGH$_2$ was incubated in 3 ml buffer (with 1 mM EDTA), pH 8.0 (or dry, adsorbed to SiO$_2$) for 2 hr at 30°C.
[b] Glutathione S-transferase B.

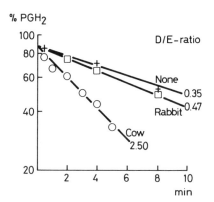

FIG. 1. Decomposition of 3 μg PGH₂ in 3 ml 0.1 M Tris, PH 8, at 20°C in the absence or presence of 2 mg serum albumin from rabbit or cow.

to silica gel yielded mainly PGD_2 (8). In our experiments, a PGE_2/PGD_2 ratio of about 1.1 was obtained (Table 1).

Reduction of Endoperoxide to PGF₂α

From Table 1 it can be deduced that a large amount of $PGF_{2\alpha}$ was obtained during incubations of PGH_2 with glutathione S-transferase and GSH. In general, and as expected, the formation of $PGF_{2\alpha}$ from the endoperoxide is often greatly increased in the presence of reducing agents. Addition of glutathione in combination with ethylenediaminetetraacetate (EDTA) as metal complexer gives hardly any increase in the amount of $PGF_{2\alpha}$, but we found that even traces of metals in distilled water can catalyze the reduction of endoperoxide (see Table 2). Therefore, it is good practice to have 1 mM EDTA in the buffer during incubations with the enzymes which form PGE or PGD. These isomerases have an absolute requirement for glutathione (see below). In incubations of PGH_2 with crude homogenates or supernatants, which always contain thiol compounds and hemoproteins, relatively large quantities of $PGF_{2\alpha}$ were invariably formed; the yield of $PGF_{2\alpha}$ was sometimes even higher after boiling the supernatant. An active principle has been described in microsomes from cow and guinea

TABLE 2. Formation[a] of PGF₂α

Addition	$PGF_{2\alpha}$ (%)
None	2
Glutathione (1.2 mg)	18
Glutathione (1.2 mg) + EDTA (0.9 mg)	4
Glutathione (0.04 mg) + ferrihem (0.5 μg)	45

[a] Conditions: incubations with 3 μg (1-¹⁴C)-PGH₂ in 1 ml 0.1 M Tris buffer (pH 8.0) for 1.5 hr at 25°C.

pig uterus catalyzing the formation of PGF$_{2\alpha}$, but this factor was resistant to boiling and therefore cannot be an enzyme (27).

Nonenzymic formation of TX and HHT

Endoperoxide, decomposing in aqueous buffer without further addition, does not give detectable quantities of TX or prostacyclin. We found, however, that the decomposition of PGH$_2$ could be modified by addition of hemin. In the presence of hemin, a large amount of HHT was found and also a certain amount of TXB$_2$ could be detected (Table 3).

One can compare this chemical reaction with the enzymic conversion occurring in blood platelets. The enzyme in platelets converts the endoperoxide into about equal quantities of HHT and TXB$_2$; but during hemin catalysis, HHT formation is much more pronounced, apparently at the cost of TXB$_2$. We also attempted to make prostacyclin from the endoperoxide by chemical treatment in aqueous medium, but until now the results have been negative. It is well-known that this reaction is performed very efficiently by aorta microsomes (ref. 12; see also Table 3). Prostacyclin can also easily be obtained from PGF$_{2\alpha}$ by relatively simple organic reactions (24).

PURIFICATION AND CHARACTERIZATION OF A PGD-FORMING ENZYME FROM RAT SPLEEN

Prostaglandins of the D type attracted only minor attention in earlier days, but starting at about 1974, various biological activities for PGD$_2$ have been described. Furthermore, PGD$_2$ has been identified in recent years as the major member of the PG family occurring in a number of systems: for instance, rat brain (1), rat mast cells (10), and mouse malignant melanoma cells (5). One of the most interesting biological activities of PGD$_2$ is its inhibitive effect on platelet aggregation in some—but not in all—mammalian species and a correlation between this activity and the capacity of a number of serum albumins to convert PGH$_2$ into PGD$_2$ (see ref. 3 and Table 1) has been suggested (25).

TABLE 3. Conversion of PGH$_2$ into HHT, TX, and prostacyclin[a]

Addition	Radioactivity (%) after TLC				
	HHT	TXB$_2$	6-keto PGF$_{1\alpha}$	PGE$_2$ + PGD$_2$	Others
None	4	0	0	94	2
Hemin (1 mg)	51	12	0	25	13
Washed bovine platelets (10 mg protein)	40	50	0	9	1
Ovine aorta microsomes (4 mg protein)	9	1	74	10	6

[a] Conditions: 5 µg endoperoxide incubated in 1 ml 0.1 M Tris. 1 mM EDTA, pH 8.0, for 15 min at 25°C with the additions indicated.

Soon after isolation of the PG endoperoxides as intermediates in the biosynthesis, we discovered an enzyme in the supernatant of rat tissues which could convert the endoperoxide specifically into PGD_2 (14). Especially rat spleen appeared to be relatively rich in this soluble (cytoplasmic) enzyme. We succeeded in purifying this D-isomerase until homogeneity. We will not discuss the purification procedure in detail: it has been described at great length in a recent paper (2). Well-known methods such as DEAE-cellulose chromatography, isoelectric focusing, and gel filtration were used. In addition, we made use of the fact that the D-isomerase needs glutathione for its action, and we successfully incorporated a glutathione-affinity chromatography step (20) in our purification procedure. We obtained this rather labile enzyme practically 100% pure according to sodium dodecylsulfate polyacrylamide slab-gel electrophoresis, and we estimate that at least a thousandfold purification was achieved compared with the crude rat spleen supernatant.

The D-isomerase had an absolute requirement for GSH, optimal concentration 10^{-4} to 10^{-3} M, and the pH optimum was between 7 and 8. The molecular weight was determined with the help of SDS-gel electrophoresis with 12% gels and with gel filtration over Sephadex G-100: values between 26,000 and 34,000 were obtained. With an adequate amount of pure enzyme [e.g., 0.9 μg (0.03 nmole) per microgram (3 nmoles) PGH_2], the endoperoxide was practically quantitatively converted into PGD_2. A yield approaching 100% is hard to reach, because as soon as PGH_2 (dissolved in a trace of methanol or acetone) is added to the enzyme in aqueous buffer, chemical decomposition into mainly PGE_2 also starts, and this reaction competes with the enzymic D-formation. It is remarkable that the D-isomerase is found in the supernatant. Thus it has a subcellular localization other than the PG endoperoxide synthase, which is membrane bound. The other endoperoxide-metabolizing enzymes—E-isomerase, TX synthase, and 6(9) oxycyclase—are all membrane bound.

PG ENDOPEROXIDE E-ISOMERASE FROM SHEEP VESICULAR GLANDS

The particulate (microsomal) fraction of sheep vesicular glands is more or less the "classical" material used for studies on PG biosynthesis. However, not until 1976 was a successful solubilization and purification of the PG endoperoxide synthase (cyclooxygenase) from this source achieved (11,21). In addition, the vesicular glands contain a glutathione-requiring enzyme which converts the endoperoxide into PGE_2, the so-called E-isomerase. This enzyme has been purified from bovine vesicular glands (16). For several years it has been our aim to solubilize and purify the E-isomerase from sheep vesicular gland microsomes. A drawback is that the E-isomerase is rather labile. Furthermore, intrinsic membrane proteins are generally more difficult to purify than soluble proteins. Purification is, of course, facilitated if a simple, rapid, and reliable assay of the enzymic activity is available. We incubated 2 μg radioactive PGH_2 (added in 4 μl methanol) in 0.4 ml buffer (pH 7.4) with 4 mM GSH and 1 mM EDTA for only 1 min at 20°C in the presence of enough E-isomerase to obtain between 30 and 70% PGE_2. The endoperoxide which was left and the PGE_2 formed were determined after rapid extraction and high performance thin-layer chromatography (HPTLC) in the cold. In this way we obtained the results of a series of incubations within 1 hr.

The purification of a membrane-bound protein can be divided into three parts (9): (a) Finding a mild detergent which solubilizes the protein without denaturation or loss of enzymic activity. (b) Separation of protein from lipid. Generally the lipid consists mainly of phospholipids, cholesterol, and some neutral lipids. Phospholipids, due to their charge and their amphiphilic character, hamper efficient purification. They can often be removed by using a sufficient excess of detergent. (c) When single protein-detergent micelles have been obtained, and provided the enzyme is still active and stable enough in the absence of phospholipid, the usual protein purification procedures such as DEAE– and CM–cellulose chromatography, isoelectric focussing, and gel filtration can often be applied. Then one obtains a pure protein–detergent complex or micelle with a detergent/protein ratio varying between 0.2 and > 4 (w/w) depending on the protein and detergent in question (9,17,19).

To solubilize the E-isomerase, we tried cholate, deoxycholate, and a number of nonionic detergents with varying values of hydrophilic–lipophilic balance (HLB) (9). It appeared that the E-isomerase was more difficult to solubilize than the PG endoperoxide synthase. Most of the synthase even remained in the supernatant with Tween-20 (HLB number, 16.7) (11) and with cholate (21), but the E-isomerase needed Triton X-100 (HLB number, 13.5) or deoxycholate for efficient solubilization (see Table 4). The table shows that deoxycholate is the strongest solubilizer, but for a number of reasons the deoxycholate superna-

TABLE 4. *Solubilization of E-isomerase from sheep vesicular gland microsomes by different detergents[a]*

Detergent	Detergent/protein ratio	Protein (%)		E-isomerase (%)	
		P	S	P	S
Tween-20	0.37	82	18	95	5
	2.0	77	23	97	3
	5.0	nd	nd	88	12
Cholate	5.0	54	46	76	24
Triton X-100	0.7	84	16	83	17
	2.9	60	40	45	55
Deoxycholate	0.37	54	46	83	17
	2.0	35	65	12	88
	2.5	23	77	16	84

[a] Pellet (P) and supernatant (S) after centrifugation for 1 hr at 100,000 $\times$ g at 2°C in the presence of 1 mM GSH and 1 mM EDTA.

tants proved to be impractical for further purification: heterogeneous micelles, rapid inactivation, and viscous solutions. Therefore, we decided to use Triton X-100 and started by measuring the stability of the E-isomerase with different concentrations of Triton X-100. The results (Fig. 2) indicate that larger amounts of Triton X-100 activated the enzyme considerably (with 2.5% detergent from 6.5 to 11 nmoles/min), but at the same time the stability on storage at 0°C decreased appreciably. Anyhow, the fact that high Triton concentrations had no inhibiting effect can be regarded as an indication that phospholipid is possibly not required for enzymic activity. This was confirmed by gel filtration on Ultrogel ACA 34 in the presence of 0.5% Triton X-100, during which the phospholipid-containing micelles were separated from the E-isomerase, which remained active in this period. During the several procedures outlined above, we subjected the different fractions to SDS-slab gel electrophoresis with 10 or 12% polyacrylamide. The preparations invariably showed many protein bands. The E-isomerase

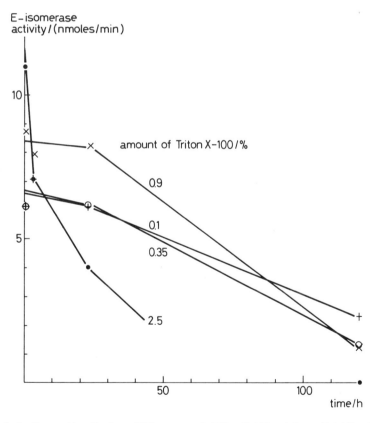

FIG. 2. Activation and inactivation of E-isomerase in Triton X-100 solutions. Solubilized microsomes (400 μg protein) were kept in 2 ml buffer at 0°C in the presence of 1 mM GSH, 1 mM EDTA, and different concentrations of Triton X-100. Aliquots of 30 μl (6 μg protein) were used for the determination of enzyme activity.

is possibly an SH-enzyme: it requires glutathione and is inhibited by p-chloromercuribenzoate (PCMB) and by N-ethylmaleimide (NEM) (6). We used [³H]NEM to label sheep vesicular gland microsomes and, after some purification, monitored the radioactivity after SDS-gel electrophoresis. It appeared that several protein bands contained radioactivity.

DETERMINATION OF THE ENDOPEROXIDE METABOLITES IN PHYSIOLOGICAL SYSTEMS

It is certainly true that studies on isolated enzymic reactions are highly informative, but the ultimate desire remains of applying the findings to the intact biological system. The *in vivo* and *in vitro* situation differs, for instance, very much with respect to substrate availability: in the test tube, mostly an excess of only one substrate is used, while it is assumed that *in vivo* the substrate concentration is rate limiting. Furthermore, it is quite possible that several substrates, inhibitors, and cofactors are active in the cell.

The intact body is extremely complicated, and a reasonable, somewhat simpler approach is to study perfused organs or suspensions or cultures of cells. It is imperative that one can assay nanogram quantities of PGs in these systems. This is possible using, for instance, bioassay, radioimmunoassay, or gas chromatography–mass spectrometry. We successfully employed the pentafluorobenzyl derivatives (esters or oximes) of the various PGs which can be determined (after purification by TLC) by gas chromatography with electron-capture detection (4,5,26). An advantage of this method is that the five different PGs which may be formed from the endoperoxide are determined in one assay and with good specificity and high sensitivity. Using suitable internal standards, reliable quantitative data can be obtained. We demonstrated with this method that prostacyclin was the major PG released from isolated perfused rabbit or rat heart (4) and that perfused rat lung excreted a mixture of prostacyclin (determined as 6-keto PGF$_{1\alpha}$) and PGD$_2$ (15). Cultures of macrophages produced a mixture of PGE$_2$ and TXB$_2$ (13), and we confirmed that pieces of aorta and cultures of endothelial cells formed mainly prostacyclin.

If we now return to what has been stated as the outset: PGs are ultimately derived from the linoleic acid in the diet (22). The kinds of studies discussed here could improve our understanding of the complicated regulatory mechanisms in which the products derived from these EFAs participate.

REFERENCES

1. Abdel-Halim, M. S., Hamberg, M., Sjöquist, B., and Änggard, E. (1977): *Prostaglandins,* 14:633–645.
2. Christ-Hazelhof, E., and Nugteren, D. H. (1979): *Biochim. Biophys. Acta,* 572:43–51.
3. Christ-Hazelhof, E., Nugteren, D. H., and Van Dorp, D. A. (1976): *Biochim. Biophys. Acta,* 450:450–461.
4. De Deckere, E. A. M., Nugteren, D. H., and Ten Hoor, F. (1977): *Nature,* 268:160–163.
5. Fitzpatrick, F. A., and Stringfellow, D. A. (1979): *Proc. Natl. Acad. Sci. USA,* 76:1765–1769.

6. Hamberg, M., and Samuelsson, B. (1973): *Proc. Natl. Acad. Sci. USA,* 70:899–903.
7. Hamberg, M., Svensson, J., and Samuelsson, B. (1975): *Proc. Natl. Acad. Sci. USA,* 72:2994–2998.
8. Hamberg, M., Svensson, J., Wakabayashi, T., and Samuelsson, B. (1974): *Proc Natl. Acad. Sci. USA,* 71:345–349.
9. Helenius, A., and Simons, K. (1975): *Bioçhim. Biophys. Acta,* 415:29–79.
10. Jackson Roberts, L., Lewis, R. A., Lawson, J. A., Sweetman, B. J., Austen, K. F., and Oates, J. A. (1978): *Prostaglandins,* 15:717.
11. Miyamoto, T., Ogino, N., Yamamoto, S., and Hayaishi, O. (1976): *J. Biol. Chem.,* 251:2629–2636.
12. Moncada, S., Gryglewski, R. J., Bunting, S., and Vane, J. R. (1976): *Nature,* 263:663–665.
13. Morley, J., Bray, M. A., Jones, R. W., Nugteren, D. H., and Van Dorp, D. A. (1979): *Prostaglandins,* 729–736.
14. Nugteren, D. H., and Hazelhof, E. (1973): *Biochim. Biophys. Acta,* 326:448–461.
15. Nugteren, D. H., Jouvenaz, G. H., and Dutilh, C. E. (1978): *Acta Biol. Med. Ger.,* 37:701–706.
16. Ogino, N., Miyamoto, T., Yamamoto, S., and Hayaishi, O. (1977): *J. Biol. Chem.,* 252:890–895.
17. Osborne, H. B., Sardet, C., and Helenius, A. (1974): *Eur. J. Biochem.,* 44:383–390.
18. Porter, N. A., Byers, J. D., Mebane, R. C., Gilmore, D. W., and Nixon, J. R. (1978): *J. Org. Chem.,* 43:2088–2090.
19. Robinson, N. C., and Tanford, C. (1975): *Biochemistry,* 14:369–378.
20. Simons, P. C., and Van der Jagt, D. L. (1977): *Anal. Biochem.,* 82:334–341.
21. Van der Ouderaa, F. J., Buytenhek, M., Nugteren, D. H., and Van Dorp, D. A. (1977): *Biochim. Biophys. Acta,* 487:315–331.
22. Van Dorp, D. A. (1969): *Naturwissenschaften,* 56:124–130.
23. Van Dorp, D. A. (1979): In: *Chemistry, Biochemistry, and Pharmacological Activity of Prostanoids,* edited by S. M. Roberts and F. Scheinmann, pp. 233–242. Pergamon Press, Oxford.
24. Whittaker, N. (1977): *Tet. Lett.,* 32:2805–2808.
25. Whittle, B. J. R., Moncada, S., and Vane, J. R. (1978): *Prostaglandins,* 16:373–388.
26. Wickramasinghe, A. J. F., and Shaw, R. S. (1974): *Biochem. J.,* 141:179–187.
27. Wlodawer, P., Kindahl, H., and Hamberg, M. (1976): *Biochim. Biophys. Acta,* 431:603–614.

Advances in Prostaglandin and Thromboxane Research,
Vol. 6, edited by B. Samuelsson, P. W. Ramwell,
and R. Paoletti. Raven Press, New York © 1980.

Characterization of Prostaglandin H_2 Synthetase

F. J. van der Ouderaa, M. Buytenhek, and D. A. van Dorp

Unilever Research Vlaardingen, 3130 AC Vlaardingen, The Netherlands

Prostaglandin (PG) endoperoxide synthetase is a membrane-bound glycoprotein catalyzing the conversion of polyunsaturated fatty acids into PG endoperoxides in two reaction steps; for example, on using arachidonic acid, PGH_2 is formed. The active enzyme has recently been obtained in a pure form by three research groups (4,5,10). Values of approximately 70,000 have been reported for the molecular weight of its polypeptide chains (4,6,10). The pure enzyme appeared to contain only traces of metals. However, it has been shown that hemin is necessary for its oxygenase activity and stimulates its peroxidase activity (5,6,10,11). In this report we present additional structural data on three different aspects of the enzyme: the hemoprotein character, the molecular weight, and the site of acetylation by acetylsalicylic acid.

HEMOPROTEIN CHARACTER

The iron content of the enzyme and the form in which it was bound were still a matter of discussion. We and other investigators found only traces of iron in the pure enzyme (6,10,11), whereas another group suggested that the enzyme would contain heme and non-heme iron in equal amounts (3,4). We carefully analyzed the amount of iron present in three enzyme preparations and, in parallel, with three reference proteins. The six protein samples were individually chromatographed on an Ultrogel ACA-34 column eluted with a buffer containing only 20 ng iron/ml. Fractions of the eluates were analyzed for iron by flameless atomic absorption spectroscopy. The results of these determinations are summarized in Table 1. The values found for the reference proteins are in agreement with those published in the literature. Only traces of iron appeared to be present in active PGH_2-synthetase preparations. The hemin requirement for the cyclooxygenase and the peroxidase activities of the enzyme are well documented (4,6,10,11). On the other hand, no restoration of the enzyme activity by addition of Fe(II) or Fe(III) (1) has been reported. However, participation of a transition metal such as iron in the reactions catalyzed by this enzyme was expected. It follows from the foregoing that it can be ruled out that non-heme iron is effective in this way. The hemin requirement of the enzyme motivated us to study enzyme–hemin interactions. Recombination of the enzyme–

TABLE 1. *Iron content (per polypeptide chain) of PG endoperoxide synthetase (PGES) and of reference proteins*

Preparation	At iron/ polypeptide[a]	Hemin (moles)/ polypeptide[b]	At non- heme iron/ polypeptide	Specific activity[c]
PGEs 1	0.14	0.10	0.04	14.0
PGEs 2	0.31	0.19	0.12	18.3
PGEs 3	0.19	0.08	0.11	11.1
Bovine serum albumin	<0.01	0	<0.01	
Catalase	0.7	0.6	0.1	
Lipoxygenase	0.9	0	0.9	

[a] Determined by atomic absorption spectroscopy.
[b] $\epsilon_{408} = 61$ mM^{-1} cm^{-1}/mole/hemin for PGES; $\epsilon_{410} = 115$ mM^{-1} cm^{-1} for catalase.
[c] Expressed as μmoles eicosatrienoic acid converted per minute per mg protein (25°C).

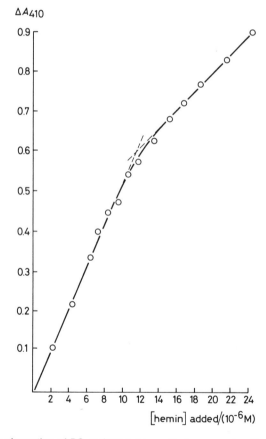

FIG. 1. Increase in absorption of PG endoperoxide synthetase as a function of added hemin, as found by difference spectroscopy carried out in tandem cells. The junction of the two lines corresponds to 11.4 μM of added hemin, which corresponds to an increase in absorbance of 0.600 at 410 mn.

hemin complex carried out in tandem cells was studied using ultraviolet–visible difference spectroscopy. The spectral differences observed are due to specific enzyme–hemin interactions. The results of these experiments are shown in Fig. 1. It can be seen that at low concentrations of added hemin, a linear increase in absorbance is found, indicating high-affinity hemin binding. Hemin–enzyme complexation was also accomplished by equilbrium ultrafiltration and equilibrium gel chromatography. Data on the heme spectra of the Fe(II) and Fe(III) holoenzyme with and without cyanide and carbon monoxide are shown in Table 2. We found no inhibition of the enzyme by carbon monoxide, in agreement with a recent observation made by Ohki et al. (7). The association of hemin to this enzyme is primarily of a hydrophobic nature. The nonionic detergent octaethyleneglycol dodecyl ether dissociates the enzyme–hemin complex at a concentration slightly above its critical micellar concentration. Enzyme inhibition can be demonstrated under these conditions. From the foregoing it had to be concluded that PGH₂-synthetase is a hemoprotein. Hemin is bound to the enzyme by hydrophobic interaction, and dissociation of hemin from the holoenzyme probably occurs during solubilization of the enzyme from the membrane.

Using an antiserum against sheep vesicular gland microsomes and a specific antiserum against the pure enzyme, it was found in a double-diffusion test that the apoenzyme and the holoenzyme are immunologically identical. This indicates that association of the apoprotein and hemin will not lead to extensive changes in the conformation of the protein.

TABLE 2. *Spectral data of PG endoperoxide synthetase*[a]

Enzyme	Absorption band		
	α	β	γ
Fe(III) enzyme			
λ			408
ϵ			61
Fe(III) enzyme + 10 mmoles CN			
λ		540	419
ϵ		5	87
Fe(III) enzyme + CO			
λ			408
ϵ			56
Fe(II) enzyme			
λ	558	530	424
ϵ	5	3	61
Fe(II) enzyme + 10 mmoles CN			
λ	560	532	428
ϵ	16	12	119
Fe(II) enzyme + CO			
λ	568	535	419
ϵ	3	3	97

[a]The millimolar absorption coefficient ϵ is expressed as mM^{-1} cm^{-1}/mole hemin; λ is given in nm.

MOLECULAR WEIGHT

Another matter of discussion concerns the molecular weight of the native enzyme. Values of 300,000 have been reported for the native enzyme solubilized in 0.1% Tween-20 using gel chromatography (4,5). On the other hand, we have found a molecular weight of 129,000 for the apoprotein excluding bound detergent by sedimentation equilibrium measurements in 0.1% Tween (10). As the nonionic detergent Tween-20 is heterogenous, we investigated the molecular weight using octyl glucoside as a pure detergent. The values obtained for the molecular weights of the detergent–enzyme complexes were corrected for the contribution of the amount of detergent bound. For this purpose we used octyl glucoside in a radioactive form. In this way we were able to correct for the contribution to the molecular weight of enzyme-bound detergent. The results of molecular weight determinations of the enzyme–detergent complexes, carried out by gel chromatography on Ultrogel ACA-34, are shown in Fig. 2. Molecular weights determined using this technique reflect the sum of protein and detergent molecular weights. Compared with Tween-20, lower amounts by weight of octyl glucoside were found to be bound to the enzyme. Correspondingly, lower molecular weights were found for the octyl glucoside enzyme complexes. The following values for the molecular weights, excluding bound detergent, were calculated from the measured molecular weights: in 3.5 and 10 mmoles/liter octyl glucoside, 132,000; in 21 mmoles/liter octyl glucoside, 151,000; and in 0.1% Tween-20,

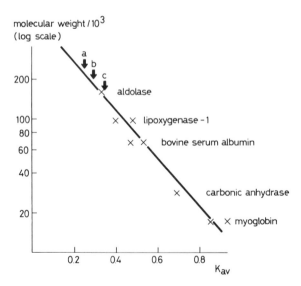

FIG. 2. Molecular weight of native PG endoperoxide synthetase as determined by gel chromatography on Ultrogel ACA-34. The calibration graph gives the molecular weights of five reference proteins versus the partition coefficient (K_{av}): (a) PG endoperoxide synthetase (PGEs) in 0.1% Tween-20; (b) PGEs in 21 mmoles/liter octyl glucoside; and (c) PGEs in 3.5 and 10 mmoles/liter octyl glucoside.

126,000. It follows from these results that dimers are obviously the smallest entities with full enzymic activity. Moreover, we concluded from these studies using different nonionic detergents at varying concentrations that a dimer is the most probable structure of the native enzyme in the membrane.

ACETYLATION BY ACETYLSALICYLIC ACID

Roth and Siok (8) suggested recently that acetylsalicylic acid acetylated the N-terminal serine residue of the enzyme as *N*-acetyl serine was found after pronase digestion of the [³H-acetyl] enzyme. Earlier, alanine had been found by us (10) as the N-terminal residue of the enzyme, whereas Roth et al. (9) found aspartic acid. In Roth's latest paper (8), it was suggested that the enzyme consisted of nonidentical polypeptide chains. We tried to eliminate the discrepancies by sequenator analysis of the native and [³H-acetyl] enzyme under carefully standardized conditions (Table 3). To exclude that variations in yields of phenyl-thiohydantoin (PTH)-amino residues were due to poor reproducibility of the sequenator, instead of being caused by N-terminal acetylation, we added in runs 2 and 3 equal amounts of myoglobin to the PGH₂-synthetase as an internal standard of sequenator performance. The myoglobin sequence does not interfere with that of the enzyme. The PTH-amino acids were quantitatively determined using high pressure liquid chromatography (1); PTH-norleucine was used as an internal standard. The yields of the myoglobin residues obtained during runs 2 and 3 were within 10% of each other. The yields of the native and [³H-acetyl] enzyme were within 15%. Considering all possible experimental variations, a better correlation could hardly be expected. The acetyl enzyme

TABLE 3. *PTH-amino acid residues from sequenator analysis of PG endoperoxide synthetase (nos. 1 and 2) and [³H-acetyl] enzyme (3)[a]*

Step	Residue found	Yield (nmoles)		
		1	2	3
1	Ala	76	40	35
2	Asp	46	++	35
3	Pro	34	48	40
4	Gly	49	33	26
5	Ala	52	33	28
6	Pro	27	42	30
7	Ala	47	31	27
8	Pro	28	36	29
9	Val	40	13	nd
10	Asn	32	+	nd
11	Pro	nd	21	nd

[a] Quantitative determination of the PTH-residues was carried out by HPLC using PTH-norleucine as an internal standard.

preparation used was quantitatively acetylated. The above results therefore indicate that the [³H-acetyl] enzyme is not N-terminally acetylated. Moreover, these results also show that the protein consists of identical subunits, as only one sequence was obtained and alanine is the N-terminal residue.

The observation by Roth and Siok (8) that an *N*-[³H-acetyl] serine was liberated from the [³H-acetyl] enzyme by pronase digestion was also made by us. However, from the literature (2) we learned that *O*-acetyl serine would undergo a rapid O → N shift under the conditions used for the digestion. Thus the *N*-[³H-acetyl]serine found most likely came from an *O*-[³H-acetyl]serine somewhere in the polypeptide chain. By thermolysin digestion of the [³H-acetyl] enzyme and by ion exchange chromatography on Aminex A5 followed by gel chromatography on Sephadex G-15, a [³H-acetyl] peptide containing phenylalanine, serine, glutamine and asparagine was found. Phenylalanine was found as the N-terminal residue by dansylation, which would be expected from the specificity of thermolysin. This means that the acetyl group is bound to a serine hydroxylic group.

In conclusion we have found that PGH₂-synthetase is a hemoprotein, devoid of non-heme iron and consists of two identical polypeptide chains. The enzyme is specifically acetylated by acetylsalicylic acid at a serine hydroxyl group in the chain.

ACKNOWLEDGMENTS

The help of Dr. J. Hofsteenge and P. Wietzes for the high pressure liquid chromatography analyses is gratefully acknowledged.

REFERENCES

1. Frank, G., and Strubert, W. (1973): *Chromatographia*, 6:522–524.
2. Guttmann, S., and Boissonnas, R. A. (1958): *Helv. Chim. Acta*, 41:1852.
3. Hemler, M. E., and Lands, W. E. M. (1977): *Lipids*, 12:591–595.
4. Hemler, M. E., Lands, W. E. M., and Smits, W. L. (1976): *J. Biol. Chem.*, 252:5575–5579.
5. Miyamoto, T., Ogino, N., Yamamoto, S., and Hayaishi, O. (1976): *J. Biol. Chem.*, 251:2629–2636.
6. Ogino, N., Ohki, S., Yamamoto, S., and Hayaishi, O. (1978): *J. Biol. Chem.*, 253:5061–5068.
7. Ohki, S., Ogino, N., Yamamoto, S., and Hayaishi, O. (1979): *J. Biol. Chem.*, 254:829–836.
8. Roth, G. R., and Siok, C. J. (1978): *J. Biol. Chem.*, 253:3782–3784 (1978).
9. Roth, G. R., Stanford, N., Jacobs, J. W., and Majerus, P. W. (1977): *Biochemistry*, 16:4244–4248.
10. Van der Ouderaa, F. J., Buytenhek, M., Nugteren, D. H., and Van Dorp, D. A. (1977): *Biochim. Biophys. Acta*, 487:315–331.
11. Van der Ouderaa, F. J., Buytenhek, M., Slikkerveer, F. J., and Van Dorp, D. A. (1979): *Biochim. Biophys. Acta*, 572:29–42.

Advances in Prostaglandin and Thromboxane Research,
Vol. 6, edited by B. Samuelsson, P. W. Ramwell,
and R. Paoletti. Raven Press, New York © 1980.

Mechanism of Oxygen Activation Involved in the Prostaglandin Synthetase Mechanism

Peter J. O'Brien and Anver D. Rahimtula

Department of Biochemistry, Memorial University of Newfoundland,
St. John's, Newfoundland A1B 3X9, Canada

We have previously shown that the prostaglandin (PG) endoperoxide synthetase of vesicular gland microsomes has a very active heme-dependent peroxidase activity as an integral part (10). The peroxidase was also found to copurify with the synthetase activity (12). Recently, evidence has been presented that the peroxidase is an integral part of the synthetase and is responsible for the conversion of PGG_2 to PGH_2 (8). Hydroperoxides including PGG_2 initiate fatty acid oxygenation (1) and are necessary for continued reaction (2). It has therefore also been suggested that the peroxidase would inhibit the synthetase activity by the removal of PGG_2 (5). However, as peroxidases in the presence of hydroperoxides can catalyze fatty acid oxygenation (9), a peroxidase mechanism may be involved. The peroxidase could therefore also be involved in PGG_2 formation. In the following, it is shown that peroxidase higher oxidation states can be observed during PGH_2 formation.

EXPERIMENTAL

Microsomes were prepared from frozen sheep vesicular gland by the method of Takeguchi (11). The seminal vesicles were homogenized in a Waring blender for 90 sec with two volumes of 0.1 M phosphate buffer pH 8.0. The homogenate was centrifuged for 10 min at $12,000 \times g$ in a Sorvall RC-2B refrigerated centrifuge. The supernatant was filtered through two layers of cheesecloth and centrifuged at $105,000 \times g$ for 75 min in a Beckman L3-50 ultracentrifuge. The microsomal pellet was collected, lyophilized, and stored in a freezer. The 100 g of seminal vesicles (wet weight) yielded about 12 g of lyophilized powder with a protein content of about 50%.

Chemicals

Arachidonic acid, hydrogen peroxide, linoleic acid, horseradish peroxidase, methemoglobin, and tryptophan were purchased from the Sigma Chemical Company. Cumene hydroperoxide was obtained from Matheson, Coleman and Bell.

Linoleic acid hydroperoxide (LAHPO) and arachidonic acid hydroperoxide (AAHPO) were made by the modified method of Gardner (3), using a final extraction described by O'Brien (6). All these chemicals were of the highest grade commercially available. PGG_2 and PGH_2 were also prepared by the method of Hamberg et al. (4).

Spectral Complexes

All spectral measurements were carried out in an Aminco DW-2a spectrophotometer set in the split-beam mode. The freeze-dried microsomes were suspended in 0.1 M Tris HCl (pH 8.2) at 5°C at a final concentration of approximately 1 mg/ml protein. After recording the base line of equal light absorption, arachidonic acid or H_2O_2 or AAHPO was added to the sample cuvette.

RESULTS AND DISCUSSION

As shown in Fig. 1, the addition of the substrate arachidonate (20:4) to sheep vesicular gland microsomes (SVGM) resulted in the immediate formation of a spectral complex absorbing at 435 nm, which decayed, and was followed by the formation of a second complex absorbing at 438 nm. A steadily increasing trough absorbing at 412 nm accompanied these changes. The addition of low concentrations of arachidonate 15 hydroperoxide or PGG_2 to the microsomes instead of arachidonate also resulted in the immediate formation of a spectral complex absorbing at 435 nm and was accompanied by a steadily increasing trough absorbing at 412 nm. No complex was observed on addition of PGH_2 to the microsomes, so that the complex is clearly formed during PGH_2 formation. The requirement of a hydroperoxide group suggests that the spectral complex is a peroxidase higher oxidation state of the heme moiety of PG endoperoxide

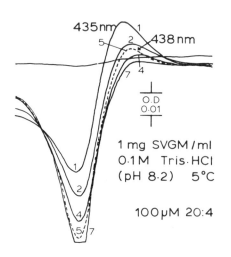

FIG. 1. Intermediate spectral complexes formed with arachidonate. The reaction conditions are described in methods. The numbers refer to successive scans every 30 sec.

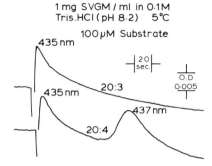

FIG. 2. Time curve for complex formation and decay. The reaction conditions are described in the text.

synthetase and analogous to the complex formed between cytochrome P450 and hydroperoxides (7). The trough is caused by the destruction of the heme by peroxide radicals and responsible for the self-catalyzed synthetase inactivation. The second complex at 438 nm could indicate the formation of a second hydroperoxide other than PGG_2. The addition of the substrate homo-γ-linolenate (see 20:3 in Fig. 2) and linolenate, α-linolenate, or γ-linolenate to microsomes also resulted in the immediate appearance of the 435-nm complex. However, as shown in Fig. 2, no second peak was observed with these fatty acids. The second peak with 20:4 could reflect the formation of another hydroperoxide.

Further evidence that the spectral complex is a higher oxidation state of the peroxidase was its immediate disappearance on the addition of the peroxidase donor tetramethylphenylenediamine (TMPD) (Fig. 3). As 1 μM TMPD was sufficient to reduce the complex formed with 10 μM arachidonate hydroperoxide (AAHPO), it is likely that 10 peroxide equivalents are needed to form the complex.

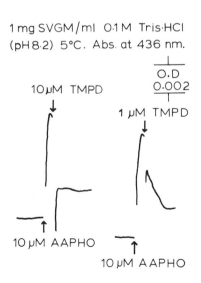

FIG. 3. The reduction of the complex formed with AAHPO by a peroxidase donor. The reaction conditions are described in the text.

The peroxide specificity of the peroxidase is broad with respect to the peroxide substrate and includes hydrogen peroxide (10). The addition of hydrogen peroxide also resulted in the rapid appearance of a 435-nm complex. The possibility that the spectral complex with arachidonate was due to hydrogen peroxide was investigated. It was found that excess catalase prevented the formation of the complex with hydrogen peroxide but did not affect the complex with arachidonate.

ACKNOWLEDGMENT

We wish to thank the Medical Research Council of Canada for financial support.

REFERENCES

1. Cook, H. W., and Lands, W. E. M. (1975): *Biochem. Biophys. Res. Commun.*, 65:464–471.
2. Cook, H. W., and Lands, W. E. M. (1976): *Nature*, 260:630–632.
3. Gardner, H. W. (1971): *Lipids*, 10:248–254.
4. Hamberg, M., Swensson, J., Wakabayashi, T., and Samuelsson, B. (1974): *Proc. Natl. Acad. Sci. USA*, 71:345–349.
5. Lands, W. E. M. (1979): *Annu. Rev. Physiol.*, 41:633–652.
6. O'Brien, P. J. (1968): *Can. J. Biochem.*, 47:1185–1191.
7. O'Brien, P. J. (1978): *Pharmacol. Ther.* 2(3):517–536.
8. Ohki, S., Ogino, N., Yamamoto, S., and Hayaishi, O. (1979): *J. Biol. Chem.*, 254:829–836.
9. Rahimtula, A., and O'Brien, P. J. (1975): *J. Agric. Food Chem.*, 23:154–158.
10. Rahimtula, A., and O'Brien, P. J. (1976): *Biochem. Biophys. Res. Commun.*, 70:893–899.
11. Takeguchi, C., Kohno, E., and Sih, C. J. (1971): *Biochemistry*, 10:2372–2376.
12. Van der Ouderaa, F. J., Buytenhek, M., Nugteren, D. H., and van Dorp, D. A. (1977): *Biochim. Biophys. Acta*, 487:315–331.

Advances in Prostaglandin and Thromboxane Research,
Vol. 6, edited by B. Samuelsson, P. W. Ramwell,
and R. Paoletti. Raven Press, New York © 1980.

Mechanism of Xenobiotic Cooxygenation Coupled to Prostaglandin H_2 Biosynthesis

Lawrence J. Marnett, Michael J. Bienkowski, William R. Pagels, and Gregory A. Reed

Department of Chemistry, Wayne State University, Detroit, Michigan 48202

Prostaglandin (PG) endoperoxide synthetase catalyzes the oxygenation of arachidonic acid (20:4) to the hydroperoxy endoperoxide, PGG_2, and the reduction of PGG_2 to the hydroxy endoperoxide, PGH_2 (4). During the oxidation of 20:4 to PGH_2, a number of substrates structurally unrelated to 20:4 undergo cooxygenation (3). Studies indicate that the cooxygenations are hydroperoxide-dependent reactions which are triggered by the interaction of PGG_2 with a peroxidase (3). As part of our studies designed to elucidate the mechanism of PG endoperoxide synthetase-dependent cooxygenation, we have investigated the oxidation of diphenylisobenzofuran (DPBF) to dibenzoylbenzene (DBB), phenylbutazone (PB) to 4-hydroxy-phenylbutazone (4-OH-PB), and 7,8-dihydroxy-7,8-dihydro-benzo[a]pyrene (BP-7,8-Diol) to 7,8-dihydroxy-7,8-dihydro-9,10-epoxy-benzo[a]pyrene (BPDE). Each of these reactions represents a different mode of oxygenation, which raises the possibility that the mechanism of cooxygenation is different for each substrate.

A mechanistically important question regards the source of the oxygen atom incorporated into the cooxidized substrate. *A priori* there are three possibilities—hydroperoxide oxygen, atmospheric oxygen, or water:

$$\text{R-OOH} + \text{S} \xrightarrow[\text{H}_2\text{O}]{\text{O}_2} \text{R-OH} + \text{S-O}$$

To test for the hydroperoxide oxygen transfer mechanism, a hydroperoxide is required, which is a substrate for the peroxidase and which can be labeled with ^{18}O. 15-Hydroperoxy-5,8,11,13-eicosatetraenoic acid (15-HPEA) was found to be equivalent to PGG_2 as a peroxidase substrate and was prepared with the requisite label by the incubation of soybean lipoxygenase with 20:4 under an $^{18}O_2$ atmosphere (Fig. 1). Reduction of the hydroperoxide to an alcohol and gas chromatographic–mass spectroscopic (GC-MS) analysis of volatile derivatives indicated an isotopic incorporation of 94 at. % excess ^{18}O.

Incubation of the [^{18}O]15-HPEA and ram seminal vesicle microsomes with either DPBF or PB led to no incorporation of ^{18}O into either DBB or 4-OH-

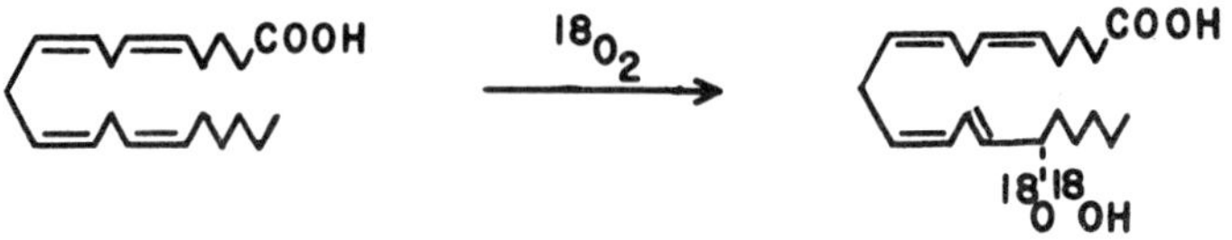

FIG. 1. Biosynthesis of ^{18}O-labeled hydroperoxide from arachidonic acid.

PB detectable by GC-MS of appropriate derivatives. In contrast, incubations performed with either $[^{16}O]15$-HPEA or $[^{16}O]PGG_2$ under an $^{18}O_2$ atmosphere led to substantial ^{18}O incorporation into both products. No incorporation was observed from $H_2{}^{18}O$. These findings are summarized in Table 1.

The stoichiometry of cosubstrate oxidized to PGG_2 added depends on the cosubstrate under investigation (Table 2). The extremely high values observed for DPBF suggest the involvement of a chain process, most likely free radical in nature. Further evidence for the importance of free radical oxidation mechanisms is the observation that PGG_2-dependent cooxygenations of DPBF, PB, and BP-7,8-Diol are inhibited by antioxidants (data not shown).

Although different cooxidizable substrates give different types of reaction products, our results suggest that the cooxygenations can be considered as free radical

TABLE 1. *Oxygen-18 investigation of hydroperoxide-dependent oxygenations catalyzed by ram seminal vesicle microsomes*

	Excess ^{18}O in product[a] labeled oxygen source (at. %)		
Substrate	$R^{18}O^{18}OH$	$^{18}O_2$	$H_2{}^{18}O$
DPBF	2.3	53 (61)[b]	0.0
PB	2.9	84 (81)	—

[a] Determined for incorporation of one atom ^{18}O.
[b] Values in parentheses indicate value obtained using PGG_2 instead of 15-HPEA.

TABLE 2. *Stoichiometry of substrate oxidized to PGG_2 added*

Substrate	Stoichiometry[a]
DPBF	2.0–3000
PB	0.3–1.0
BP-7,8-Diol	< 0.1

[a] Ratio of cosubstrate oxidized to PGG_2 added. All incubations were performed at constant substrate concentrations and varying PGG_2 concentration.

oxidations. The initiator, which is presently unidentified, arises as a result of the interaction of PGG_2 with a peroxidase in ram seminal vesicle microsomes (2). This oxidizing agent may either be hydroperoxide or enzyme derived. If it is hydroperoxide derived, it would be an alkoxy or peroxy radical formed from PGG_2. If it is enzyme derived, it would most likely be one of the higher oxidation states exhibited by peroxidases and generally termed compounds I and II (1).

ACKNOWLEDGMENT

Financial support by the National Institutes of Health (GM 23642) is gratefully acknowledged.

REFERENCES

1. Dunford, H. B., and Stillman, J. S. (1976) *Coord. Chem. Rev.,* 19:187–251.
2. Egan, R. W., Paxton, J., and Kuehl, F. A., Jr. (1976): *J. Biol. Chem.,* 251:7329–7335.
3. Marnett, L. J., Wlodawer, P., and Samuelsson, B. (1975): *J. Biol. Chem.,* 250:8510–8517.
4. Ohki, S., Ogino, N., Yamamoto, S., and Hayaishi, O. (1979): *J. Biol. Chem.,* 254:829–836.

Advances in Prostaglandin and Thromboxane Research,
Vol. 6, edited by B. Samuelsson, P. W. Ramwell,
and R. Paoletti. Raven Press, New York © 1980.

Direct and Indirect Involvement of Radical Scavengers During Prostaglandin Biosynthesis

Robert W. Egan, Paul H. Gale, George C. Beveridge, *Lawrence J. Marnett, and Frederick A. Kuehl, Jr.

*Merck Institute for Therapeutic Research, Rahway, New Jersey 07065; and * Wayne State University, Detroit, Michigan 48202*

It has been established that substances which can act as radical scavengers and reducing agents are capable of stimulating prostaglandin biosynthesis under certain conditions and of depressing it under others (2,6,8,9). For example, phenol stimulated the cyclooxygenase-dependent oxidation of arachidonic acid from 250 nmoles O_2/mg protein to about 500 nmoles O_2/mg protein when administered at 500 μM. However, at successively higher phenol concentrations, this stimulation became less and eventually gave way to inhibition, until at 10 mM there was virtually no reaction.

Several other substances also known to be radical-scavenging reducing agents were then studied in similar fashion (Table 1). N,N-Dimethyl phenylene diamine (DMPD) showed half-maximal stimulation at 8 μM. As with phenol, this stimulation became less pronounced at higher concentrations, achieving 50% inhibition (ID_{50}) of the control reaction at 279 μM. The same is qualitatively true for guaiacol at 18 and 340 μM, butylated hydroxy anisole at 30 and 160 μM, and aminopyrine, at 50 and 18,000 μM, respectively. Phenol, of course, stimulated and then inhibited. Hence there is a dual action of these substances on cyclooxygenase, depending on their concentration and potency. Stimulation at lower concentrations may be attributed to enzyme preservation, as we have described previously (2). On the other hand, the inhibitory phase at higher concentrations may be explained by the observations that small quantities of hydroperoxides are necessary to initiate the cyclooxygenase reaction (4). At high enough concentrations, these reducing agents would chemically lower the hydroperoxide levels, and the reaction would never get going. These effects are listed as indirect because neither would necessarily involve the enzyme itself. Both could, instead, entail reaction with effectors of the enzyme, an oxidant in the case of stimulation and hydroperoxides in the case of inhibition.

In contrast, some actions of these agents on cyclooxygenase must be interpreted as direct interactions with the enzyme. Table 2 lists the potency of a variety of inhibitors of cyclooxygenase in the presence and absence of 500 μM phenol (1). The first three nonsteroidal agents, indomethacin, flurbiprofen, and ibuprofen

TABLE 1. *Dual effects on cyclooxygenase*[a]

Compound	Half-maximal stimulation (μM)	ID_{50} values (μM)
DMPD	8	279
Guaiacol	18	340
Butylated hydroxyanisole	30	160
Aminopyrine	50	18,000
Phenol	200	4,500

[a] With 100 μM arachidonic acid substrate.

inhibited at low concentrations. As expected, when phenol, a stimulator of the reaction, was added, they became somewhat less effective as the two competing effects opposed each other. In complete contrast, the *N*-phenylanthranilic acids from meclofenamic down were relatively poor inhibitors of the cyclooxygenase in the absence of phenol, but when phenol was added, they became significantly more effective. This effect on fenamate inhibition can also be demonstrated with the other stimulators of cyclooxygenase besides phenol. In order to produce a differential effect like this between the fenamates and nonfenamates, there must be direct interaction between phenol and the enzyme. This is yet another mode of involvement of these substances in prostaglandin biosynthesis, a direct one, in addition to the indirect effect already described.

The *in vivo* action of these inhibitors from indomethacin to niflumic acid is clearly to depress prostaglandin biosynthesis. On the other hand, the *in vivo* effects of radical-scavenging reducing agents are not so immediately obvious. Radical scavenging leads to increased prostaglandin levels *in vitro* and would thereby either increase or leave unchanged those levels *in vivo*. On the other hand, if suppression of the hydroperoxide initiator prevails, then prostaglandins would be depressed in both instances. Whether radical scavenging or hydroperoxide suppression would predominate within a given cell could be inferred from the level of endogenous antioxidant or radical-scavenging reducing agent. For

TABLE 2. *Inhibition of cyclooxygenase by nonsteroidal anti-inflammatory agents*

Inhibitor	ID_{50} values (μM)	
	− Phenol	+ Phenol
Indomethacin	0.2	0.3
Flurbiprofen	0.2	0.4
Ibuprofen	2.2	3.1
Meclofenamic acid	10	0.1
Mefenamic acid	150	6.3
Flufenamic acid	390	8.5
Niflumic acid	605	18

example, the cyclooxygenase in a cell with a high level of endogenous reducing agent might already be maximally stimulated, and the addition of an agent such as phenol could, therefore, only lead to inhibition. On the other hand, cells with a low level of factors would be susceptible to stimulation and could elicit this effect when treated with exogenous radical-scavenger. Consequently, the effects of additives could vary dramatically among cell types, depending on the endogenous level of comparable substances.

Indeed, both stimulation and inhibition have been found at the cellular level (3,5). An endogenous factor, uric acid, was recently described as a stimulator of the bovine cyclooxygenase (7). We find that it also stimulates the ram cyclooxygenase and depresses the peroxidase-dependent electron paramagnetic signal. When appropriate quantities of uric acid and phenol are added together to this enzyme, the combination will inhibit in spite of the fact that when each was added separately at the same level, they both stimulated. This is certainly suggestive evidence that what we propose *in vivo* may well exist and may explain some of the observations in cellular systems.

REFERENCES

1. Egan, R. W., Humes, J. L., and Kuehl, F. A., Jr. (1978): *Biochemistry,* 17:2230–2234.
2. Egan, R. W., Paxton, J., and Kuehl, F. A., Jr. (1976): *J. Biol. Chem.,* 251:7329–7335.
3. Flanders, L., Boroski, P., Palicharla, P., and Fretland, D. (1978): *Fed. Proc.,* 37:385.
4. Hemler, M. E., Graff, G., and Lands, W. E. M. (1978): *Biochem. Biophys. Res. Commun.,* 85:1325–1331.
5. Lindgren, J. A., Claesson, H. E., and Hammerström, S. (1977): *Prostaglandins,* 13:1093–1102.
6. Marnett, L. J., and Wilcox, C. L. (1977): *Biochem. Biophys. Acta,* 487:222–230.
7. Ogino, N., Yamamoto, S., Hayaishi, O., and Tokuyama, T. (1979): *Biochem. Biophys. Res. Commun.,* 87:184–191.
8. Panganamala, R. V., Gavino, V., and Cornwell, D. G. (1979): *Prostaglandins,* 17:155–162.
9. Smith, W. L., and Lands, W. E. M. (1971): *J. Biol. Chem.,* 246:6700–6702.

Advances in Prostaglandin and Thromboxane Research,
Vol. 6, edited by B. Samuelsson, P. W. Ramwell,
and R. Paoletti. Raven Press, New York © 1980.

Interaction of Arachidonic Acid and Heme Iron in the Synthesis of Prostaglandins

*D. A. Peterson, *J. M. Gerrard, **G. H. R. Rao, *E. L. Mills,
and *,**J. G. White

*Departments of *Pediatrics and **Laboratory Medicine and Pathology, University of
Minnesota, Minneapolis, Minnesota 55455*

The prostaglandin (PG) endoperoxide synthetase or cyclooxygenase enzyme which converts arachidonic acid to PGG_2 (2–4) is a hemoprotein, and heme is essential for its activity (6–8,17–19). It is probable that the iron in heme is at the active site of the enzyme and is critically involved in fatty acid oxidation. We have, therefore, explored reactions between iron and arachidonic acid and between heme and arachidonic acid to probe the mechanism of fatty acid oxidation by the cyclooxygenase enzyme.

INTERACTION OF FE^{2+} AND ARACHIDONIC ACID

Rao et al. (12) first observed that nitroblue tetrazolium (NBT) together with vitamin E inhibits arachidonic acid oxidation by platelets when concentrations of the individual reagents are used which are relatively ineffective by themselves. While inhibiting this reaction, NBT is itself reduced, presumably by trapping a radical required for the reaction. Rao et al. (13) then made the observation that ferrous sulfate alone could oxidize arachidonic acid and convert it to peroxides measured by absorption at P_{232} or using the thiobarbituric acid reaction. When ferrous sulfate, arachidonic acid, and oxygen are reacted in the presence of NBT, NBT prevents production of these arachidonic acid peroxides and is itself reduced (10). The Fe^{2+} is oxidized to Fe^{3+}. In a short incubation (30 sec) the reaction is optimum using a 1:1 molar ratio of arachidonic acid and Fe^{2+}, suggesting that one molecule of iron interacts with one molecule of arachidonic acid. In longer incubations, the arachidonic acid, which is itself unchanged during the reaction, is required in a much smaller concentration than the Fe^{2+}, suggesting that it can be reutilized. Results using other fatty acids show that both the carboxylic acid group and a double bond are essential to the reaction. It was, therefore, suggested that arachidonic acid interacts with Fe^{2+} at two sites, one site to bind the carboxyl group and a second site where oxygen bound to the Fe^{2+} can interact with the fatty acid double bond. We hypothesize that a radical generated on the arachidonic acid during its association with Fe^{2+}

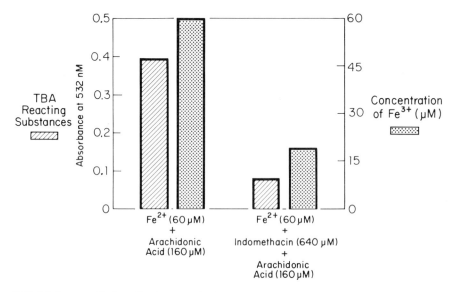

FIG. 1. Influence of indomethacin on production of thiobarbituric acid (TBA) reacting substances and conversion of Fe^{2+} to Fe^{3+} when arachidonic acid is reacted with Fe^{2+}. Arachidonic acid and Fe^{2+} were reacted in 1 ml of 40% ethanol for 1 min. When indomethacin was used, it was premixed with the Fe^{2+} for 30 sec. TBA reacting substances and conversion of Fe^{2+} to Fe^{3+} were evaluated as described in ref. 11.

and oxygen is trapped by NBT, preventing subsequent arachidonic acid peroxidation, similar to NBT inhibition of the cyclooxygenase reaction (9,11). However, in the presence of the enzyme, vitamin E is required, perhaps to penetrate to the hydrophobic reaction site and transfer the radical to NBT.

To further evaluate the similarity between arachidonic acid oxidation by Fe^{2+} and the cyclooxygenase enzyme, we used agents which are known to inhibit the conversion of arachidonic acid to PGG_2, including indomethacin, ibuprofen, and tolmetin. All three agents inhibited arachidonic acid oxidation by Fe^{2+} (11); however, the concentrations needed were higher than that used *in vivo* (Fig. 1). Nevertheless, the concentration of Fe^{2+} required for the oxidation of AA is relatively high since the reaction in the enzyme is much more efficient than the reaction with Fe^{2+} alone. Therefore, a relatively high concentration of indomethacin and other antiinflammatory agents is to be expected. If it were possible to adjust the iron concentration down to the level of the enzyme in cells, then the concentration of indomethacin might be reduced to levels which can inhibit the enzyme *in vivo*. These studies, therefore provide important support for the mechanism of arachidonic acid oxidation by Fe^{2+} being similar to the mechanism of the cyclooxygenase reaction.

INTERACTION OF HEME AND ARACHIDONIC ACID

Since it is heme iron that is required for the cyclooxygenase reaction (6–8, 17–19), we next evaluated heme interaction with arachidonic acid. First, we applied the concept developed concerning oxidation of arachidonic acid by Fe^{2+}, namely, that the arachidonic acid interacts with Fe^{2+} at two sites. Since the heme iron has only two available ligands, one below and the other above the porphyrin ring, the arachidonic acid would have to attach to the Fe^{2+} ligand on one side of the heme and wind around the protoporphyrin ring; the C_{11} double bond would then interact with oxygen bound to the second available ligand on the other side of the heme. We built a molecular model and found that this was sterically possible. Indeed, much of the stereospecificity in the conversion of arachidonic acid to PGG_2 in biological systems can be explained by this model (Fig. 2). Thus closure of the ring at C_{8-12} with C_7 alpha to the ring and C_{13} beta to the ring; and addition of the O_2 across C_{9-11}, alpha to the ring, would be required by the model. Furthermore, if the enzyme deter-

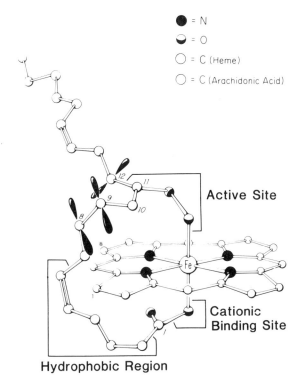

Active Site

Cationic Binding Site

Hydrophobic Region

FIG. 2. Proposed model for the interaction of arachidonic acid with heme. The cationic binding site is shown where the carboxylate residue of arachidonic acid attaches to the Fe^{2+} ligand below the plane of the porphyrin ring. The hydrophobic region is where the acyl chain fits between carbons 1 and 8 of the porphyrin ring of protoporphyrin IX. These carbons have methyl groups which create a groove into which the acyl chain of arachidonic acid fits. For reasons of clarity these methyl groups, as well as the other side chains on the porphyrin ring, are not shown on the diagram. At the active site, oxygen bound to the ligand of the Fe^{2+} above the plane of the heme adds on to C_{11} of arachidonic acid. The *p* orbitals of the resulting radical at C_{12} and the π orbitals of the double bond at C_{8-9} are shown by the *teardrop-shaped symbols*.

mined the site of the second O_2 addition at C_{15}, the model would require abstraction of the S hydrogen at C_{13} and formation of the C_{13-14} double bond as trans, as occurs in natural PGs (1,2). The prediction of four of the six stereospecific steps by this model lends credence to its similarlity to the biological reaction.

The model includes the cationic binding site (the ligand of the iron on one side of the heme where the carboxylate group attaches), the hydrophobic region where the acyl group curls around the protoporphyrin ring, and the active site (the other side of the protoporphyrin ring where the iron bound to oxygen interacts with the double bond at C_{11})—three ingredients of the interaction of arachidonic acid and enzyme, as suggested by Shen and Sherrer (1,14–16). In previous models of the enzyme, attempts were made to interact inhibitors such as indomethacin with both cationic and active sites. However, indomethacin may inhibit by binding only at the cationic site and in the hydrophobic region, without needing to interfere at the active site per se, and indeed, indomethacin could not interact with both cationic and active sites in this model. Perhaps this is the explanation for the ability of indomethacin to inhibit the cyclooxygenase but not the peroxidase activity of the PG endoperoxide synthetase enzyme.

A useful model should help our understanding of previously unexplained findings. One such enigma is the stimulatory role of lipid peroxides on PG synthesis (5). Recent data (D. A. Peterson and J. M. Gerrard, *unpublished*) shows that lipid peroxides can reduce heme. Since the reaction shown by the model would require reduction of the ferric-heme usually added to the reaction to ferrous heme, lipid peroxides might enhance cyclooxygenase activity by reducing the heme iron.

SUMMARY

The reaction of ferrous iron and oxygen to oxidize arachidonic acid has been studied to aid in understanding the mechanism of PGG_2 formation. Based on these results we have presented a novel concept of heme–arachidonic acid interaction in PG synthesis.

ACKNOWLEDGMENTS

Supported by U.S.P.H.S. Grants HL-11880, AM-06317, HL-06314, CA-12607, CA-08832, CA-11996, GM-AM-22167, HL-20695, HL-16833, and AM-15317, as well as a grant from the Leukemia Task Force. Dr. Gerrard is the recipient of an Established Investigatorship from the American Heart Association.

REFERENCES

1. Gund, R., and Shen, T. Y. (1977): *J. Med. Chem.,* 20:1146–1150.
2. Hamberg, M., and Samuelsson, B. (1967): *J. Biol. Chem.,* 242:5336–5343.

3. Hamberg, M., and Samuelsson, B. (1967): *J. Biol. Chem.,* 242:5344–5354.
4. Hamberg, M., and Samuelsson, B. (1967): *Proc. Natl. Acad. Sci. USA,* 71:3400–3404.
5. Hemler, M. E., Cook, H. W., and Lands, W. E. M. (1979): *Arch. Biochem. Biophys.,* 193:340–345.
6. Hemler, M. E., and Lands, W. E. M. (1976): *J. Biol. Chem.,* 251:5575–5579.
7. Miyamoto, T., Ogino, N., Yamamoto, S., and Hayaishi, O. (1976): *J. Biol. Chem.,* 251:2629–2636.
8. Ogino, N., Ohki, S., Yamamoto, S., and Hayaishi, O. (1978): *J. Biol. Chem.,* 253:5061–5068.
9. Peterson, D. A., and Gerrard, J. M. (1979): *Med. Hypothesis,* 5:683–697.
10. Peterson, D. A., Gerrard, J. M., Rao, G. H. R., Krick, T. P., and White, J. G. (1978): *Prostaglandins Med.,* 1:304–318.
11. Peterson, D. A., Gerrard, J. M., Rao, G. H. R., and White, J. G. (1979): *Prostaglandins Med.,* 2:97–108.
12. Rao, G. H. R., Gerrard, J. M., Eaton, J. W., and White, J. G. (1978): *Photochem. Photobiol.,* 28:845–850.
13. Rao, G. H. R., Gerrard, J. M., Eaton, J. W., and White, J. G. (1978): *Prostaglandins Med.,* 1:55–70.
14. Scherrer, R. A. (1974): In: *Antiinflammatory Agents: Chemistry and Pharmacology,* Vol. 1, edited by R. A. Scherrer and M. W. Whitehouse, pp. 29–43. Academic Press, New York.
15. Shen, T. Y. (1967): *Top. Med. Chem.,* 1:29–78.
16. Shen, T. Y., and Winter, C. A. (1977): *Adv. Drug Res.,* 12:87–245.
17. Van Der Ouderaa, F. J., Buytenhek, M., Nugteren, D. H., and Van Dorp, D. A. (1977): *Biochim. Biophys. Acta,* 487:315–331.
18. Van Der Ouderaa, F. J., Buytenhek, M., Slikkerveer, F. J., and Van Dorp, D. A. (1979): *Biochim. Biophys. Acta,* 572:29–42.
19. Yoshimoto, A., Ito, H., and Tomita, K. (1970): *J. Biochem. (Tokyo),* 68:487–499.

Advances in Prostaglandin and Thromboxane Research,
Vol. 6, edited by B. Samuelsson, P. W. Ramwell,
and R. Paoletti. Raven Press, New York © 1980.

Identification of Prostaglandin D_2-Isomerase in Rat Basophilic Leukemia and Rat Mast Cells

B. A. Jakschik, M. M. Steinhoff, and L. H. Lee

*Department of Pharmacology, Washington University School of Medicine,
St. Louis, Missouri 63110*

Basophils and mast cells play an important role in immediate hypersensitivity reactions. The major cyclooxygenase product produced by these cells is prostaglandin D_2 (PGD_2) (1,2). The almost exclusive formation of this PG by these cells suggests the presence of a specific, efficient PGD_2 isomerase.

METHODS

Rat basophilic leukemia (RBL-1) cells were grown in Eagle's minimum essential medium with 15% heat-inactivated fetal calf serum, L-glutamine, antibiotic-antimycotic mixture and gentamycin. The cells were washed prior to experiments with 50 mM sodium phosphate buffer, 1 mM ethylenediaminetetraacetic acid and 0.1% gelatin, pH 7. Rat mast cells, obtained from washings of the peritoneal and thoracic cavity were purified on bovine serum albumin gradients (93–98% purity). Both cell types were homogenized (Tekmar tissumizer and tight Dounce) and centrifuged at $9,000 \times g$, 20 min, cold, to remove debris and granules. The supernatant was centrifuged at $150,000 \times g$ for 2 hr. The $150,000 \times g$ pellet (microsomes) and supernatant (soluble fraction) were used for incubations with [^{14}C]arachidonic acid (AA) or [^{14}C]PGH_2. The incubation mixture was acidified, pH 3.2 to 3.5 and extracted with ethyl acetate, and chromatography was performed in the organic phase of ethyl acetate:2,2,4-trimethylpentane: acetic acid:water (110:50:20:100). The radioactive bands were detected by scanning or radioautography after dipping the plate into 0.4% Omnifluor in 2-methylnaphthalene. Quantitation was achieved by scraping and liquid scintillation counting.

RESULTS AND DISCUSSION

Incubations of RBL-1 microsomes with [^{14}C]AA alone yielded $8.9 \pm 0.9\%$ $PGF_{2\alpha}$, $17.5 \pm 2\%$ PGE_2, and $9.1 \pm 1.4\%$ PGD_2 ($n = 14$). Addition of epinephrine led to an increase in cyclooxygenase activity and reduced glutathione significantly enhanced PGD_2 formation. Maximum conversion to PGD_2 was obtained with both cofactors present (6.1 ± 0.4% $PGF_{2\alpha}$, 7.1 ± 0.4% PGE_2, and 35.6 ± 3.6% PGD_2, $n = 21$). This marked enhancement of PGD_2 synthesis was not observed with oxidized glutathione or another sulfhydryl compound such as cysteine. The presence of a glutathione-dependent PGD_2 isomerase in the RBL-1 microsomal fraction was confirmed by incubations with [¹⁴C]PGH₂ bypassing the cyclooxygenase. With microsomes and [¹⁴C]PGH₂ alone, we observed the formation of 23.1 ± 2.4% $PGF_{2\alpha}$, 41.7 ± 3.2% PGE_2, and 12.8 ± 1.5% PGD_2 ($n = 14$). Addition of reduced glutathione and epinephrine yielded 13.1 ± 1.6% $PGF_{2\alpha}$, 28.5 ± 5.3% PGE_2, and 37.5 ± 6% PGD_2 ($n = 12$). Incubations of boiled microsomes with [¹⁴C]PGH₂ with or without cofactors gave results similar to those observed with buffer controls. Therefore, the RBL-1 microsomes do not only contain cyclooxygenase activity, but also a glutathione-dependent PGD_2 isomerase.

Since other investigators have reported PGD_2 isomerase activity in the soluble fraction of rat tissue, we also incubated the RBL-1 soluble fraction with [¹⁴C]PGH₂. It was found that PGD_2 isomerase activity was also present in this fraction. In the presence of reduced glutathione and epinephrine [¹⁴C]PGH₂ was converted to 3.6 ± 0.4% $PGF_{2\alpha}$, 43.9 ± 10.8% PGE_2, and 37.7 ± 7.9% PGD_2. This represents a twofold increase in PGD_2 over buffer controls. Therefore, in RBL-1 cells, PGD_2-isomerase activity is present both in the microsomal and soluble fraction.

When mast cell microsomes were incubated with [¹⁴C]AA, cyclooxygenase activity was found in this fraction but no PGD_2-isomerase. Incubations with [¹⁴C]PGH₂ confirmed the absence of PGD_2-isomerase in the microsomal fraction and localized this enzyme in the soluble fraction. Similar to the RBL-1 enzyme, the mast cell PGD_2-isomerase was glutathione dependent. Without glutathione present, PGH₂ was converted to 4.4 ± 0.2% $PGF_{2\alpha}$, 41.1 ± 0.7% PGE_2, and 14.0 ± 1.6% PGD_2 ($n = 3$). Addition of glutathione yielded 2.4 ± 0.2% $PGF_{2\alpha}$, 8.2 ± 0.8% PGE_2, and 56.6 ± 5.8% PGD_2 ($n = 3$). This shows that the PGD_2 isomerase is very efficient, since PGH₂ is converted quantitatively to PGD_2. This efficiency is also observed in whole cell preparation when the endoperoxide which is formed endogenously by cyclooxygenase, a membrane-bound enzyme, is converted almost exclusively to PGD_2.

The observation that PGD_2-isomerase in RBL-1 cells is found both in the microsomal and soluble fraction is in contrast to the data obtained from normal rat mast cells and other rat tissues. The question arises whether this localization of the enzyme is a characteristic of a malignant cell line or typical for basophils.

ACKNOWLEDGMENTS

This work was supported by NIH 5-R01-HL 21874-02 and 5-P30-CA 16217-03.

REFERENCES

1. Jakschik, B. A., Lee, L. H., Shuffer, G., and Parker, C. W. (1978): *Prostaglandins,* 16:733–748.
2. Roberts, L. J., II, Lewis, R. A., Lawson, J. A., Sweetman, B. J., Austin, K. F., and Oates, J. A. (1978): *Prostaglandins,* 15:717 (abstract).

Advances in Prostaglandin and Thromboxane Research,
Vol. 6, edited by B. Samuelsson, P. W. Ramwell,
and R. Paoletti. Raven Press, New York © 1980.

New Approach to the RIA of Prostaglandins and Related Compounds Using Iodinated Tracers

F. Dray, K. Gerozissis, B. Kouznetzova, S. Mamas, P. Pradelles,
and G. Trugnan

Analytic Radioimmunology Unit, INSERM, Pasteur Institue, 75724 Paris 15, France

Since the discovery of the structure of prostaglandins (PGs) E_1 and $F_{1\alpha}$ by Bergström and Sjovall in the 1960s (2), the list of PGs and related substances has continued to increase not only in number, but also in diversity of biological action. These substances are present in biological media in very low concentrations (10^{-9}–10^{-11} M); some (the endoperoxides, thromboxane A_2, prostacyclin), having very short half-lives, may be synthetized and metabolized *in vitro.* Their study therefore poses certain technical difficulties. The analytical tool chosen must fulfill criteria of high sensitivity, precision, reproducibility, specificity, and ease of adaptation to a wide range of biological media. In addition, the technique should be simple, so that large series of assays may be carried out easily. Of the various techniques which have been used, there are two which best fit the criteria discussed above:

(a) Mass spectrometry combined with gas chromatography (GC-MS), which is the more specific (8).

(b) Immunological assay using PG antiserum as specific binder, which is the more sensitive (3–5,11–13). In competition assays, the tracer is tritiated and is available commercially with a high specific activity (70–150 Ci/mmole). In some biological conditions, PG concentrations are too low and a more sensitive assay is desirable. A first attempt was made using PG covalently bound to bacteriophage T_4 as a tracer. This yielded a highly sensitive assay for $PGF_{2\alpha}$ ($\sim$ 1 pg), but the application to plasma was difficult due to nonspecific binding (1). Simultaneously, we developed a radioimmunoassay (RIA) using an iodinated derivative of PG.

RIA of PGs was first carried out in 1970 by Levine and Van Vunakis (13) to measure PGE_1 and $PGF_{2\alpha}$. Since then the number of RIAs for PGs, their metabolites and analogs, and thromboxanes and their derivatives has increased greatly and become highly diversified, both in terms of techniques for the production of antisera and radioactive tracers and in the separation of free from bound antigen. Successful assay depends upon several factors:

Preparation and selection of specific immune sera,

Preparation of radioactive tracers with high specific activity (iodinated tracers),

Method of extraction and purification of the sample analyzed,

Radioimmunological procedure (incubation, separation, measurement),

Validation of the assay, and

Increase in RIA sensitivity by structural modification of the substance assayed.

PREPARATION AND SELECTION OF IMMUNE SERA

Preparation of the Immunogen

To act as immunogens, PGs are covalently linked to an antigenic carrier. The chemical reaction selected must enable an adequate number of molecules to be bound to the carrier and maintain the structural integrity of the molecule (except for the group involved in the covalent bond with the antigenic carrier). In our experiments, we used bovine serum albumin (BSA) as the carrier; the free carboxyl function of the hapten, activated by a carbodiimide, forms a peptide bond with the free NH_2 groups of the antigenic carrier (4). Under our conditions (Table 1), in most experiments 15 to 20 moles PG were bound per mole BSA.

Immunization

Animals were administered the PG–BSA conjugate according to a method originally proposed by Vaitukaitis et al. (19). Each rabbit received 30 to 40 subcutaneous injections of the conjugate (about 200 μg) dissolved in 1 ml physiological buffered saline and emulsified in an equal volume of Freund's complete adjuvant. Five animals were immunized in each series. Booster injections, given 2 months after the primary injections, were carried out following the same schedule. Subsequent booster injections were given depending on the development of antibody titer. These subsequent booster injections, using smaller

TABLE 1. *Preparation of PG immunogen[a]*

	Reagent	Quantity (mg)	Volume (ml)	Medium	Reaction time
Step 1 (COOH activation)	PG + ^{3}H-PG +	10	10	Sodium carbonate	
	EDCl[b]	10		pH 5.5	1 hr
Step 2 (coupling)	+ BSA	20	10	Sodium carbonate pH 5.5	Overnight

[a] All reactions are carried out at room temperature. Conjugate is dialyzed against distilled water for 24 hr at +4°C. Number of PG residues per molecule of albumin is estimated on the basis of isotopic dilution.

[b] 1-Ethyl-3-(3-dimethyl-amino-propyl)-carbodiimide-HCl.

amounts of antigen, were carried out when the antibody titer fell from a maximum value. Animals were bled every 10 days after the fourth week of immunization.

Study of Binding Parameters

The course of the immune response may be followed by measuring the titer of the antiserum, defined as the dilution giving 50% binding of the radioactive tracer. When the titer of the serum was high enough, its sensitivity, affinity, and specificity were tested. The best bleedings were kept separately or pooled. They were stored either at +4°C after addition of 0.02% sodium azide or at −20°C after dilution in an equal volume of glycerol. Table 2 shows the specificity of certain selected antisera.

PREPARATION OF RADIOIODINATED TRACERS OF PGs

A PG derivative which was a substrate for iodination was first synthesized. In our experiments the sample was coupled to histamine (His) (in a few cases tyramine and tyrosine methyl ester were used) (6,14,17,18). A peptide bond was formed between the free NH_2 group of histamine and the free carboxyl group of PG (Table 3).

The chloramine T method, developed by Hunter and Greenwood (10) was used for iodination of PG–histamine derivatives (Table 4).

A comparison of the sensitivities obtained using tritiated tracers and iodinated tracers for certain antisera is given in Table 5. With the exception of the $PGF_{1\alpha}$ and $PGF_{2\alpha}$ assays, use of the iodinated tracer increased the sensitivity of the assay, as well as of the titer of the antiserum.

EXTRACTION AND PURIFICATION OF BIOLOGICAL SAMPLES

Sampling of biological fluids (blood, urine, amniotic fluid, etc.) or tissues should be carried out according to a standard procedure adapted for each biological medium. Biosynthesis and metabolism of PGs in the sample must be inhibited. In the case of urine, for example, each miction was collected in a clean vessel and immediately transferred to a bottle at 4°C containing meclofenamic acid. The total volume was measured after 24 hr and a fraction stored at −20°C.

Extraction

A 2-ml urine sample was pipetted into a centrifuge tube containing about 1,800 dpm of appropriate ^3H tracer for calculation of extraction recovery. After acidification to pH 3.5 with citric acid, the PGs were extracted from the sample with three volumes of a mixture of cyclohexane and ethyl acetate (1:1, v/v). After 15 min of vigorous shaking, and centrifugation at 250 × g, the organic

TABLE 2. Cross-reactions of PG antisera[a]

	Inhibitors									
Antiserum	E_1	E_2	$F_{1\alpha}$	$F_{2\alpha}$	DHK E_2	DHK $F_{2\alpha}$	TXB_2	6-K-$F_{1\alpha}$	19-OH-$F_{2\alpha}$	19-OH-E_2
E_1	100	15	0.2	<0.1	—	<0.1	—	—	—	—
E_2	3	100	<0.1	0.1	0.1	<0.1	—	—	—	—
$F_{1\alpha}$	0.1	<0.1	100	7	<0.1	<0.1	—	—	<0.1	<0.1
$F_{2\alpha}$	0.3	0.8	29	100	<0.1	4	—	—	<0.1	<0.1
DHK E_2	<0.5	<0.5	<0.5	<0.5	100	7	—	—	—	—
DHK $F_{2\alpha}$	<0.1	<0.1	<0.1	<0.1	<0.1	100	—	—	—	—
TXB_2	<0.1	<0.1	—	<0.1	<0.1	<0.1	100	—	<0.1	<0.1
6-K-$F_{1\alpha}$	6	2	18	11	—	0.3	<0.1	100	0.2	<0.1
19-OH-F_α	—	—	4	2	—	—	—	—	100	<0.1
19-OH-E	35	23	—	<0.2	—	—	—	—	—	100

[a] Cross-reactivities are calculated on the basis of the quantity (pg) necessary for 50% tracer displacement. DHK, 13,14-dihydro-15-keto.

TABLE 3. *Preparation of PG-His[a] derivative*

	Reagent	Quantity (μmole)	Volume (ml)	Medium	Reaction time
Step 1 (COOH activation)	PG + EDCI[b]	28.6 52	0.5	Ethanol/water (1:1, v/v)	1 hr
Step 2 (Coupling)	+ His + ^{3}H-His	90 (10 μCi)	0.5	Water	Overnight

[a] All reactions are carried out at room temperature. PG–His derivative is purified by TLC (silica gel) in *n*-butanol/acetic acid/water system (75:10:25, v/v). Concentration of PG–His is determined on the basis of isotopic dilution.
[b] 1-Ethyl-3-(3-dimethyl-amino-propyl)-carbodiimide-HCl.

phase was pipetted into a conical siliconized tube. The extraction was repeated, and the two extracts were pooled and evaporated to dryness under nitrogen. The extract was redissolved in 0.2 ml benzene/ethyl acetate/methanol (60:40:10, v/v) (solvent 1) and 0.8 ml benzene/ethyl acetate (60:40, v/v) (solvent 2).

Purification

The PGs were purified by passage over a silicic acid column: 500 mg silicic acid was equilibrated in 2 ml of solvent 2 and washed first with 5 ml benzene/ethyl acetate/methanol (60:40:20, v/v) (solvent 3) and then with 1.5 ml solvent 2. The extract was placed on the column and the PGs were eluted by three successive solvents:

Elution 1: 6 ml solvent 2 to extract the less polar lipids, pigments, PGA, PGB, and 13,14-dihydro-15-keto-PGE$_1$ and E$_2$.

TABLE 4. *Iodination procedure[a]*

Product	Volume (μl)	Concentration and buffer
PG–His	10	~ 1 nmole
Phosphate buffer	10	0.5 M, pH 7.4
Na[125]I	2	100 Ci/ml
Chloramine T	2	2.5 mg/ml in phosphate buffer

[a] Reaction time, 20 sec; stopped with sodium metabisulfite (32 μg). ^{125}I-PG–His is purified by TLC (silica gel) in chloroform/water (60:30:5, v/v). Radioactive spot is located by autoradiography, and iodinated product is eluted from silica gel by ethanol and stored at $-20°C$ until use.

TABLE 5. Sensitivities of PG antisera using tritiated and iodinated tracers

Tracer	Antisera							
	E_1	E_2	$F_{1\alpha}$	$F_{2\alpha}$	DHK E_2	DHK $F_{2\alpha}$	TXB_2	6-K-$F_{1\alpha}$
³H-PG								
Sensitivity[a]	32	5	15	3.5	54	8	14	94
Specific radioactivity (Ci/mmole)	90	117	79	178	66	85	125	20
Final dilution of antiserum	1/45,000	1/75,000	1/15,000	1/90,000	1/3,600	1/45,000	1/24,000	1/13,500
¹²⁵I-PG–His[b]								
Sensitivity	18	2.5	29	7	33	5	8	15
Final dilution antiserum	1/300,000	1/150,000	1/25,000	1/105,000	1/15,000	1/150,000	1/45,000	1/168,000

[a] Quantity of PG (pg) necessary to give 50% displacement of B_o; for all assays, the final dilution of the antiserum was adjusted to obtain 50–40% initial binding.

[b] Specific radioactivity of ¹²⁵I–labeled PG–His tracers was estimated to 2,000 Ci/mmole.

Elution 2: 13 ml solvent 4 (benzene/ethyl acetate/methanol, $60:40:2$, v/v) to extract PGE_1 and PGE_2 and also 13,14-dihydro-15-keto-$PGF_{1\alpha}$ and $F_{2\alpha}$.

Elution 3: 4 ml solvent 3 to extract PGs F_α and 19-OH-PGE and F.

Under these conditions, thromboxane B_2 (TXB_2) and 6-keto-$PGF_{1\alpha}$ were eluted in the last two waves. Each eluate was evaporated under nitrogen and redissolved in an adequate quantity of buffer for RIA. A portion was used to calculate recovery for the extraction and purification processes.

RADIOIMMUNOLOGICAL REACTION

The method varies depending on whether an iodinated or a tritiated tracer is used.

RIA Using a Tritiated Tracer

To 5-ml polystyrene tubes were added successively 0.1 ml tritiated tracer (about 7,500 dpm), 0.1 ml PG standard or biological extract, and 0.1 ml of a dilution of the antiserum such that the initial binding in the absence of standard or unknown PG is 40–50% of the total radioactivity. All the reagents were diluted in phosphate-buffered saline at pH 7.4, 0.1 M, 0.9% NaCl, 0.1% gelatin. The tubes were incubated overnight at 4°C. Separation of the free fraction from that bound to the antiserum was carried out at 0°C by the addition of 1 ml charcoal–dextran. After incubation for 12 min in a melting ice bath, the tubes were centrifuged for 15 min at $2,000 \times g$. The supernatant (bound fraction) was transferred to scintillation vials and counted in a liquid scintillation counter for 4 min. The standard curve was determined by plotting the log of the dose (pg/tube) on the abscissa against the value (%) of the ratio B/B_0 (B being the amount of radioactivity bound to the antibody) on the ordinate. The results were then calculated by computer.

RIA Using Iodinated Tracers

The technique is basically the same as for tritiated tracers, with the following modifications: 14,000 dpm iodinated tracer was added to each tube, and the buffer used contained 0.3% bovine gamma globulin instead of gelatin. Free and bound radioactivity was separated by adding 0.3 ml polyethylene glycol 6000 at 0°C to each tube (25 g/100 ml distilled water), mixing well, and centrifuging at +4°C for 15 min at $2,000 \times g$. The supernatant was decanted, and the pellet (the bound fraction) was counted for 1 min in a gamma counter.

STUDY OF THE VALIDITY OF THE ASSAY

The radioimmunological technique is based on competition for antibody sites between the radioactive tracer and the standard or endogenous PG. An inhibition of the binding of the tracer is measured, increasing with the amount of unlabeled PG present. It is essential to ensure that only those molecules for which the antiserum is specific are capable of entering into competition with the tracer, and also to ensure that no antibodylike substances are present in the biological sample being assayed. Various tests may be carried out to check the validity of the assay; these include addition of known amounts of standard PGs, inhibition and stimulation studies, and comparison with other analytical techniques [bioassay, GC-MS, thin-layer chromatography combined with incorporation of radioactive precursor (TLR) or high performance liquid chromatography combined with RIA (HPLC-RIA)].

Two examples are given here: comparison of the amounts of TXB_2 formed during platelet aggregation as measured by RIA, GC-MS, and TLR (14) and the assay for 6-keto-$PGF_{1\alpha}$, $PGF_{2\alpha}$, and PGE_2-like material in human urine using HPLC-RIA.

In the first case, RIA of TXB_2 was performed using ^{125}I-TXB_2–histamine and GC-MS analysis using a glass capillary column coupled to an LKB 2091 apparatus for mass spectroscopy. The determination of ^{14}C-TXB_2 was based on the method of Flower et al. (7). The data are shown in Table 6. Concordance of results using GC-MS and RIA for washed human platelets has allowed us to use RIA as a rapid screening test of TXB_2 synthesis in other biological materials. Although the TLR method is limited by its specificity (i.e., TLC resolution), the results shown here were in good accordance with the two other methods.

In the HPLC-RIA method, biological extracts, purified as described above,

TABLE 6. Amounts of TXB_2 formed during arachidonic acid-induced aggregation of washed human platelets as measured by RIA, GC-MS and TLR[a]

Sample	RIA	GC-MS	TLR
1	1.85	2.02	2.15
2	1.91	1.76	1.64
3	2.18	1.73	1.96
4	2.08	1.58	2.01
5	2.41	2.90	2.17
6	2.18	1.48	1.99
7	1.63	2.18	1.22
8[b]	0.027	0.04	UND[c]
9[b]	0.025	0.03	UND[c]

[a] TXB_2 data in μg/ml of ethanol extracts. Platelets, 0.5 ml 8×10^5 platelets/μl. Each value represents the mean of three separate determinations.
[b] Samples 8 and 9 were incubated in the presence of indomethacin (1.4×10^{-4} M).
[c] UND, undetected.

were injected onto a column of μBondapack C_{18} (Waters) with elution conditions allowing separation of several PGs and their derivatives (Fig. 1A). After collection of the eluates, the content of the tubes was evaporated and RIA was carried out on each. This procedure eliminated difficulties otherwise encountered due to cross-reacting antisera and demonstrated the presence of PG-like substances. Figure 1A shows the profile of 6-keto-PFG$_{1\alpha}$ equivalents assayed in human urine.

At least four products were assayed, of which one (retention time 7 to 8 min) corresponds to standard 6-keto-PGF$_{1\alpha}$. The three others, one of which was present in concentrations as high as those of 6-keto-PGF$_{1\alpha}$, have not thus far been identified. The existence of other chemical forms of 6-keto-PGF$_{1\alpha}$ such as the hemiketal proposed by several authors (9,16) may explain this. We have demonstrated that during the synthesis of the tracer ^{125}I-6-keto-PGF$_{1\alpha}$-His (13), there are two forms in equilibrium *(unpublished data)*. In the case of PGF$_{2\alpha}$, one major immunoreactive component was eluted from the HPLC column with the same retention time as the PGF$_{2\alpha}$ standard, whereas the PGE$_2$ immunoreactive component comigrated with the PGE$_2$ standard.

SENSITIZATION OF THE RIA BY STRUCTURAL MODIFICATION OF THE SUBSTANCE TO BE ASSAYED

The slope of the dose-response curves obtained in the RIA of PGE$_1$ using an iodinated tracer was less steep than that obtained with the tritiated tracer. This modification of affinity was brought about by the introduction of a peptide bond between the COOH group of the PG and the NH$_2$ of histamine, as can be demonstrated by the parallelism obtained using ^{3}H-PGE$_1$-His as tracer (Fig. 2). These results led to a study of the effects of blocking the COOH function on recognition by the antiserum. We proposed that the system could be rendered less heterologous by modifying the structure of the ligand so as to bring it closer to that of the tracer. With the COOH blocked by methylation by diazomethane, an increase in sensitivity of the RIA without significant modification of the specificity of the antisera was noted in several instances (15). An example of this is shown in Table 7.

COMMENTS

The PG-His are stable derivatives which are easily prepared and purified; iodination with Na^{125}I under classical conditions gives a monoiodinated derivative, the specific radioactivity of which can reach the theoretical maximum (i.e., 2,000 Ci/mmole) if an appropriate chromatographic procedure is adapted.

In some RIA systems, an increased sensitivity was obtained with iodinated tracers, although in others the sensitivity was better with the tritiated tracer. A possible explanation for this fact is that the structure of the iodinated tracer

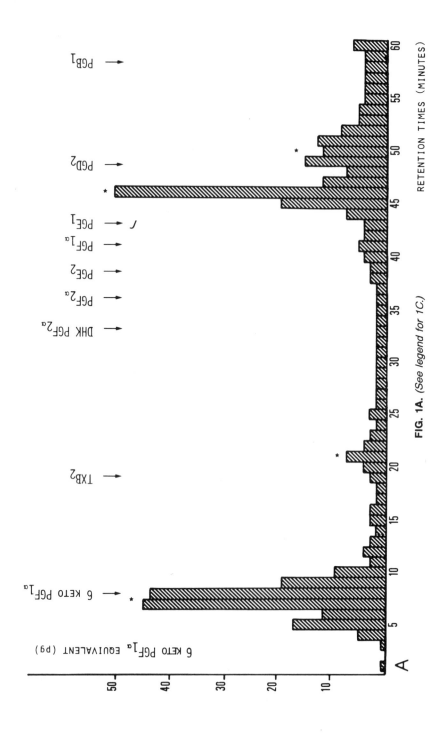

FIG. 1A. (See legend for 1C.)

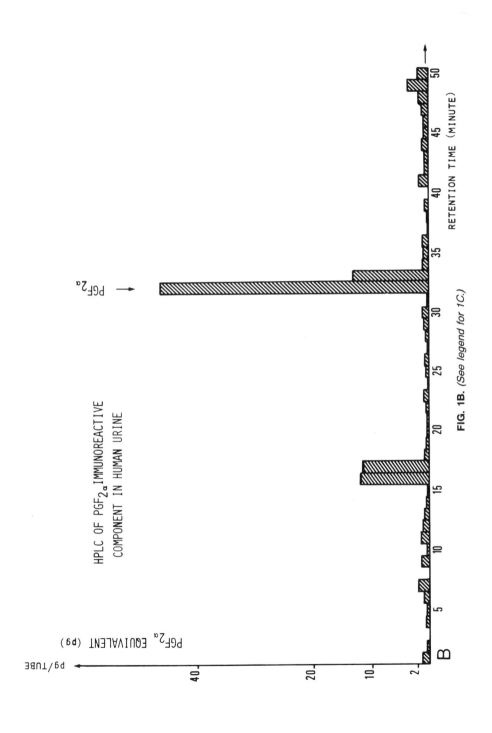

HPLC OF $PGF_{2\alpha}$ IMMUNOREACTIVE COMPONENT IN HUMAN URINE

FIG. 1B. (See legend for 1C.)

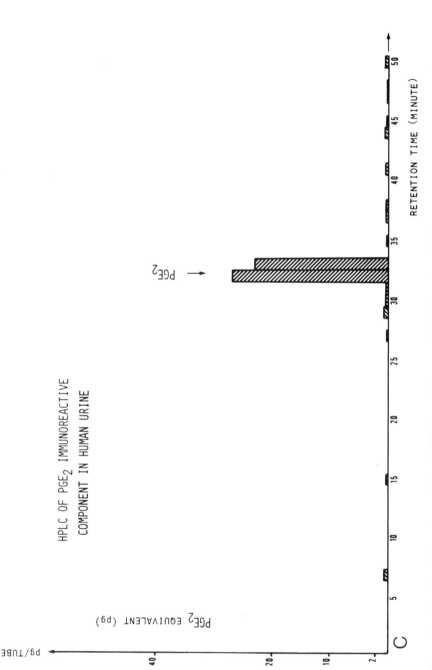

FIG. 1. Separation of various PGs and metabolites by HPLC applied to analysis of the 6-keto-PGF₁α (**A**), PGF₂α (**B**), and PGE₂ (**C**) immunoreactive component in human urine *(stars)*. Conditions: instrument, Waters Associates; packing, μBondapack C₁₈; column, 3.9 mm × 30 cm; flow rate, 1 ml/min; solvents A, acetonitrile/water (5:95, v/v), B, acetonitrile/water (95:5, v/v). Model 660 solvent programmer for 1 hr, curve 8. Starting solvent, 17% B in A; final solvent, 100% B.

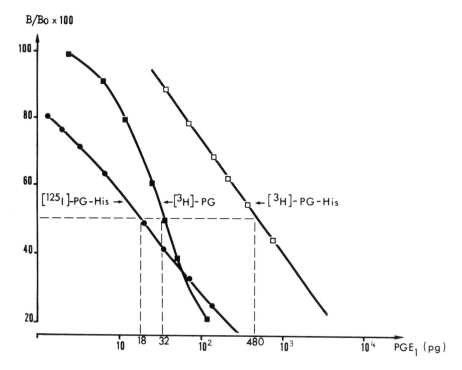

FIG. 2. Inhibition of the binding of various PGE_1 tracers to PGE_1 antiserum by unlabeled PGE_1.

may be close to that of the immunogen, and thus an endogenous substance is needed for competition. It appears that the iodinated RIA is greatly improved by the use of methylated, rather than standard PG as the competing ligand.

GC-MS is currently favored by most authors in the validation of radioimmunological methods. HPLC analysis combined with RIA can greatly contribute to validation by resolving the uncertainty caused by the use of antibodies with multiple specificities; we have here demonstrated its use in the revealing of some PG-like substances which compete for binding sites on anti-PG antisera.

TABLE 7. *Concentration of PG required (pmole/ml) to give 50% displacement of B_o using different tracers and inhibition*

Tracer/inhibitor	System					
	PGE_1	PGE_2	$PGF_{1\alpha}$	$PGF_{2\alpha}$	DHK PGE_2	DHK $PGF_{2\alpha}$
[125]I-labeled PG–His/PG	0.17	0.025	0.82	0.20	0.95	0.09
[125]I-labeled PG–His/PG–ME[a]	0.09	0.028	0.14	0.08	0.26	0.09

[a] ME, methyl ester.

REFERENCES

1. Andrieu, J. M., Mamas, S., and Dray, F. (1974): *Prostaglandins,* 6:15–22.
2. Bergström, S., Ryhage, R., Samuelsson, B., and Sjovall, J. (1963): *J. Biol. Chem.,* 238:3555–3558.
3. Caldwell, B. V., Burstein, S., Brock, W. A., and Speroff, L. (1971): *J. Clin. Endocrinol. Metab.,* 33:171–175.
4. Dray, F., Charbonnel, B., and Maclouf, J. (1975): *Eur. J. Clin. Invest.,* 5:311–318.
5. Dray, F., Maron, E., Tillson, S. A., and Sela, M. (1972): *Anal. Biochem.,* 50:399–408.
6. Dray, F., Pradelles, P., Maclouf, J., Sors, H., and Bringuier, A. (1978): Presentation at Winter Prostaglandin Conference, Sarasota, Florida, January 28–31.
7. Flower, R. J., Chering, M. S., and Cushman, D. W. (1973): *Prostaglandins,* 4:325–329.
8. Green, K. (1973): *Adv. Biosci.,* 9:91–108.
9. Hawkins, H. J., Smith, J. B., Nicolaou, K. C., and Eling, T. E. (1978): *Prostaglandins,* 16:871–884.
10. Hunter, W. N., and Greenwood, F. C. (1962): *Nature,* 194:495–496.
11. Jaffe, B. M., Smith, J. W., Newton, W. T., and Parker, C. W. (1971): *Science,* 171:494–496.
12. Kirton, K. T., Cornette, J. C., and Barre, K. L. (1972): *Biochem. Biophys. Res. Commun.,* 47:903–909.
13. Levine, L., and Van Vunakis, H. (1970): *Biochem. Biophys. Res. Commun.,* 41:1171–1177.
14. Maclouf, J., Pradel, M., Pradelles, P., and Dray, F. (1976): *Biochem. Biophys. Acta,* 431:139–146.
15. Maclouf, J., Sors, H., Pradelles, P., and Dray, F. (1978): *Anal. Biochem.,* 87:169–176.
16. Pace-Asciak, C. (1976): *J. Am. Chem. Soc.,* 98:2348–2349.
17. Sors, H., Maclouf, J., Pradelles, P., and Dray, F. (1977): *Biochim. Biophys. Acta,* 486:553–564.
18. Sors, H., Pradelles, P., Dray, F., Rigaud, M., Maclouf, J., and Bernard, P. (1978): *Prostaglandins,* 16:277–290.
19. Vaitukaitis, J., Robbins, J. B., Nieschlag, E., and Ross, T. (1971): *J. Clin. Endocrinol.,* 33:988–990.

Advances in Prostaglandin and Thromboxane Research,
Vol. 6, edited by B. Samuelsson, P. W. Ramwell,
and R. Paoletti. Raven Press, New York © 1980.

Radioimmunologic Determination of 15-Keto-13,14-Dihydro-PGE$_2$: A Method for Its Stable Degradation Product, 11-Deoxy-15-Keto-13, 14-Dihydro-11β,16-Cyclo-PGE$_2$

Elisabeth Granström and *Hans Kindahl

*Department of Chemistry, Karolinska Institute, S-104 01 Stockholm 60; and *Department of Obstetrics and Gynecology, Swedish University of Agricultural Sciences, S-750 07 Uppsala, Sweden*

Very few assay methods have been developed for the major circulating metabolite of prostaglandin E$_2$ (PGE$_2$), 15-keto-13,14-dihydro-PGE$_2$, and little information on concentrations of this compound in biologic material is available (2–4,6–9). The reason is probably the instability of this metabolite in aqueous media, which seriously affects particularly radioimmunoassays for the compound.

EXPERIMENTAL AND RESULTS

The half-life and various fates of 15-keto-13,14-dihydro-PGE$_2$ were studied in different environments. A major degradation product was identified as 11-deoxy-13,14-dihydro-15-keto-11β,16-cyclo-PGE$_2$ (Fig. 1; see also refs. 1 and 5), which was rapidly formed at alkaline pH by dehydration of the β-ketol system in the ring and subsequent immediate cyclization. This compound also seemed to be the ultimate degradation product of the PGE$_2$ metabolite in water and alcoholic solutions. The half-life of 15-keto-dihydro-PGE$_2$ was about 3 days in room temperature at pH 7.4.

In plasma, the fate of 15-keto-13,14-dihydro-PGE$_2$ was somewhat different. Its half-life was considerably shorter (about 8 hr at room temperature), and after complete degradation, only about 50% could be identified as the bicyclic product. The remainder was covalently bound to proteins, mainly albumin. Blocking of sulfhydryl groups did not prevent this binding to proteins.

Since it was difficult to prevent degradation of 15-keto-13,14-dihydro-PGE$_2$, the opposite solution of the assay problem was chosen instead; a radioimmunoassay was developed for the bicyclic degradation product and used for measurements of 15-keto-dihydro-PGE$_2$ after it had been completely converted into this product. The lower limit of detection of the assay was 12 pg, and the

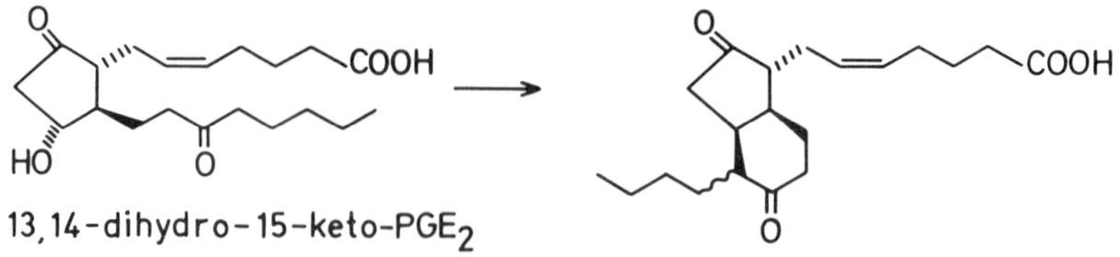

13,14-dihydro-15-keto-PGE₂

11-deoxy-13,14-dihydro-15-keto-
-11ß,16 ξ - cyclo-PGE₂

FIG. 1. Structure of the major degradation product of 15-keto-13,14-dihydro-PGE₂.

antibody was very specific for the hapten, cross-reacting less than 0.1% with all common PGs and their metabolites. An exception was 15-keto-13,14-dihydro-PGE₂ itself. The antibody showed an apparent cross-reaction of 6% with this compound. However, most of this was probably caused by formation of the bicyclic derivative during the assay.

The assay could not be used for unextracted plasma samples. Albumin seriously affected the assay, due to the covalent binding of the compound, as mentioned above. Standard curves run in buffer differed considerably from those run in plasma or albumin. Thus prior to assay, plasma samples had to be extracted and purified on microcolumns of silicic acid before conversion of the 15-keto-dihydro metabolite into the bicyclic degradation product.

The assay was used for determination of elevated 15-keto-dihydro-PGE₂ levels during intravenous infusion of PGE₂ in sheep and of decreased metabolite levels during aspirin treatment in man. Samples that did not contain proteins or could be strongly diluted prior to assay did not have to be extracted: thus direct radioimmunoassay (after conversion into the bicyclic product) was performed on perfusates from guinea pig lung before, during, and after perfusion with PGE₂ and on lymph from the hindleg of rabbits after scalding injury to the paw.

ACKNOWLEDGMENT

This study was supported by grants from the World Health Organization.

REFERENCES

1. Beal, R. F., Babcock, J. C., and Lincoln, F. H. (1967): In: *Prostaglandins. Nobel Symposium 2*, edited by S. Bergström and B. Samuelsson, pp. 219–230. Almqvist and Wiksell, Uppsala, Sweden.
2. Gréen, K., and Granström, E. (1973): In: *Prostaglandins in Fertility Control*, Vol. 3, edited by S. Bergström, pp. 55–61. Karolinska Institutet, Stockholm.
3. Hubbard, W. C., and Watson, J. T. (1976): *Prostaglandins*, 12:21–35.
4. Levine, L. (1977): *Prostaglandins*, 14:1125–1139.
5. Lincoln, F. H., Schneider, W. P., and Pike, J. E. (1973): *J. Org. Chem.*, 38:951–956.
6. Mitchell, M. D., Sors, H., and Flint, A. P. F. (1977): *Lancet*, 2:558.
7. Peskar, B. A., Holland, A., and Peskar, B. M. (1974): *FEBS Lett.*, 43:45–48.
8. Samuelsson, B., and Gréen, K. (1974): *Biochem. Med.*, 11:298–303.
9. Tashjian, A. H., Jr., Voelkel, E. F., and Levine, L. (1977): *Prostaglandins*, 14:309–317.

Advances in Prostaglandin and Thromboxane Research,
Vol. 6, edited by B. Samuelsson, P. W. Ramwell,
and R. Paoletti. Raven Press, New York © 1980.

Radioimmunoassay for 13,14-Dihydro,15-Keto-Prostaglandin E_2 in Human Plasma: Applications and Artifacts

Stewart A. Metz, Maureen G. Rice, and R. Paul Robertson

Division of Clinical Pharmacology, Veterans Administration Medical Center,
Seattle, Washington 98108, U.S.A.

Radioimmunoassays (RIAs) for prostaglandin E (PGE) are inherently limited by the short half-life of PGE *in vivo,* thus making a single plasma sample a poor indicator of PGE synthesis. Furthermore, plasma levels can be spuriously elevated by generation of PGE by blood elements during collection or storage of samples. It has been anticipated that measurement of 13,14-dihydro,15-keto-PGE_2 (DHK-PGE_2), the major circulating metabolite of PGE_2, would obviate these problems, since its half-life is considerably longer than that of PGE_2, and it is not expected that this metabolite would be generated *in vitro.* We report herein our experience using a RIA for DHK-PGE_2, emphasizing the features of the sensitivity, specificity, and clinical applicability of this method.

METHODS

The RIA system is essentially that as originally described by Levine (1), who generously provided us with the antiserum directed against DHK-PGE_2. The specificity of this antiserum has been previously characterized (1). In our hands, $100 \pm 4\%$ ($\bar{x} \pm$ SE) of added DHK-PGE_2 standard is recovered from plasma samples. The assay sensitivity is 10 pg/tube; 500 λ of unextracted human plasma is routinely used in the assay. *In vivo* studies were performed in normal male volunteers. Blood samples were obtained via an indwelling catheter, placed in prechilled glass tubes containing ethylenediaminetetraacetic acid (EDTA), quickly centrifuged, and stored at $-20°C$; the samples were measured by the RIA within 2 weeks. For studies of the effect of clotting, aliquots of blood samples from eight normal volunteers were placed either into chilled EDTA tubes or into tubes lacking anticoagulant so that the sample was allowed to clot at room temperature. Hemolysis was induced in other aliquots of anticoagulated blood by vigorous shaking or addition of distilled water. The effect of storage was studied by measuring DHK-PGE_2 levels in human plasma which had been stored at $-20°C$ for a variable duration.

RESULTS

During 60 to 75-min infusions of PGE_2, increments of DHK-PGE_2 could be detected in plasma within 5 min and reached peak levels of approximately 100 times (0.03 $\mu g/kg/min$ of PGE_2 infused) or 500 times (0.15–0.30 $\mu g/kg/min$) base-line values. In one of the low-dose studies, plasma PGE levels were measured, and no increments were detectable. After discontinuation of the high-dose infusion, metabolite levels declined with an approximate half-life of 16 min.

Since adrenergic stimulation has been reported to stimulate PGE synthesis in animals, we examined the effects of epinephrine infusions (6 $\mu g/min \times 2$ hr) in six normal subjects. DHK-PGE_2 levels rose from apparent basal values of 54 ± 17 pg/ml to a peak of 236 ± 43 pg/ml ($p < 0.02$) during the first 60 min of the infusion but then declined toward base-line despite continuation of the infusion. Basal and stimulated i-DHK-PGE_2 values correlated closely with basal ($r = 0.51$; $p < 0.01$) or stimulated ($r = 0.73$, $p < 0.001$) levels of free fatty acid (FFA) during the epinephrine infusions, suggesting that a significant portion of basal and stimulated DHK-PGE_2 immunoreactivity was a result of interference by the high molar concentration of FFA in plasma. This formulation was further supported by virtual obliteration of the epinephrine-induced rise in both FFA and DHK-PGE_2 by pretreatment with any of three antilipolytic substances (sodium salicylate, propranolol, or nicotinic acid). In contrast, indomethacin did not modify rises in either FFA or "DHK-PGE_2." Dilutions of plasma containing high levels of FFA and "DHK-PGE_2" induced by epinephrine caused a displacement curve which was not parallel to the standard curve, suggesting that the assay was not measuring true DHK-PGE_2 in these samples. Furthermore, solutions of oleic acid bound to albumin displaced tracer in the RIA and thus were "read" as DHK-PGE_2.

In samples from eight subjects, clotting caused a marked increase of apparent DHK-PGE_2 (plasma, 52 ± 16; serum, 5,795 ± 1,219 pg/ml). DHK-PGE_2 immunoreactivity increased linearly with time in normal human plasma during storage ($r = 0.92$). Displacement curves using serial dilutions of such stored or clotted human blood samples revealed nonparallelism with the standard curve but resembled that seen using plasma rich in FFA. Hemolysis did not increase DHK-PGE_2 levels.

DISCUSSION

This RIA for DHK-PGE_2 in unextracted human plasma is capable of detecting 500-fold increases in DHK-PGE_2 levels during a PGE_2 infusion when one would expect at most two- to threefold increments in venous PGE levels (2). The augmented sensitivity of this method compared to that of PGE_2 measurements was also seen in studies of the PGE_2-producing VX_2 tumor by Tashjian et al. (3).

However, there are important limitations to this method. The expected increase in DHK-PGE$_2$ levels during epinephrine and its blockade by a PG synthesis inhibitor (sodium salicylate) or by propranolol could have been interpreted to mean that beta-adrenergic stimulation augments PGE$_2$ synthesis in man. However, several subsequent studies all support the concept that changes in FFA levels *in vivo* interfere in the RIA due to cross-reaction of fatty acids with the antiserum or displacement by FFA of DHK-PGE$_2$ bound to albumin. The presence of an analogous artifact induced by clotting and storage of samples suggests that fatty acids are released from platelet or white cell membrane phospholipids *in vitro* and lead to spurious increments in DHK-PGE$_2$ levels. Since many disease states (e.g., stress) and drugs (e.g., salicylates) not only may affect rates of PGE synthesis, but may also concomitantly alter circulating FFA levels, it is apparent that these artifacts present a major problem in the application of this method to studies of physiologic responses or pathologic states. Further purification of samples to exclude FFA is clearly needed for this and possibly other RIAs for PG metabolites, which currently use unextracted human plasma. However, such refinement should allow DHK-PGE$_2$ measurements by RIA to serve as a markedly improved clinical and research tool.

ACKNOWLEDGMENTS

We thank Dr. Lawrence Levine for his help and generous supply of antiserum. The work was supported by the Veterans Administration.

REFERENCES

1. Levine, L. (1977): *Prostaglandins,* 14:1125–1139.
2. Robertson, R. P., and Chen, M. (1977): *Trans. Assoc. Am. Phys.,* 90:353–365.
3. Tashjian, A. H., Jr., Voelkel, E. F., and Levine, L. (1977): *Prostaglandins,* 14:309–317.

Advances in Prostaglandin and Thromboxane Research,
Vol. 6, edited by B. Samuelsson, P. W. Ramwell,
and R. Paoletti. Raven Press, New York © 1980.

Radioimmunoassay of Serum Thromboxane B_2: A Simple Method of Assessing Pharmacologic Effects on Platelet Function

C. Patrono, G. Ciabattoni, F. Pugliese, E. Pinca, G. Castrucci, A. De Salvo, M. A. Satta, and M. Parachini

Department of Pharmacology, Catholic University, 00168 Rome, Italy

A variety of methods are currently employed to evaluate the effects of drugs on human platelet function. These include a graphic recording of platelet aggregation (8) measurement of cyclooxygenase products—prostaglandins (PGs) and/or thromboxanes (TXs)—in platelet-rich plasma (PRP), in superfusates of isolated platelets or in incubates of platelet microsomes (6,10,12), and indirect measurement of unacetylated platelet cyclooxygenase (2). Although all these methods can provide pharmacologically as well as clinically relevant information, they suffer from one or more of the following limitations: (a) they require a relatively large volume of blood; (b) they remove platelets from their physiologic milieu, i.e., whole blood; (c) they generally assess the inhibition of a measured parameter of platelet function in response to variable concentrations of a variety of exogenously added stimuli; (d) they may require lengthy and sophisticated techniques.

In an attempt to overcome these limitations, we have developed a relatively simple method, based on two well-known observations: (a) when whole blood is allowed to clot, prothrombin is activated to thrombin, within minutes, thereby initiating platelet aggregation and secretion; (b) aggregation of washed human platelets by thrombin is accompanied by release of large amounts of arachidonic acid metabolites, the main products originating via the cyclooxygenase pathway being TXB_2 and hydroxyheptadecatrienoic acid (HHT) (4).

The method is described in detail elsewhere (11). Essentially, it exploits the generation of endogenous thrombin, occurring during the clotting of whole blood at 37°C, and the subsequent release of platelet TXB_2. This release is a time- and temperature-dependent process, which can be monitored by a direct radioimmunoassay (RIA) of the separated serum TXB_2 concentrations. Figure 1 depicts the standard curve of the assay, and Table 1 lists the immunologic specificity of the anti-TXB_2 serum. Both the time course of TXB_2 release and the total amount released can be assessed by letting multiple 1-ml aliquots of the same blood sample clot simultaneously and separating the serum at varying intervals. However, in order to evaluate the effects of drugs on this process, a standard

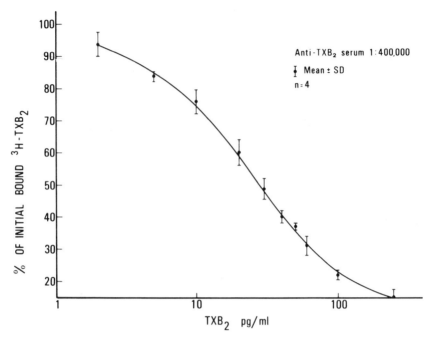

FIG. 1. Standard curve for TXB₂. ³H-TXB₂ (New England Nuclear: 150 Ci/mmole, 10,000 dpm) and anti-TXB₂ serum were appropriately diluted in order to obtain a 45% binding after 16 hr of incubation at 4°C, in the absence of unlabeled TXB₂. The percent change in initial binding is plotted as a function of the concentration of unlabeled TXB₂. Each point represents the mean ± SD of values found in four successive assays.

TABLE 1. *Immunological specificity of anti-TXB₂ serum*

Substance measured	IC_{50}[a] (ng/ml)	Relative cross-reaction (%)
TXB₂	0.05	100
PGD₂	5	1.0
6-keto-PGF₁α	16	0.31
PGF₂β	24	0.21
PGE₂	27	0.19
PGF₂α	33	0.15
PGA₂	1,400	0.004
13,14DH-15K-PGF₂α [b]	2,100	0.002
13,14DH-15K-PGE₂ [b]	5,200	0.001

[a] Concentration required to displace 50% of bound ³H-TXB₂.

[b] 13,14-Dihydro-15-keto-PGF₂α and -PGE₂.

TABLE 2. *Serum TXB$_2$ concentrations measured after clotting multiple 1-ml aliquots of the same blood sample in the presence of antiplatelet drugs*[a]

Drug	TXB$_2$ concentration (ng) at dose (μg/ml) of					
	0	0.5	2	10	50	100
Vehicle	298 ± 7					
Aspirin		54 ± 3	5.4 ± 2	0.8 ± 0.09		
Diflunisal				157 ± 14	76 ± 2	36 ± 1
Dipyridamole				209 ± 6	209 ± 19	138 ± 5

[a] Values are means ± SD.

30-min interval can be employed, thus allowing serum TXB$_2$ concentration to reach a plateau. The same method can be used for *in vitro* and *ex vivo* drug evaluation. In the former case, a single 30-ml blood sample is drawn and 1-ml aliquots are transferred into glass tubes containing varying concentrations of the drug(s) to be tested or the vehicle alone. This allows three drugs to be compared at three dose levels, in triplicate. One such experiment comparing the inhibitory effects of aspirin, diflunisal, and dipyridamole is reported in Table 2. A distinct advantage of this method over other *in vitro* assays for platelet cyclooxygenase inhibitors such as the use of platelet microsomes or superfused platelets is provided by its inherent integration of enzyme inhibitory potency with variable protein binding of different drugs. It was earlier shown by Gryglewski (3) that such integration can more closely relate the *in vitro* potency estimates to the *in vivo* situation.

For *ex vivo* drug evaluation, 1–3-ml blood samples are drawn before and 1, 2, 3, 4, 6, and 24 hr after a single oral dose and allowed to clot for 30 min. Figure 2 depicts the inhibitory effects of dipyridamole, L 8027, sulfinpyrazone, and aspirin on platelet TXB$_2$ production as assessed on separate occasions in the same healthy volunteer. Besides showing the variable potency pattern and duration of the inhibitory effect of the different drugs, the data presented indicate a high degree of intra-assay and interassay reproducibility (coefficient of variation: 10 and 17%, respectively) of the biologic response measured. In contrast with the other three drugs, a single 75-mg dose of dipyridamole caused no statistically significant changes of serum TXB$_2$ concentrations. This might suggest that such a dose produces blood levels of dipyridamole lower than those required to reduce serum TXB$_2$ when added *in vitro* (see Table 2) or to obtain a disaggregating effect when locally infused in the venous blood of rabbits (7). Previously reported discrepancies between *in vitro* and *in vivo* effects of this drug are reviewed by Packham and Mustard (9).

Measurement of serum PGE$_2$ concentrations by means of a specific RIA revealed that at the single dosage tested, L 8027 behaves as a cyclooxygenase, rather than TX-synthetase inhibitor, in that it reduced serum PGE$_2$ and TXB$_2$ concentrations to a similar extent. Aspirin stands as a unique drug in causing

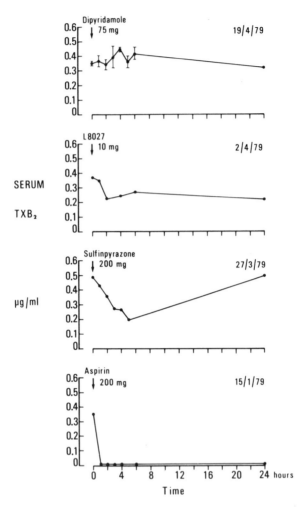

FIG. 2. Time course for the inhibitory effect of a single oral dose of dipyridamole (75 mg), L 8027 (10 mg), sulfinpyrazone (200 mg), and aspirin (200 mg) on TXB₂ formation during whole blood clotting. All studies were performed on the same healthy man (34 years old) on different dates. In the dipyridamole study, each point represents the mean of triplicate 1-ml aliquots of the same blood sample; bars represent one SD from the mean.

a complete and long-lasting suppression of platelet TXB₂ production. We have recently characterized the time and dose dependence of the inhibitory effect of oral aspirin in healthy subjects (11). Our data indicate that a single oral dose of 2 mg/kg given every 72 hr is adequate to maintain a constant inhibition of platelet TXB₂ production ≥ 90% and suggest that such a therapeutic regimen might represent a more rational approach to its use as an antithrombotic agent (11). Burch et al. (1) have recently demonstrated that a daily 160-mg aspirin dose is indeed an effective antithrombotic regimen in patients who had arterio-venous shunts for chronic dialysis. In view of the recent report of Jaffe and Weksler (5) that human endothelial cell cyclooxygenase is as sensitive to aspirin as the enzyme in platelets, the intermittent regimen that we have proposed, by exploiting the different rate of recovery of endothelial PGI_2 versus platelet TXA_2 synthesis, might represent the only way to produce a selective inhibition of platelet function with but a transient disturbance of endothelial function.

In conclusion, RIA of serum TXB_2 appears to represent a valuable and rela-tively simple tool to study the clinical pharmacology of antiplatelet drugs.

ACKNOWLEDGMENTS

We are indebted to Dr. B. A. Peskar for considerable help and advice in the development of the RIA for TXB_2 and to Dr. J. E. Pike (Upjohn Company) for several gifts of TXB_2. This study was supported in part by a C.N.R. grant (Progetto Finalizzato Tecnologie Biomediche, Subprogetto CHIM-2).

REFERENCES

1. Burch J. W., Harter H., Stanford N., Delmez J., and Majerus P. W. (1979): *Clin. Res.,* 27:509A.
2. Burch J. W., Stanford N., and Majerus P. W. (1978): *J. Clin. Invest.,* 61:314–319.
3. Gryglewski R. J. (1974): In: *Prostaglandin Synthetase Inhibitors,* edited by H. J. Robinson and J. R. Vane, pp. 33–52. Raven Press, New York.
4. Hamberg M., Svensson J., and Samuelsson B. (1974): *Proc. Natl. Acad. Sci. USA,* 71:3824–3828.
5. Jaffe E. A., and Weksler B. B. (1979): *J. Clin. Invest.,* 63:532–535.
6. Kocsis J. J., Hernandovich J., Silver M. J., Smith J. B., and Ingerman C. (1973): *Prostaglandins,* 3:141–144.
7. Moncada S., and Korbut R. (1978): *Lancet,* 1:1286–1289.
8. O'Brien J. R. (1968): *Lancet,* 1:779–783.
9. Packham M. A., and Mustard J. F. (1977): *Blood,* 50:555–573.
10. Patrono C., Ciabattoni G., and Grossi-Belloni D. (1975): *Prostaglandins,* 9:557–568.
11. Patrono C., Ciabattoni G., Pinca E., Pugliese F., Castrucci G., De Salvo A., Satta M. A., and Peskar B. A. (1980): *Thromb. Res. (in press).*
12. Smith J.B., and Willis A. L. (1971): *Nature [New Biol.,]* 231:235–237.

Advances in Prostaglandin and Thromboxane Research,
Vol. 6, edited by B. Samuelsson, P. W. Ramwell,
and R. Paoletti. Raven Press, New York © 1980.

A Radioimmunoassay for 6-Keto-Prostaglandin $F_{1\alpha}$

Laurence M. Demers and Dennis D. Derck

*Department of Pathology, Milton S. Hershey Medical Center, Pennsylvania State University,
Hershey, Pennsylvania 17033*

Radioimmunoassays (RIAs) for the primary prostaglandins PGE and PGF (1) and their 13,14-dihydro,15-keto metabolites have been developed and used to determine blood, urine, and tissue levels under various physiological and pathological conditions (4). With the recent discovery of prostacyclin (PGI_2), the newest member of the PG class of compounds, considerable information is already available on blood and tissue levels under various physiological and pathological conditions (5). The bulk of our information on PGI_2 stems from bioassay methodology using the rat stomach strip and bovine coronary artery preparations as described by Vane and colleagues (3). PGI_2 formation is rapidly followed within minutes by chemical breakdown to 6-keto-$PGF_{1\alpha}$. Direct measurements of PGI_2 in blood or tissues is virtually impossible due to its instability. Thus measurements of 6-keto-$PGF_{1\alpha}$, the principal metabolite of PGI_2, is necessary in order to assess meaningful changes in PGI_2 metabolism and turnover.

This chapter describes the development and evaluation of a radioimmunoassay for 6-keto-$PGF_{1\alpha}$ in blood and urine and its preliminary application in cancer patients.

EXPERIMENTS AND RESULTS

Antibody Preparation

The 6-keto-$PGF_{1\alpha}$ antibody was developed in rabbits using an immunogen prepared by coupling bovine serum albumin to 6-keto-$PGF_{1\alpha}$ using the standard carbodiimide coupling technique (1). Suitable antibody with appropriate titer (generally 1:1,500) for radioimmunoassay was obtained within 3 months of initial injection. Antibodies prepared against the 6-keto-$PGF_{1\alpha}$–albumin conjugate showed minimal cross-reactivity with potentially interfering substances (Table 1).

TABLE 1. *Specificity of 6-keto-PGF$_{1\alpha}$ antiserum*

Compound	Relative cross-reaction (%)
6-keto-PGF$_{1\alpha}$	100.0
PGF$_{2\alpha}$	4.53
PGE$_1$	2.87
PGE$_2$	2.34
PGA$_1$	0.11
15-keto-PGE$_2$	0.03
PGA$_2$	0.03
13,14-Dihydro,15-keto PGF$_{2\alpha}$	0.02
13,14-Dihydro,15-keto PGE$_2$	0.02
15-keto-PGE$_1$	0.01

Radiolabeled 6-Keto PGF$_{1\alpha}$

Tritium-labeled 6-keto-[9-^{3}H] PGF$_{1\alpha}$ was custom prepared for us by the Amersham Corporation from [9-^{3}H] PGF$_{2\alpha}$ methyl ester. Treatment of the PGF$_{2\alpha}$ methyl ester with iodine and sodium bicarbonate yielded a 5-iodo-9-deoxy-6,9-epoxy-PGF$_{1\alpha}$ methyl ester which was treated with base to give [9-^{3}H] PGI$_2$. Reaction of the PGI$_2$ with acid yielded the 6-keto-[9-^{3}H] PGF$_{1\alpha}$, which was purified by thin-layer chromatography. The material had 98% radiochemical purity following chromatography on silica gel with a chloroform: methanol: acetic acid: water (90:9:1:0.65) solvent system. The purified labeled compound obtained had a specific activity of 5.9 Ci/mmole.

STANDARD CURVE AND SAMPLE ANALYSIS

Extraction and preparation of samples for 6-keto-PGF$_{1\alpha}$ radioimmunoassay are essentially the same as for conventional PG radioimmunoassay (1). Samples with trace added for recovery estimations are extracted into ethyl acetate and then subjected to silicic acid chromatography for partial purification and separation from free fatty acids and other potential interfering substances. When the assay was performed with simple extraction without the liquid chromatography step, nonspecific interference was consistently noted, differing from sample to sample and yielding high, spurious results. Thus a liquid column chromatography step is recommended prior to radioimmunoassay. In our procedure, the silicic acid column was first equilibrated with benzene: ethyl acetate (60:40). The sample is then added to the column in a benzene: ethyl acetate: methanol (60:40:10) mixture. Benzene (1 ml) was then put on the column to remove the free fatty acids and other lipids. This was followed by 6 ml of a benzene: ethyl acetate (60:40) solvent system, which was discarded. Collection of the 6-keto-PGF$_{1\alpha}$ fraction was then achieved by putting 12 ml of a benzene: ethyl acetate: methanol (60:40:20) mixture on the column which eluted the 6-keto-PGF$_{1\alpha}$. Recovery

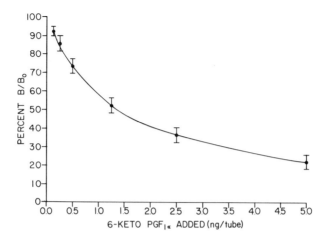

FIG. 1. Reproducibility of standard curves for 6-keto-PGF$_{1\alpha}$. Each point represents the mean and SD of B/B_0 for six standard curves.

following extraction and column chromatography averaged 71%. The collection was dried down at this point under a gentle stream of nitrogen and reconstituted in 1 ml of ethanol. Aliquots were taken for recovery analysis and radioimmunoassay. The radioimmunoassay was performed with a standard curve ranging from 100 pg to 5 ng of 6-keto-PGF$_{1\alpha}$ per tube. Standard curve reproducibility over six assays had a mean coefficient of variation of 6.61%. Reproducibility results from six standard curves are shown in Fig. 1. A typical 6-keto-PGF$_{1\alpha}$ radioimmunoassay protocol is shown in Fig. 2. Separation of antibody bound from free 6-keto-PFG$_{1\alpha}$ was achieved with dextran-coated charcoal and the bound fraction counted on a Searle Delta 300 liquid scintillation counter. The standard curve was plotted and unknowns calculated using Logit transformation of B/B_0 on a Hewlett-Packard 9831 programable desk-top calculator. A typical standard curve is plotted as B/B_0 before and after Logit transformation as shown in Fig. 3.

Precision studies were performed on four pools for within assay and between-assay reproducibility. These results are shown in Table 2. Intraassay precision data were based on performing 10 replicates of controls A and B within the same assay. Interassay precision was based on performing in duplicate controls C and D over 10 separate assays.

Analytical recovery studies with the 6-keto-PGF$_{1\alpha}$ radioimmunoassay were performed as shown in Fig. 4. Additions of 6-keto-PGF$_{1\alpha}$ in concentrations ranging from 125 to 2,500 pg per tube were made to a human serum pool and the radioimmunoassay performed on each sample. Excellent recovery (91.7%) was obtained, with a correlation of 0.994.

Parallelism results obtained with the serum 6-keto-PGF$_{1\alpha}$ radioimmunoassay are shown in Fig. 5. Over the concentration range investigated in this study,

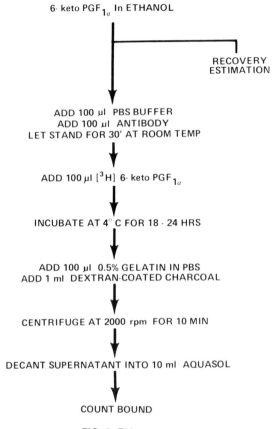

6- keto PGF₁ₐ In ETHANOL

RECOVERY
ESTIMATION

ADD 100 μl PBS BUFFER
ADD 100 μl ANTIBODY
LET STAND FOR 30' AT ROOM TEMP

ADD 100 μl [³H] 6- keto PGF₁ₐ

INCUBATE AT 4° C FOR 18 - 24 HRS

ADD 100 μl 0.5% GELATIN IN PBS
ADD 1 ml DEXTRAN-COATED CHARCOAL

CENTRIFUGE AT 2000 rpm FOR 10 MIN

DECANT SUPERNATANT INTO 10 ml AQUASOL

COUNT BOUND

FIG. 2. RIA protocol.

using volumes of ethanolic extract ranging from 25 to 400 μl, excellent parallelism was achieved with an intercept of −0.03 ng/tube and a slope of 1.03. Considering the wide range of 6-keto-$PGF_{1\alpha}$ levels present in blood, dilutions can be approximately made without appreciable loss in accuracy.

Although several clinical studies using this assay are under way, we have recently applied the assay to determine blood levels of 6-keto-$PGF_{1\alpha}$ in a cancer population (2). In a population of 80 control subjects considered free of disease by clinical and laboratory criteria, the blood 6-keto-$PGF_{1\alpha}$ levels by RIA were consistently less than 125 pg/ml. In a cancer population with various type malignancies (carcinoma of the lung, breast and colon, lymphoma, sarcoma), the 6-keto-$PGF_{1\alpha}$ levels ranged from a low of 77 pg/ml to a high of over 6,000 pg/ml. Tumors are often extremely vascular, and since PGI_2 is synthesized by vascular endothelium, it is not totally surprising to see elevated levels of this PGI_2 metabolite in the blood of solid tumor cancer patients. Whether this

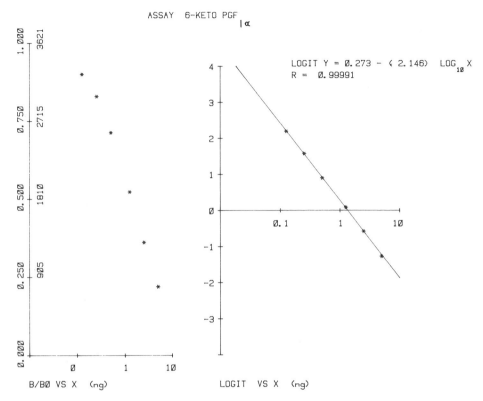

FIG. 3. 6-Keto-PGF$_{1\alpha}$ standard curves. **Left:** Plot of B/B_o V.S. log dose. **Right:** Logit transformation of B/B_o V.S. log dose.

assay has potential as a tumor marker used either to follow tumor regression with radio- or chemotherapy or as a diagnostic tool for the presence of cancer awaits further study. Application of this assay to urine samples yielded a range of 100 to 1,200 ng/24 hr in a control population.

TABLE 2. *Intra- and interrun precision for 6-keto-PGF$_{1\alpha}$ RIA*

Matrix	Mean (ng/ml)	SD (ng/ml)	Coefficient of variation (%)
Intra-assay			
control A	4.06	0.33	8.04
control B	9.52	1.05	11.05
Interassay			
control C	5.35	0.54	10.10
control D	20.52	2.53	12.32

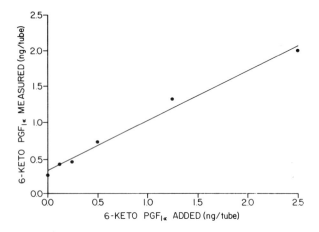

FIG. 4. Recovery of 6-keto-PGF$_{1\alpha}$ added to serum.

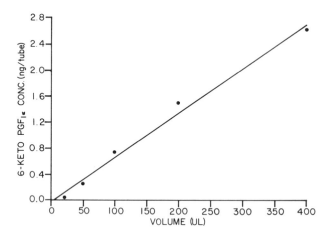

FIG. 5. Parallelism of serum 6-keto-PGF$_{1\alpha}$ RIA.

DISCUSSION

We describe here a RIA for blood and urine 6-keto-PGF$_{1\alpha}$ using a tritium-labeled tracer with acceptable specific activity for assay. Antibodies developed in rabbits to an albumin 6-keto-PGF$_{1\alpha}$ conjugate in Freund's complete adjuvant were highly specific and minimized the need to separate the 6-keto-PGF$_{1\alpha}$ from the PGE and PGF series prior to RIA. Dextran-coated charcoal was an acceptable means of separating antibody bound from free trace following first antibody incubation. Precision and accuracy studies revealed an assay with totally acceptable specificity with good recovery qualities and acceptable parallelism over the range of several dilutions.

Although application of this assay to human clinical studies has just begun, the 6-keto-$PGF_{1\alpha}$ assay shows promise as a possible tumor marker in cancer patients (2). Elevated levels of blood 6-keto-$PGF_{1\alpha}$ are found in a highly significant proportion of cancer patients. Present studies are continuing. We are looking into blood levels of patients with various hypertensive disorders. This assay may have application in sorting out deficiencies or excesses in endothelial cell PGI_2 production.

SUMMARY

We describe a highly specific RIA for blood and urine 6-keto-$PGF_{1\alpha}$, the principal metabolite of PGI_2. The method requires extraction and column chromatography prior to assay and uses a tritium trace for assay monitoring. Dextran-coated charcoal is used to separate bound from free trace. Acceptable standard curve reproducibility over six assays had a mean correlation of 0.991 with a coefficient of variation of 6.61%. Good precision and accuracy data were generated with this assay, and normal human blood levels in 80 control subjects was less than 125 pg/ml. Significant elevations of blood 6-keto-$PGF_{1\alpha}$ were found in a high proportion of cancer patients with various solid tumor malignancies.

ACKNOWLEDGMENT

Standards for antibody preparation and RIA calibrators were generous gifts from Dr. John Pike of the Upjohn Company.

REFERENCES

1. Demers, L. M. (1979): In: *Laboratory Medicine, Vol 1,* edited by G. Race, pp. 1–15. Harper & Row, New York.
2. Demers, L. M., Schweitzer, J., Lipton, A., Harvey, H., and White, D. (1979): *Clin. Res.* 27:383A.
3. Dusting, G. J., Moncada, S., and Vane, J. R. (1977): *Prostaglandins,* 13:3–16.
4. Granström, E., and Kindahl, H. (1978): In: *Advances in Prostaglandin and Thromboxane Research,* edited by J. C. Frolich, pp. 119–211. Raven Press, New York.
5. Moncada, S., and Vane, J. R. (1977): In: *Biochemical Aspects of Prostaglandins and Thromboxanes,* edited by N. Kharasch and J. Fried, pp. 155–177. Academic Press, New York.

Advances in Prostaglandin and Thromboxane Research,
Vol. 6, edited by B. Samuelsson, P. W. Ramwell,
and R. Paoletti. Raven Press, New York © 1980.

Radioimmunoassay of Urinary Prostaglandins

M. Korteweg, *J. De Boever, D. Vandevivere, and G. Verdonk

*Laboratory of Gerontology, Dietetics, and Nutrition Research, and * Department of Obstetrics and Gynecology, Faculty of Medicine, State University of Ghent, B-9000 Ghent, Belgium*

Direct radioimmunoassay (RIA) of prostaglandin E_2-like (i-PGE$_2$) and PGF$_{2\alpha}$-like material (i-PGF$_{2\alpha}$) is possible when urine is free of protein, seminal, or menstrual fluid. The method can be used for the study of urinary PG excretion during starvation, as the effect of fasting on PG excretion is not exceeded by PG variations during the menstrual cycle.

MATERIALS AND METHODS

Three healthy, nonobese volunteers collected urine for several menstrual cycles to test the method. Hormone assays were accomplished at the Department of Obstetrics and Gynecology. Obese patients were admitted to the hospital and placed on 2,500 kJ/day diets containing 400 mg sodium/day. After 4 days, a total starvation period of 3 weeks started. Patients were allowed to drink water *ad libitum* and were given ample amounts of water-soluble vitamins (no minerals). A readaption period of 1 week of low caloric intake (2,500 kJ/day, 400 mg sodium/day) followed fasting. At different times during and at the end of each period, urine was collected for 24 hr. Sodium and potassium were determined by flame photometry. The absence of protein was checked with a Combur test strip (Boehringer), and urine was examined microscopically to eliminate collections containing sperm. Urine was kept at $-20°C$ until PG assays were performed, which were accomplished by RIA using a second antibody technique. PGE$_2$(5,6,8,11,12,14,15(n)-^{3}H) 4.4 to 6.3 TBq/mmole was purchased from Amersham, England; and PGE$_2$ antiserum from the Pasteur Institute, Paris. PGE$_2$ was a gift of Upjohn. Goat anti-rabbit serum, rabbit normal serum, and reagents for PGF$_{2\alpha}$ assay were obtained from Clinical Assays (Travenol Laboratories, Inc.).

Sufficient inhibition (60 to 90%) was obtained when 100 μl of urine was used for the assay. After the addition of Isogel/Tris working buffer (Clinical Assays): (300 μl/tube for PGE$_2$, 360 μl/tube for PGF$_{2\alpha}$), 50 μl of ^{3}H-PGF$_{2\alpha}$ or ^{3}H-PGE$_2$ was added, followed by 50 μl of antiserum. The tubes were mixed and allowed to incubate for 1 hr at 37°C for PGF$_{2\alpha}$ assay and for 2 hr at 4°C for PGE$_2$ assay. Normal rabbit serum (100 μl) and goat anti-rabbit serum

(100 μl) were added to all tubes and incubated for at least 18 hr at 4°C. After centrifugation the supernatant was discarded with a syringe, taking care not to touch the precipitate at the bottom. The precipitate was dissolved in 1 ml 0.1 N NaOH by mixing on a vortex mixer and decanted into a mini scintillation vial; 4 ml of scintillation fluid (Aqualuma, Lumac Systems AG) was then added. The vials were counted twice for 4 min.

RESULTS

Table 1 shows $PGF_{2\alpha}$ and PGE_2 levels obtained either with direct RIA or after dialysis of the extract of 5 ml of urine (extraction with dimethoxymethane/ethanol (3:1, v/v; recovery, 46%).

Not only may seminal fluid influence the assay (Fig. 1, female F1), but the presence of menstrual fluid or cervical mucus may also cause higher levels. As shown in Table 2, their presence in high amounts (1 drop/ml of urine) influences the results. However, the increase of i-PGE_2 around the time of ovulation seems not to be caused by the presence of cervical mucus because of the lower levels of i-$PGF_{2\alpha}$ at that time (Fig. 1). Another menstrual cycle is documented with data on sodium and potassium excretion, hormonal pattern, and PG levels in urine and serum (Fig. 2). The variation of PG serum levels during the menstrual cycle is probably due to changes in factors present in blood at that moment of the cycle or due to differences at the platelet site. In urine, i-$PGF_{2\alpha}$/24 hr declines during the follicular phase. During the mucus period, i-PGE_2 starts to rise or shows spikes. One or two spikes are also found for i-$PGF_{2\alpha}$ during that period. Higher i-$PGF_{2\alpha}$ levels were found at or just after ovulation. As the changes in PG excretion due to starvation exceed the variations during the cycle, the urine collected during total starvation can be used for the investigation of the changes due to fasting. Serum PG levels were found to rise during food restriction and/or the first days of total starvation (3). After this initial rise they return to prestarvation values when calorie restriction or total starvation is prolonged, and they tend to increase again during refeeding.

TABLE 1. PGs in urine as measured by RIA

Method	i-$PGF_{2\alpha}$/tube (pg)	i-PGE_2/tube (pg)
Direct RIA of urine (vol/tube, μl)		
50	62	11
100	136	18
200	299	36
RIA of extracted urine (corrected for recovery)	1,137 pg/ml	174 pg/ml

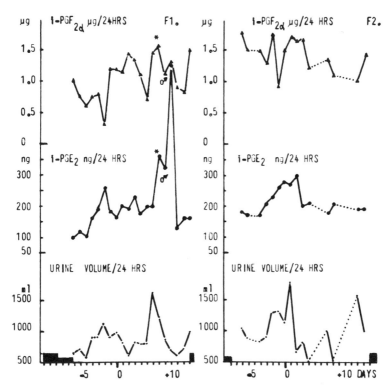

FIG. 1. i-PGE$_2$ and i-PGF$_{2\alpha}$ material excreted per 24 hr during the menstrual cycle of volunteers F1 and F2. Day 0, day of ovulation. *, stress. ♂, collection period with intercourse. Note the higher levels found in urine collected the day after ♂.

TABLE 2. *Influence of cervical mucus and menstrual fluid on PG levels*

Method	i-PGF$_{2\alpha}$/100 µl (pg)	i-PGE$_2$/100 µl (pg)
Direct RIA of 100 µl of:		
Control urine A	185	35
Control urine A + cervical mucus	248	82
Control urine B	89	13
Control urine B + clear cervical mucus	200	138
Control urine C	163	19
Control urine C + menstrual fluid	3612	439
RIA of extracted urine C + menstrual fluid (corrected for recovery)	3357	417

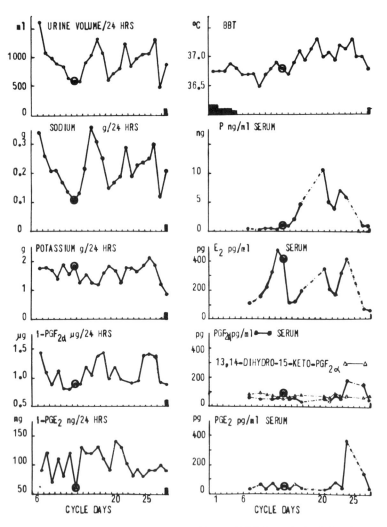

FIG. 2. Excretion of urine, sodium, potassium, i-PGF$_{2\alpha}$ and i-PGE$_2$ per 24 hr during the menstrual cycle. Serum levels of progesterone, extradiol, PGF$_{2\alpha}$, and PGE$_2$ of the same cycle. Peaks of luteinizing hormone (92 mIU/ml) and follicle-stimulating hormone (33 mIU/ml) on day 13 of the cycle.

To investigate the relation of this phenomenon with changing kidney conditions, sodium, potassium, i-PGE$_2$, and i-PGF$_{2\alpha}$ excretion were measured. The excretion patterns of two patients are shown in Fig. 3.

DISCUSSION

The i-PGE$_2$ and i-PGF$_{2\alpha}$ excretion/24 hr found with direct RIA is consistent with the values reported by others (2,4). During starvation the urinary i-PGE$_2$

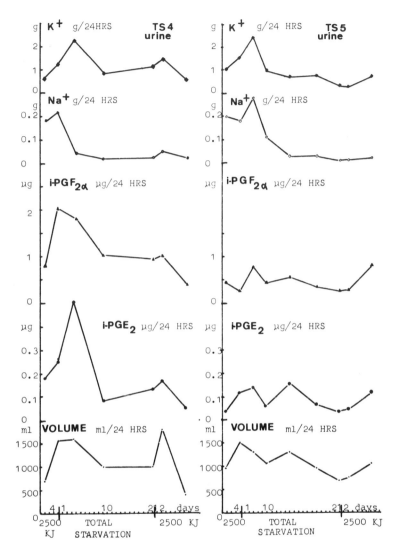

FIG. 3. Urine, sodium, potassium, i-PGE₂, and i-PGF₂α excretion per 24 hr during food restriction, total starvation, and refeeding.

and i-PGF$_{2\alpha}$ excretion moves in parallel with urine volume and sodium and potassium excretion. The same parallelism was found by Bowden et al. (1) in their study on the effect of posture and circadian rhythm. This parallelism is less pronounced during the menstrual cycle.

The described method is very useful in clinical studies because of ease and rapidity, and the points of interest revealed with this method may be studied in detail with highly specific, but more complicated, techniques.

ACKNOWLEDGMENTS

This work was supported by the F.G.W.O. (No. 30077.76) and the F.K.F.O. (No. 10420). We wish to thank Upjohn for the gift of PGE$_2$ and M. Dhont from the Department of Obstetrics and Gynecology for the analyses of luteinizing and follicle-stimulating hormones.

REFERENCES

1. Bowden, R. E., Ware, J. H., DeMets, D. L., and Keiser, H. R. (1977): *Prostaglandins,* 14:151–161.
2. Gill, J. R., Frölich, J. C., Bowden, R. E., Taylor, A. A., Keiser, H. R., Seyberth, H. W., Oates, J. A., and Bartter, F. C. (1976): *Am. J. Med.,* 61:43–51.
3. Korteweg, M., Christophe, A., and Verdonk, G. (1976): In: *Advances in Prostaglandin and Thromboxane Research, Vol. 2,* edited by B. Samuelsson and R. Paoletti, p. 879. Raven Press, New York.
4. Zia, P., Zipser, R., Speckart, P., and Horton, R. (1978): *J. Lab. Clin. Med.,* 92:415–422.

Advances in Prostaglandin and Thromboxane Research,
Vol. 6, edited by B. Samuelsson, P. W. Ramwell,
and R. Paoletti. Raven Press, New York © 1980.

Biologic and Methodologic Variables Affecting Urinary Prostaglandin Measurement

G. Ciabattoni, *F. Pugliese, E. Pinca, *G. A. Cinotti, A. De Salvo,
M. A. Satta, and C. Patrono.

*Department of Pharmacology, Catholic University, 00168 Rome; and *Department of
Medicine II, Polyclinic Umberto I, University of Rome, Rome, Italy*

Considerable attention has focused in recent years on the pathophysiology of the renal prostaglandin (PG) system (see ref. 2 for a review). In view of major limitations inherent to the measurement of unmetabolized PGs in renal venous plasma, i.e., very low levels, possible platelet contribution and invasive procedure, their measurement in urine has gained general acceptance following the original report by Frölich et al. (3) suggesting their renal origin in healthy women. Radioimmunoassay (RIA) offers some distinct advantages over gas chromatography–mass spectrometry (GC–MS) for such measurements because of higher sensitivity and the potential for handling large number of samples. However, large discrepancies can be found in the recent literature on "normal" PG excretion rates as measured by RIA as compared to GC–MS (see ref. 1). This has generated skepticism of the general validity of RIA measurements. In an attempt to define the nature of such discrepancies, we have investigated a number of methodologic and biologic variables possibly affecting urinary PG measurement.

STORAGE OF URINE

The influence of duration and temperature of storage on urinary PGE_2 and $PGF_{2\alpha}$ concentrations was studied by RIA techniques recently described (1). As shown in Fig. 1, a variable time- and temperature-dependent decrease of PGE_2 concentrations was observed on storage of both male and female urine before extraction. With respect to urine immediately extracted after voiding, a significant drop to 82% ($p < 0.025$) in apparent PGE_2 concentrations was observed when urine was stored 3 hr at 4°C before extraction, with a further decrease to 56% ($p < 0.025$) of control levels by 24 hr. In contrast, no statistically significant changes were measured in urine immediately frozen and kept (up to 1 month) at −20°C until extracted nor in chromatographed extracts kept (up to 3 months) at −20°C until assayed. Figure 2 similarly depicts the behavior of urinary $PGF_{2\alpha}$ on storage. It thus appears that immediate freezing of urine

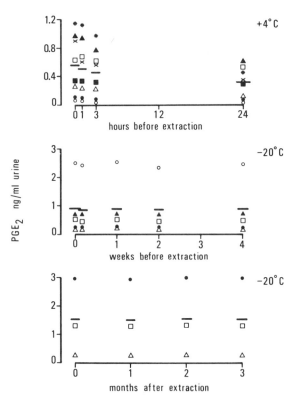

FIG. 1. Time and temperature dependence of urinary PGE_2 concentrations on storage. Different symbols represent individual urine samples; horizontal bars represent average concentrations.

and storage at $-20°C$ before extraction represents a necessary prerequisite in order to obtain reliable estimates of urinary PG concentrations. As an alternative, a known amount of standard PGE_2 and $PGF_{2\alpha}$ should be added to one-half of the urinary sample immediately after voiding, in order to monitor the variable losses occurring during storage, extraction, and chromatographic separation.

ANALYSIS OF URINE

Although employing radioactivity and requiring expensive counting equipment, RIA relies on a biologic reaction, i.e., an antigen–antibody reaction. It can therefore be regarded as a sophisticated form of bioassay, substituting the classical smooth muscle strip with soluble antibody as reactant. Given a particular antibody, the specificity of the reaction depends on a constant, i.e., the affinity and conformation of binding sites, and a variable, i.e., the composition of the biologic fluid to be examined and its degree of purification. Urine differs from other biologic fluids in containing perhaps the most complex mixture of arachidonic acid metabolites, in addition to a number of factors possibly interfering with any antigen–antibody reaction. We have previously demonstrated (1)

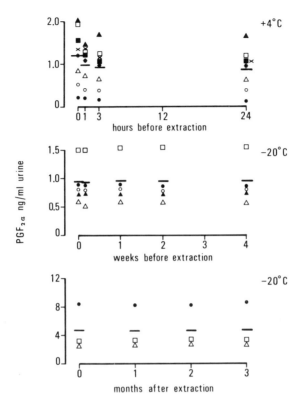

FIG. 2. Time and temperature dependence of urinary $PGF_{2\alpha}$ concentrations on storage. Different symbols represent individual urine samples; horizontal bars represent average concentrations.

the inadequacy of classical criteria of specificity such as cross-reactivity and dilution studies to validate urinary measurements, inasmuch as different anti-PGE_2 sera meeting such requirements may yield completely different estimates of PGE_2-like immunoreactivity (LI). In order to characterize the nature of urinary PGE_2-LI, we have developed a thin-layer chromatographic (TLC) technique, assessing its pattern of distribution with different solvent systems and different antisera (4). Besides demonstrating the heterogeneous nature of urinary PGE_2-LI, as assessed by some anti-PGE_2 sera, our findings clearly indicate that even antibodies of low affinity and specificity can "specifically" recognize urinary PGE_2, provided that a TLC step is included in the purification procedure. To rely on the binding characteristics of a particular antiserum rather than on the degree of purification of the sample can be completely misleading and account for large discrepancies in urinary PG concentrations. Alternatively, consistency of data obtained with two different antisera or with an independent method of analysis such as GC–MS (Table 1) can add enormously to the validation of RIA measurements.

TABLE 1. *Comparison of the analysis of human urine for PGE$_2$ and PGF$_{2\alpha}$ by GC-MS[a] and by RIA employing different anti-PG sera*

Comparison	Correlation coefficients[b]	
	PGE$_2$	PGF$_{2\alpha}$
GP 356 vs. GC-MS	0.97	
	(9)	
GP 356 vs. Pasteur Institute[c]	0.98	
	(10)	
GP 705 vs. GC-MS		0.93
		(9)
GP 705 vs. GP 2		0.90
		(19)

[a] Performed by Dr. S. Nicosia (Department of Pharmacology, University of Milan).
[b] Numbers in parentheses refer to number of samples.
[c] Gift of Dr. M. J. Dunn.

CONTRIBUTION FROM EXTRARENAL SOURCES

The overall validity of estimating renal PG synthesis by urinary PG determinations relies on a crucial assumption, i.e., that the lower urogenital tract does not contribute substantial amounts of unmetabolized PGs to urine. On the basis of the available evidence, the validity of such an assumption seems to be limited to women, since seminal fluid may contribute a highly variable fraction of the measured urinary PGs in men (5). In fact, two characteristics of seminal fluid PG content, i.e., very high concentrations (10^5 to 10^6 times higher than urine) and a very high PGE/PGF ratio (6), can easily account for the consistently higher urinary PGE excretion rate and higher PGE/PGF ratio found in men as compared to women (1). In contrast, we have recently shown that the PGE$_2$/PGF$_{2\alpha}$ ratio in renal venous plasma is in favor of PGF$_{2\alpha}$, with no appreciable difference between men and women (5). The presence of only 5–10 μl of seminal fluid over a 24-hr urine collection is sufficient to increase the apparent urinary PGE$_2$ concentration by two to five times and shift the PGE$_2$/PGF$_{2\alpha}$ ratio in favor of PGE$_2$. On this account, it is our opinion that urinary PG measurements (by any method) should be limited to women (unless urine is taken by a catheter).

VARIABLE PG EXCRETION RATE DURING THE MENSTRUAL CYCLE

In order to assess the reproducibility of urinary PG measurements in successive days, we studied the 24-hr excretion rates of a healthy volunteer (24 years old), who agreed to collect urine every other day for two menstrual cycles, with and without addition of known amounts of standard PGs to calculate overall recovery. The results are reported in Table 2 and show a high degree of variation in both cycles, with higher values in the second cycle, perhaps due to a more

TABLE 2. *Mean (± SD) excretion rates of PGE₂ during two menstrual cycles of a healthy woman, without and with standard PGE₂ added to urine for overall recovery*

	Number of collections	Urinary PGE$_2$ (ng/day)	Coefficient of variation (%)
Cycle I, no PGE$_2$ added	16	169 ± 107	63
Cycle II, 0.5 μg PGE$_2$ added immediately after voiding	13	214 ± 117	55

accurate evaluation of overall recovery by added PGs. No apparent pattern was observed in either cycle. It is obvious that such a spontaneous variation precludes meaningful studies to be performed on successive days to evaluate the effect of drugs or diet on the renal PG system. In an attempt to overcome this major limitation, we have investigated the reproducibility of PG excretion rate, when measured in a 2-hr (7–9 A.M.) urine collection performed on successive days under controlled conditions of recumbency and hydration (5 ml water/ kg body weight). As shown in Fig. 3, the results obtained in two healthy women indicate a considerably lower degree of variation, probably adequate to allow meaningful physiologic and pharmacologic studies to be performed on successive days.

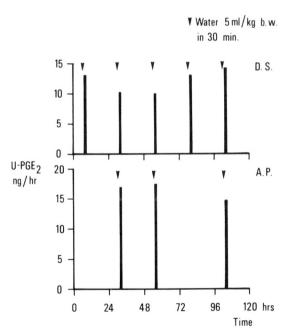

FIG. 3. Reproducibility of urinary PGE$_2$ excretion rate as assessed in 2-hr collections following constant water intake in two healthy women.

CONCLUSIONS

In conclusion, a number of methodologic as well as biologic variables, which we have attempted to characterize, should be taken into proper consideration when interpreting urinary PG measurements in humans. Failure to do so may only generate random numbers eventually supporting conflicting theories.

ACKNOWLEDGMENT

This study was supported by a grant from Consiglio Nazionale delle Ricerche (Progetto Finalizzato Tecnologie Biomediche, Subprogetto CHIM-2).

REFERENCES

1. Ciabattoni, G., Pugliese, F., Spaldi, M., Cinotti, G. A., and Patrono, C. (1979): *J. Endocrinol. Invest.*, 2:173–182.
2. Dunn, M. J., and Hood, V. L. (1977): *Am. J. Physiol.*, 233:F169–F184.
3. Frölich, J. C., Wilson, T. W., Sweetman, B. J., Smigel, M., Nies, A. S., Carr, K., Watson, J. T., and Oates, J. A. (1975): *J. Clin. Invest.*, 55:763–770.
4. Patrono, C., Ciabattoni, G., Cinotti, G. A., Pugliese, F., De Salvo, A., and Castrucci, G. (1978): *Prostaglandins,* 15:700–701.
5. Patrono, C., Wennmalm, A., Ciabattoni, G., Nowak, J., Pugliese, F., and Cinotti, G. A. (1979): *Prostaglandins (in press).*
6. Templeton, A. A., Cooper, I., and Kelly R.W. (1978): *J. Reprod, Fertil.,* 52:147–150.

Advances in Prostaglandin and Thromboxane Research,
Vol. 6, edited by B. Samuelsson, P. W. Ramwell,
and R. Paoletti. Raven Press, New York © 1980.

Radioimmunoassay of the Main Urinary Metabolite of Prostaglandin $F_{2\alpha}$ in Normal Subjects After Oral Administration of Prostaglandins E_2 and $F_{2\alpha}$

Satoshi Kitamura and Yoko Ishihara

Third Department of Internal Medicine, Faculty of Medicine, University of Tokyo, Hongo, Bunkyo-ku, Tokyo, 113, Japan

Granström identified the main urinary metabolite of prostaglandin $F_{2\alpha}$ ($PGF_{2\alpha}$-MUM) as 5α, 7α-dihydroxy-11-keto-tetranorprosta-1,16-dioic acid (1). Because of the rapid metabolism of $PGF_{2\alpha}$, the level of $PGF_{2\alpha}$-MUM appears to reflect more precisely the endogenous synthesis of $PGF_{2\alpha}$ than does the $PGF_{2\alpha}$ level in blood plasma. In 1977 we performed radioimmunoassays of $PGF_{2\alpha}$-MUM in normal subjects (3) and found that an oral administration of aspirin resulted in a significant decrease of $PGF_{2\alpha}$-MUM in both sexes. In the present investigation we performed radioimmunoassays of $PGF_{2\alpha}$-MUM in normal subjects after the oral administration of PGE_2 and $PGF_{2\alpha}$.

MATERIALS AND METHODS

Eleven healthy males and 15 females volunteered for this study. They ranged in age from 23 to 45 years. They were prohibited from taking any medicines, including aspirinlike anti-inflammatory drugs, from drinking alcohol, and from engaging in strenuous exercise. Female volunteers were prohibited from collecting urine samples for 2–3 days before and after menstruation. Urine was collected during 24 hr from 8 A.M. to 8 A.M. on the next day; the 1 to 2 ml of a urine sample was taken into a tube, kept in a freezer at −20°C until analyzed, and diluted 10-fold just before radioimmunoassay. After collecting the control urine samples, one or two capsules containing 0.5 mg of PGE_2 or $PGF_{2\alpha}$ were given immediately after the beginning of 24-hr urine sampling. Radioimmunoassay of $PGF_{2\alpha}$-MUM was carried out by the method of Ohki et al. (5). The $PGF_{2\alpha}$-MUM radioimmunoassay kit and capsules of PGE_2 and $PGF_{2\alpha}$ were generously provided by Ono Pharmaceutical Co., Osaka, Japan. Glutathione (Tathion) was purchased from Yamanouchi Pharmaceutical Co., Tokyo.

RESULTS

Figure 1 shows mean values and standard deviations (SD) of the 24-hr excretion of $PGF_{2\alpha}$-MUM after oral administration of 0.5 or 1.0 mg of PGE_2 and $PGF_{2\alpha}$, with $PGF_{2\alpha}$-MUM values on the ordinate. In the control, mean values ($\pm$ SD) of $PGF_{2\alpha}$-MUM in males and females were 29.7 $\pm$ 4.8 and 15.6 $\pm$ 2.1 μg, respectively. Mean values ($\pm$ SD) of $PGF_{2\alpha}$-MUM in males and females after oral administration of 0.5 mg of PGE_2 were 91.9 $\pm$ 15.2 and 95.1 $\pm$ 19.3 μg, respectively, and those with an added 0.6 g of glutathione were 94.9 $\pm$ 14.1 μg for males. Mean values ($\pm$ SD) of $PGF_{2\alpha}$-MUM in males after oral administration of 1 mg of PGE_2 were 171.9 $\pm$ 2$_5$.4 μg. Values for males and females after oral administration of 0.5 mg of $PGF_{2\alpha}$ were 178.3 $\pm$ 26.9 and 184.4 $\pm$ 22.8 μg, respectively, and those in males after oral administration of 1 mg of $PGF_{2\alpha}$ were 334.4 $\pm$ 23.2 μg.

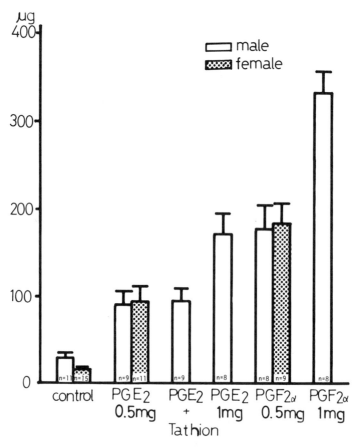

FIG. 1. Excretion of $PGF_{2\alpha}$-MUM in normal subjects for 24 hr after oral administration of PGE_2 and $PGF_{2\alpha}$.

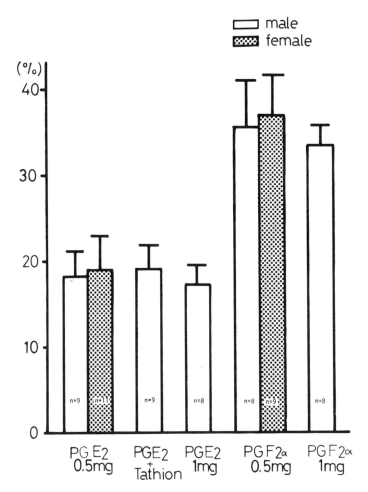

FIG. 2. Percent excretion of PGF$_{2\alpha}$-MUM in normal subjects after oral administration of PGE$_2$ and PGF$_{2\alpha}$.

Figure 2 shows the percent excretion of PGF$_{2\alpha}$-MUM in males and females after oral administration of 0.5 or 1 mg of PGE$_2$ and PGF$_{2\alpha}$. Mean percents excretion ($\pm$ SD) of PGF$_{2\alpha}$-MUM in males and females after oral administration of 0.5 mg of PGE$_2$ were 18.2 ± 3.0 and 19.0 ± 3.9, respectively; and those in males with 0.6 g of glutathione and after oral administration of 1 mg of PGE$_2$ were 18.9 ± 2.8 and $17.2 \pm 2.3\%$, respectively. There were no significant differences among these values. Mean percents excretion ($\pm$ SD) of PGF$_{2\alpha}$-MUM in males and females after oral administration of 0.5 mg of PGF$_{2\alpha}$ and in males after oral administration of 1 mg of PGF$_{2\alpha}$ were 35.7 ± 5.4 and 36.9 ± 4.6, and $33.4 \pm 2.3\%$, respectively, and showed no significant differences.

Figure 3 shows mean ($\pm$ SD) hourly percents excretion of PGF$_{2\alpha}$-MUM,

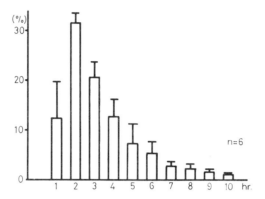

FIG. 3. Percent excretion of PGF$_{2\alpha}$-MUM every hour assuming 24-hr excretion as 100%.

assuming 24-hr excretion to be 100%. They reached a maximum 2 hr after oral administration of 0.5 mg of PGF$_{2\alpha}$.

Figure 4 shows the mean ($\pm$ SD) cumulative percents excretion of PGF$_{2\alpha}$-MUM at every hour after oral administration of 0.5 mg of PGF$_{2\alpha}$ in three males and three females (A) and of 0.5 mg of PGE$_2$ in two females (B). It is obvious from this graph that the values almost reach a plateau 5 to 6 hr after oral administration of PGs.

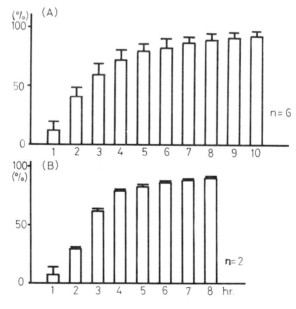

FIG. 4. Cumulative percent excretion of PGF$_{2\alpha}$-MUM every hour after oral administration of 0.5 mg PGF$_{2\alpha}$ **(A)** and PGE$_2$ **(B).**

DISCUSSION

The antiserum used in this experiment did not show significant cross-reaction with either natural PGs or metabolites in blood. A slight cross-reaction was found in the main urinary metabolites of PGE$_1$ and PGE$_2$, as had been identified by Hamberg et al. (2).

Mean values of PGF$_{2\alpha}$-MUM increased 6 times in males and 12 times in females after oral administration of 0.5 mg of PGF$_{2\alpha}$, and 11.3 times in males after oral administration of 1 mg of PGF$_{2\alpha}$. Although PGF$_{2\alpha}$-MUM increased almost twice on doubling of the dose of oral administration of PGF$_{2\alpha}$, the percents excretion of PGF$_{2\alpha}$-MUM after oral administration of 0.5 and 1 mg of PGF$_{2\alpha}$ were between 33 and 37%, and there was no significant difference among these values. Mean values of PGF$_{2\alpha}$-MUM increased three times in males and six times in females after oral administration of 0.5 mg of PGE$_2$. Although PGF$_{2\alpha}$-MUM increased almost twice on doubling of the dose of PGE$_2$, the percent excretion of PGF$_{2\alpha}$-MUM was 17 to 19% showing no significant difference.

These results may suggest that in the human body there is a conversion of PGE$_2$ into PGF$_{2\alpha}$. In 1973 Leslie and Levine (4) demonstrated the presence of 9-keto-PG-reductase (9K-PGR) in rat lung tissues, especially in cytoplasmic fractions, which catalyzed conversion between PGF$_{2\alpha}$ and PGE$_2$. It is therefore suggested that the administered PGE$_2$ is converted into PGF$_{2\alpha}$ by 9K-PGR and is metabolized into PGF$_{2\alpha}$-MUM, and that radioimmunoassay of PGF$_{2\alpha}$-MUM is a valuable method of estimating total production of PGF$_{2\alpha}$.

ACKNOWLEDGMENT

This work was supported by a Grant-in Aid for Scientific Research from the Ministry of Education, Science and Culture of Japan (A-337030, C-357280).

REFERENCES

1. Granström, E., and Samuelsson, B. (1971): *J. Biol. Chem.,* 241:5254–5263.
2. Hamberg, M., Svensson, J., Hedqvist, P., Strandberg, K., and Samuelsson, B. (1976): *Advances in Prostaglandin and Thromboxane Research, Vol. 1,* edited by B. Samuelsson and R. Paoletti, pp. 495–501. Raven Press, New York
3. Kitamura, S., Ishihara, Y., and Kosaka, K. (1977): *Prostaglandins,* 14:961–965.
4. Leslie, C. A., and Levine, L. (1973): *Biochem. Biophys. Res. Commun.,* 52:717–724.
5. Ohki, S., Hanyu, T., Imaki, K., Nakazawa, N., and Hirata, F. (1974): *Prostaglandins,* 6:137–148.

Advances in Prostaglandin and Thromboxane Research,
Vol. 6, edited by B. Samuelsson, P. W. Ramwell,
and R. Paoletti. Raven Press, New York © 1980.

Diglyceride Lipase: A Pathway for Arachidonate Release from Human Platelets

R. L. Bell, Nancy Stanford, Donald A. Kennerly, and Philip W. Majerus

Division of Hematology–Oncology, Departments of Internal Medicine and Biological Chemistry, Washington University School of Medicine, St. Louis, Missouri 63110

In platelets, as in other cells, prostaglandins and other products of arachidonate metabolism are not stored, but are synthesized after appropriate stimulation of the cell (12). The arachidonate in platelets is esterified in the 2-position of membrane phospholipids; therefore, the first step in arachidonate metabolism is hydrolysis of the fatty acid. When platelets are stimulated by thrombin or other appropriate agonists, there is a burst of arachidonate release, resulting in 5 to 10 nmoles of arachidonate metabolites formed per 10^9 platelets in less than 1 min (7). The release of fatty acids is specific for arachidonate; only traces of other fatty acids are released (2). It has been presumed that this release is accompanied by hydrolysis of arachidonate from phosphatidyl choline and phosphatidyl inositol by action of a phospholipase A_2 (2,3,14,15). We and others have attempted to study this putative phospholipase A_2 with little success (6,16). Two main problems remain unresolved. (a) No arachidonate-specific phospholipase A_2 has been found. The small amount of phospholipase A_2 activity in platelets has no specificity for the 2-position fatty acid. (b) The *amount* of activity found in crude extracts of platelets (≤ 0.1 nmole arachidonate release/min/10^9 cells) was insufficient to account for the 5 to 10 nmoles of arachidonate metabolites formed.

We have previously proposed a different pathway to account for arachidonate release from human platelets, and this is shown in Fig. 1 (1). The first step in this pathway is the conversion of phosphatidyl inositol to 1,2-diglyceride by the action of an inositol phosphodiesterase (phospholipase C). The 1,2-diglyceride thus liberated is metabolized by a diglyceride lipase that releases free arachidonate. The phosphatidyl inositol-specific phospholipase C was described in platelets by Rittenhouse-Simmons (13) and by Mauco et al. (10). Rittenhouse-Simmons also showed that the phospholipase C was inhibited when platelets were incubated with dibutyryl cyclic adenosine monophosphate prior to stimulation by thrombin (13). We have discovered a diglyceride lipase activity in a particulate fraction of human platelets that can release sufficient arachidonate to account for prostaglandin synthesis (1). The other reactions shown in Fig.

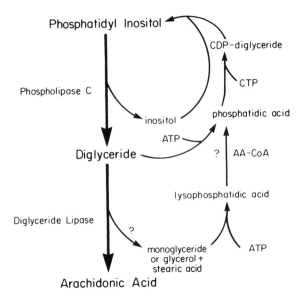

FIG. 1. Proposed pathway for arachidonate release from platelets.

1 are those of the widely studied "phosphatidyl inositol effect," wherein increased $^{32}PO_4$ labeling of phosphatidic acid and phosphatidyl inositol has been observed in a variety of secreting tissues when they are stimulated (11). We propose that these reactions serve to regenerate substrate phosphatidyl inositol for later agonist stimulation in these tissues. Whether phosphatidyl inositol is regenerated in platelets after thrombin stimulation has not yet been elucidated.

EVIDENCE THAT ARACHIDONATE IS DERIVED FROM PHOSPHATIDYL INOSITOL

Most studies of fatty acid release from platelets have determined release by radiochemical methods rather than by measurement of the mass of fatty acid. These studies suggested that several unsaturated fatty acids could be incorporated into platelet lipids but that only arachidonate or other cyclooxygenase substrate fatty acids were released on stimulation by thrombin or other agonists (2). In these studies, Bills et al. observed that the substrate arachidonate was derived primarily from phosphatidyl choline, although some was from phosphatidyl inositol, as suggested by Schoene and Iacono (15). When fatty acid release after thrombin stimulation of platelets is measured directly by gas liquid chromatography, primarily arachidonate is released. The only other fatty acid released on thrombin stimulation is a small amount of stearate. In order to measure arachidonate accumulation, the acetylenic eicosatetrayanoic acid that blocks arachidonate metabolism must be added. Under these conditions 3 to 6 nmoles arachidonate are released per 10^9 platelets along with 0.3 to 0.6 nmole stearate.

When the arachidonate metabolism inhibitor is omitted, 0.3 to 0.6 nmole of both arachidonate and stearate are released. The significance of these findings is that platelet phosphatidyl inositol contains primarily arachidonate and stearate (9).

That phosphatidyl inositol is the source of arachidonate was shown directly by measuring the depletion of platelet phosphatidyl inositol after thrombin stimulation. In these experiments platelets were incubated with thrombin for varying periods and the reaction was stopped by addition of chloroform/methanol/ethylenediaminetetraacetic acid/KCl to extract phosphatidyl inositol as described by Cohen et al. (5). The lipid extract was hydrolyzed in 6 N HCl in sealed, evacuated tubes for 48 hr at 120°C. The liberated inositol was analyzed as the trimethylsilyl derivative by gas liquid chromatography. ^{3}H-inositol-labeled phosphatidyl inositol (0.1 nmole) was added per 10^9 platelets as an internal standard to measure recovery of inositol. We find that platelet phosphatidyl inositol is rapidly depleted after thrombin stimulation (Fig. 2). Unstimulated platelets contain approximately 18 nmoles of phosphatidyl inositol/10^9 cells. Within 30 sec after addition of thrombin, phosphatidyl inositol levels fell by 50%, an amount that can provide sufficient substrate for arachidonate metabolism even without any new phosphatidyl inositol synthesis. We therefore conclude that most or all of the arachidonate metabolized by platelets is derived from phosphatidyl inositol. This conclusion is supported by recent experiments of Broekman et al. (4), who measured the change in total phospholipid content after thrombin stimulation of platelets and found that while phosphatidyl inositol decreased, no changes occurred in phosphatidyl choline, phosphatidyl ethanolamine, sphingomyelin, phosphatidyl serene, or cardiolipin. We propose that the release of radioactive arachidonate from phospholipids other than phosphatidyl inositol may reflect secondary shifts of arachidonate into phosphatidyl inositol as this phospholipid is regenerated after agonist stimulation.

The rapid hydrolysis of phosphatidyl inositol is accompanied by an appropriate transient accumulation of 1,2-diglyceride, as shown by Rittenhouse-Simmons

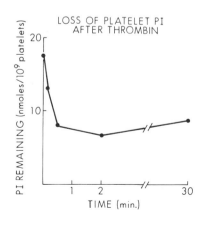

FIG. 2. Time course of phosphatidyl inositol loss induced by thrombin. Each point is the average of results from two separate experiments.

(13). Within 15 sec of addition of thrombin, 1 nmole diglyceride accumulates/ 10^9 platelets; by 2 min the diglyceride has disappeared. The time course of diglyceride appearance compared to phosphatidyl inositol loss suggests a precursor product relationship. Further, the rapid loss of diglyceride suggests that this moiety is rapidly metabolized. Marcus et al. (9) reported that platelet phosphatidyl inositol has a unique fatty acid composition, approximately 90% of the fatty acids being either stearate or arachidonate. It follows that a diglyceride formed from phosphatidyl inositol would have the same fatty acids composition. We determined the composition of the transiently formed diglyceride by extracting platelet lipids 15 sec after thrombin treatment using ether/petroleum ether/ acetic acid (80:20:1). We isolated diglyceride by silicic acid column chromatography and preparative thin-layer chromatography. The diglyceride obtained was hydrolyzed and the fatty acids methylated and analyzed by gas liquid chromatography. In three experiments we found 1 to 1.2 nmoles of arachidonate and 1 to 1.3 nmoles stearate/10^9 platelets. No other fatty acids were detected. The diglyceride was further shown to be 1,2-diglyceride, since it was converted to ^{32}P-phosphatidic acid when it was used as a substrate for *E. coli* diacylglycerol kinase with [γ-^{32}P] adenosine triphosphate. Since the 1,2-diglyceride produced after inositol phosphodiesterase action contains only arachidonate in the 2-position, this could explain the specificity of arachidonate release without any fatty acid specificity required by the diglyceride lipase.

DIGLYCERIDE LIPASE

We recently described a diglyceride lipase that has sufficient activity to account for arachidonate release from transient diglyceride (1). We used 1,2-diglyceride labeled with either ^{14}C-arachidonate or ^{14}C-oleate in the 2-position as substrate for diglyceride lipase. The activity was found only in a particulate fraction of platelets. The enzyme displays a broad pH activity curve, with the maximum at pH 7. Arachidonoyl and oleoyl diglyceride were hydrolyzed equally well, indicating that the specificity of arachidonate release from platelets does not reside in this enzyme. A substrate concentration curve (1) indicates that the enzyme can hydrolyze 30 nmoles of arachidonate/min/10^9 platelets. The enzyme is stimulated by reduced glutathione and inactived by *p*-chloromercuribenzoate and *N*-ethyl maleimide, suggesting that it has a sulfhydryl group required for activity. When the diglyceride lipase assay was carried out using doubly labeled substrate (^{3}H-glycerol-labeled, ^{14}C-arachidonoyl-labeled diglyceride), we found 1 mole of arachidonate liberated per mole of glycerol at all time points. Therefore, in this particulate fraction, there is no evidence for any monoglyceride product. However, in intact cells it is possible that the products of the reaction are free arachidonate and 1-monostearin, since free stearic acid is not released in large quantities. The activity of the diglyceride lipase is shown in Fig. 3. The enzyme is unlike other lipases such as lipoprotein lipase and hormone-sensitive lipase in that triglyceride is not cleaved at a significant rate. Monoglyceride is cleaved rapidly (data not shown).

PHOSPHATIDYL INOSITOL PHOSPHODIESTERASE (PHOSPHOLIPASE C)

Unlike the diglyceride lipase, the phosphatidyl inositol phosphodiesterase is found in the soluble fraction of disrupted platelets. The enzyme is stimulated by deoxycholate and requires calcium ions for activity. The enzyme is specific for phosphatidyl inositol (Fig. 3), neither phosphatidyl choline nor phosphatidyl ethanolamine is hydrolyzed. The enzyme formed 70 nmoles of 1,2-diglyceride/ 10^9 cells, more than sufficient to account for arachidonate metabolism in platelets.

SUMMARY

We have described a new pathway for the initiation of prostaglandin synthesis. The two enzymes involved are a phosphatidyl inositol phosphodiesterase (phospholipase C) and a diglyceride lipase with unique properties. The diglyceride

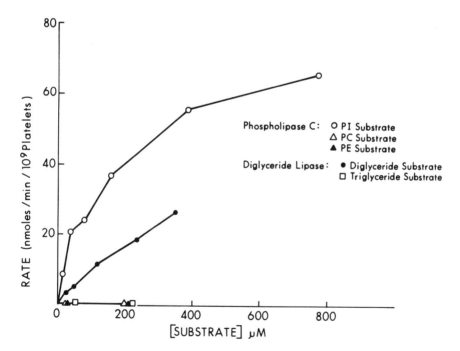

FIG. 3. Enzyme activities involved in arachidonate release. Phospholipase C activities are derived from liberated ^{3}H-inositol, ^{14}C-choline, and ^{14}C-ethanolamine from the corresponding phospholipids. Fatty acid release indicating diglyceride or triglyceride lipase activity was assayed as described by Bell et al. (1).

lipase does not have fatty acid specificity, rather the release of only cyclooxygenase substrate fatty acids is ensured by the restricted fatty acid composition of inositol phospholipids. Thus since phosphatidyl inositol contains only arachidonate in the 2-position and the diglyceride is formed solely from phosphatidyl inositol, only arachidonate is released by the diglyceride lipase. Unlike the putative phospholipase A_2 previously proposed to initiate platelet arachidonate metabolism, these enzymes have sufficient activity to account for the process. Hokin and Hokin (8) first described the phenomenon of increased phosphatidyl inositol turnover that accompanies stimulation of a variety of secretory tissues and nerves. The function of the phosphatidyl inositol turnover has never been explained. We speculate that the phenomenon reflects prostaglandin synthesis or other metabolism of arachidonate in these tissues, as phosphatidyl inositol is replenished after stimulation by the reactions shown in Fig. 1.

ACKNOWLEDGMENTS

This research was supported by Grants HLBI 14147 (Specialized Center for Research in Thrombosis) and HLBI 16634 from the National Institutes of Health, and by a Medical Scientist Training Program Award GM 07200 (to D.A.K). This work was presented in part at the Deuel Conference on Lipids, March, 1979, Carmel, California.

REFERENCES

1. Bell, R. L., Kennerly, D. A., Stanford, N., and Majerus, P. W. (1979): *Proc. Natl. Acad. Sci. USA*, 76:3238–3241.
2. Bills, T. K., Smith, J. B., and Silver, M. J. (1977): *J. Clin. Invest.* 60:1–6.
3. Blackwell, G. J., Duncombe, W. G., Flower, R. J., Parsons, M. F., and Vane, J. R. (1977): *Br. J. Pharmacol.*, 59:353–366.
4. Broekman, M. J., Ward, J. W., and Marcus, A. J. (1979): *Clin. Res.*, 27:459a.
5. Cohen, P., Broekman, M. J., Verkely, A., Lisman, J. W. W., and Derksen A. (1971): *J. Clin. Invest.*, 50:762–772.
6. Derksen, A., and Cohen, P. (1975): *J. Biol. Chem.*, 250:9342–9347.
7. Hamberg, M., Svensson, J., and Samuelsson, B. (1974): *Proc. Natl. Acad. Sci. USA*, 71:3824–3828.
8. Hokin, M. R., and Hokin, L. E. (1953): *J. Biol. Chem.*, 203:967–977.
9. Marcus, A. J., Ullner, H. L., and Safier, L. B. (1969): *J. Lipid Res.*, 10:108–114.
10. Mauco, G., Chap, H., and Douste-Blazy, L. (1979): *FEBS Lett.*, 100:367–370.
11. Michell, R. H. (1975): *Biochem. Biophys. Acta*, 415:81–147.
12. Piper, P., and Vane, J. (1971): *Ann. NY Acad. Sci.*, 180:363–383.
13. Rittenhouse-Simmons, S. (1979): *J. Clin. Invest.*, 63:580–587.
14. Russell, F. A., and Deykin, D. (1976): *Am. J. Hematol.*, 1:59–70.
15. Schoene, N. W., and Iacono, J. M. (1975): *Fed. Proc.*, 34:257.
16. Trugman, G., Benezirt, G., Manier, M., and Polonovski, J. (1979): *Biochim. Biophys. Acta*, 573:61–72.

Advances in Prostaglandin and Thromboxane Research,
Vol. 6, edited by B. Samuelsson, P. W. Ramwell,
and R. Paoletti. Raven Press, New York © 1980.

Release of Arachidonic Acid and Its Conversion to Prostaglandins in Various Diploid Cell Types in Culture

Peter Polgar, *William H. J. Douglas, *Louis Terracio,
and Linda Taylor

*Boston University School of Medicine, and *Tufts University School of Medicine
Boston, Massachusetts 02118*

Prostaglandins (PGs) are cell-to-cell messengers produced by eukaryotic cells, often in response to extracellular stimuli (1,8). Under physiologic conditions, the synthesis of these messengers occurs consequent to the freeing of the precursor fatty acids from lipid stores (5), followed by the conversion of these precursors to PG-like molecules via endoperoxide formation (7). Results from a number of laboratories studying the mechanisms controlling the synthesis of these molecules have made it clear that at least three critical determinants exist in PG synthesis. These are the activation of phospholipase, the action of cyclooxygenase-peroxidase, and the action of the individual PGs isomerases, and reductases (4). Because the quantity and kind of PG produced by the given cell is critical to the message it emits, elucidation of the action of these enzyme systems is important. Our own aims have been to elucidate the role of these mechanisms (fatty acid uptake, release, and conversion to PGs) on the cellular level. In this report, we chose to study normal diploid cells that vary in the kind of PGs they produce. We looked at cellular incorporation and release of arachidonic acid and its subsequent conversion to PGs. The effector molecules for these studies included ascorbic acid, a reducing agent with peroxide activity on phospholipids, bradykinin, a vasoactive hormone, and serum, a mixture of physiologically active factors.

RESULTS AND DISCUSSION

Table 1 illustrates PG production by pulmonary artery endothelial and smooth muscle cells, prostate epithelial cells, and lung fibroblasts. Under the culture condition described, the endothelial cells are actively producing 6-keto-$PGF_{1\alpha}$ with some thromboxane B_2 (TXB_2). Prostate cells produce predominantly PGE_2. Smooth muscle and fibroblastic cells are much less active, producing 1/100 the 6-keto-$PGF_{1\alpha}$ and PGE_2.

TABLE 1. *PG production by four diploid cell types in culture*[a]

Cell type	PG production (ng/ml medium)			
	6-keto $F_{1\alpha}$	E_2	$F_{2\alpha}$	TXB_2
Lung fibroblast	0.170	0.203	0.175	0.175
Smooth muscle	0.350	0.187	0.175	0.175
Endothelial	40	0.196	0.175	2.5
Prostate epithelial	0.350	15	0.175	0.175

[a] The cultures were maintained in 20-cm^2 dishes at 37°C in air containing 5% CO_2. Cell density was at 2×10^6 cells/dish. PG content in the culture medium, which contained 2% fetal bovine serum (FBS), was determined 5 hr after exposure to the cells. The radioimmunoassay (RIA) was run directly on the culture medium. The standard curves for each RIA were also run with an equivalent aliquot of the same medium, which had not been exposed to the cells. The antibody for $PGF_{2\alpha}$ was purchased from Boehringer Mannheim Corp., New York; PGE_2 was prepared in our laboratory; 6-keto-$PGF_{1\alpha}$ and TXB_2 were a gift from Immunalysis, Inc., Milton, Massachusetts. Labeled PGE_2, F_2, and TXB_2 were purchased from NEN Corp., Boston. ^{3}H-6-keto-$PGF_{1\alpha}$ was a gift from Dr. D. Ahern, NEN Corp., Boston. The fibroblasts are human embryo lung fibroblasts (IMR-90) from Institute Medical Research, Camden, New Jersey. The smooth muscle cells were prepared from rabbit pulmonary artery (6). The endothelial cells originated from calf pulmonary artery (6). The prostate cells were obtained from rat prostate (11). All points were determined in duplicate. Variation did not exceed 15%.

In all four cell types the incorporation of ^{3}H-arachidonic acid was similar with respect to the velocity of incorporation and the type of lipid labeled (P. Polgar and L. Taylor, *unpublished results*). Typically, maximum uptake is in the vicinity of 90% within 7 hr of exposure. Uptake is linear during the first 2 hr and then begins to reach a plateau. The majority of the label (85%) is incorporated into phospholipid, and the remaining label is found in neutral lipid (10).

When the labeled cells are washed and challenged with various effectors, radioactivity is released into the medium. Tables 2 and 3 illustrate the release of label from the four cell types in response to 2% serum and 2% serum plus 15 mM ascorbic acid. Two of the cell types, smooth muscle cells and fibroblasts, respond to ascorbic acid with a large increase of release of the label. When this radioactivity was subjected to thin-layer chromatography (TLC), however, it was found that relative to the serum effect, in the smooth muscle cells the percent of released label converted to PGs decreases, though the total amount of radioactivity converted to PGs increases. In fibroblasts both release and conversion to PGs is stimulated by ascorbic acid. "Old" (late passage) and "young" (early passage) fibroblasts respond equally to ascorbic acid relative to the serum effect, although "old" cells generally convert less of their released radioactivity to PGs (Table 2; and Polgar and Taylor, *unpublished*). Ascorbic acid does

TABLE 2. Response of smooth muscle cells and fibroblasts to serum and ascorbic acid[a]

	Smooth muscle cells		Fibroblasts (PDL 21)		Fibroblasts (PDL 54)	
	2% FBS	2% FBS + 15 mM Asc.	2% FBS	2% FBS + 15 mM Asc.	2% FBS	2% FBS + 15 mM Asc.
Incorporation radioactivity released (%)	1.7	39	3.8	29	4.6	49
Radioactivity released (cpm)	14,502	332,704	28,437	217,016	33,113	352,722
Radioactivity released as PG (%)	11	1	3	16	1	6
Radioactivity running as PG (cpm)	1,595	33,270	853	44,301	331	21,163

[a] The same cell types were used and maintained as in Table 1. Culture plates (20 cm^2) were prelabeled with ^{3}H-arachidonic acid (specific activity, 62–100 Ci/mmole; NEN Corp., Boston) for 5 hr. The culture medium containing the unincorporated label was then removed from each culture dish, and the culture was washed once with Hank's balanced salt solution. Fresh culture medium containing the given effectors was then added to the culture plate. Five hr later the medium containing the released counts was removed, and an aliquot was used to determine radioactivity. Presence of PGs in the medium was determined by TLC (10). Asc., ascorbic acid; PDL, Population doubling level. The PGs were gifts from Dr. J. Pike, Upjohn Co., Kalamazoo, Michigan.

TABLE 3. *Response of endothelial and prostate epithelial cells to serum and ascorbic acid[a]*

	Endothelial cells		Prostate epithelial cells	
	2% FBS	2% FBS + 15 mM Asc.	2% FBS	2% FBS + 15 mM Asc.
Incorporated radioactivity released (%)	1.5	1.6	4.0	4.1
Radioactivity released (cpm)	12,715	13,563	29,609	30,350
Radioactivity running as PG (%)	43	34	20	12
Radioactivity running as PG (cpm)	5,467	4,611	5,922	3,642

[a] For details see footnote to Table 2. Culture medium contained 2% FBS or 2% FBS + ascorbic acid (Asc.).

not affect the release of radioactivity from endothelial or prostate epithelial cells and decreases the percent of that radioactivity converted to PGs. Ascorbic acid, then, increases the release of arachidonic acid from two of the cell types tested but decreases the ability of three of the cell types to convert the label to PGs. Only in the lung fibroblast does ascorbic acid stimulate both the release of label and the conversion of the label to PGs.

The effect of bradykinin on the release of arachidonic acid and its conversion to PGs was tested in the two cell types most responsive to this hormone. Table 4 shows that bradykinin increased only slightly the release of radioactivity from these cells. However, the conversion of that radioactivity to PGs was stimulated in both cell types.

Thus, though incorporation of the precursor fatty acid, arachidonic acid, into cellular lipid stores is similar in the cell types tested, the release of the label varies with the cell type and the effector molecule. The conversion of

TABLE 4. *Response of endothelial and fibroblastic cells to bradykinin[a]*

	Endothelial cells		Fibroblasts	
	Medium	Medium + BK	Medium	Medium + BK
Incorporated radioactivity released (%)	1	2.1	2.4	3.2
Radioactivity released (cpm)	8,476	17,801	17,960	23,946
Radioactivity running as PG (%)	50	72	2	39
Radioactivity running as PG (cpm)	4,238	12,817	360	9,339

[a] For details, see footnote to Table 2. BK, bradykinin (5 μg/ml).

the released label to PGs also varies with the cell type and effector molecule, although each cell type appears programed to produce certain types of PGs. In addition, as has been shown in other systems (2,3), certain effectors such as bradykinin appear to channel the released fatty acid or perhaps activate the cyclooxygenase and/or synthetase enzyme systems. In sum, our results suggest that the release of arachidonic acid and its conversion to PGs may be under separate controls depending on cell type and effector molecule.

ACKNOWLEDGMENTS

This work was supported by Grants AG-00455 and HL-19717 from the National Institutes of Health.

REFERENCES

1. Harris, R. H., Ramwell, P. W., and Gilmer, P. J. (1979): *Ann. Rev. Physiol.,* 41:653–658.
2. Hong, S. C., and Levine, L. (1976): *J. Biol. Chem.,* 251:5814–5816.
3. Hsueh, W., Isakson, P. C., and Needleman, P. (1977): *Prostaglandins,* 13:1073–1089.
4. Lands, W. E. M. (1979): *Ann. Rev. Physiol.,* 41:633–652.
5. Lands, W. E. M., and Samuelsson, B. (1968): *Biochim. Biophys. Acta,* 164:426–429.
6. Polgar, P., Taylor, L., and Downing, D. (1979): *Prostaglandins,* 18:43–52.
7. Samuelsson, B. (1976): In: *Advances in Prostaglandin and Thromboxane Research,* Vol. 1, edited by S. Samuelsson and R. Paoletti, pp. 1–6. Raven Press, New York.
8. Samuelsson, B., Goldyne, M., Granstrom, E., Hamberg, M., Hammarstrom, S., and Malsten, C. (1978): *Ann. Rev. Biochem.,* 47:997–1029.
9. Taylor, L., Polgar, P., MacAteer, J., and Douglas, W. H. J. (1979): *Biochem. Biophys. Acta,* 572:502–509.
10. Taylor, L. (1979): *Ph.D. dissertation,* Boston University School of Medicine.
11. Terracio, L., Douglas, W. H. J., and Glass, H. (1979): *37th Annual Proc. Electr. Microsc. Soc. Am.,* p. 138–139.

Advances in Prostaglandin and Thromboxane Research,
Vol. 6, edited by B. Samuelsson, P. W. Ramwell,
and R. Paoletti. Raven Press, New York © 1980.

Effects of Divalent Cations on Prostaglandin Biosynthesis and Phospholipase A₂ Activation in Rabbit Kidney Medulla Slices

A. Raz and A. Erman

Department of Biochemistry, The George S. Wise Center for Life Sciences, Tel Aviv University, Tel Aviv, Israel

Prostaglandin (PG) formation requires the hydrolysis of esterified arachidonic acid (AA) from tissue lipids (1,4,5). AA is particularly abundant among the fatty acids in the 2-position of phospholipids (7) from which it could be hydrolyzed by the action of phospholipase A_2. Renal PG biosynthesis was reported to be depressed in a Ca^{2+} free media (6). The studies reported here determine the selectivity of several divalent cations for stimulation of kidney medulla PG generation and examine the relationship between the activity of the cations in stimulating PG biosynthesis and in inducing release of fatty acids from medulla slices.

METHODS AND MATERIALS

Kidney Slices Preparation and Incubation

Rabbits, local strain, were sacrificed by an injection into the heart; both kidneys were removed and medulla slices quickly prepared. The slices were incubated at 37°C for 10 to 120 min in Tris-HCl buffer (0.1 M, pH 8.0).

Determination of PG Products and Fatty Acids

Following incubation, an aliquot of the medium was assayed for PGE_2 content by bioassay on rat stomach strip (9), while the remainder of the medium was acidified to pH 3.5, extracted with ethyl acetate and the lipid extract separated by thin-layer chromatography (t.l.c.). The fatty acids zone was extracted, subjected to methylation, and its composition determined by g.l.c. (3).

Materials

PGs (E_2, D_2, $F_{2\alpha}$, A_2) were kindly supplied by Dr. U. Axen and Dr. J. E. Pike of the Upjohn Co. (Kalamazoo, Michigan). Fatty acids standards were obtained from Supelco. All other reagents were analytical grade.

RESULTS AND DISCUSSION

Calcium ions stimulated PGE_2 generation up to 3- to 5-fold in a time- and dose-dependent manner. PGE_2 generation was linear up to 30 min and reached a plateau at 60 to 90 min. Selectivity of the calcium stimulatory effect on medullary PG biosynthesis was evaluated in studies with other divalent cations (Fig. 1). Ca^{2+}, Mn^{2+}, and Sr^{2+} showed dose-dependent stimulation of PGE_2 production. In contrast, Ba^{2+}, Co^{2+}, and Mg^{2+} ions were without effect at concentrations of 2 mM or lower and showed only very small stimulation at higher concentrations.

In an attempt to elucidate the enzymatic step at which the cations exert their effect, we also examined their effect on release of fatty acids from the medullary slices. The results (Table 1) indicated complete correlation between the effects of the divalent cations to stimulate medullary PG production and to release lineoleic acid (LL) and AA. Ca^{2+}, Mg^{2+}, and Sr^{2+} ions dose dependently stimulated the release of PGE_2, AA, and LL; except for a small increase in oleic acid, the release of other fatty acids was unaffected by these divalent cations. As both AA and LL acids are mainly found in the 2-position of phospholipids, it appears that these cations stimulate PGE_2 biosynthesis by stimulating a phospholipase A_2 reaction that provides the PG precursor, AA. Noteworthy is the fact that kidney medulla phospholipase A_2 shows a different cation specificity than that observed previously for phospholipase A_2 from venoms and other toxins where inhibition by Ba^{2+} and Sr^{2+} is seen (2,10).

The properties and selective products of cation-dependent phospholipase A_2 activation contrast with the nonselective lipolysis induced by extracellular serum

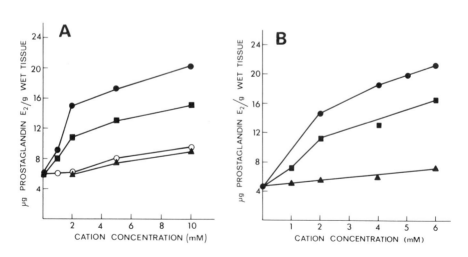

FIG. 1. Effects of divalent cations on PG biosynthesis. Medulla slices (0.2 g) were incubated with shaking at 37°C for 60 min in the presence of different concentrations of **A:** Mg^{2+} (▲–▲), Co^{2+} (○–○), Mn^{2+} (■–■), or Ca^{2+} (●–●); **B:** Ba^{2+} (▲–▲), Sr^{2+} (■–■), or Ca^{2+} (●–●).

TABLE 1. Release of fatty acids and PGE$_2$ from medulla slices by divalent cations and bovine serum albumin

Addition to incubation medium	Fatty acids released (µg/g wet tissue)					total 20:4[a]	PGE$_2$ released (µg/g wet tissue)
	16:0	18:0	18:1	18:2	20:4		
—	58 ± 2	24 ± 1	28 ± 1	12 ± 1.4	3.1 ± 0.2	8.7	6.6 ± 0.3
BSA	77 ± 3	49 ± 2	56 ± 2	29 ± 1	9.3 ± 0.4	14.4	6.1 ± 0.4
2 mM CaCl$_2$	61 ± 2	25 ± 1	33 ± 1	22 ± 2	7.1 ± 0.4	18.3	13.2 ± 0.5
2 mM CaCl$_2$ + BSA	75 ± 3	47 ± 2	63 ± 2	38 ± 2	16.6 ± 0.6	26.7	12.0 ± 0.6
5 mM CaCl$_2$	60 ± 2	25 ± 1	38 ± 2	27 ± 2	9.4 ± 0.6	25.5	18.9 ± 0.6
5 mM CaCl$_2$ + BSA	77 ± 2	50 ± 3	69 ± 3	44 ± 3	21.6 ± 1.4	34.3	15.5 ± 0.7
2 mM MnCl$_2$	61 ± 2	28 ± 2	31 ± 2	19 ± 1	5.2 ± 0.5	13.8	9.0 ± 0.6
2 mM MnCl$_2$ + BSA	81 ± 3	46 ± 3	60 ± 2	33 ± 2	13.3 ± 0.8	20.0	7.9 ± 0.4
5 mM MnCl$_2$	56 ± 3	27 ± 2	37 ± 2	22 ± 2	6.9 ± 0.5	19.7	15.1 ± 0.7
5 mM MnCl$_2$ + BSA	74 ± 2	48 ± 3	65 ± 3	34 ± 2	13.9 ± 0.9	26.4	14.7 ± 0.8
5 mM MgCl$_2$	61 ± 2	25 ± 1	29 ± 1	12 ± 0.5	4.2 ± 0.3	10.4	7.3 ± 0.5
5 mM MgCl$_2$ + BSA	79 ± 2	46 ± 1	59 ± 2	32 ± 2	10.9 ± 0.7	17.1	7.3 ± 0.4
2 mM SrCl$_2$	57 ± 3	24 ± 1	27 ± 1	18 ± 2	4.9 ± 0.3	12.5	8.9 ± 0.6
2 mM SrCl$_2$ + BSA	71 ± 3	51 ± 3	53 ± 3	34 ± 2	16.0 ± 0.8	23.5	8.8 ± 0.5
5 mM SrCl$_2$	60 ± 3	27 ± 2	29 ± 2	23 ± 2	7.8 ± 0.6	19.7	14.0 ± 0.8
5 mM SrCl$_2$ + BSA	76 ± 3	48 ± 2	56 ± 3	37 ± 3	18.0 ± 0.9	27.6	11.3 ± 0.7

[a] Total amount of arachidonate released from tissue lipids during the incubation is equal to the isolated amounts of free arachidonate and PGE$_2$. The amount of "µg PGE$_2$ released" can be converted to "µg arachidonate released" by multiplication by the factor 304/352 (m.w. arachidonate/m.w. PGE$_2$). The total amount of arachidonate released thus equals "µg 20:4" + "µg PGE$_2$" × 304/352.

Medulla slices (200 mg) were incubated at 37°C for 60 min in 0.1 M Tris buffer pH 8.0. Cations were added at 2 or 5 mM final concentration and bovine serum albumin (BSA) at 2 mg/ml. The medium was analyzed for PGE$_2$ and fatty acids as described in Methods section. Values given are mean ± S.E.M. of 6 experiments.

albumin which promotes the hydrolysis of all fatty acids (Table 1). Albumin-mediated lipolysis and cation-stimulated lipolysis apparently work by independent mechanisms, since the additive effects of both stimulants were observed in incubations with albumin and Ca^{2+}, Mn^{2+}, or Sr^{2+}. Furthermore, cation-stimulated lipolysis is accompanied by significant increase in PGE_2 production, whereas albumin causes a slight decrease in the release of PGE_2. This difference indicates that AA release by divalent cations (but not by albumin) is coupled in some measure to the subsequent conversion of this acid to PGs. In this respect, the cation-stimulated phospholipase A_2 activity resembles the hormone-sensitive lipase described previously (4,8).

SUMMARY

The divalent cations Ca^{2+}, Mg^{2+}, Co^{2+}, Mn^{2+}, Sr^{2+}, and Ba^{2+} were compared for their stimulatory or inhibitory effect on PG formation in rabbit kidney medulla slices. Calcium, manganese, and strontium ions stimulated PG generation up to 3- to 5-fold in a time- and dose-dependent manner ($Ca^{2+} > Mn^{2+} \sim Sr^{2+}$) while the magnesium and cobalt ions were without significant effects. Stimulatory effects of Ca^{2+}, Mn^{2+}, and Sr^{2+} on the medullary generation of PGE_2 was found to correlate with their stimulatory effects on the release of AA and LL acids from tissue lipids. The release of other fatty acids was unaffected. As both AA and LL acids are predominantly found in the 2-position of phospholipids, the stimulation by these cations appears to be mediated via stimulation of phospholipase A_2 activity.

REFERENCES

1. Bills, T. and Smith, B. (1976): *Biochim. Biophys. Acta,* 424:303–314.
2. Chiung Chang, C., Jai Su, M., Don Lee, J., and Eaker, D. (1977): *Arch. Pharmacol.,* 299:155–161.
3. Erman, A., and Raz, A. (1979): *Biochem. J. (in press).*
4. Hsueh, W., Isakson, P. C., and Needleman, P. (1977): *Prostaglandins,* 13:1073–1091.
5. Isakson, P. C., Raz, A., Denney, S. E., Wyche, A., and Needleman, P. (1977): *Prostaglandins,* 14:853–871.
6. Kalisker, A., and Dyer, D. C. (1972): *Eur. J. Pharmacol.,* 19:305–309.
7. Morgan, T. H., and Hanahan, D. J. (1963): *Arch. Biochim. Biophys.,* 103:54–65.
8. Schwartzman, M., and Raz, A. (1979): *Biochem. Biophys. Acta,* 572:363–369.
9. Vane, J. R. (1957): *Br. J. Pharmacol. Chemotherap.,* 12:344–350.
10. Wells, M. A. (1972): *Biochemistry,* 11:1030–1041.

Advances in Prostaglandin and Thromboxane Research,
Vol. 6, edited by B. Samuelsson, P. W. Ramwell,
and R. Paoletti. Raven Press, New York © 1980.

Synthesis and Biological Activities of Arachidonic and α- and β-Alkyl-Substituted Arachidonic Acid Derivatives

C. D. Liang, John S. Baran, James E. Miller, D. H. Steinman, and R. N. Saunders

Department of Chemical Research, G. D. Searle & Co., Chicago, Illinois 60680

5,8,11,14-Eicosatetraenoic acid **1a** (AA), 8,11,14-eicosatrienoic acid, and 5, 8,11,14,17-eicosapentaenoic acid possess a variety of physiological activities, presumably due to their conversion to prostaglandin (PG) hormones. These essential polyunsaturated fatty acids have been reported to act as vasodilators (5,14), vasoconstrictors (15), promote or inhibit platelet aggregation (1,11), produce antisecretory effects (3), increase myocardial contractility (6), and possess antiarrhythmic activity (7). In addition, α- and β-substituted 8,11,14-eicosatrienoic acids have been enzymatically converted to the corresponding PGs (12). Other unsaturated fatty acids which were not substrates for cyclooxygenases but nevertheless influenced the relative pathway of AA to its metabolites were 5,8,11,14-eicosatetraenoic acid (4), C-5, C-8, C-11-eicosatrienoic acid (13), and 5,8,11, 14,17-eicosapentaenoic acid (8).

Two types of fatty acid dioxygenases were found in acetone powder preparation of sheep vesicular gland by Lands et al. (10). One type, latent form (Ea), was found stimulated by phenol but was suppressed by the functions of glutathione peroxidase. The other type, basal form (Eb), was not affected by glutathione peroxidase. It is also known that phenol and other cyclooxygenase stimulators have differential effects on two classes of cyclooxygenase inhibitors. The fenamates themselves are weak inhibitors of cyclooxygenase alone but are much more potent in the presence of phenol, while the effectiveness of the more potent inhibitors i.e., ibaprofen, indomethacin, and flurbiprofen are reduced in the presence of phenol (2).

For the above reasons, phenol esters of AA and alkylated AA were prepared and their activities in prevention of spontaneous platelet aggregation in the male retired breeder rat were compared (9).

SYNTHESIS OF AA DERIVATIVES

(R), (S)-Methyl AA **2b** and *(R), (S)*-ethyl AA **2d** were obtained by the alkylation of AA ethyl ester **1b**. The lithium ester enolate of AA ethyl ester was

generated by the dropwise addition of **1b** in tetrahydrofuran to a dilute THF solution of lithium *N*-diisopropylamide at −78°C with vigorous stirring, followed by addition of alkyl iodide. The nuclear magnetic resonance of the alkylation products of AA ester and AA ester were compared, and no sign of the isomerization of the double bonds was found. It was found, however, that a highly diluted solution of AA anion is essential for this alkylation. Alkylation **2a** with methyl iodide, under identical conditions for the synthesis of **2a,** gave the α,α-methyl AA ethyl ester **3a,** in an overall yield of 60%. The polyunsaturated fatty acids

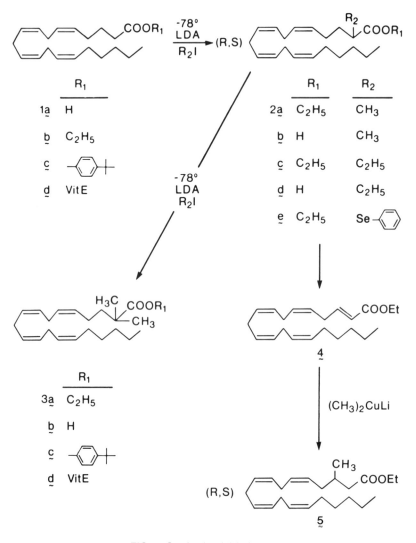

FIG. 1. Synthesis of AA derivatives.

2b, 2d, and **3b** were obtained by the cleavage of the corresponding esters with lithium iodide and collidine at 120°C, careful acidification of the reaction mixture with aqueous acid, and their extraction with ether.

Treatment of the lithium enolate of **1b** with diphenyl diselenide at −78°C yielded 2-phenylselenoarachidonate ethyl ester **2e.** Oxidation of **2e** with sodium periodate at 20°C was followed by rapid elimination to the Δ^2-AA ethyl ester **4.** Conjugate addition of dimethyl copper lithium to **4** gave a quantitative yield of *(R),(S)*-3-methyl-AA ethyl ester **5.** The polyunsaturated fatty acids **1a** and **3b** were converted to the corresponding anhydrides by treating them with dicyclohexylcarbodiimide in CH_2Cl_2. When the anhydrides were stirred in with 4-*tert*-butyl-phenol or vitamin E, the esters **1c, 1d, 3c** and **3d** were obtained.

IN VITRO HUMAN PLATELET AGGREGATION

Using standard *in vitro* turbidometric method, AA has been demonstrated to induce irreversible platelet aggregation in human citrated platelet-rich plasma at final concentrations as low as 0.4 mM. 2,2-Dimethyl AA **3b** when added to the platelet-rich plasma, displays a dose-related reduction in the arachidonate-induced platelet aggregation. At final concentration of 0.6 mM, **3b** reduces the aggregatory response induced by a 0.67 mM arachidonate concentration by 50%. Furthermore, **3b** at a concentration of 1.0 mM was found to inhibit the second phase of aggregation induced by epinephrine (10 μM) or adenosine diphosphate (2 μM).

EFFECTS OF AA DERIVATIVES ON PLATELET AGGREGATION IN THE RAT

Platelets from male retired breeder rats (COBS CD1) have been observed to form spontaneous aggregates by the Wu and Hoak aggregate ratio technique (16). This phenomenon is not observed with nonbred rats of the same sex, age, and supplier. Acetylsalicylic acid, sulfinpyrazone, and dipyridamole will prevent the formation of these platelet aggregates in a dose-related fashion in this model (9). When evaluated 3 hr after a single oral administration, these compounds may be ranked in order of decreasing potency as follows: sulfinpyrazone, dipyridamole, and acetylsalicylic acid with the ED_{50} of 4.1, 6.8, and 7.7 mg/kg, respectively.

All compounds listed in Table 1 were dissolved in polyethylene glycol 400 and administered to retired breeder rats intragastrically. Three hr after a single administration of the above compounds, the rats were anesthetized and blood was removed into two syringes, as described by Wu and Hoak (16). Dose–response relationships in the prevention of platelet aggregate formation in this technique were determined for each of the above compounds. A ranking of the potency of these compounds in decreasing order of the calculated ED_{50} is given in Table 1. (The incorporation of ^{14}C-2,2-dimethyl-arachidonic acid **3b** into lipid fractions was investigated. It was found that *in vivo* **3b** is a poor

TABLE 1. *Normalization of platelet activity in the male retired breeder rat*

Compound	MED (mg/kg/rat)
Arachidonic acid, *p-t*-butylphenol ester	1.1
2,2-Dimethyl arachidonic acid, *p-t*-butylphenol ester	2.2
Arachidonic acid, vitamin E ester	10
Vitamin E	10
2,2-Dimethylarachidonic acid	13
Arachidonic acid	15
2,2-Dimethylarachidonic acid ethyl ester	20
Linoleic acid, *p-t*-butylphenol ester	Inactive at 20
Stearic acid, *p-t*-butylphenol ester	Inactive at 20
p-t-butylphenol	Inactive at 2 and 10

substrate for incorporation into phospholipid. Only 5% of the radioactive **3b** was found in a phospholipid subclass.)

SUMMARY

In the male retired breeder rat, arachidonic acid **1a** and 2,2-dimethylarachidonic acid **3a** exhibited plasma platelet disaggregation as measured after 3 hr after the compounds were administered intragastrically at 15 and 13 mg/kg/rat mean effective dose (MED), respectively.

The corresponding *p-t*-butylphenol ester of the acids showed a remarkable potentiation of platelet disaggregation. The MED for *p-t*-butylphenol ester of AA was 1.1 mg/kg/rat.

REFERENCES

1. Dyerberg, J., Bang, H. O., Stofferson, E., Moncada, S., and Vane, J. R. (1978): *Lancet,* 2:117–119. [Also see leading reference, McGiff, J. C. (1979): *Fed. Proc.,* 38:64–65.]
2. Egan, R. W., Humes, J. L., and Kuehl, F. A. Jr. (1978): *Biochemistry,* 17:2230–2234.
3. Frame, M. M., Main, I. H. M., and Melarange, R. A. (1977): *Proc. Phys. Soc.,* 270:79–80.
4. Hammarström, S. (1977): *Biochem. Biophys. Acta,* 487:517–519.
5. Kulkarni, P. S., Roberts, R., and Needleman, P. (1976): *Prostaglandins,* 12:337–353.
6. Mentz, P., and Forster, W. (1977): *Prostaglandins,* 14:173–179.
7. Mest, H. J., Blass, K. E., and Forster, W. (1977): *Prostaglandins,* 14:163–172.
8. Needleman, P., Raz, A., Minkes, M. S., Ferrendelli, J. A., and Sprecher, H. (1979): *Proc. Natl. Acad. Sci. USA,* 76:944–948.
9. Saunders, R. N., Burns, T. S., Stelzer, M. R., and Waskawic, E. R. (1977): *Anim. Sci.,* 27:757–761.
10. Smith, W. L., and Lands, W. E. M. (1972): *Biochemistry,* 11:3276–3285.
11. Uzunova, A. D., Ramey, E. R., and Ramwell, P. W. (1977): *Prostaglandins,* 13:995–1002.
12. van Dorp, D. A., and Christ, E. J. (1975): *Rec. Trav. Chim.,* 94:247–276.
13. van Evert, W. C., Nugteren, D. H., and van Dorp, D. A. (1978): *Prostaglandins,* 15:267–272.
14. Wennmalm, Å. (1977): *Prostaglandins,* 13:809–810.
15. Wicks, T. C., Rose, J. C., Johnson, M. J., Ramwell, P. W., and Kot, P. A. (1976): *Circ. Res.,* 38:167–171.
16. Wu, K. K., and Hoak, J. C. (1974): *Lancet,* 2:924–926.

Advances in Prostaglandin and Thromboxane Research,
Vol. 6, edited by B. Samuelsson, P. W. Ramwell,
and R. Paoletti. Raven Press, New York © 1980.

Activation of Arachidonic Acid Turnover in Adrenal Phospholipids by ACTH, A23187, and Ca^{2+}

M. P. Schrey and R. P. Rubin

Department of Pharmacology, Medical College of Virginia, Richmond, Virginia

A role for membrane-bound phospholipases during ligand–receptor-mediated cell activation has been established in recent years (6). Previous studies from our laboratory which utilized an exogenous radiolabeled phospholipid substrate to measure changes in enzyme activity (2) and radioimmunoassay to measure prostaglandin (PG) levels (4) have demonstrated that adrenocorticotropic hormone (ACTH) induces a Ca^{2+}-dependent increase in phospholipase A$_2$ (PLA$_2$) activity and PG synthesis in cat adrenocortical cells (5). Moreover, ACTH was able to enhance the conversion of ^{3}H-arachidonic acid (AA) to PGs (3). The present investigation employs both ^{14}C-AA incorporation into phospholipids and radiolabeled PLA$_2$ substrate to provide further information for the existence of a Ca^{2+}-dependent cortical PLA$_2$. Special attention is paid to a rapid and specific turnover of arachidonate within a phosphatidylinositol (PI) pool during activation of steroidogenesis by ACTH which is independent of changes in *de novo* PI synthesis.

When cat cortical cells were incubated with ^{14}C-AA in the presence of ACTH (200 μU), incorporation of label specifically into PI was increased to 177% of unstimulated values within 2 min (Table 1). By contrast, incorporation of label into phosphatidylcholine, phosphatidylserine, and phosphatidylethanolamine was unaffected by ACTH (Table 1). The effect on label incorporation into PI was maximal at 2 min and thereafter declined to around half maximal levels after 30 min. Significant increases in ^{14}C-AA incorporation were observed with as little as 2 μU ACTH (129 ± 5% of control), and the dose response paralleled that of cortisol release. The PI effect was dependent on the presence of extracellular Ca^{2+} and could be mimicked by A23187 (5 μM). The ionophore increased ^{14}C-AA incorporation into PI (230 ± 13% of control) more effectively than did ACTH (170%) but resembled ACTH in its specificity for PI. Other peptide hormones (insulin, 10^{-8} M, luteinizing hormone, 10^{-8} M, vasopressin, 10^{-9} M) and dibutyryl cyclic adenosine monophosphate (1 mM) failed to promote AA incorporation into cortical phospholipids. ACTH elicited no change in label incorporation when ^{14}C-saturated fatty acid (palmitate) (Table 1), ^{14}C-glycerol,

TABLE 1. *Effect of ACTH on incorporation of* ^{14}*C-AA or* ^{14}*C-palmitic acid into adrenocortical cell phospholipid*[a]

Phospholipid	Relative change in fatty acid incorporation (% of control)	
	AA	Palmitic acid
Phosphatidylcholine	100 ± 4	98 ± 6
Phosphatidylinositol	177 ± 5	97 ± 5
Phosphatidylserine	96 ± 5	108 ± 6
Phosphatidylethanolamine	103 ± 12	126 ± 17

[a] Isolated cells (4×10^5) were incubated at 37°C for 2 min in 500 μl culture medium containing labeled fatty acid in the presence or absence of ACTH (200 μU). The incubation was terminated by addition of 3 ml of chloroform/methanol (1:2, v/v) and the lipid extracted overnight. The extracted phospholipids were separated by thin-layer chromatography and quantitated by liquid scintillation spectrometry.

or ^{3}H-inositol were employed as precursor, which suggests that stimulated incorporation of ^{14}C-AA was not a consequence of *de novo* synthesis of PI. Chlorpromazine (100 μM) and *p*-bromophenacylbromide (10 μM), agents known to suppress PLA_2 activity, reduced the ACTH-induced PI effect from 177% to 101 and 103%, respectively. In cells prelabeled with ^{14}C-AA, a significant loss of label from the PI fraction was observed with ACTH ($13 \pm 3\%$) and A23187 ($23 \pm 6\%$) after 2 min.

We have also identified a Ca^{2+}-requiring PLA_2 in a subcellular fraction of lysed cortical cells using exogenous phospholipid substrate (autoclaved *E. coli*), which constitutes evidence that the enzyme is localized to cell membranes. Moreover, increasing Ca^{2+} concentrations induced a dose-dependent release of nonesterified ^{14}C-AA from this subcellular fraction of prelabeled cells which paralleled Ca^{2+} activation of PLA_2. Thus Ca^{2+} concentrations from 0 to 20 mM elicited a linear increase in release of free ^{14}C-AA to a maximum of $128 \pm 2\%$ of control at 20 mM Ca^{2+} ($p < 0.025$). Similarly, PLA_2 activity increased in a linear fashion from 4 ± 1 to $21 \pm 4\%$ hydrolysis/mg protein/hr in the concentration range of 0.1 to 10 mM Ca^{2+}.

The parallel actions of Ca^{2+} on ^{14}C-AA release and on PLA_2 activity in this membrane fraction provide supportive evidence for the existence of a Ca^{2+}-stimulated deacylation reaction catalyzed by PLA_2. The deacylation reaction appears to be followed by a rapid, selective reacylation of lysoPI, as evidenced by the enhanced incorporation of ^{14}C-AA into PI during the action of ACTH or A23187. This deacylation–reacylation sequence may not only be important for initiating reactions concerned with PG synthesis, but may also be a pivotal mechanism for altering the architecture of cortical membrane phospholipids during activation of the adrenal cortex by ACTH. The critical role of Ca^{2+} in the diverse actions of ACTH (1) may be attributable, at least in part, to the effects of this cation on the deacylation–reacylation cycle.

ACKNOWLEDGMENT

This work was supported by U.S. Public Health Service Grant AM-18066.

REFERENCES

1. Halkerston, I. D. K. (1975): In: *Advances in Cyclic Nucleotide Research,* Vol. 6, edited by P. Greengard and G. A. Robison, pp. 99–136. Raven Press, New York.
2. Laychock, S. G., Franson, R. C., Weglicki, W. B., and Rubin, R. P. (1977): *Biochem. J.,* 164:753–756.
3. Laychock, S. G., and Rubin, R. P. (1975): *Prostaglandins,* 10:529–540.
4. Laychock, S. G., and Rubin, R. P. (1976): *Prostaglandins,* 11:753–767.
5. Rubin, R. P., and Laychock, S. G. (1978): *Ann. N.Y. Acad. Sci.,* 307:377–390.
6. Vogt, W. (1978): In: *Advances in Prostaglandin and Thromboxane Research,* Vol. 3, edited by C. Galli, G. Galli, and G. Porcellati, pp. 89–95. Raven Press, New York.

Advances in Prostaglandin and Thromboxane Research,
Vol. 6, edited by B. Samuelsson, P. W. Ramwell,
and R. Paoletti. Raven Press, New York © 1980.

Role of Phospholipase in the Regulation of Prostaglandin E_2 Biosynthesis by Rabbit Renomedullary Interstitial Cells in Tissue Culture: Effects of Angiotensin II, Potassium, Hyperosmolality, Dexamethasone, and Protein Synthesis Inhibition

Randall M. Zusman and C. Alan Brown

Cellular and Molecular Research Laboratory, Cardiac Unit, Medical Services, Massachusetts General Hospital, Boston, Massachusetts 02114

Within the kidney a minimum of five sites—the mesangial cells of the glomerulus, epithelial cells of Bowman's capsule, endothelial cells of the vasculature, epithelial cells of the collecting duct, and interstitial cells of the renal medulla and papilla—are capable of converting arachidonic acid to prostaglandins (PGs), thromboxane, and/or prostacyclin (3). Although many physiologic and pharmacologic agents stimulate the release of PGs from the kidney (1), researchers have been unable to study the regulation of cellular PG biosynthesis because of the lack of a suitable homogeneous cell population for the study of arachidonic acid metabolism. The isolation of rabbit renomedullary interstitial cells in tissue culture provided a model system for the study of cellular PG synthesis (4). These cells grow in monolayer in tissue culture and synthesize large quantities of PGE_2. Angiotensin II, bradykinin, and arginine vasopressin stimulate PGE_2 synthesis by renomedullary interstitial cells by increasing the rate of arachidonic acid release from the cellular arachidonic acid storage pool (4). The finding that mepacrine, a phospholipase inhibitor, decreases polypeptide hormone-stimulated PG synthesis has led to the conclusion that a phospholipase catalyzes the deacylation of phospholipids and results in arachidonic acid release with subsequent synthesis of PGE_2 (5). Increasing the osmolality of the incubation medium or removing potassium from the medium stimulates PGE_2 synthesis, whereas dexamethasone inhibits PGE_2 synthesis. Cycloheximide, an inhibitor of protein synthesis, decreases angiotensin II-stimulated PGE_2 synthesis but does not change the effects of hyperosmolality, dexamethasone, or potassium on arachidonic acid release or PGE_2 synthesis (6). These results suggest that the stimulation of arachidonic acid release by polypeptide hormones is due to phospholipase activation and is dependent on *de novo* protein synthesis. The effects of potassium, hyperosmolality, and dexamethasone are also due to changes in the rate of arachidonic acid release but are independent of protein synthesis.

The purpose of this study was to measure the phospholipase activity of the cells both under basal conditions and in response to angiotensin II, hyperosmolality, dexamethasone, and potassium-free media, and to determine the cellular source of arachidonic acid released in response to these agents.

METHODS

Rabbit renomedullary interstitial cells were grown in tissue culture as previously described (4). Experiments were performed in Krebs bicarbonate buffer; the potassium concentration was 3 mEq/liter unless stated otherwise, and a final osmolality was adjusted to 300 mOsm/liter with mannitol. Each incubation period was 1 hr at 37°C in an atmosphere of 95% air–5% CO_2.

Phospholipase Assay

The substrate for the phospholipase assay was prepared by incubating the cells overnight with tritium-labeled arachidonic acid (New England Nuclear, 62 Ci/mmole) and unlabeled arachidonic acid (NuChek Prep, Elysian, Minnesota). The phospholipid fraction of the cellular lipids was isolated by thin-layer chromatography. After the cells were exposed to the experimental variable for 1 hr, they were washed with fresh Krebs bicarbonate buffer and lysed by mild sonication in 1 ml of buffer. The calcium content of the buffer was raised to 5 mEq/liter and 100 pmoles of arachidonic acid-containing phospholipid was added to the solution. After incubation for 1 hr at 37°C, the free arachidonic acid was separated from the phospholipid substrate by extraction into chloroform (2), and the amount of arachidonic acid released was determined by scintillation counting of the radiolabeled lipids released.

The cellular source of arachidonic acid released in response to angiotensin II, potassium-free medium, hyperosmolality, or dexamethasone was determined by incubating the cells overnight with tritium-labeled arachidonic acid, washing the cells with fresh media prior to initiating the experiment, exposing the cells to the experimental agent or conditions, extracting the cellular lipids, and separating the phospholipid and triglyceride fractions by thin-layer chromatography (2).

RESULTS

The experimental data are summarized in Tables 1 and 2. Angiotensin II, 2 nM, stimulated phospholipase activity from 422 ± 13 to 1641 ± 76 fmoles arachidonic acid released/μg protein/hr (mean $\pm$ SEM, $N = 6$, $p < 0.01$); neither potassium-free media, hyperosmolality, nor dexamethasone affected cellular phospholipase activity.

TABLE 1. *Effects of angiotensin II, potassium-free media, hyperosmolality, and dexamethasone on PGE$_2$ synthesis, phospholipase activity, and arachidonic acid storage pool in rabbit renomedullary interstitial cells in tissue culture*[a]

Experimental conditions	PGE$_2$ synthesis (pmoles/μg protein/hr)	Phospholipase activity (fmoles arachidonic acid released/μg protein/hr)	Arachidonic acid storage pool (pmoles/ug protein)	
			Phospholipids	Triglycerides
Basal	1.8 ± 0.4	422 ± 13	17.17 ± 0.14	15.13 ± 0.39
Angiotensin II (2 nM)	27.1 ± 1.4[b]	1641 ± 76[b]	14.14 ± 0.29[b]	15.14 ± 0.24
Potassium (0 mEq/liter)	3.2 ± 0.5[b]	395 ± 29	16.22 ± 0.18[b]	15.09 ± 0.23
Hyperosmolality (1,200 mOsm/liter)	7.9 ± 0.7[b]	441 ± 31	15.83 ± 0.18[b]	14.75 ± 0.26
Dexamethasone (500 nM)	1.0 ± 0.2[b]	419 ± 18	17.54 ± 0.11[b]	14.70 ± 0.31

[a] Rabbit renomedullary interstitial cells were incubated for 1 hr in Krebs' bicarbonate buffer (potassium concentration, 3 mEq/liter, osmolality, 300 mOsm/liter); PGE$_2$ synthesis was measured by radioimmunoassay (4); phospholipase activity was measured as the rate of release of arachidonic acid from a radiolabeled arachidonic acid-containing phospholipid substrate; the distribution of arachidonic acid in the cellular lipid storage pool was measured by thin-layer chromatographic separation of the lipids extracted from cells incubated with tritium-labeled arachidonic acid. Each value represents the mean ± SEM ($N=6$).

[b] Statistically significant ($p < 0.01$) compared to basal values.

TABLE 2. Effects of cyclohexamide, mepacrine, and indomethacin on angiotensin II-stimulated PGE_2 synthesis, phospholipase activity, and arachidonic acid storage pool in rabbit renomedullary interstitial cells in tissue culture[a]

Experimental conditions	PGE_2 synthesis (pmoles/μg protein/hr)	Phospholipase activity (fmoles arachidonic acid released/μg protein/hr)	Arachidonic acid storage pool (pmoles/μg protein)	
			Phospholipids	Triglycerides
Angiotensin II (2 nM)	27.1 ± 1.4	1641 ± 76	14.14 ± 0.29	15.14 ± 0.24
+ cycloheximide (35 μM)	8.6 ± 1.1[b]	974 ± 37[b]	15.79 ± 0.19[b]	14.87 ± 0.29
+ mepacrine (100 μM)	13.7 ± 1.4[b]	806 ± 66[b]	16.18 ± 0.25[b]	14.94 ± 0.38
+ indomethacin (100 μM)	0.21 ± 0.03[b]	1601 ± 57	14.77 ± 0.60	14.98 ± 0.27

[a] PGE_2 synthesis, phospholipase activity, and the distribution of arachidonic acid in the cellular storage pool were measured as described in footnote a of Table 1. The cells were preincubated with cycloheximide, mepacrine, or indomethacin for a minimum of 2 hr prior to incubation with angiotensin II. Each value represents the mean ± SEM ($N=6$).

[b] Statistically significant ($p < 0.01$) compared to the value obtained after incubation with angiotensin II alone.

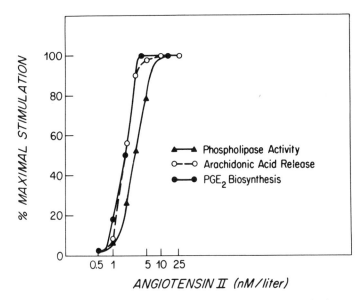

FIG. 1. Effect of angiotensin II on phospholipase activity, arachidonic acid release, and PGE₂ synthesis. PGE₂ synthesis and arachidonic acid release were measured as previously reported (4,5). Phospholipase activity was measured as described in the text as the rate of phospholipolysis of an arachidonic acid-containing phospholipid substrate.

Angiotensin II, potassium-free media, and hyperosmolality stimulated the loss of arachidonic acid from the phospholipid storage pool, whereas dexamethasone prevented the loss of arachidonic acid from phospholipids. Neither angiotensin II, potassium-free media, hyperosmolality, nor dexamethasone affected the amount of arachidonic acid stored in the triglyceride cellular lipid pool.

Cycloheximide and mepacrine inhibited angiotensin II-stimulated phospholipase activity and the loss of arachidonic acid from the phospholipid pool. Indomethacin inhibited PGE₂ synthesis but had no effect on phospholipase activity or the release of arachidonic acid from phospholipids. When cycloheximide was added to the phospholipase assay media after exposure of the cells to angiotensin II, no decrease occurred in phospholipase activity; the addition of mepacrine at that point inhibited phospholipase significantly. Thus cycloheximide is an inhibitor of the stimulation of phospholipase activity and mepacrine is an inhibitor of the phospholipase.

The dose–response relationship for angiotensin-stimulated PGE₂ synthesis, arachidonic acid release and phospholipase activity shows the close relationship of these parameters in this system (Fig. 1).

DISCUSSION

We conclude that angiotensin II-stimulated arachidonic acid release and PGE₂ synthesis are due to the stimulation of cellular phospholipase activity and the subsequent increased rate of phospholipolysis. This step is dependent on *de novo* protein synthesis. Potassium-free media, hyperosmolality, and dexamethasone also affect the rate of arachidonic acid release from the cellular phospholipid storage pool; however, these agents have no affect on phospholipase activity nor are their effects dependent on *de novo* protein synthesis. It is possible that these agents affect the accessibility of phospholipids in the plasma membrane to phospholipase action.

REFERENCES

1. Dunn, M. J., and Hood, V. L. (1977): *Amer. J. Physiol.,* 233:F169–F184.
2. Itaya, K., and Ui, M. (1965): *J. Lipid Res.,* 6:16–20.
3. Smith, W. L., and Bell, T. G. (1978): *Am. J. Physiol.,* 235:F451–F457.
4. Zusman, R. M., and Keiser, H. R. (1977): *J. Clin. Invest.,* 60:215–223.
5. Zusman, R. M., and Keiser, H. R. (1977): *J. Biol. Chem.,* 252:2069–2071.
6. Zusman, R. M., and Keiser, H. R. (1980): *Kidney Int.,* 17 *(in press).*

Advances in Prostaglandin and Thromboxane Research,
Vol. 6, edited by B. Samuelsson, P. W. Ramwell,
and R. Paoletti. Raven Press, New York © 1980.

Role of Extracellular Arachidonate in Regulation of Prostaglandin Biosynthesis in Cultured 3T3 Fibroblasts

K. A. Chandrabose, R. W. Bonser, and P. Cuatrecasas

The Molecular Biology Department, The Wellcome Research Laboratories, Research Triangle Park, North Carolina 27709

De novo synthesis of prostaglandins (PGs) requires the presence of specific precursor fatty acid molecules, which must be released from endogenous esterified membrane lipids. This process (i.e., release of arachidonic acid by phospholipases) is generally regarded as being the rate-limiting step in PG biosynthesis (4). Using a mouse fibroblast cell line in culture, the experiments described here show that the extent of endogenous phospholipase activity can be considerably underestimated unless a product (arachidonate) trap such as serum albumin (2,3) is used, because the released arachidonate is immediately re-esterified into cell lipids. Physiological stimuli which activate PG biosynthesis by stimulating phospholipase activity also stimulate the process of re-esterification, a process which acts to deplete the substrate available for PG synthesis. Such stimuli thus act both to initiate and terminate a rapid flux of the fatty acid substrate from the cell monolayer to medium and back to the cell. Evidence is presented that suggests the true substrate for PG biosynthesis is the free fatty acid that is released into the external medium and that there is no apparent coupling (or substrate transfer) between the phospholipase and PG synthetase systems (3).

EFFECT OF SERUM ALBUMIN ON ARACHIDONATE RELEASE AND STIMULATED PG BIOSYNTHESIS

We have previously shown that 3T3 cells respond to thrombin and bradykinin by activation of phospholipases and PG biosynthesis (1). Isakson et al. (3) demonstrated in isolated perfused rabbit hearts that the quantity of arachidonate released was considerably underestimated if the perfusing buffer did not contain a fatty acid trap such as albumin. 3T3 cells labeled with [1-C^{14}] arachidonate overnight (to minimize pools of lipids differing in specific activity) show strikingly different responses to various stimuli in the absence and presence of albumin (Fig. 1). In the presence of albumin, much more radioactivity is released as

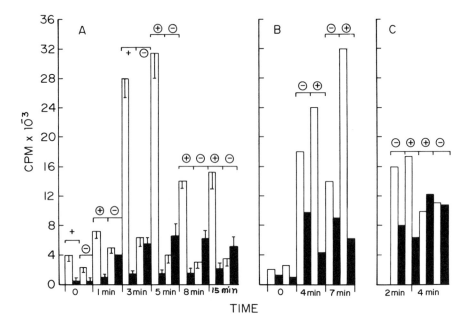

FIG. 1. A: Effect of albumin on the incorporation of ^{14}C-arachidonate into PGE$_2$. Swiss 3T3 cells, obtained from the American Type Culture Collection, were tested for mycoplasma once every four passages by Microbiological Associates. Cells were seeded at a density of 10^6 in a 9-cm petri dish in Dulbeco's modified Eagles medium (DMEM) with 10% fetal calf serum. The medium was changed on the third day and the confluent monolayer (7–7.5 × 10^6 cells/dish) was labeled on the fifth day after seeding. [1-C^{14}] Arachidonate, specific activity 55 μCi/μmole (Amersham), was used at 0.1 μCi/ml of medium. On the sixth day the cell monolayer was washed three times with phosphate-buffered saline (PBS), and 10 ml serum-free DMEM was added to one set of dishes. DMEM made 4% with fatty acid-free albumin (Sigma Chemicals, St. Louis) was added to an identical set of dishes. Bradykinin acetate was then added at a concentration of 1 μg/ml to all dishes, which were incubated at 37°C in a gyratory shaker for the indicated periods. At the end of incubation periods the medium was withdrawn and the monolayer was washed with 5 ml of PBS; the wash and medium were combined and lyophilized. The dry residue was extracted and analyzed for PGs by radiochromatography as previously described (1). Symbols used: +, medium containing 4% albumin; −, medium with no albumin; □, cpm in arachidonate fraction; ■, cpm in PGE$_2$. The inhibition of PGE$_2$ synthesis by 4% albumin medium was also confirmed by radioimmunoassay. **B:** Effect of unlabeled arachidonate on the incorporation of radioactivity to PG. The conditions were as described in **A**, except that 10^{-5} M unlabeled arachidonate (sonicated in DMEM) was added at the same time as bradykinin. The increase in radioactivity in the arachidonate fraction, as well as the decreased incorporation into PGs, was dose dependent from 10^{-4} to 10^{-6} M of unlabeled arachidonate. In a typical experiment, endogenous stimulation with bradykinin for 5 min produced 21.9 ng of PGE$_2$ (measured by radioimmunoassay) per 5 × 10^6 cells; when 10^{-5} M unlabeled arachidonate was present in the incubation medium, the yield of PGs was 1,660 ng. The specific activity of PGE$_2$ in these experiments was 45 cpm/ng in the absence of unlabeled arachidonate and 0.16 cpm/ng with 10^{-5} M arachidonate. **C:** Absence of effects of unlabeled palmitate on the incorporation of label into PG. The protocol was identical to that of **B**, except that 10^{-5} M unlabeled palmitate was substituted for arachidonate. The cells also synthesize PGF$_{2\alpha}$ and 6-keto PGF$_{1\alpha}$ but at much lower concentrations than E$_2$. The same patterns are observed with these two PGs.

free arachidonate, as shown by Isakson et al. (3) in perfused heart and in MC-5-cells by Hong and Levine (2). Such sequestration of arachidonate by albumin drastically reduces the radioactivity incorporated into PGs (Fig. 1), an observation not reported previously. This observation alone suggests the rather important concept that it is the extracellular arachidonate (including that on the external surface of the cell, accessible to albumin) which is the sole precursor for PG biosynthesis. Since in the absence of albumin (Fig. 1A) only a very small fraction of the *total* radioactivity known to be released is actually converted into PG and the quantity of free arachidonate in the medium is also low, it is obvious that most of the released fatty acid must be taken up and esterified very rapidly. Analysis of the cell monolayers in these experiments shows that there is no accumulation of cell-bound, free arachidonate throughout the time course of the experiment in the presence or absence of albumin.

STIMULATION IN THE PRESENCE OF UNLABELED ARACHIDONATE

Addition of excess unlabeled arachidonate to the medium produces qualitatively the same pattern as observed with albumin (Fig. 1B). The data indicate that the labeled, released pool is mixing freely with the unlabeled arachidonate outside the cell and, in accordance with the hypothesis outlined above, forms the substrate pool for PG biosynthesis. This is supported by the fact that along with the decreased incorporation of arachidonate radioactivity into PGs in the presence of unlabeled exogenous arachidonate, the specific radioactivity of the PGs produced is decreased considerably and the yield is quantitatively greater (Fig. 1B). PG biosynthesis can thus proceed from the extracellular pool, totally independent of the potential substrate in cellular lipid precursors in the absence or presence of a stimulus. The substrate specificity of the reactions under study is demonstrated by the fact that unlabeled palmitate is essentially without effect if it is substituted for exogenous arachidonate (Fig. 1C).

STIMULATED UPTAKE OF ARACHIDONATE FROM THE MEDIUM

Since it appeared that in the absence of albumin considerably larger quantities of arachidonate were released on stimulation than could actually be detected (Fig. 1), and since synthesis remained constant over longer periods of time if comparable amounts of arachidonate were supplied to unstimulated cells, the possibility existed that stimuli might affect not only the release, but also the cell reuptake of arachidonate. Experiments to show direct effects on the uptake of labeled fatty acid are especially difficult because the stimuli release unlabeled, endogenous substrate which dilutes the isotopic tracer, [1-C^{14}] arachidonate, employed to measure uptake by the cell. The masses involved are so small that accurate estimates and corrections, even by gas-liquid chromatography, have been too difficult and imprecise. Therefore, the concentration of the isotopic

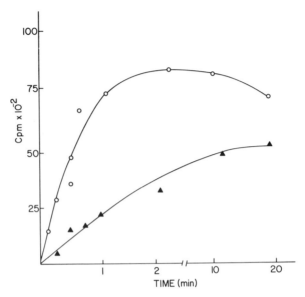

FIG. 2. Effect of thrombin on the rate of uptake (esterification) of exogenous arachidonate by cell monolayers. Confluent 3T3 monolayers were washed three times with PBS and 10 ml of serum-free DMEM, 1-C^{14}-arachidonate (specific activity, 5.5 μCi/μmole) and thrombin (1 U/ml) were added simultaneously. At the indicated times the medium was aspirated, the monolayer was washed three times with PBS, and chilled ($-60°$C) methanol was added to cell monolayers. The cells were then scraped and total lipids extracted and counted. Symbols: ▲, control dishes with no thrombin; ○, 1 U/ml of thrombin present.

pool in the medium was increased, so that any endogenous contribution would only have negligible effects on dilution of the outside pool. Under these conditions it is clear that a stimulus can markedly increase the rate of incorporation (re-esterification) of arachidonate into cells (Fig. 2).

When the cells are stimulated by thrombin, the radioactivity associated with the arachidonic acid fraction in the medium (in the absence of albumin) declines with virtually identical kinetics as PG biosynthesis (Fig. 3), suggesting that the free arachidonate remaining in the medium determines both the rate and extent of PG biosynthesis. The rate of synthesis declines sharply at the time when virtually all the free arachidonate disappears, presumably in large part by re-esterification.

SUMMARY

The stimuli that activate phospholipase releasing substrate fatty acids for PG biosynthesis also activates the reuptake of liberated fatty acids by the cell. The substrate released by these stimuli is accessible to albumin in 3T3 cells, and it is therefore presumably released into the extracellular space before it undergoes enzymatic conversion. Added exogenous arachidonate competes freely

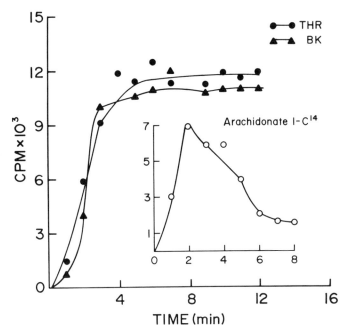

FIG. 3. Time course of PGE_2 production from endogenous substrate. 3T3 cell monolayers labeled as described in the legend to Fig. 1 were stimulated with thrombin (1 U/ml) and bradykinin (1 μg/ml) in the absence of albumin. The medium was removed at the indicated times, processed and analyzed for PG. Inset shows free arachidonate remaining in the medium at the indicated times.

with endogenous arachidonate released by a stimulus, suggesting no apparent coupling mechanism between phospholipase and cyclooxygenase enzyme systems.

REFERENCES

1. Chandrabose, K. A., Lapetina, E. G., Schmitges, C. J., Siegel, M. I., and Cuatrecasas P. (1978): *Proc. Natl. Acad. Sci. USA,* 75:214–217.
2. Hong, S. L., and Levine, L. (1976): *J. Biol. Chem.,* 251:5814–5816.
3. Isakson, P. C., Raz, A., Denny, S. E., Wyche, A., and Needleman, P. (1977): *Prostaglandins,* 14:853–871.
4. Lands, W. E. M., and Samuelsson, B. (1968): *Biochim. Biophys. Acta,* 164:426–429.

Advances in Prostaglandin and Thromboxane Research,
Vol. 6, edited by B. Samuelsson, P. W. Ramwell,
and R. Paoletti. Raven Press, New York © 1980.

Time-synchronized Activation of Lipolysis and Fatty Acids Reacylation by Bradykinin and Angiotensin II in the Perfused Rabbit Kidney

A. Raz and M. Schwartzman

Department of Biochemistry, The George S. Wise Center of Life Sciences, Tel Aviv University, Tel Aviv, Israel

Bradykinin (BK) and angiotensin II (AII) evoke the release of prostaglandins (PGs) from the perfused kidney, heart, and other tissues (1,5–7). PG production is preceded by hormone stimulation of intracellular lipolysis which is selective for the release of only AA in an amount 2- to 5-fold in excess of that converted to PGs (3,4,9). Excess AA released by the hormones but not converted to PGs is apparently reacylated into tissue lipids (9). The purpose of this investigation was to determine whether the effect of the hormones is limited to the selective hydrolysis of esterified AA or whether the hormones also activate fatty acid reacylation.

METHODS AND MATERIALS

Perfusion of Kidneys and Lipid Analysis of Kidney Effluent

Ureter-obstructed rabbit kidneys were prepared and perfused with Krebs-Henseleit buffer pH 7.4 at the rate of 15 ml/min (8). Effluent samples were acidified to pH 3.5 and extracted with ethyl acetate. The extract was dried over Na_2SO_4 and aliquots separated by thin-layer chromatography (t.l.c.). The PGE_2 and fatty acids were isolated from the t.l.c. plates and determined by bioassay and g.l.c. respectively (9).

Materials

Male rabbits 2 to 2.5 kg were employed. PGs $F_{2\alpha}$, E_2, D_2, and A_2 were kindly supplied by Dr. J. E. Pike of the Upjohn Co. (Kalamazoo, Michigan). All other materials were purchased from commercial sources.

RESULTS AND DISCUSSION

Stimulation by BK or AII (Fig. 1A and B) resulted in a 10- to 20-fold increase in PGE_2 release with no change or a small increase (10 to 15%) in AA release.

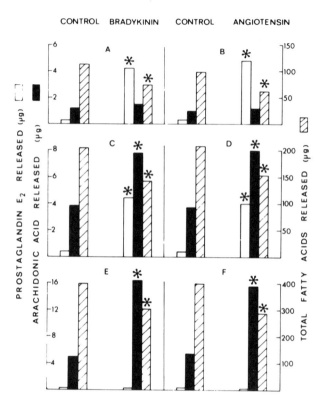

FIG. 1. Release of PGE₂, AA, and total fatty acids from perfused, ureter-obstructed, rabbit kidneys. Kidney effluent samples were collected for 4 min prior to (control) and immediately after bolus injection of bradykinin (0.5 μg) or AII (1 μg). Results in each experiment were normalized so that a value of 1 was assigned to the prehormone level of release. Percent of change after hormone stimulation was calculated for each parameter, and these values were averaged and analyzed by a Student *t*-test. The symbol * indicates posthormone values that are significantly different (p < 0.05) from control values. Perfusion was done with Krebs buffer (A,B) or Krebs buffer containing bovine serum albumin (fatty acid-poor, 1 mg/ml) before (C,D) or after (E,F) preinfusion of indomethacin (1 μg/ml, 15 min).

In contrast, there was a pronounced decrease of 35 to 50% in the release of total fatty acids after administration of the hormones. Experiments in which fatty acid-free bovine serum albumin was added to the perfusing media provide clear differentiation between the hormone-induced changes in PGE₂ and AA release and the changes in total fatty acids release (Fig. 1C and D). Albumin increases the basal release of all fatty acids by approximately 2-fold. Bolus injection of either hormone produces a 2- to 2.5-fold increase in the release of AA and a concomitant decrease of 25 to 30% in the release of total fatty acids. Upon hormone stimulation, blockade of PG biosynthesis by indomethacin resulted in a higher increase in the release of AA (Fig. 1E and F) that was approximately equal to the combined release of PGE₂ and AA in the absence of indomethacin. Although the results shown (Fig. 1) were obtained with Ureter-obstructed kidneys, the same pattern of results was also seen in experiments

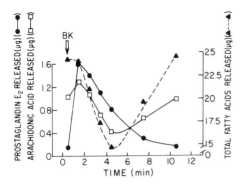

FIG. 2. Changes in the rate of release of PGE_2, AA, and total fatty acids from perfused rabbit kidney following stimulation by BK (0.5 µg). Experimental details were the same as in Fig. 1A and B and are given in the text and legend to Fig. 1. After collection of control effluent for 1 min, BK was administered *(arrow)* and 1-min effluent collections were continued for 12 min.

with normal rabbit kidneys except that both basal and hormone-stimulated release of PGE_2 and AA were considerably lower, as seen previously (8). BK and AII appear to activate a selective phospholipase A_2 which releases only arachidonate and a nonselective reacylation reaction that leads to increased esterification of intracellular free fatty acids into cellular lipids. The lipolysis and reacylation processes together with the PG synthetase system comprise the PG generation cycle. Experiments were performed to qualitatively and quantitatively determine the time course for activation of the lipolytic and reacylation processes. Experimental design was as described above (Fig. 1) but effluent collections were made for 1-min periods. A clear time lag exists between the activation of AA release (and its immediate partial conversion to PG products) and the subsequent activation of the reacylation process (Fig. 2). This difference in timing of approximately 1 min is apparently crucial in order to provide sufficient time for AA to be available as substrate to the cyclooxygenase. The possible nature of substances that could participate in the control of this synchronized lipolysis-reacylation cycle is the subject of current investigation in our laboratory.

SUMMARY

BK and AII administered to the isolated perfused rabbit kidney activate two sequential enzymatic processes: 1) a selective release of the PG precursor, AA with concomitant, partial conversion of arachidonate to PGE_2. 2) Activation of a reacylation process which leads to decreased release of all fatty acids in the perfusate. There is a lag time of approximately 1 min between initial activation of the arachidonate-specific deacylation reaction that is coupled to PG generation, and subsequent activation of the reacylation process.

ACKNOWLEDGEMENT

This work was supported by a research grant from the US-Israel Bi-National Fund.

REFERENCES

1. Blumberg, A. L., Denny, S. F., Marshall, G. R., and Needleman, P. (1977): *Am. J. Physiol.*, 232:H305–H310.
2. Folch, J., and Lees, M. (1957): *J. Biol. Chem.*, 226:497–504.
3. Hsieh, W., Isakson, P. C., and Needleman, P. (1977): *Prostaglandins*, 13:1073–1091.
4. Isakson, P. C., Raz, A., Denny, S. E., Wyche, A., and Needleman, P. (1977): *Prostaglandins*, 19:853–871.
5. McGiff, J. C., Terragno, N. A., Malik, K. V., and Lonigro, A. J. (1972): *Circ. Res.*, 31:36–43.
6. Needleman, P., Key, S. L., Denny, S. E., Isakson, P. C., and Marshall, G. R. (1975): *Proc. Natl. Acad. Sci. USA*, 72:2060.
7. Needleman, P., Marshall, G. R., and Sobel, B. E. (1975): *Circ. Res.*, 37:802–808.
8. Nishikawa, K., Morrison, A. R., and Needleman, P. (1977): *J. Clin. Invest.*, 59:1143–1150.
9. Schwartzman, M., and Raz, A. (1979): *Biochim. Biophys. Acta*, 572:363–369.

Advances in Prostaglandin and Thromboxane Research,
Vol. 6, edited by B. Samuelsson, P. W. Ramwell,
and R. Paoletti. Raven Press, New York © 1980.

Thrombin and Bradykinin Modulate Prostaglandin Synthetase Independently of Phospholipase

R. W. Bonser, K. A. Chandrabose, and P. Cuatrecasas

Department of Molecular Biology, Wellcome Research Laboratories,
Research Triangle Park, North Carolina 27709

Prostaglandins (PGs) have been implicated in many physiological processes (3), yet they are not stored to any appreciable extent in any tissue (6). Their presence and actions therefore reflect *de novo* synthesis and release. It is the availability of free arachidonic acid (AA), the substrate for PG synthetase, that limits PG biosynthesis (5,8). AA is found in cells mostly esterified in the form of membrane phospholipids, and it is generally accepted that activation of phospholipase A_2 is necessary for release of substrate. Stimulated PG production by vasoactive agents such as bradykinin and angiotensin II in perfused kidneys (7) has been suggested to involve the activation of a tightly coupled phospholipase–PG synthetase system. The stimulus activates a phospholipase-releasing AA which is immediately made available to the PG synthetase.

We have studied PG biosynthesis using a fibroblast cell line in culture. These cells release large amounts of PG when stimulated with bradykinin (BK) or thrombin (Th). We have found that on stimulation, PGs are synthesized from exogenous AA at a rate which far exceeds nonstimulated exogenous AA utilization. Furthermore, this large increase in PG production cannot be explained simply by the contribution from endogenous AA metabolism. We present evidence which suggests that BK and Th stimulate PG synthetase independently of phospholipase.

MATERIALS AND METHODS

Swiss 3T3 fibroblasts were purchased from the American Type Culture Collection and were cultured in Dulbecco's modified Eagle's minimum essential medium with 10% fetal calf serum, penicillin, and streptomycin. Cells seeded at an initial density of 1×10^6 cells/10-cm dish were grown for 2 days. The cell monolayers were washed twice with 5 ml minimum essential medium (MEM) and then incubated with 10 ml MEM containing AA, with and without BK (1 μg/ml) or Th (1 U/ml). At various times an aliquot of the medium was withdrawn, diluted appropriately, and PG measured by the radioimmunoassay procedure described by Jaffe et al. (4).

RESULTS AND DISCUSSION

Table 1 shows that Th stimulates PG production from exogenous AA in 3T3 cells. In the presence of 1×10^{-6} M AA, the rate of PG biosynthesis is virtually doubled. Preincubation with Th for 5 min prior to the addition of AA considerably reduces the rate of PG production. Figure 1 demonstrates more clearly the stimulation by Th and also by BK. Stimulation with BK or Th increases the rate of PG biosynthesis in the presence of 1×10^{-5} M AA from 6 to 54 ng/min and 47 ng/min, respectively. It is also apparent from Fig. 1 that the increase in PG production is not due simply to the contribution from endogenous AA metabolism. Stimulated PG production from both exogenous and endogenous AA remains linear for 3 min, with the rate then falling rapidly. The transient nature of the stimulus on endogenous AA metabolism in cultured cells has been reported (2), but to our knowledge a similar effect has not been described for exogenous AA metabolism.

The major PG produced by these cells is PGE_2. PGE_2 can be formed nonenzymatically from the PG endoperoxide PGH_2. PGH_2 is formed from AA by the enzyme cyclooxygenase; therefore, it is not unreasonable to assume that the increase in PGE_2 is simply a reflection of increased cyclooxygenase activity.

The efficient utilization of exogenous AA for PG biosynthesis in the presence of a stimulus argues against the tightly coupled phospholipase–cyclooxygenase system proposed by Schwartzman and Raz (7). The only way to explain the observations we have made in terms of a tightly coupled system is to propose that exogenous AA is rapidly cycled through a pool of phospholipid via a reacylation–deacylation reaction sequence. However, there is no evidence to date which proves the existence of such a highly dynamic pool of phospholipid.

TABLE 1. *Effect of Th on PG synthesis from exogenous AA in 3T3 cells*[a]

Preincubation conditions	Additions		PGE_2 (cpm)
	Thrombin	Arachidonic acid	
None	+	+	42,000
None	−	+	22,000
5 min + Th		+	16,000
5 min − Th		+	24,000

[a]Cell monolayers were incubated for 1.5 min in the presence of 1×10^{-6} M $[1 - {}^{14}C]$AA, with and without Th. Radioactively labeled PGE_2 was isolated by thin-layer chromatography using the procedure described by Chandrabose et al. (1).

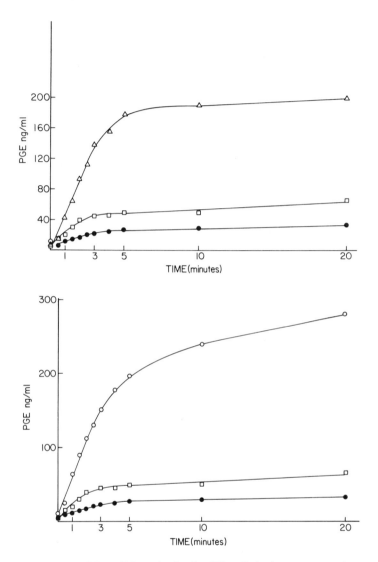

FIG. 1. Effect of Th and BK on PG production by 3T3 cells in the presence of exogenous AA. *Top:* ●, AA (1×10^{-5} M); □, Th (1 U/ml); △, AA (1×10^{-5} M) + Th (1 U/ml). *Bottom:* ●, AA (1×10^{-5} M); □, BK (1 μg/ml); ○, AA (1×10^{-5} M) + BK (1 μg/ml).

Therefore, we believe the stimulated production of PG in 3T3 cells from exogenous AA reflects a direct effect of the stimulus on the cyclooxygenase enzyme.

SUMMARY

Thrombin and bradykinin stimulate prostaglandin production from exogenous arachidonic acid in 3T3 cells. The increase in PG production cannot be explained simply by the contribution from endogenous AA metabolism. The rates of stimulated PG production from exogenous and endogenous AA both remain linear for 3 min, then fall rapidly. It is suggested that BK and Th may act by directly stimulating cyclooxygenase independently of phospholipase.

REFERENCES

1. Chandrabose, K. A., Lapetina, E. G., Schmitges, C. J., Siegel, M. I., and Cuatrecasas, P. (1978): *Proc. Natl. Acad. Sci. USA,* 75:214–217.
2. Hong, S. C. L., Polsky-Cynkin, R., and Levine, L. (1976): *J. Biol. Chem.,* 251:776–780.
3. Horton, E. W. (1972): *Monogr. Endocrinol.,* 7:1–197.
4. Jaffe, B. M., Behrman, H. R., and Parker, C. W. (1973): *J. Clin. Invest.,* 52:398–405.
5. Kunze, N., and Vogt, W. (1971): *Ann. N.Y. Acad. Sci.,* 180:123–125.
6. Piper, P. J., and Vane, J. R. (1971): *Ann. N.Y. Acad. Sci.,* 180:363–385.
7. Schwartzman, M., and Raz, A. (1979): *Biochim. Biophys. Acta,* 472:363–369.
8. Vonkeman, H., and Van Dorp, D. A. (1968): *Biochim. Biophys. Acta,* 164:430–432.

Advances in Prostaglandin and Thromboxane Research,
Vol. 6, edited by B. Samuelsson, P. W. Ramwell,
and R. Paoletti. Raven Press, New York © 1980.

Glucocorticoids and the Prostaglandin System in Adipose Tissue

Carmen Vigo, G. P. Lewis, and Priscilla J. Piper

Department of Pharmacology, Institute of Basic Medical Sciences, Royal College of Surgeons of England, Lincoln's Inn Fields, London WC2A 3PN, United Kingdom

Prostaglandin (PG) formation has been demonstrated in adipose tissue following nervous and hormonal stimulation (7,15). Release of PGs from adipose tissue was found to be inhibited by cyclooxygenase inhibitors (2) and by glucocorticoids (8). However, it was also observed that some PG formation continued in the tissue in the presence of the steroids (3). This finding was difficult to understand in view of the fact that the glucocorticoids were found to interfere with the action of phospholipase A_2 on membrane phospholipids (1,5,10). In a recent discussion of the mode of action of glucocorticoids on the PG system in adipose tissue (9), it was concluded that PGs can be synthesized from the arachidonic acid derived from both phospholipids and neutral lipid triglyceride.

This view agrees with an earlier observation (4) that the PG synthesized in isolated fat cells could be derived from the arachidonic acid released from triglycerides during lipolysis. This finding might well explain the continued formation of PGs in fat tissue in the presence of glucocorticoids but not in the presence of cyclooxygenase inhibitors.

In an attempt to clarify the mechanisms of action of the steroids, we decided to use the simpler system represented by fat cell ghosts from which the fat droplets and much of the cytoplasm has been removed. When the ghosts were stimulated with adrenocorticotropic hormone (ACTH), PGE_2 and $F_{2\alpha}$ were released. The precursor of these PGs, arachidonic acid, was found to be mainly present in the phospholipid (90%), while 8.5% was in the neutral lipid and 1.5% was unbound. When the ghosts were stimulated in the presence of glucocorticoids, the mobilization of endogenous arachidonic acid from the phospholipids was inhibited, while that from neutral lipid was enhanced. This finding is also consistent with the continued formation of PGs from the neutral lipid of whole fat tissue in the presence of glucocorticoids. This also agrees with the earlier observation (13) that glucocorticoids facilitate release of free fatty acids by decreasing glucose uptake into fat. The reduction in glucose uptake results in a decreased incorporation of ^{14}C from glucose into CO_2 and fat. It may therefore be through their effects on glucose metabolism that glucocorticoids restrict lipid synthesis and, via triglyceride, stimulate fatty acid release. This phenomenon also occurs in other extrahepatic tissues such as skin and lymphoid tissue. Such a control over glucose metabolism might be the basis of a general function of glucocorticoids with respect to lipid, proteins, and perhaps other metabolities regulating the balance between synthesis and breakdown. These effects are considerably enhanced in the presence of other compounds such as epinephrine or ACTH.

In fat cell ghosts, arachidonic acid release from the phospholipids was reduced, indicating that phospholipase A_2 was in some way being inhibited by the glucocorticoids. We have therefore studied the mechanisms by which this enzyme can be inhibited. Differential scanning calorimetry and assays of phospholipase A_2 activity were used as tools to distinguish between drugs which interact with the phospholipids and those which interact directly with the enzyme. Multibilayer liposomes were prepared from dipalmitoyl lecithin, and purified phospholipase A_2 from pig pancreas and naja naja venom were used. Hydrolysis of the liposomes induced by the phospholipase A_2 was studied at the transition temperature of dipalmitoyl lecithin (41°C), where enzyme activity is optimal, using a spectrophotometric method or chemical assays of the lysophospholipids formed, as well as the remaining dipalmitoyl lecithin (11).

Irregularities in lipid packing in the bilayer of liposomes strongly enhances phospholipase activity and these packing faults exist at the transition temperature of the lipid. The activity of this enzyme can therefore be inhibited by drugs which interact with the phospholipids in the membrane and alter the transition temperature or by molecules which directly interact with the enzyme. Cholesterol lowers the transition temperature, reduces the heat absorbed at transition (6), and also inhibits phospholipase A_2 activity on liposomes prepared from dipalmitoyl lecithin–cholesterol (12). Furthermore, this activity was reversed by filipin, a polyene antibiotic which interacts with cholesterol and restores the phase transition of the phosphatidylcholine molecules. It seems likely, therefore, that cholesterol inhibits the phospholipase by interacting with the phospholipids.

Mepacrine and phentermine did not interact with dipalmitoyl lecithin liposomes as determined by differential scanning calorimetry, but reduced the rate of hydrolysis induced by purified phospholipase A_2 by a direct interaction with the enzyme. On the other hand, the general anesthetics ethrane, halothane, and trichloroethylene inhibited the enzyme by interacting with the dipalmitoyl lecithin. These anesthetics increase the fluidity of the membrane, lowering the transition temperature significantly. However, they also appeared to interact directly with the enzyme, because the inhibitory effect was not overcome by assaying phospholipase A_2 at the new transition temperature. It has been suggested that some local anesthetics inhibit phospholipase A_2 by competing for Ca^{2+} (14,16). In our own experiments even when the Ca^{2+} concentration was increased 10-fold (10 mM), the effect of the anesthetics was not reversed.

Our studies using the glucocorticoids hydrocortisone, dexamethasone, and beta methasone, in concentrations from 1 μg to 2 mg steroid/mg lipid, failed to reveal any effect of the drugs on membrane fluidity or any direct effect on the rate of hydrolysis of dipalmitoyl liposomes by phospholipase A_2.

Further mechanisms must therefore be sought to explain the action of glucocorticoids.

REFERENCES

1. Blackwell, G. J., Flower, R. J., Nijkamp, F. P., and Vane, J. R. (1978): *Br. J. Pharmacol.*, 62:79–89.
2. Bowery, B., and Lewis, G. P. (1973): *Br. J. Pharmacol.*, 47:305–314.
3. Chang, J., Lewis, G. P., and Piper, P. J. (1977): *Br. J. Pharmacol.*, 59:425–432.
4. Christ, E. J., and Nugteren, D. H. (1970): *Biochim. Biophys. Acta*, 218:296–307.
5. Gryglewski, R. J. (1976): *Pharmacol. Res. Commun.*, 8:337–348.
6. Ladbrooke, B. D., Williams, R. M., and Chapman, D. (1968): *Biochim. Biophys. Acta*, 150:333–340.
7. Lewis, G. P., and Matthews, J. (1970): *J. Physiol.*, 207:15–30.
8. Lewis, G. P., and Piper, P. J. (1975): *Nature*, 254:308–311.
9. Lewis, G. P., and Piper, P. J. (1978): *Biochem. Pharmacol.*, 27:1409–1412.
10. Lewis, G. P., Piper, P. J., and Vigo, C. (1979): *Br. J. Pharmacol.*, 66:99P.
11. Lewis, G. P., Piper, P. J., and Vigo, C. (1979): *Br. J. Pharmacol.*, 66:500–501.
12. Lewis, G. P., Piper, P. J., and Vigo, C. (1979): *Br. J. Pharmacol.*, 66:453 P.
13. Munck, A. (1962): *Biochim. Biophys. Acta*, 57:312–326.
14. Scherphof, G. L., Scarpa, A., and Van Toorenenbergen, A. (1972): *Biochim. Biophys. Acta*, 270:226–240.
15. Shaw, J. E., and Ramwell, P. W. (1968): *J. Biol. Chem.*, 243:1498–1503.
16. Waite, M., and Sisson, P. (1972): *Biochemistry*, 11:3098–3105.

Advances in Prostaglandin and Thromboxane Research,
Vol. 6, edited by B. Samuelsson, P. W. Ramwell,
and R. Paoletti. Raven Press, New York © 1980.

Biosynthesis of Thromboxanes

Sven Hammarström and Ulf Diczfalusy

Department of Chemistry, Karolinska Institutet, S-104 01 Stockholm, Sweden

A labile derivative of arachidonic acid, formed by human platelets, was discovered by trapping experiments with nucleophilic reagents (5). The compound, thromboxane A_2, is a powerful inducer of platelet aggregation and vasoconstriction (5). The previously described rabbit aorta contracting substance (9) consists mainly of thromboxane A_2 (10). The biosynthesis of thromboxanes from arachidonic acid involves two enzymes, prostaglandin (PG) endoperoxide synthase (cyclooxygenase), which converts arachidonic acid to PGH_2 (8), and thromboxane synthase, which isomerizes PGH_2 to thromboxane A_2 (7,11). This chapter deals with some characteristics of the latter enzyme.

RESOLUTION OF THROMBOXANE SYNTHESIZING ENZYMES (7)

Incubation of microsomes from human platelets with PGG_2 yielded 12-hydroxy-5,8,10-heptadecatrienoic acid (HHT), thromboxane B_2, PGE_2, and $PGF_{2\alpha}$. The former two products were obtained in greatest yield. $PGF_{2\alpha}$ was formed mainly by $SnCl_2$ reduction of excess substrate at the end of the incubation. Platelet microsomes also converted arachidonic acid and PGH_2 to thromboxane B_2, whereas cytosol, α-granules, dense bodies, and plasma membranes did not. The thromboxane synthesizing enzymes were released from the microsomes by treatment with Triton X-100. Upon chromatography on DEAE-cellulose, PG endoperoxide synthase was eluted with the 10 mM application buffer and thromboxane synthase with 0.2 M buffer (Table 1). Unless otherwise indicated, the experiments below were performed using partially purified enzyme obtained in this way.

INHIBITORS OF THROMBOXANE SYNTHASE

A number of compounds have been reported to inhibit thromboxane synthesis in vitro (2). Inhibitors, evaluated by a radiochemical assay of thromboxane synthase are listed in Table 2. Some of these substances are PGH_2 analogs which have biological effects similar to those of thromboxane A_2. Others also inhibit cyclooxygenase or have additional side effects.

TABLE 1. *Resolution of cyclooxygenase and thromboxane synthase by DEAE-cellulose chromatography[a]*

Eluate	Substrate	Products
I (0.01 M K-PO$_4$, pH 7.4, with 0.1% Triton X-100)	20:4 PGH$_2$	PGE$_2$, HHT none
II (0.02 M K-PO$_4$, pH 7.4, with 0.1% Triton X-100)	20:4 PGH$_2$	none none
III (0.2 M K-PO$_4$, pH 7.4, with 0.1% Triton X-100)	20:4 PGH$_2$	none thromboxane A$_2$, HHT

[a] Platelet microsomes were solubilized with 0.5% Triton X-100, and the 100,000 × g supernatant was applied to a DEAE-cellulose column.

TABLE 2. *Inhibitors of thromboxane synthase[a]*

Inhibitor	ID$_{50}$ (μM)
9,11-Azo-15-hydroxyprosta-5,13-dienoic acid	2
9,11-Epoxymethano-15-hydroxyprosta-5,13-dienoic acid	20
2-Isopropyl-3-nicotinyl-indole (L-8027)	10
Sodium-*p*-benzyl-4-[-1-oxo-2-(4-chlorobenzyl)-3-phenylpropyl] phenyl phosphonate (N-0164)	24
Imidazole	150

[a] Platelet microsomes were preincubated with inhibitors for 15 sec at 24°C, [1 − ^{14}C]PGH$_2$ was added, and the incubation was continued for 1 min. Percent conversion to thromboxane B$_2$ was determined by thin-layer chromatography.

FORMATION OF C-17 ACIDS FROM PG ENDOPEROXIDES

HHT and thromboxane B$_2$ are the major arachidonic acid metabolites in platelets, formed via the cyclooxygenase pathway (4). These products are also formed by platelet microsomes and partially purified preparations of thromboxane synthase (7). During experiments with inhibitors of thromboxane synthesis, it was observed that HHT formation was also inhibited (1). Figure 1 shows a plot of the inhibition of thromboxane B$_2$ versus the inhibition of HHT synthesis. The virtually identical inhibition by five structurally unrelated compounds strongly suggested that the same enzyme catalyzed the formation of HHT and thromboxane B$_2$. The possibility that thromboxane A$_2$ decomposes to a mixture of HHT and thromboxane B$_2$ was investigated by incubating PGH$_2$ for a short (10 sec) and a longer (2 min) period with enzyme. The substrate concentration was chosen such that all PGH$_2$ had been converted after 10 sec. The reactions were stopped by addition of methanol to convert thromboxane A$_2$ to 11-*O*-methyl thromboxane B$_2$. Table 3 shows the product compositions obtained. A

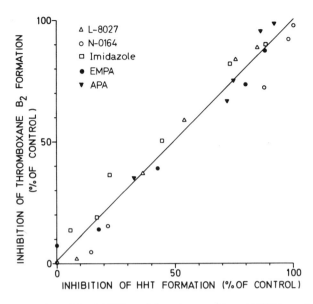

FIG. 1. Linear regression of the inhibition of thromboxane B_2 and HHT formation from PGH_2 by platelet microsomes. EMPA, 9,11-epoxymethano-15-hydroxyprosta-5,13-dienoic acid; APA, 9,11-azo-15-hydroxyprosta-5,13-dienoic acid. (From ref. 8.)

TABLE 3. *Transformation of thromboxane (TXA$_2$)*
to TXB$_2$ and independent formation of HHT

Incubation time (sec)	Radioactivity distribution (%)		
	TXA$_2$ [b]	TXB$_2$	HHT
10	21	22	55
120	<3	42	55

[a] Determined as 11-*O*-methyl TXB$_2$.

decrease of thromboxane A_2 and a corresponding increase of thromboxane B_2 was observed between the 10-sec and the 2-min incubations. In contrast, there was no change in the amount of HHT between the two incubations. Therefore, thromboxane A_2 did not appear to be an intermediate in HHT biosynthesis.

STRUCTURAL REQUIREMENTS FOR THROMBOXANE SYNTHESIS

Incubations of PGH_1 with partially purified thromboxane synthase gave only small amounts of thromboxane B_1. PGH_1 was, however, efficiently transformed to 12-hydroxy-8,10-heptadecadienoic acid (HHD) (1). L-8027 and imidazole inhibited the conversions of PGH_1 to HHD and of PGH_2 to HHT similarly

(Fig. 2). Unlabeled PGH_2 also competed with $[1-^{14}C]PGH_1$ in the transformation to C-17 acids (Fig. 3). These experiments suggest that thromboxane synthase catalyzes the formation of HHD from PGH_1 and of thromboxane A_2 plus HHT from PGH_2 (3). Trapping experiments with methanol did not provide evidence that thromboxane A_1 was formed and preferentially converted to HHD. Therefore, the Δ^5-double bond in PGH_2 seems essential for enzymatic synthesis of thromboxanes. To further investigate this possibility, cis-Δ^4-$[^3H_8]PGH_1$ was synthesized from 4,8,11,14-eicosatetraenoic acid (Fig. 4). This positional isomer of PGH_2 was converted to Δ^4-HHD but not significantly to Δ^4-thromboxane B_1 (Table 4), suggesting a high structural specificity for isomerization to thromboxanes (3).

The enzymatic conversion of endoperoxides to thromboxanes may involve initial protonation of the oxygen atom at C-9 and cleavage of the O-O bond (Fig. 5). The subsequent reactions comprise a cleavage of the C-11 to C-12 bond and formation of two new C-O bonds (the oxygen at C-9 is attached to C-11 and the oxygen at C-10 is attached to C-12). The Δ^5-double bond

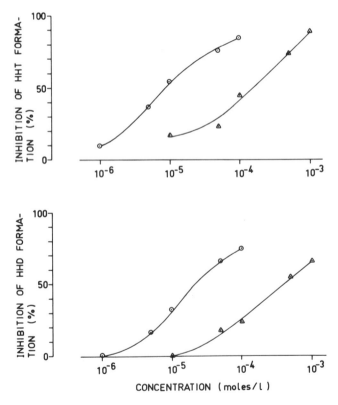

FIG. 2. Dose-inhibition curves for the conversion of PGH_1 and PGH_2 to HHD and HHT by platelet microsomes. ⊙, L-8027; △, imidazole (from ref. 3).

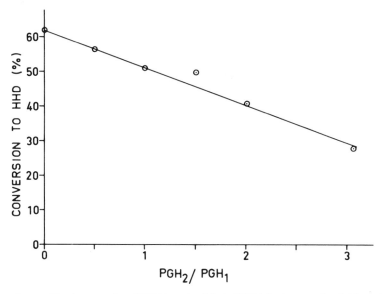

FIG. 3. Competition between [1-¹⁴C]PGH₁ and unlabeled PGH₂ for human platelet thromboxane synthase (from ref. 3).

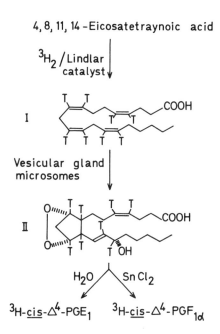

FIG. 4. Synthesis of *cis*-Δ⁴-[³H₈]PGH₁. I: 4, 8,11,14-*(all cis)*-[³H₈]-eicosatetraenoic acid; II: *cis*-Δ⁴-[³H₈]PGH₁ (from ref. 3).

TABLE 4. *Conversions of PG endoperoxides by thromboxane synthase*

Substrate	Conversion to C-17 acid (%)	Conversion to thromboxane (%)	C-17 acid/ thromboxane
[1 − ¹⁴C]PGH₁	66.5	1.6	42[b]
cis − Δ⁴ − [³H₈]PGH₁	89.5[a]	2.2[b]	41
[1 − ¹⁴C]PGH₂			2.3 ± 0.3[c]
[1 − ¹⁴C]PGG₂			1.6 ± 0.2[d]

[a] Corrected for loss of two tritium atoms.
[b] Radioactive material cochromatographing with thromboxane B₂.
[c] Mean ± SD; $n = 17$.
[d] Mean ± SD; $n = 15$.

may be required for exact positioning of the substrate at the active site of the enzyme to allow the latter reactions. This would lead to accumulation of intermediate I from endoperoxides lacking a Δ⁵-double bond and rearrangement of I to C-17 acids plus malondialdehyde.

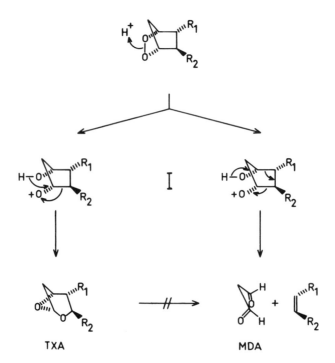

FIG. 5. Hypothetical mechanism for the conversion of PG endoperoxides to C-17 hydroxy acids and thromboxanes by one enzyme.

CONVERSIONS OF PGG$_2$ (6)

Incubations of PGG$_2$ with thromboxane synthase yielded two products, less polar than HHT and thromboxane B$_2$, respectively, on thin-layer chromatography. Reduction by SnCl$_2$ converted these products to HHT and thromboxane B$_2$, whereas dehydration by lead tetraacetate afforded 12-keto-5,8,10-heptadecatrienoic acid and 15-keto-thromboxane B$_2$. Methanol trapping yielded 11-O-methylthromboxane B$_2$ after SnCl$_2$ reduction of a less polar compound. Based on these results, the products obtained from PGG$_2$ were identified as 12-hydroperoxy-5,8,10-heptadecatrienoic acid (HPHT) and 15-hydroperoxythromboxane A$_2$ (HPTXA$_2$). HPTXA$_2$ induces platelet aggregation and contractions of rabbit aorta (S. Hammarström, *to be published*). Figure 6 summarizes the transformations of PGG$_2$, PGH$_2$, Δ^4-PGH$_1$, and PGH$_1$ by thromboxane synthase. The four substrates are all converted to C-17 hydroxy acids but only PGG$_2$ and PGH$_2$ are isomerized to thromboxanes.

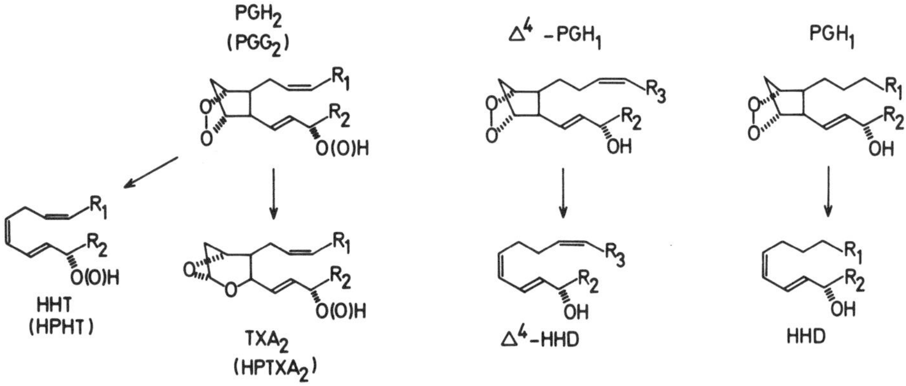

FIG. 6. Transformations of PG endoperoxides by thromboxane synthase: R$_1$,-(CH$_2$)$_3$COOH; R$_2$,-(CH$_2$)$_4$CH$_3$; and R$_3$,-(CH$_2$)$_2$COOH.

ACKNOWLEDGMENT

This work was supported by a grant from the Swedish Medical Research Council (project 03X-217).

REFERENCES

1. Diczfalusy, U., Falardeau, P., and Hammarström, S. (1977): *FEBS Lett.,* 84:271–274.
2. Diczfalusy, U., and Hammarström, S. (1977): *FEBS Lett.,* 82:107–110.

3. Diczfalusy, U., and Hammarström, S. (1979): *FEBS Lett.* 105:291–295.
4. Hamberg, M., and Samuelsson, B. (1973): *Proc. Natl. Acad. Sci. USA,* 70:899–903.
5. Hamberg, M., Svensson, J., and Samuelsson, B. (1975): *Proc. Natl. Acad. Sci. USA,* 72:2994–2998.
6. Hammarström, S. (1979): *J. Biol. Chem., (in press).*
7. Hammarström, S., and Falardeau, P. (1977): *Proc. Natl. Acad. Sci. USA,* 74:3691–3695.
8. Miyamoto, T., Ogino, N., Yamamoto, S., and Hayaishi, O. (1976): *J. Biol. Chem.,* 251:2629–2636.
9. Piper, P. J., and Vane, J. R. (1969): *Nature,* 223:29–35.
10. Svensson, J., Hamberg, M., and Samuelsson, B. (1975): *Acta Physiol. Scand.,* 94:222–228.
11. Yoshimoto, T., Yamamoto, S., Okuma, M., and Hayaishi, O. (1977): *J. Biol. Chem.,* 252:5871–5874.

Advances in Prostaglandin and Thromboxane Research,
Vol. 6, edited by B. Samuelsson, P. W. Ramwell,
and R. Paoletti. Raven Press, New York © 1980.

Effects of Platelet Aggregation and Adenosine 3':5'-Monophosphate on the Synthesis of Thromboxane B_2 in Human Platelets

Jan Åke Lindgren, Hans-Erik Claesson, Hans Kindahl,
and Sven Hammarström

Department of Chemistry, Karolinska Institutet, S-104 01 Stockholm, Sweden

Elevation of platelet adenosine 3':5'-monophosphate (cyclic AMP) inhibits aggregation (10,12) and formation of thromboxane (TX) B_2 (2,6–8,11). Several reports have shown that cyclic AMP can prevent TXB_2 synthesis by inhibition of arachidonic acid release from platelet phospholipids (2,6,7,11). In addition, it has previously been proposed that cyclic AMP inhibits prostaglandin (PG) endoperoxide synthase (E.C. 1.14.99.1) (8). However, others have been unable to reproduce these results (2,6,11). It was therefore of interest to reinvestigate the effect of cyclic AMP on the conversion of arachidonic acid to TXB_2. PGI_2 was used to raise cyclic AMP levels in platelets (4,13). The results suggest that platelet PG endoperoxide synthase is activated during aggregation and that the activating process could be reversed by cyclic AMP.

MATERIALS AND METHODS

Platelet-rich plasma (PRP) and platelet-poor plasma (PPP) were prepared from human blood (1). The donors were healthy and had not taken any drug for at least 10 days. All experiments were performed at 37°C. To restore calcium in plasma, samples were preincubated for 1 min with $CaCl_2$ (final concentration, 2.5 mM). Platelet aggregation was continuously followed in a Payton dual-channel aggregometer (Payton Associated Ltd., Ontario, Canada). TXB_2 was determined by radioimmunoassay (5), and cyclic AMP was analyzed by the protein-binding technique of Gilman (3).

RESULTS

Effect of PGI_2 on TXB_2 Formation from Arachidonic Acid

Preincubation of PRP with PGI_2 (25 ng/ml) for 15 sec had no effect on TXB_2 synthesis in the presence of low (25–100 µg/ml) arachidonic acid concen-

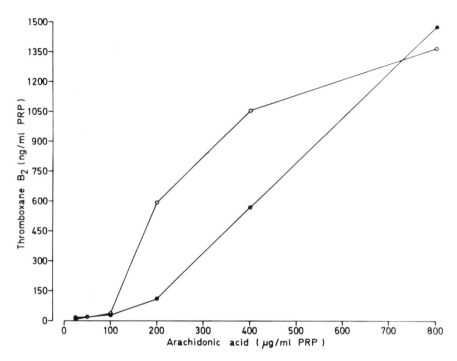

FIG. 1. Arachidonic acid-induced TXB₂ formation in absence and presence of PGI₂. PRP (0.5 ml) was preincubated for 1 min at 37°C with CaCl₂ (2.5 mM) and for another 15 sec with or without PGI₂ (25 ng/ml). After incubation for 5 min with arachidonic acid (25–800 μg/ml), indomethacin was added (final concentration, 10 μM), and the samples were rapidly frozen for TXB₂ analyses. Control, ○, PGI₂, ●.

trations (Fig. 1). These low concentrations of fatty acid did not induce platelet aggregation in controls (samples incubated without PGI₂). Aggregation was induced (not shown) and TXB₂ levels were substantially elevated at ≥200 μg arachidonic acid/ml. PGI₂ decreased TXB₂ formation with 50% or more at 200 or 400 μg arachidonic acid/ml but had no effect on the synthesis of TXB₂ at a substrate concentration of 800 μg/ml. PGI₂ prevented platelet aggregation at all concentrations of arachidonic acid.

Effects of PGI₂ or Colchicine on Levels of Cyclic AMP, Arachidonic Acid-Induced Aggregation, and TXB₂ Synthesis

PRP was preincubated in an aggregometer with PGI₂ (0–1,000 ng/ml; 15 sec) or colchicine (0–2 mM; 1 min) prior to addition of arachidonic acid (250 or 1,000 μg/ml). PGI₂ induced a dose-related increase in cyclic AMP levels (Fig. 2), while colchicine had no effect on this parameter (Fig. 3). Both agents caused parallel dose-dependent inhibition of platelet aggregation and formation of TXB₂ at 250 μg arachidonic acid/ml (Figs. 2A and 3A). At 1,000 μg arachi-

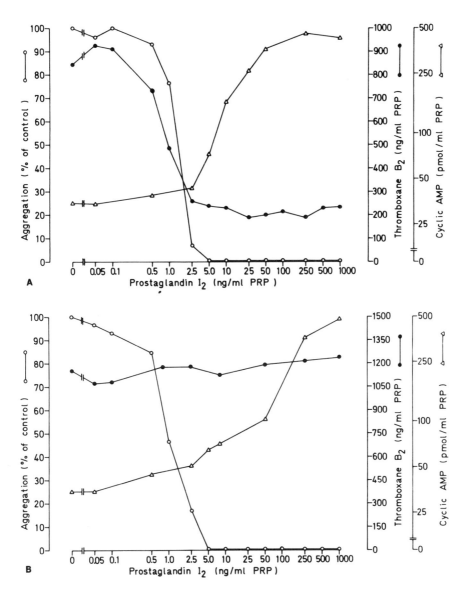

FIG. 2. Effects of PGI₂ on cyclic AMP concentrations and arachidonic acid-induced aggregation and TXB₂ synthesis. PRP (0.5 ml) was preincubated for 1 min in an aggregometer at 37°C with CaCl₂ (2.5 mM) and for 15 sec with PGI₂ (0–1,000 ng/ml). Thereafter, samples were incubated for 5 min with 250 μg arachidonic acid/ml **(A)** or 1,000 μg arachidonic acid/ml **(B)**. Platelet aggregation was monitored continously. After addition of indomethacin (10 μM), the samples were rapidly frozen for TXB₂ determinations. To identically incubated samples were added 0.5 ml 10% (w/v) trichloroacetic acid for measurements of cyclic AMP levels.

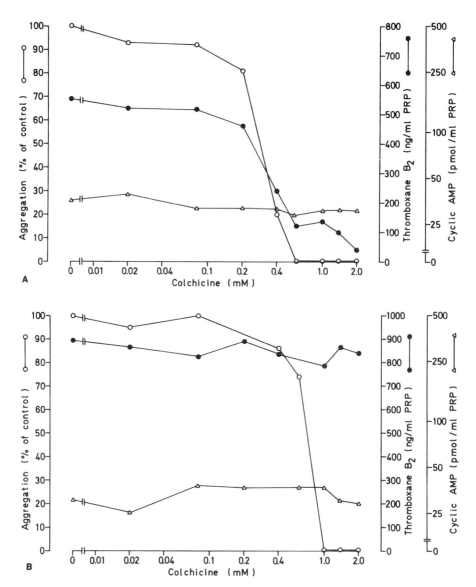

FIG. 3. Effects of colchicine on cyclic AMP levels and arachidonic acid-induced aggregation and TXB₂ synthesis. PRP (0.5 ml) was preincubated for 1 min in an aggregometer at 37°C with CaCl₂ (2.5 mM) and colchicine (0–2 mM). Thereafter, the samples were incubated for 5 min with 250 μg arachidonic acid/ml **(A)** or 1,000 μg arachidonic acid/ml **(B)**. Platelet aggregation was monitored continously. After addition of indomethacin (10 μM), the samples were rapidly frozen for TXB₂ determinations. To identically incubated samples were added 0.5 ml 10% (w/v) trichloroacetic acid for measurements of cyclic AMP levels.

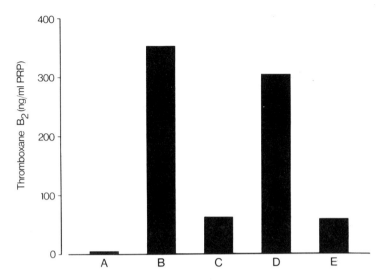

FIG. 4. Effects of PGI₂ on conversion of arachidonic acid to TXB₂ after ADP-induced aggregation. Aliquots of PRP (1 ml) were preincubated for 2 min at 37°C with CaCl₂ (2.5 mM) and thereafter incubated as indicated: A, 10 μM ADP (5 min); B, 400 μg arachidonic acid/ml (5 min); C, 50 ng PGI₂/ml (15 sec) + 400 μg arachidonic acid/ml (5 min); D, 10 μM ADP (5 min) + 400 μg arachidonic acid/ml (5 min); E, 10 μM ADP (5 min) + 50 ng PGI₂/ml (15 sec) + 400 μg arachidonic acid/ml (5 min). After incubation, 0.5 ml of samples were removed and mixed with 0.5 ml 10% (w/v) trichloroacetic acid for analyses of cyclic AMP levels. To the remaining 0.5-ml aliquots were added indomethacin (10 μM), and the samples were rapidly frozen for determinations of TXB₂.

donic acid/ml, sufficient concentrations of PGI₂ or colchicine inhibited platelet aggregation (Figs. 2B and 3B). However, no inhibition of TXB₂ synthesis was observed at this substrate concentration.

Effects of PGI₂ on Cyclic AMP Levels and Conversion of Arachidonic Acid to TXB₂ After ADP-Induced Aggregation

Platelet aggregation was induced in PRP by adenosine diphosphate (ADP) (10 μM) prior to incubation with PGI₂ (0 or 50 ng/ml) for 15 sec and arachidonic acid (400 μg/ml) for another 5 min. PGI₂ inhibited TXB₂ formation also when added after ADP-induced platelet aggregation (Fig. 4). Cyclic AMP levels were elevated in PGI₂-treated samples (two- to four fold increase; not shown).

DISCUSSION

The present results show that both platelet aggregation and the conversion of arachidonic acid (250 μg/ml) to TXB₂ in platelets were inhibited by PGI₂-induced elevation of cyclic AMP levels in PRP (Figs. 1 and 2A). Colchicine inhibited platelet aggregation and caused a similar inhibition of TXB₂ formation

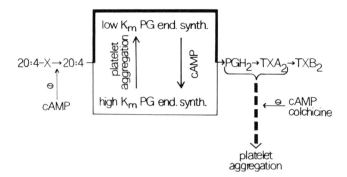

FIG. 5. Hypothetical scheme for the effects of platelet aggregation and cyclic AMP on thromboxane synthesis in platelets. 20:4-x, arachidonic acid bound in the phospholipid pool: end. synth., platelet endoperoxide synthase.

but did not alter cyclic AMP concentrations (Fig. 3A). This suggests that inhibition of platelet aggregation (with or without elevation of cyclic AMP) prevents synthesis of TXB_2. The parallel dose-dependent inhibition of platelet aggregation and TXB_2 formation obtained with both PGI_2 and colchicine (Figs. 2A and 3A) gives further evidence for this hypothesis. The results also suggest that platelet PG endoperoxide synthase is activated during aggregation.

At a higher concentration of arachidonic acid (1,000 μg/ml), PGI_2 and colchicine inhibited platelet aggregation but had no effect on the synthesis of TXB_2 (Figs. 2B and 3B). This shows that cyclic AMP inhibits platelet aggregation at several steps and that at least one of these is beyond the synthesis of PG endoperoxides and TXs (1,9,11). The inhibition at low, but not at high, substrate concentrations suggests a K_m change of the PG endoperoxide synthase.

Elevation of cyclic AMP levels by PGI_2 in ADP-aggregated platelets decreased the formation of TXB_2 from arachidonic acid (Fig. 4). This indicates that the negative effect of cyclic AMP on TXB_2 synthesis is not exclusively due to inhibition of platelet aggregation.

In summary, the results suggest that platelet aggregation activates PG endoperoxide synthase (Fig. 5), probably by decreasing the K_m of the enzyme. This activation is prevented by platelet aggregation inhibitors (e.g., cyclic AMP and colchicine). Furthermore, cyclic AMP seems to reverse the activation process. Further experiments regarding the relationship between aggregation and platelet endoperoxide synthase activity are in progress.

ACKNOWLEDGMENTS

We thank Ms. Margareta Hovgard and Ms. Eva Ohlson for their skillful technical assistance. This work was supported by a grant from the Swedish Medical Research Council (project 03X-217).

REFERENCES

1. Claesson, H-E. and Malmsten, C. (1977): *Eur. J. Biochem.,* 76:277–284.
2. Gerrard, J. M., Peller, J. D., Krick, T. P., and White, J. G. (1977): *Prostaglandins,* 14:39–50.
3. Gilman, A. G. (1970): *Proc. Natl. Acad. Sci. USA,* 67:305–312.
4. Gorman, R. R., Bunting, S., and Miller, O. V. (1977): *Prostaglandins,* 13:377–388.
5. Granström, E., Kindahl, H., and Samuelsson, B. (1976): *Anal. Lett.,* 9:611–627.
6. Lapetina, E. G., Schmitges, C. J., Chandrabose, K., and Cuatrecasas, P. (1977): *Biochem. Biophys. Res. Commun.,* 76:828–835.
7. Lindgren, J. Å., Claesson, H-E., Kindahl, H., and Hammarström, S. (1979): *FEBS Lett.,* 98:247–250.
8. Malmsten, C., Granström, E., and Samuelsson, B. (1976): *Biochem. Biophys. Res. Commun.,* 68:569–576.
9. Miller, O. V., and Gorman, R. R. (1976): *J. Cyclic Nucleotide Res.,* 2:79–87.
10. Mills, D. C. B., and Smith, J. B. (1971): *Biochem. J.,* 121:185–196.
11. Minkes, M., Stanford, N., Chi, M. M.-Y., Roth, G. J., Raz, A., Needleman, P., and Majerus, P. W. (1977): *J. Clin. Invest.,* 59:449–454.
12. Marquis, N. R., Vigdahl, R. L., and Tavormina, P. A. (1969): *Biochem. Biophys. Res. Commun.,* 36:965–972.
13. Tateson, J. E., Moncada, S., and Vane, J. R. (1977): *Prostaglandins,* 13:389–397.

Advances in Prostaglandin and Thromboxane Research,
Vol. 6, edited by B. Samuelsson, P. W. Ramwell,
and R. Paoletti. Raven Press, New York © 1980.

Thromboxane A$_2$ and Prostaglandin H$_2$ Form Covalently Linked Derivatives with Human Serum Albumin

J. Maclouf, H. Kindahl, E. Granström, and B. Samuelsson

Department of Chemistry, Karolinska Institutet, S-104 01 Stockholm, Sweden

Platelets transform the prostaglandin (PG) endoperoxides into the highly unstable thromboxane (TX) A$_2$ ($t_{1/2} = 32$ sec in buffer, pH 7.4) which is hydrolyzed to the stable hemiacetal derivative, TXB$_2$ (4). In platelet-rich plasma (PRP), the yield of TXB$_2$ from PGH$_2$ is low (7) in comparison with platelets suspended in buffer (2). In those conditions, the low occurrence of TXB$_2$ may be due to a degradation of PGH$_2$ into PGD$_2$ by albumin (5) and to the recently hypothesized reaction of TXA$_2$ with plasma proteins (1). In this work, we present evidence that human serum albumin (HSA) reacts with TXA$_2$ and with PGH$_2$ to form covalently bound derivatives.

RESULTS AND DISCUSSION

PRP was incubated with [1-^{14}C]PGH$_2$. The platelet-poor plasma was dialyzed against 8 M urea and against a large volume of buffer. About 35% of the added radioactivity remained bound to proteins and was neither extractable at pH 3 by a resin (XAD-2) known to remove arachidonic acid derivatives nor by organic solvents, therefore demonstrating the formation of a covalent bond between PGH$_2$-generated metabolites and plasma proteins. Plasma was labeled as above: filtration on a Sephadex G-200 column showed a homogenous peak of radioactivity bound to proteins that corresponded to the filtration volume of standard HSA. Noncovalently bound material was further extracted by XAD-2. The labeled protein showed an isoelectric point of 4.7 to 5.1 [theoretical value for HSA: 4.6–5.3 (6)]. A very specific anti-HSA antiserum was coupled to Sepharose, and the labeled plasma was subjected to affinity chromatography. A radioactive protein was retained that was still immunoreactive with the anti-HSA antiserum.

Washed platelets in the presence of HSA were stimulated by PGH$_2$. High levels of TXB$_2$ were detected during the first few seconds and were followed by a rapid disappearance of material (Fig. 1). The levels were proportional to the amount of added PGH$_2$. The phenomenon was abolished in the presence of TX synthase inhibitors. Since TXB$_2$ is stable in PRP (1), the disappearing

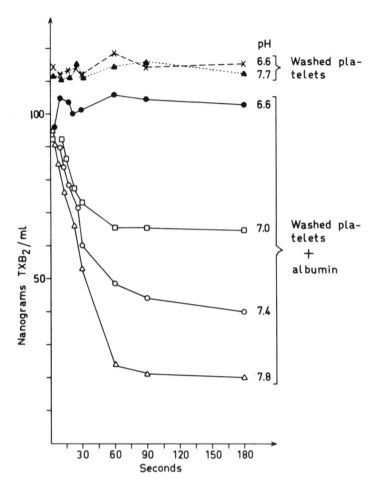

FIG. 1. Washed platelets in the presence of albumin transform increasing amounts of PGH₂ (1–150 μg/ml; 0,1 μg/ml; 5 μg/ml; Δ, 50 μg/ml; x, 150 μg/ml; *solid lines*) into TXB₂ in a concentration-dependent fashion. The concentration of HSA was 45 mg/ml; PGH₂ concentrations are indicated in the figure. The burst of TXB₂ is suppressed by TX synthase inhibitors: either imidazole, 100 μg/ml (x-----x) or 9,11-azoprosta-5,13-dienoic acid, 7 μg/ml (0----0). In these last two experiments, the PGH₂ concentration was 1 μg/ml. Note the logarithmic scale on ordinate.

material is its unstable precursor (i.e., TXA_2). An incubation was repeated as above using $[1-^{14}C]PGH_2$. As can be seen in Fig. 2, at pH 7.7, the decrease of TXB_2 was symmetrical to the increase of protein-bound radioactivity. When the pH of incubation was slightly lowered (pH 6.3 vs. 7.7), TXB_2 values remained constantly elevated, whereas there was nearly no increase in bound radioactivity. The higher concentration of protons had therefore suppressed the reaction of TXA_2 with HSA and also accelerated the conversion of generated TXA_2 into TXB_2 (2). However, PGH_2 itself showed a covalent binding to HSA of 38% of added radioactivity at pH 7.7 and still 33% at pH 6.3. Therefore, the TXA_2

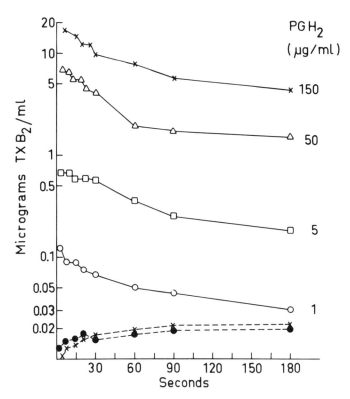

FIG. 2. Effect of pH on TXB_2 formation (pH 7.7, — ○ —; ph 6.3 — □ —) and on protein-bound material (pH 7.7 --- ○ ---; pH 6.3, --- □ ---). [1-^{14}C]PGH_2, 1 µg/ml; HSA, 45 mg/ml. Reaction quenching was as in Fig. 1. Radioactive material bound to protein was analyzed after dialyzing each aliquot. Arbitrary units were chosen for protein-bound radioactivity: the increase of protein-bound label from 5 sec to 5 min was called 100%.

reaction with HSA seemed more sensitive to pH variation than PGH_2. As can be expected, the half-life of PGH_2 was considerably reduced in the presence of HSA ($t_{1/2} = 1$ min) as compared to buffer at pH 7.7 ($t_{1/2} = 170$ sec).

Our results demonstrate that the presence of HSA deeply alters the fate of both PGH_2 and TXA_2. Further, the reaction of these compounds with HSA prevent their detection using the classical analytical methods. The choice of TXB_2 as an indicator of TXA_2 synthesis from platelets has therefore to be reassessed when the incubation is performed in plasma.

ACKNOWLEDGMENTS

This work was supported by grants from the World Health Organization. J. M. was awarded a fellowship by the Swedish Medical Research Council and the Institut National de la Santé et de la Recherche Médicale, France.

The skillful technical assistance of Ms. Eva Ohlson is gratefully acknowledged.

REFERENCES

1. Fitzpatrick, F. A., and Gorman, R. R. (1977): *Prostaglandins,* 14:881–883.
2. Folco, G., Granström, E., and Kindahl, H. (1977): *FEBS Lett.,* 82:321–324.
3. Granström, E., Kindahl, H., and Samuelsson, B. (1976): *Anal. Lett.,* 9:611–627.
4. Hamberg, M., Svensson, J., and Samuelsson, B. (1975): *Proc. Natl. Acad. Sci. USA,* 72:2994–2998.
5. Hamberg, M., and Fredholm, B. B. (1976): Biochim. Biophys. Acta, 431:189–193.
6. Malamud, D., and Drysdale, J. M. (1978): *Anal. Biochem.,* 86:620–647.
7. Malmsten, C., Hamberg, M., Svensson, J., and Samuelsson, B. (1975): *Proc. Natl. Acad. Sci. USA,* 72:1446–1450.

Advances in Prostaglandin and Thromboxane Research,
Vol. 6, edited by B. Samuelsson, P. W. Ramwell,
and R. Paoletti. Raven Press, New York © 1980.

Heparin Potentiates Synthesis of Thromboxane A_2 in Human Platelets

*W. H. Anderson, S. F. Mohammad, H. Y. K. Chuang,
and R. G. Mason

*Departments of Pathology and *Pharmacology and Therapeutics, University of South
Florida College of Medicine, Tampa, Florida 33612*

Heparin is widely used as an anticoagulant for the prevention or treatment of a variety of thromboembolic disorders. However, it has been reported in several studies that intravenous administration of heparin may result in marked thrombocytopenia in certain patients (3,5,9). Heparin has also been shown to cause potentiation of platelet aggregation and the release reaction by a variety of agents *in vitro*. It has been suggested that this effect of heparin on platelet function is a consequence of heparin-induced release of products from platelet granules (2,11). The mechanism whereby heparin causes thrombocytopenia in some patients or enhancement of platelet aggregation and the release reaction in others is not known. The present studies were undertaken to elucidate mechanisms whereby heparin alters platelet function.

MATERIALS AND METHODS

Blood, obtained from adult human donors who denied receiving medication for at least 1 week preceding the venipuncture, was processed for preparation of platelet-rich plasma (PRP) and platelet-poor plasma (PPP) following techniques described earlier (6). Platelet aggregation was determined photometrically by use of a dual-channel aggregometer (6).

Thromboxane A_2 (TXA_2) production was determined by a bioassay on a spirally cut segment of rabbit aorta as described by Piper and Vane (8), suspended in a 1.0-ml perfused microbath (1).

PRP anticoagulated with acid/citrate/dextrose was centrifuged at 1,100 × g for 10 min; the platelet pellet was resuspended in 2 to 3 drops of Ringers/citrate/dextrose (RCD, pH 6.5) and diluted to one-quarter the original PRP volume with citrated PPP. ^{3}H-arachidonic acid was added and incubated for 60 min at 37°C. The platelet suspension was then diluted threefold with RCD. Albumin (0.5 ml, 300 mg/ml) was added to the bottom of the centrifuge tube, and platelets were isolated at the albumin–RCD interface by centrifugation at 1,100 × g for 10 min, resuspended in citrated PPP, and then allowed to incorporate ^{14}C-serotonin following the method described elsewhere (6). Generally, 90% of ^{14}C-serotonin was taken up by platelets. Heparin from ox lung (The Upjohn Co., Kalamazoo, Michigan) or porcine mucosa (Sigma Chemical Co., St. Louis, Missouri) was used without further purification.

RESULTS

Heparin (5 U/ml) added to citrated PRP did not cause aggregation of platelets but potentiated aggregation induced by a variety of agents. Figure 1 illustrates the aggregation of platelets exposed to adenosine diphosphate (ADP) and arachidonic acid both in the presence and absence of heparin.

Since the metabolic fate of arachidonic acid in platelets is known to some extent, the effect of heparin on the ability of platelets to metabolize arachidonic acid and to produce TXA$_2$ was explored further. Addition of increasing concentrations of arachidonic acid to PRP produced a dose-dependent increase of TXA$_2$ (Fig. 2).

Pretreatment of PRP with imidazole (500 μg/ml), an inhibitor of TXA$_2$

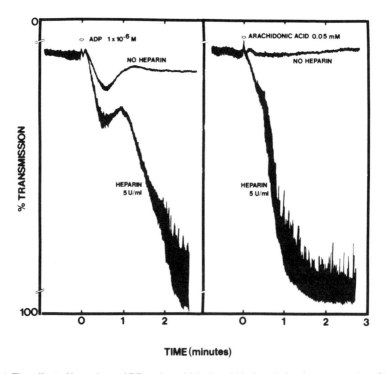

FIG. 1. The effect of heparin on ADP and arachidonic acid-induced platelet aggregation. Citrated PRP was incubated with or without heparin at 37°C for 5 min. Aggregation was initiated with ADP (10⁻⁶M) or arachidonic acid (0.05 mM), and the change in light transmission was recorded by a Payton dual-channel aggregation module.

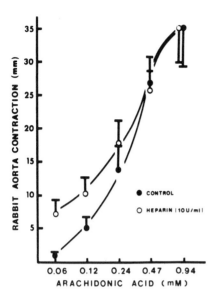

FIG. 2. Effect of heparin on contractile responses of rabbit aorta to PRP in which platelet aggregation was induced by addition of varying concentrations of arachidonic acid. Citrated PRP with or without heparin was incubated for 5 min, and aggregation was initiated by addition of increasing concentrations of arachidonic acid. After a 60-sec incubation period, a 200-μl aliquot of this mixture was removed and added to a microbath containing a segment of rabbit aorta (see text). Data presented are means ($\pm$ SEM) of six separate experiments.

synthetase, prevented arachidonic acid-induced platelet aggregation, the release reaction, and the production of a substance which contracts the rabbit aorta. The presence of heparin in the reaction mixture prior to the addition of arachidonic acid resulted in a dose-dependent potentiation of TXA₂ production (Fig. 3).

When doubly labeled platelets were exposed to ADP in either the presence or absence of heparin, determination of radioactivity released from platelets into the supernatant at different time intervals revealed a concomitant increase of ³H and ¹⁴C in the presence of heparin (Table 1). Heparin by itself neither caused aggregation of platelets nor release of ³H or ¹⁴C.

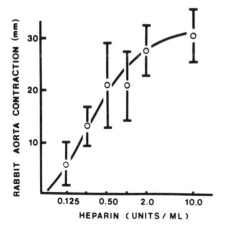

FIG. 3. Dose-dependent effect of heparin on the contractile response of rabbit aorta to PRP incubated with arachidonic acid. To citrated PRP, arachidonic acid (0.05 mM) was added and incubated for 60 sec in the presence of heparin (0.125–10 U/ml). A 200-μl aliquot of this mixture was removed rapidly and added to a microbath containing a segment of rabbit aorta (see text). Data are presented as means ($\pm$ SEM) of five separate experiments.

TABLE 1. *Effect of heparin on ³H-arachidonic acid and ¹⁴C-serotonin release from human platelets*[a]

Time (sec)	Control		Heparin (10 U/ml)	
	^{14}C (cpm)	^{3}H (cpm)	^{14}C (cpm)	^{3}H (cpm)
0	452	557	384	494
15	275	268	393	310
30	271	295	419	341
60	206	269	506	374
120	469	394	2228	1214
180	1142	708	2257	1243

[a] Platelets were labeled with ^{3}H-arachidonic acid and ^{14}C-serotonin (see text) and aggregated with ADP (10^{-5} M). At the time points indicated, the contents of the aggregometer tube were transferred to a microcentrifuge tube, and centrifuged at 5,000 $\times$ g for 15 sec. A 200-μl aliquot was removed rapidly and counted in a scintillation counter for 10 min using Omniflour scintillation cocktail.

DISCUSSION

Studies on the effect of heparin on platelets have produced diverse and often conflicting observations. Heparin has been shown to (a) cause aggregation of platelets by itself, (b) potentiate aggregation and the release reaction by certain aggregating agents, or (c) inhibit platelet aggregation (11). Under the experimental conditions used in this study, platelet aggregation was not observed when heparin was added to citrated PRP. However, the presence of heparin in citrated PRP resulted in potentiation of aggregation and the release reaction when platelets were exposed to various aggregating agents (Fig. 1). Since potentiation of aggregation was also observed with arachidonic acid, and in view of convincing reports that arachidonic acid is metabolized by platelets to produce TXA₂ (4,10), it was tempting to speculate that heparin stimulates production of TXA₂. Observations summarized in Figs. 2 and 3 and Table 1 appear to support this assumption.

Heparin or arachidonic acid, alone or in combination, showed no effect on the rabbit aorta. However, heparin, which potentiated aggregation of platelets induced by arachidonic acid (Fig. 1), also caused increased contraction of the rabbit aorta (Figs. 2 and 3). Since this contraction has been shown to be specific for TXA₂ under the conditions described, these observations suggest that heparin caused increased production of TXA₂. This conclusion is based on the fact that the presence of imidazole, a specific inhibitor of TXA₂ synthetase (7), in the mixture inhibited the production of the substance that contracts the rabbit aorta.

Studies with doubly labeled platelets showed a concomitant release of both ^{3}H and ^{14}C in response to ADP. Due to the limitations of methodology, we were unable to determine whether membrane bound ^{3}H or ^{14}C from platelet granules was released first. This reaction proceeds at a fast pace once platelet aggregation has been initiated. Therefore, the precise mechanism whereby heparin potentiates aggregation and the release reaction in platelets remains unknown.

Heparin potentiates platelet aggregation and the release reaction and, in the presence of an aggregating agent, also causes an increased production of TXA$_2$. It is possible that these interrelated effects of heparin may be responsible, at least in part, for thrombocytopenia observed in patients receiving this anticoagulant.

ACKNOWLEDGMENTS

Part of this work was supported by Grants HL22583 and HL24026 of the National Institutes of Health, Grant PDT 79 of American Cancer Society, and grant 939 from the Council for Tobacco Research-U.S.A., Inc.

REFERENCES

1. Anderson, W. H., Krzanowski, J. J., Polson, J. B., and Szentivanyi, A. (1979): *Biochem. Pharmacol.,* 28:2223–2226.
2. Eika, C. (1972): *Scand. J. Haematol.,* 9:248–257.
3. Fratantoni, J. C., Pollet, R., and Granlick, H. R. (1975): *Blood,* 45:395–401.
4. Gerrard, J. M., and White, J. G. (1978): *Prog. Hemostasis Thromb.,* 4:87–125.
5. Hammerschmidt, D. E. (1976): *N. Engl. J. Med.,* 295:1200.
6. Mohammad, S. F., Whitworth, C., Chuang, H. Y. K., Lundblad, R. L., and Mason, R. G., (1976): *Proc. Natl. Acad. Sci. USA,* 73:1660–1663.
7. Needleman, P., Raz, A., Ferrendelli, J. A., and Minkes, M. (1977): *Proc. Natl. Acad. Sci. USA,* 74:1716–1720.
8. Piper, P. J., and Vane, J. R. (1969): *Nature,* 223:2935.
9. Rhodes, G. R., Dixon, R. H., and Silver, D. (1973): *Surg. Gynecol. Obstet.,* 136:409–416.
10. Samuelsson, B., Goldyne, M., Granstrom, E., Hamberg, M., Hammerstrom, S., and Malmsten, C. (1978): *Ann. Rev. Biochem.,* 47:997–1029.
11. Zucker, M. (1977): *Fed. Proc.,* 36:4749.

Advances in Prostaglandin and Thromboxane Research,
Vol. 6, edited by B. Samuelsson, P. W. Ramwell,
and R. Paoletti. Raven Press, New York © 1980.

In Vivo Inhibition of Thromboxane Biosynthesis by Hydralazine

James E. Greenwald, Lan K. Wong, Michael Alexander, and
Joseph R. Bianchine

Department of Pharmacology, The Ohio State University, College of Medicine,
Columbus, Ohio 43210

We have previously shown that hydralazine, diazoxide, and dipyridamole are selective thromboxane A_2 (TXA_2) inhibitors (2). However, the concentrations that produce significant inhibition *in vitro* are considerably greater than the therapeutic blood levels of these drugs in man. This discrepancy may be due to the presence of active metabolites and/or the ability of certain tissues to selectively sequester these drugs, thus increasing the effective concentration of the drug at the site of action. Therefore, the following experiments were designed to test whether a concentration reported to lower blood pressure in hypertensive rabbits had an effect on platelet TXA_2 production. Since these drugs have a direct relaxant effect on vascular smooth muscle, we also investigated their ability to modify arachidonic acid (AA) metabolism in vascular tissues.

METHODS

Platelet TXA_2 Inhibition in Response to Hydralazine

Three male rabbits were administered hydralazine, 3.2 mg/kg, i.m., every 8 hr for 3 days to achieve on effective blood concentration of approximately 2 mg/kg, a dose reported to lower blood pressure in hypertensive rabbits (1). Blood samples were obtained at predrug administration to determine control levels of TXB_2 production in platelet-rich plasma (PRP) as well as being drawn once each treatment day. A final sample was drawn at 30 hr, approximately 10 half-lives, after the last dose of hydralazine. Blood samples were collected and prepared and PRP prostaglandin (PG) production was determined as previously described (2).

Rabbit Aorta PG Production

Rabbit aortic rings (60–90 mg) were incubated with ^{14}C-AA (1 μg) and 50 mM Tris/HCl (pH 7.5) in a 0.5-ml reaction volume in the presence and absence

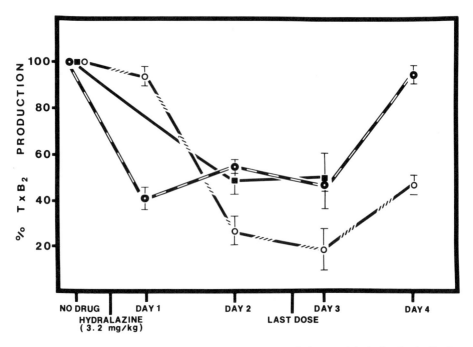

FIG. 1. Intramuscular administration of hydralazine (3.2 mg/kg) every 8 hr in 3 animals. Each point represents the mean ± standard deviation of four separate determinations.

of 0.25 mM hydralazine for 5 min at 37°C. Samples were analyzed as mentioned above, but thin-layer chromatographic plates were developed in ethyl acetate/ hexane/acetic acid/water (58:26:6:60).

As can be seen in Fig. 1, after an acute dose of hydralazine, only one rabbit showed a decrease in its platelet TXB₂ production. However, after four maintenance doses of hydralazine, all rabbits displayed a marked inhibition of platelet TXB₂ production. A final TXB₂ determination was made 10 half-lives after the last hydralazine administration. If hydralazine was the reason for a decrease in platelet TXB₂ production, this last determination should indicate a regain of platelet TXB₂ synthetic capabilities. As evidenced in Fig. 1, the TXB₂ biosynthetic capabilities in two rabbits were indeed returning to normal.

In a second group of experiments, the effect of hydralazine on rabbit aorta AA metabolism was investigated. A typical radiochromatogram of an aortic incubation in the presence of 0.25 mM hydralazine is seen in Fig. 2. The quantitation of 6-keto PGF₁α, the stable metabolite of prostacyclin (PGI₂), is displayed in Table 1. The quantitation was achieved by scraping this zone of radioactivity followed by scintillation counting.

Finally, it should be pointed out that when the platelet or tissue samples were washed free of drug before the incubation with AA, no inhibition of TXA₂ in platelets or stimulation of PGI₂ in the aorta could be detected.

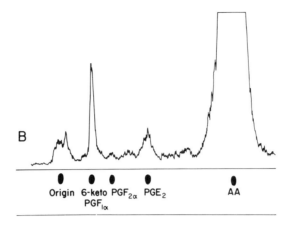

FIG. 2. Representative radiochromatogram of rabbit aortic ring incubation with [^{14}C]-arachidonic acid in the presence of 0.25 mM hydralazine.

TABLE 1. *Effect of 0.25 mM hydralazine on rabbit aortic 6-keto PGF$_{1\alpha}$ production*

Experiment	6-keto-PGF$_{1\alpha}$ (pmoles/mg tissue)	Change from control (%)
Control	1.31 ± 0.21 [a]	
Hydralazine (0.25 mM)	2.74 ± 0.42 [b]	110

[a] $n = 8$.
[b] $n = 8$.

Hydralazine is a smooth muscle vasodilator and antihypertensive agent whose mechanism of action has not yet been fully elucidated. Our experiments demonstrate this drug's ability to stimulate PGI_2, the most potent endogenous vasodilator, and its ability to inhibit TXA_2 production, the most potent endogenous vasoconstrictor. These data suggest to us that a PG-mediated antihypertensive mechanism is involved in the action of this drug. Currently we are investigating the biochemical events which lead to this drug–enzyme interaction.

REFERENCES

1. Bretherton, K. N., Day, A. J., and Skinner, S. L. (1977): *Atherosclerosis,* 27:79–87.
2. Greenwald, J. E., Wong, L. K., Rao, M., Bianchine, J. R., and Panganamala, R. V. (1978): *Biochem. Biophys. Res. Commun.,* 84:1112–1118.

Advances in Prostaglandin and Thromboxane Research,
Vol. 6, edited by B. Samuelsson, P. W. Ramwell,
and R. Paoletti. Raven Press, New York © 1980.

Thromboxane B₂ Production and Lipid Peroxidation in Human Blood Platelets

L. C. Best, P. B. B. Jones, M. B. McGuire, and R. G. G. Russell

Department of Human Metabolism and Clinical Biochemistry, Sheffield University Medical School, Sheffield, S10 2RX, United Kingdom

Human platelet aggregation is thought to be closely associated with the biosynthesis of prostaglandins. The unstable intermediates of platelet prostaglandin metabolism, prostaglandin endoperoxides and thromboxane (TX) A_2 are potent inducers of aggregation (3) and are also formed during aggregation in response to several agents, including arachidonic acid, thrombin, and collagen (1). Because of the instability of these intermediates, the most convenient approach for assessing platelet prostaglandin production is the measurement of the more stable, biologically inactive end products [e.g., malondialdehyde (MDA), TXB_2, and hydroxyheptadecatrienoic acid (HHT)].

The formation of TXB_2 and MDA were measured in human platelet suspensions by radioimmunoassay (2) for TXB_2 and by the fluorimetric thiobarbituric acid reaction for MDA.

Platelet TXB_2 and MDA production were studied in relation to aggregation under a wide variety of conditions in order to assess the role of TX biosynthesis in the control of platelet function.

Exogenous sodium arachidonate was converted to TXB_2 and MDA in a dose-dependent fashion by platelet-rich plasma, Sepharose 2B gel-filtered platelets and by bovine platelet microsomes. The binding of arachidonate to plasma proteins necessitated the use of high concentrations of arachidonate to produce TXB_2 and MDA in platelet-rich plasma. Platelet aggregation induced by collagen or by thrombin was also associated with a large rise in TXB_2 and MDA levels (Fig. 1). In the case of collagen, the aggregation response was preceded by a rise in TXB_2. Epinephrine-induced aggregation was also accompanied by a rise in TXB_2 and MDA production, although the levels attained were always lower than those produced by arachidonate, collagen, or thrombin. Adenosine/diphosphate (ADP) resulted in low, and often undetectable, levels of TXB_2 and MDA, suggesting either that TX production was not essential for ADP-induced platelet aggregation or that the amounts of TX required were below the detection limits of the assay. When platelets were preincubated for 10 min with aspirin (a cyclooxygenase inhibitor) or with imidazole or 1-N-butyl imidazole (TX synthetase inhibitors), TXB_2 and MDA in response to arachidonate or collagen

297

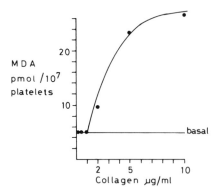

FIG. 1. Production of TXB₂ and MDA accompanying aggregation induced by collagen.

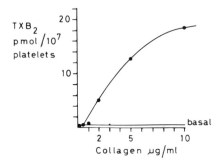

were inhibited in parallel. In addition, aggregation in response to arachidonate was inhibited, although aggregation in response to collagen persisted in the absence of TXB_2 or MDA, suggesting that collagen could induce aggregation by a TX-independent pathway.

In general, the results indicated that TXB_2 and MDA were produced in approximately equimolar quantites and were probably both formed by the TX synthetase enzyme. However, at high concentrations of exogenous arachidonate, higher levels of thiobarbiturate-positive substances ("MDA") were found. This may be due to nonspecific oxidation products of arachidonate which are detected by the MDA assay.

The production of measurable quantities of TXB_2 and MDA in platelets was not a prerequisite for aggregation. In addition, increased TXB_2 formation was often detected in the absence of aggregation. Thus platelet TX biosynthesis may exert a regulating role in platelet function rather than being part of a common final pathway leading to aggregation.

ACKNOWLEDGMENTS

We would like to thank the Wellcome Trust for financial support for this work and Dr. J. B. Smith (Cardeza Foundation) for supplying the antiserum to TXB_2.

REFERENCES

1. Blackwell, G. J., Duncombe, W. G., Flower, R. J., Parsons, M. F., and Vane, J. R. (1977): *Br. J. Pharmacol.,* 59:353–366.
2. Ferraris, J. B., Smith, J. B., and Silver, M. J. (1977): *Thromb. Haemost.,* 38:20.
3. Hamberg, M., Svensson, J., and Samuelsson, B. (1975): *Proc. Natl. Acad. Sci. USA,* 72:2994–2998.

Advances in Prostaglandin and Thromboxane Research,
Vol. 6, edited by B. Samuelsson, P. W. Ramwell,
and R. Paoletti. Raven Press, New York © 1980.

PGD₃ Is the Mediator of the Antiaggregatory Effects of the Trienoic Endoperoxide PGH₃

M. O. Whitaker, P. Needleman, A. Wyche, *F. A. Fitzpatrick,
and †H. Sprecher

*Department of Pharmacology, Washington University School of Medicine, St. Louis,
Missouri 63110; *Department of Physical and Analytical Chemistry, The UpJohn Company,
Kalamazoo, Michigan 49001; and †Department of Physiological Chemistry, Ohio
State University, Columbus, Ohio 43210*

5,8,11,14,17-Eicosapentaenoic acid (C20:5, EPA) is converted to the endoperoxide prostaglandin (PG) H_3 by sheep seminal vesicle (SSV) cyclooxygenase (3). In contrast to PGH_2 which aggregates human platelet-rich plasma (PRP), PGH_3 does not cause aggregation and, furthermore, inhibits aggregation by subsequently added agonists (3). In this investigation we found that PGD_3 formed from the nonenzymatic breakdown of PGH_3 is sufficient qualitatively to account for the inhibition produced by the endoperoxide. An inhibitor of platelet adenyl cyclase activity unmasks the aggregatory effect of PGH_3, and an antisera directed against PGD shows PGD_3 to be the PG responsible for the inhibition.

MATERIALS AND METHODS

PGD_3 was prepared by incubation of EPA with SSVs, acidification with 2 N formic acid, and extraction with hexane/diethyl ether (1:4). The extract was concentrated and eluted through a silicic acid column, and the polar eluate was applied to silica gel plates. The zone which comigrated with authentic PGD_2 standard was scraped and extracted twice with methanol. Estimation of concentration was made from ^{14}C-labeled endoperoxide marker included in the preparation.

Platelet inhibition studies were carried out by incubating PGs in PRP for 1 min prior to addition of arachidonic acid (125 μg).

The half-time of breakdown of endoperoxides was determined by assaying the ability of aliquots of incubate of endoperoxide in PRP to contract perfused rabbit aorta strips. The products formed from breakdown were determined by incubation of ^{14}C-labeled endoperoxide in PRP for 10 min, followed by extraction, separation, and counting of products on silica gel thin-layer chromatography plates.

2',5-Dideoxyadenosine (DDA), which was shown by Haslam et al. (2) to be an inhibitor of adenylate cyclase, was incubated for 2 min with platelets at a final concentration of 100 μM prior to aggregation studies.

An antiserum-binding PGD_2 was prepared using methods that have been described (1) and incubated for 2 min with platelets prior to aggregation studies.

RESULTS AND DISCUSSION

EPA is converted by SSV cyclooxygenase to the endoperoxide, PGH_3, which inhibits aggregation and elevates cyclic adenosine monophosphate (cAMP) concentration in human PRP. In plasma, PGH_3 breaks down to yield PGD_3 and PGE_3, and it has been suggested (4) that the inhibition by PGH_3 is caused by one or both of these breakdown products. We found that PGE_3 did not affect arachidonic acid induced aggregation in human PRP, but that, surprisingly, PGD_3 is a more potent inhibitor of aggregation and elevator of platelet cyclic AMP than is PGD_2.

Given the relatively rapid $t_{1/2}$ of breakdown of PGH_3 that we observed and the percent PGD_3 formed on breakdown, it can be calculated (Table 1) that in the 1-min preincubation time used in the aggregation studies, the amount of PGH_3 giving 50% inhibition would degrade to give 1.9 ng of PGD_3, which is almost identical to the amount of PGD_3 alone that would be required to give this degree of inhibition. We showed that the adenylate cyclase inhibitor DDA abolishes the inhibitory effect of PGI_2 on platelets by maintaining cyclic AMP at basal levels. Similarly, it abolishes the inhibition due to PGD_3, and in DDA-treated human platelets, PGH_3 now causes weak, reversible aggregation, although it cannot produce full irreversible aggregation like PGH_2. Thus PGH_3 appears to be a weak aggregating agent; but this effect is normally masked by its very rapid breakdown to PGD_3, which potently inhibits platelet function. These experiments do not exclude the possibility that, as well as being aggregatory, PGH_3 might be capable of stimulating platelet adenylate cyclase itself.

However, platelets incubated with an antisera to PGD_2 can no longer be inhibited by PGD_3 demonstrating that the antisera cross-reacts with PGD_3

TABLE 1

Parameter	2-Series PG	3-Series PG
$t_{1/2}$ breakdown of endoperoxide in PRP at 37°C (sec)	350 ± 35	90 ± 8
PGD formed from endoperoxide at 100% breakdown (%)	24 ± 6	20 ± 2
Inhibition of rate of human PRP aggregation IC$_{50}$ (ng)		
PGH	NR	26 ± 6
PGD	6 ± 1	2.1 ± 0.5
Calculated amount of PGD formed after 1 min of breakdown in PRP (ng)	—	1.9

and prevents it from having an inhibitory effect on the platelets. In the presence of this antisera, a dose of PGH₃ that inhibits nontreated platelets no longer causes inhibition. This demonstrates conclusively that it is PGD₃, not the PGH₃ itself, that is responsible for the inhibitory effects associated with the endoperoxide.

REFERENCES

1. Fitzpatrick, F. A., and Bundy, G. L. (1978): *Proc. Natl. Acad. Sci., USA,* 75:2689–2693.
2. Haslam, R. J., Davidson, M. M. L., Fox, J. E. B., and Lynham, J. A. (1978): *Thrombus Haemostas,* 40:232–240.
3. Needleman, P., Minkes, M., and Raz, A. (1976): *Science,* 193:163–165.
4. Needleman, P., Raz, A., Minkes, M. S., Ferrendelli, J. A., and Sprecher, H. (1979): *Proc. Natl. Acad. Sci. USA,* 76:944–948.

Advances in Prostaglandin and Thromboxane Research,
Vol. 6, edited by B. Samuelsson, P. W. Ramwell,
and R. Paoletti. Raven Press, New York © 1980.

Inhibition of Platelet Aggregation by Novel Benzoylpyrrole Derivatives

Seizi Kurozumi, Akira Ohtsu, Kenji Hoshina, Makiko Jimba, Keiji Komoriya, Tatsuyuki Naruchi, Toshio Wakabayashi, Yoshinobu Hashimoto, and Sachio Ishimoto

Teijin Institute for Bio-medical Research, 4-3-2 Asahigaoka, Hino, Tokyo 191, Japan

It is generally agreed that adhesion and aggregation of platelets play an important role on arterial thrombus formation, and antiplatelet therapy has recently been recognized as a possible preventive therapy for thrombosis.

Novel N-substituted 3-benzoyl-2,5-dimethylpyrrole (BDP) derivatives were found to have an antiplatelet effect by *in vitro* screening of platelet aggregation induced by arachidonic acid (AA).

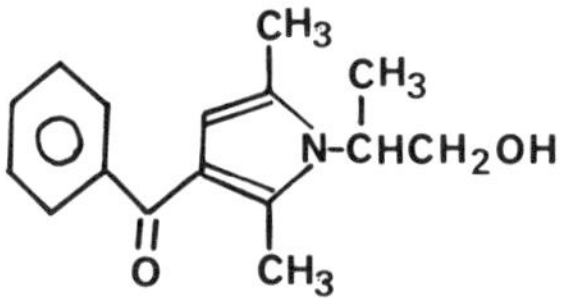

FIG. 1. Chemical structure of TEI-2117.

In Table 1, the inhibitory effect of 2-(3-benzoyl-2,5-dimethylpyrrol-1-yl)propanol (TEI-2117) on AA-induced human platelet aggregation is shown. One μg/ml of the compound exhibited a remarkable inhibitory effect which was stronger than that of indomethacin (IM). In collagen-induced human platelet aggregation, it showed an effect equipotent with IM. On the other hand, in epinephrine-induced aggregation, it inhibited only secondary aggregation at 1.0 μg/ml. In adenosine diphosphate-induced primary aggregation, it had no effect at 10 μg/ml. From these results, it was considered that the compound might have some effect on prostaglandin (PG) biosynthesis *in vitro*.

Experiments were carried out on the inhibitory effect of our compound on PG endoperoxide formation by bovine seminal vesicle microsomes (BSVM), which was bioassayed according to Vane (1), by superfusion of rabbit aorta (RbA), rabbit mesentric artery (RbM), rat stomach strip, and rat colon. A 28 μM dose of TEI-2117 inhibited 50% of the PG endoperoxide formation (IC_{50} = 28 μM), which was 10 times weaker than that of IM (IC_{50} = 3μM). Furthermore, we investigated the effect of this compound on thromboxane formation

TABLE 1. *Inhibitory effects of TEI-2117 on platelet aggregation induced by various stimulants*

Aggregation inducer	Concentration	Platelet	IC_{50} (μg/ml)
AA	0.33 mM	human	0.5
Collagen	3.0 μg/ml	human	6.0
Epinephrine	20 μg/ml	human	1.0[a]
ADP	10 μM	rabbit	no effect[b]

[a] Secondary aggregation.
[b] Primary aggregation.

from PG endoperoxides by horse platelet microsome. No effect was seen with concentrations up to 1 mM.

To assess structure–activity relationship of BDP derivatives, compounds having several substituents at the 1-position of the pyrrole ring were synthesized and examined on their inhibitory effects on PGE_2 biosynthesis and on guinea pig platelet aggregation induced by AA. In the derivatives of which R is an alkyl, phenyl, or benzyl group, relatively stronger inhibitory effects were observed. However, there was no close correlation between PG biosynthesis and AA-induced aggregation.

The effect of TEI-2117 on the AA-induced releasing reaction in the whole cell of rabbit platelet was investigated by the following procedure. A mixture of AA and rabbit platelet-rich plasma (PRP) were incubated at 37°C for 30 sec, and the RbA contracting activity of the resulting broth was bioassayed. TEI-2117 inhibited contractions of both RbA and RbM, in a dose-dependent manner, with an IC_{50} of ca. 0.15 μM. The effect was stronger than that of IM (IC_{50} = 0.75 μM).

In the *ex vivo* experiments, guinea pig PRP was prepared from the blood collected by heart puncture 1 hr after 10–100 mg/kg, p.o. or s.c., administration of BDP. As shown in Table 2, TEI-2117 was found to inhibit AA- and collagen-

TABLE 2. *Inhibitory effects of TEI-2117 on AA- and collagen-induced platelet aggregation ex vivo*

Compound	Dose (mg/kg)	Route	N	Inhibition (%) AA[a]	Collagen[b]
TEI-2117	10	p.o.	2	3	3
	30	p.o.	3	23	42
	100	p.o.	12	70	37
	1	s.c.	3	15	45
	10	s.c.	3	99	79
Aspirin	30	p.o.	2	50	32
	100	p.o.	6	77	41

[a] 0.03 mM.
[b] 5 μg/ml.

TABLE 3. *Biological profile of TEI-2117*

Platelet Aggregation	
in vitro (human)	
AA	TEI-2117 > IM
Collagen	TEI-2117 = IM
Epinephrine (secondary)	TEI-2117 = IM
Epinephrine (primary)	no effect
ADP (primary)	no effect
ex vivo (guinea pig)	
AA	IM > TEI-2117 ≈ ASA[a]
Collagen	IM > TEI-2117 ≈ ASA
PG synthesis (by BSVM)	IM > TEI-2117
RbACS[b] release from platelet	TEI-2117 > IM
Carrageenan paw edema	IM ≫ TEI-2117

[a] Acetylsalicylic acid.
[b] Rabbit aorta contracting substance.

induced platelet aggregation in a dose-dependent manner, and its activity was equipotent to aspirin. Other BDP derivatives (100 mg/kg) were orally administered to guinea pigs. Although these derivatives had the *in vitro* inhibitory activity in AA- and collagen-induced platelet aggregation, some of these compounds with no N-α-methyl and no functional group in N-substitutent, diminished the activity in *ex vivo* assay.

We note that the novel BDP derivative, TEI-2117, showed the most remarkable inhibitory activity in AA-induced platelet aggregation, the effect being stronger than that of IM (Table 3). Although its inhibitory profile on platelet aggregation was similar to that of nonsteroidal anti-inflammatory drugs, its mode of action on AA metabolism was different from that of IM. The compound inhibited PG endoperoxide formation more weakly than IM, whereas it inhibited the release of RbA contracting substances more strongly than IM. Furthermore, oral or subcutaneous administration of 100 mg/kg of TEI-2117 resulted in no reduction of carrageenan-induced paw edema.

Although further detailed studies on the mechanism of action on platelets must yet be done, the novel BDP derivative described here had a promising antiplatelet activity both *in vitro* and *ex vivo*, and its mode of action on platelets cannot be explained only by the regulation of AA metabolism.

ACKNOWLEDGMENT

The authors express sincere thanks to Prof. M. Katori of Kitasato University for his kind suggestion and assistance in the bioassay of AA metabolites.

REFERENCES

1. Vane, J. R. (1964): *Br. J. Pharmacol.*, 23:360–373.

Advances in Prostaglandin and Thromboxane Research,
Vol. 6, edited by B. Samuelsson, P. W. Ramwell,
and R. Paoletti. Raven Press, New York © 1980.

Altered Arachidonic Acid Metabolism in Platelets Inhibited by Onion or Garlic Extracts

Amar N. Makheja, Jack Y. Vanderhoek, Robert W. Bryant, and J. Martyn Bailey

Department of Biochemistry, George Washington University Medical Center, Washington, D.C. 20037

The presence of platelet inhibitors in onion and garlic has been reported previously by a number of workers (1,2,6,7) and by us (4,5). We have isolated antiplatelet inhibitors from the homogenates of fresh onion and found them to inhibit both platelet aggregation and thromboxane synthesis. An ethanolic extract of onion was first partitioned into petroleum ether, and the aqueous phase was then extracted with chloroform and evaporated. The oily chloroform residue was further fractionated into six fractions by silicic acid column chromatography (4,5). The relative effects of these six fractions on aggregatory responses to adenosine diphosphate (ADP) are shown in Fig. 1. These extracts produced a dose-dependent inhibition of ADP- or arachidonic acid-induced platelet aggregation. The ID_{50} (i.e., median dose required to inhibit platelet aggregation by 50%) of the extracts, as well as those of onion and garlic oils obtained from commercial sources, are shown in Table 1. The results indicated that most of the antiplatelet activity was present in the nonpolar volatile components of onion and garlic.

The relationship between the effects of platelet inhibitors present in all fractions and the synthesis of thromboxane B_2 and other metabolites from platelets incubated with [1-^{14}C]arachidonic acid was examined. Washed platelet suspensions were incubated with labeled arachidonic acid in the presence and absence of onion extract or indomethacin. The products were analyzed by thin-layer chromatography and autoradiography using previously described procedures (3). The results are illustrated in Fig. 2. The most striking effect of the addition of onion or garlic extract was the almost complete suppression of thromboxane B_2 synthesis and the appearance of a new metabolite in the region of the hydroxy fatty acid. Formation of this metabolite was unaffected by further addition of indomethacin but was inhibited in the presence of 5,8,11,14-eicosatetraynoic acid. This metabolite appears to arise from the platelet-lipoxygenase pathway.

The new metabolite was isolated and converted to the methyl ester–tetramethyl silane (TMS) ether and analyzed by gas chromatography–mass spectroscopy.

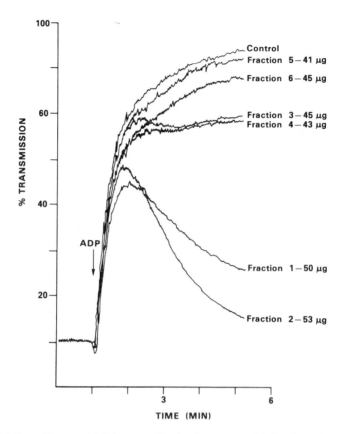

FIG. 1. Inhibition of human platelet aggregation by chromatographic fractions of onion extract. Freshly prepared platelet-rich plasma (300 μl) was incubated for 1 min with ethanol (0.5 μl, control) or the indicated concentrations of fractions 1–6 (Table 1) in ethanol. Aggregation was initiated by addition of ADP (1.2 μg in saline, 1.5 μl).

The major component had a retention time (2.6 min) which differed from hydroxyheptatrienoic acid (HHT), 1.0 min, and hydroxyeicosatetraynoic acid (HETE), 1.7 min, on SP-2250 column packing at 210°C. From its mass spectrum (Fig. 3), this metabolite was tentatively identified as 10-hydroxy-11,12-epoxy-5,8,14-eicosatrienoic acid (10,11,12-HEPA). The identities of cleavage fragments were confirmed by the mass ion shifts seen with the methyl ester D_9–TMS derivatives.

These results indicate that two members of the allium family commonly used in the diet contain similar compounds which inhibit platelet aggregation by alterations in both the platelet cyclooxygenase and lipoxygenase pathway. The relationship of these metabolic changes to the observed changes in platelet function and the chemical characterization of the active principles in onion and garlic are currently the subject of further investigation.

TABLE 1. *Platelet inhibitory activity of different fractions*[a]

FRACTIONS		WT. OF ETHANOL SOLUBLE EXTRACT mg	I_{50}/ml PRP µg	TOTAL UNITS	TOTAL RECOVERED UNITS %
CHLOROFORM EXTRACTS	1	40.0	137	292	13.7
	2	16.2	132	123	5.7
	3	12.7	181	70	3.3
	4	13.9	204	68	3.2
	5	6.2	610	10	0.5
	6	64.5	570	113	5.3
PET. ETHER EXTRACT		169.0	116	1460	68.3
STEAM-DISTILLED	ONION OIL	—	94	—	—
	GARLIC OIL	—	95	—	—

[a]One unit is the amount required to produce 50% aggregation in 1 ml platelet-rich plasma measured in a standardized aggregation assay system (4,5).

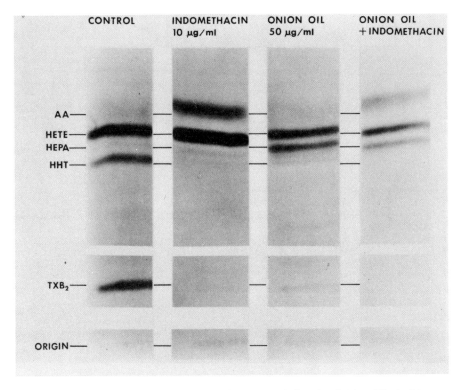

FIG. 2. Influence of onion inhibitor on arachidonate metabolism in platelets. Washed human platelets were incubated into [1-14C]arachidonic acid in the presence and absence of onion oil and indomethacin in the indicated proportions and concentrations. The products were separated by thin-layer chromatography and radioautographed (3). AA, arachidonic acid; TXB$_2$, thromboxane B$_2$.

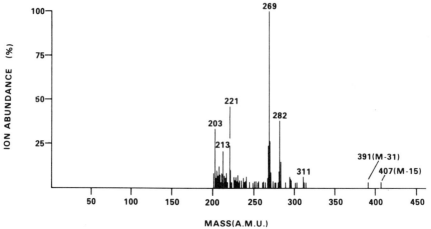

STRUCTURE AND CLEAVAGE PATTERN OF HEPA

FIG. 3. Identification of platelet lipoxygenase product formed in the presence of onion extract as 10,11,12-HEPA. Mass spectrum of a new lipoxygenase product, 10,11,12-HEPA, obtained in the presence of onion oil as illustrated in Fig. 2.

REFERENCES

1. Baghurst, K. I., Raj, M. J., and Truswell, A. S. (1977): *Lancet,* 1:101.
2. Bordia, A. (1978): *Atherosclerosis,* 30:355–360.
3. Bryant, R. W., Feinmark, S. J., Makheja, A. N., and Bailey, J. M. (1978): *J. Biol. Chem.,* 253:8134–8142.
4. Makheja, A. N., Vanderhoek, J. Y., and Bailey, J. M. (1979): *Lancet,* 1:781 (letter).
5. Makheja, A. N., Vanderhoek, J. Y., and Bailey, J. M. (1979): *Prostaglandins Med.,* 413–424.
6. Phillip, C., and Poyster, N. L. (1978): *Lancet,* 1:1051–1052.
7. Weisenberger, H., Grube, H., Koening, E., and Pelzer, H. (1972): *FEBS Lett.,* 26:105–108.

Advances in Prostaglandin and Thromboxane Research,
Vol. 6, edited by B. Samuelsson, P. W. Ramwell,
and R. Paoletti. Raven Press, New York © 1980.

Effect of Oral Aspirin Dose on Platelet Aggregation and Arterial Prostacyclin Synthesis: Studies in Humans and Rabbits

E. F. Ellis, P. S. Jones, K. F. Wright, *D. W. Richardson, and C. K. Ellis

*Departments of Pharmacology and *Medicine, Medical College of Virginia, Richmond, Virginia 23298*

Aspirin (ASA) inhibits platelet aggregation and prostaglandin synthesis by irreversibly acetylating the cyclooxygenase enzyme. While inhibition of cyclooxygenase-dependent platelet aggregation may be a clinically desirable effect of ASA, simultaneous inhibition of the cyclooxygenase-dependent vascular synthesis of the antiaggregatory vasodilator prostacyclin (PGI_2) may not be desirable. In order to determine if one can achieve selective inactivation of platelet cyclooxygenase using oral doses of aspirin, we studied human and rabbit platelet aggregation and rabbit aortic synthesis of PGI_2 before and 3 hr after various doses of oral ASA.

Platelet aggregation stimulated by arachidonic acid (AA) was used as an indicator of platelet cyclooxygenase integrity. Vascular cylooxygenase integrity was assessed by assaying for aortic production of PGI_2. Inhibition of adenosine diphosphate (ADP)-induced platelet aggregation was used as the bioassay for vascular synthesis of PGI_2. Therefore, ASA inhibition of platelet cyclooxygenase is demonstrated by a decreased platelet aggregation in response to AA (Figs. 1 and 3), while ASA inhibition of arterial cyclooxygenase is shown by a decreased inhibition of ADP-induced platelet aggregation (Fig. 2).

In rabbits, we found that the lower dose of ASA (30 mg/kg) produced a major inhibition of platelet aggregation (Fig. 1) and a minor inhibition of PGI_2 synthesis (Fig. 2), while higher doses of ASA inhibited both platelet aggregation and vascular PGI_2 synthesis. We next studied the effect of various doses of oral ASA on human platelet aggregation (Fig. 3) and found that a dose equivalent to approximately one-quarter of a 300 mg ASA tablet (1.1 mg/kg) consistently produced a major inhibition of cyclooxygenase-dependent platelet aggregation in a pattern similar to the loss of rabbit platelet aggregation, where rabbit vascular PGI_2 synthetic capacity was not much inhibited. With both the 1.1 mg/kg human dose and the 30 mg/kg rabbit dose of ASA there is a major inhibition of the peak platelet aggregation induced by lower doses of AA, although substan-

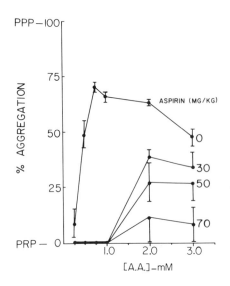

FIG. 1. AA-stimulated aggregation of platelet-rich plasma (PRP) from control and ASA-treated rabbits. Blood for preparation of PRP was drawn immediately before and 3 hr after ASA was given by a stomach tube. Technically, increased aggregation is indicated by increased light transmission, as measured with the aggregometer. Control, no aspirin ($n = 17$); 30 mg/kg ($n = 4$); 50 mg/kg ($n = 4$); 70 mg/kg ($n = 4$). Values in all figures are means ± SEM.

tial aggregation remains when the highest doses of AA are used. In additional experiments on six humans, we found that 1.1 mg/kg ASA inhibited epinephrine- and collagen-stimulated platelet aggregation by 61 and 78%, respectively, but had no effect on aggregation induced by 10 or 30 μM ADP.

In another series of rabbit experiments, we demonstrated that *in vivo,* it takes the arterial vasculature over 24 hr to return to control PGI_2 synthetic capacity following a single, high dose of oral ASA. In rabbits sacrificed at 13 and 24 hr after 70 mg/kg ASA, PGI_2 synthesized by the aorta inhibited 10 μM ADP-induced platelet aggregation by 22 and 62%, respectively, the pre-ASA value being 92%. Extrapolation of the data indicates that vascular cyclooxygenase

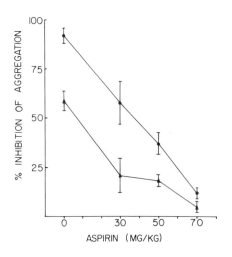

FIG. 2. Inhibition of ADP-induced aggregation by PGI_2 synthesized by aortic tissue from control and ASA-treated rabbits. Aortic tissue was obtained 3 hr after ASA administration. PRP was prepared from rabbits receiving no drugs. Control, no aspirin ($n = 4$); 30 mg/kg ($n = 4$); 50 mg/kg ($n = 4$); ●, 10 μM ADP, ▲, 30 μM ADP.

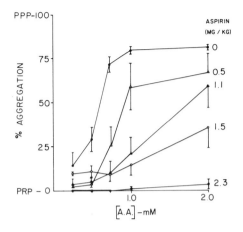

FIG. 3. AA-stimulated aggregation of PRP from control and ASA-treated humans. Blood for preparation of PRP was drawn immediately before and 3 hr after ASA ingestion. Control, pre-ASA ($n = 23$); 0.5 mg/kg ($n = 5$); 1.1 mg/kg ($n = 6$); 1.5 mg/kg ($n = 5$); and 2.3 mg/kg ($n = 5$).

activity would return to pre-ASA control levels at approximately 27 to 30 hr after a high dose of ASA.

In conclusion we speculate that in humans approximately one-quarter of an ASA tablet, which strongly inhibits cyclooxygenase-dependent aggregation, may not inhibit vascular cyclooxygenase-dependent PGI_2 synthesis to any great extent and may be a more efficacious use of ASA as an antithrombotic agent.

ACKNOWLEDGMENTS

This work was supported by a grant-in-aid from the American Heart Association, with funds contributed in part by the American Heart Association, Virginia Affiliate; a grant-in-aid from Virginia Commonwealth University; and Grant # HL-07309, National Heart, Lung, and Blood Institute, NIH. We thank The Upjohn Company for the prostaglandins and Ms. J. McKinney for secretarial assistance.

Advances in Prostaglandin and Thromboxane Research,
Vol. 6, edited by B. Samuelsson, P. W. Ramwell,
and R. Paoletti. Raven Press, New York © 1980.

Differential Inhibition of Prostacyclin Production and Platelet Aggregation by Aspirin in Humans

Giulio Masotti, Giorgio Galanti, Loredana Poggesi, Rosanna Abbate, and Gian Gastone Neri Serneri

Istituto di Patologia Medica II dell'Università di Firenze, Florence, Italy

Aspirin has been found to be a powerful inhibitor of platelet aggregation by blocking cyclooxygenase (7–9). It has been shown that endothelial cells synthesize prostacyclin (PGI_2) (2–4), a substance that causes vasodilatation and potent inhibition of platelet aggregation. Therefore, the use of aspirin in the prevention of thrombosis might not be devoid of risks, because it inhibits not only thromboxane A_2, but also PGI_2 production. The present investigation was undertaken to compare the effects in man of different doses of aspirin on platelet aggregation and PGI_2 production by the vessel wall 3 min after ischemia of the arm.

MATERIALS AND METHODS

Twenty-three healthy volunteers (11 males and 12 females) 18 to 30 years of age were studied. PGI_2 production, platelet aggregation, and malondialdehyde (MDA) formation were investigated before and 2, 12, 24, 48, and 72 hr after aspirin dosing.

PGI_2 was assayed by Vane's cascade superfusion technique (10) as modified by Ferreira and De Souza Costa (1) and adapted by us to the assay in circulating blood (5). Assay tissues were bovine coronary artery (BCA), rat stomach strip (RSS), and chick rectum (CR). Synthetic PGI_2 (kindly supplied by Dr. Vane, The Wellcome Research Laboratories, Beckenham, U.K.) was used as a standard reference.

Platelet aggregation was investigated in a Born apparatus. Platelet-rich plasma (PRP) was aggregated by adenosine monophosphate (ADP, 2 μM final concentration), epinephrine (10 μM final concentration), and collagen (Stago) (5 μg/ml final concentration).

MDA formation by platelet buttons from 1 ml of PRP stimulated by thrombin (5 U/ml) was assayed according to Okuma et al. (6).

RESULTS

Effects of Aspirin on Platelet Aggregation and MDA Production

MDA production was completely inhibited 2 hr after 2 mg/kg of aspirin. Epinephrine- and collagen-induced platelet aggregation were only slightly affected. A dose of 2.5 mg/kg reduced ADP-, epinephrine-, and collagen-induced platelet aggregation by 25, 35.6, and 35%, respectively. The inhibition of platelet aggregation was almost maximal for all three inducers 2 hr after the administration of 3.5 mg/kg of aspirin (Fig. 1). Further increases in the dose (5, 8, and 10 mg/kg) only provoked a minor increase of the inhibition, not proportional to the increase of the dose (Fig. 1). Whatever dosage was used, aspirin never completely inhibited platelet aggregation, regardless of the aggregating agent. Concerning the duration of aspirin-induced inhibition of platelet aggregation, after 3.5 mg/kg of aspirin epinephrine-induced aggregation was still inhibited by 35% after 72 hr, ADP-induced aggregation by 22.5% and collagen-induced aggregation by 18%. Seventy-two hr after 5 mg/kg aspirin, platelet aggregation was slightly more inhibited (Fig. 2). MDA production was still markedly inhibited 72 hr after 3.5 to 10 mg/kg.

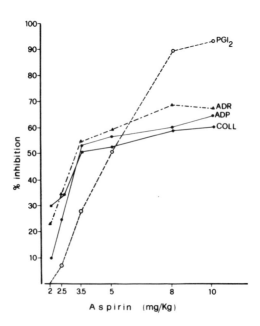

FIG. 1. Effect of increasing doses of aspirin on PGl₂ production and platelet aggregation 2 hr after administration. Mean values of the different patient groups treated with increasing doses of aspirin are reported.

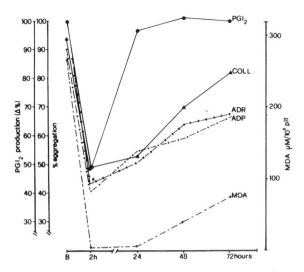

FIG. 2. Duration of the effect of one dose of aspirin (5 mg/kg) on platelet aggregation induced by collagen (COLL), epinephrine (ADR), and ADP, and on the production of PGI_2 and MDA. Mean values of four cases.

Effects of Aspirin on PGI_2 Production by Ischemia

A dose of 2.5 mg/kg resulted in a slight inhibition of PGI_2 production 2 hr after administration, whereas doses of 3.5 and 5 mg/kg induced an average inhibition of 30 and 50% after 2 hr. Almost complete inhibition of PGI_2 production occurred after 8 mg/kg (90% of inhibition) (Fig. 1). Twenty-four hr after aspirin, PGI_2 production reversed in all subjects after doses of 2, 3.5, and 5 mg/kg (Fig. 2).

DISCUSSION

These findings show that production of PGI_2 by the vessel wall, MDA production by platelets, and platelet aggregation were affected in different degrees by increasing doses of aspirin. Moreover, the duration of inhibition of vessel wall cyclooxygenase was also remarkably different, compared to that of platelet cyclooxygenase. These findings allow for the determination of the dose of aspirin that achieves a significant and long-lasting inhibition of platelet aggregation with only a slight and short inhibition of PGI_2 production. Aspirin doses of 3.5 mg/kg of aspirin at 3-day intervals seem to induce an almost maximal platelet aggregation without significantly affecting PGI_2 production by the vessel wall. Higher doses inhibit PGI_2 production while increasing platelet aggregation only slightly. The identification of the aspirin dose giving maximum antiaggregating action and minimum PGI_2 inhibition can be useful in the prevention of thrombosis. The administration of doses much greater than the optimal one could be the explanation for the poor results sometimes seen in the prophylaxis of arterial thrombosis with aspirin.

ACKNOWLEDGMENT

We thank The Wellcome Research Laboratories, Beckenham, U.K., for providing the PGI$_2$ standard.

REFERENCES

1. Ferreira, S. H., and De Souza Costa, F. (1976): *Eur. J. Pharmacol.*, 39:379.
2. Gryglewski, R. J., Bunting, S., Moncada, S., Flower, R. J., and Vane, J. R. (1976): *Prostaglandins*, 12:685.
3. Moncada, S., Gryglewski, R. J., Bunting, S., and Vane, J. R. (1976): *Nature*, 263:663.
4. Moncada, S., Higgs, E. A., and Vane, J. R. (1977): *Lancet*, 1:18.
5. Neri Serneri, G. G., Masotti, G., Poggesi, L., and Galanti, G. (1978): In: *Fifth International Congress on Thromboembolism*, Bologna, p. 45 (abstr.).
6. Okuma, M., Steiner, M., and Baldini, M. (1970): *J. Lab. Clin. Med.*, 75:283.
7. Roth, G. J., and Majerus, P. W. (1975): *J. Clin. Invest.*, 56:624.
8. Roth, G. J., Stanford, N., and Majerus, P. W. (1975): *Proc. Natl. Acad. Sci. USA*, 72:3073.
9. Smith, J. B., and Willis, A. L. (1971): *Nature*, 231:235.
10. Vane, J. R. (1964): *Br. J. Pharmacol.*, 23:360.

Advances in Prostaglandin and Thromboxane Research,
Vol. 6, edited by B. Samuelsson, P. W. Ramwell,
and R. Paoletti. Raven Press, New York © 1980.

Serine-Esterase (Protease) Inhibitors Block Stimulus-Induced Mobilization of Arachidonate in Platelets

Maurice B. Feinstein, Jack Y. Vanderhoek,* and Ronald Walenga

*Department of Pharmacology, University of Connecticut Health Center,
Farmington, Connecticut 06032*

Prostaglandin endoperoxides and thromboxane A_2 (TXA_2) formed by the metabolism of arachidonic acid can induce platelets to aggregate and to release the contents of secretory granules. Normally, little if any free arachidonic acid exists in unstimulated platelets; therefore, the rate-limiting step in arachidonate metabolism is its release from phospholipids by various stimulating agents. The mechanism for stimulus-induced release of arachidonate is not well understood, but two routes appear possible: (a) via phospholipase A_2 action on phospholipids (1) and (b) involvement of the sequential action of a phospholipase C-type enzyme to produce diglyceride (3), which can be attacked by lipases to release free fatty acids (4).

We previously reported (2) that the serine-esterase (protease) inhibitor phenylmethanesulfonyl fluoride (PMSF) blocked the formation of malonyldialdehyde (MDA) and TXA_2 (bioassayed as rabbit aorta contracting substance) and the oxygen burst in platelets that were stimulated with collagen or thrombin. These effects of PMSF were not simply due to inactivation of thrombin. In this paper we report on a number of other active-site specific inhibitors of serine-esterases (proteases) which can also block stimulus-induced mobilization of arachidonate (Fig. 1): e.g., acetylbenzenesulfonyl fluoride, p-toluenesulfonyl chloride and fluoride (tosyl chloride and fluoride), 5-dimethylaminonaphthalene-1-sulfonyl fluoride (dansyl fluoride), 2-nitro-4-carboxyphenyl-N,N-diphenylcarbamate (NCDC), and p-nitrophenyl anthranilate.

In order to study the effects of serine-esterase (protease) inhibitors on arachidonate metabolism, platelets were incubated in plasma at 37°C with ^{14}C-arachidonic acid for 1 hr to permit its incorporation into phospholipids. The platelets were subsequently washed with Tris–HCl (pH 8.0) buffered salt solution to remove extracellular arachidonate and then resuspended in buffered saline in the presence or absence of serine-esterase (protease) inhibitors. The latter were

---

* *Present address:* Department of Biochemistry, George Washington University, Washington, D.C., 20052

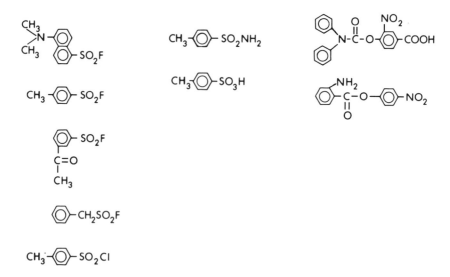

FIG. 1. Serine-esterase (protease) inhibitors which block stimulus-induced mobilization of platelet arachidonic acid. The tosyl sulfonamide and sulfonic acid derivatives are inactive.

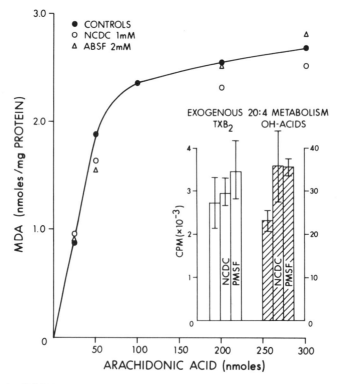

FIG. 2. Lack of inhibition of arachidonic acid metabolism in platelets treated with serine-esterase (protease) inhibitors.

added dissolved in small volumes of dimethyl sulfoxide. Controls contained the same volume of solvent. MDA was measured in aliquots of the platelet suspensions by the thiobarbituric acid method. The remainder of the platelet suspensions were extracted with chloroform–methanol and the radioactive phospholipids and arachidonate metabolites were separated by thin-layer chromatography and measured as previously described (5). The metabolism of exogenously added ^{14}C-arachidonate in the presence of serine-esterase (protease) inhibitors was also studied.

A number of platelet-stimulating agents were employed in these experiments, all of which induce the release of phospholipid arachidonate and the formation of its various metabolites. These included proteolytic enzymes (thrombin, trypsin, papain), proteins or peptides (collagen, polylysine, melittin, gamma globulin-coated latex beads), and certain thiol reagents (N-ethylmaleimide and ethylmercurithiosalicylate). It is presumed that the protein- and peptide-stimulating agents act on the surface membrane of the platelet, whereas evidence favors an intracellular Ca^{2+}-releasing action for the ionophore and the SH-reagents.

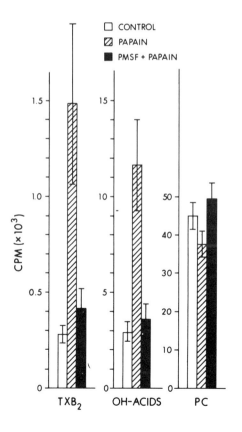

FIG. 3. Inhibition of papain- (cysteine-activated) induced mobilization of platelet arachidonate from phosphatidyl choline and TXB_2 and hydroxyacid formation by PMSF (1mM).

RESULTS

All of the serine-esterase (protease) inhibitors (Fig. 1) produced a concentration-dependent inhibition of the stimulus-induced formation of MDA but were essentially without effect on the metabolism of exogenous arachidonic acid (Fig. 2). Each of the platelet-stimulating agents mentioned above could be inhibited. Figures 3 and 4 show typical effects on TXB_2 and hydroxyacid and MDA formation, as well as the inhibition of stimulus-induced fall in phosphatidyl choline ^{14}C-arachidonate. In several cases we determined that the serine-esterase (protease) inhibitors did not directly inactivate the protease-stimulating agents. Papain was protected from sulfonation of its active-site cysteine by the addition of cysteine to the buffer solution. It was also established that trypsin was not inactivated by dansyl fluoride or NCDC during the duration of platelet exposure to the enzyme (5 min), in agreement with published data that these inhibitors inactivate trypsin very slowly. The nonsulfonating sulfonamide or sulfonic acid derivatives of PMSF, tosyl fluoride, and dansyl fluoride (Fig. 1) were inactive, or much less so than the parent compounds. Although this suggests that sulfona-

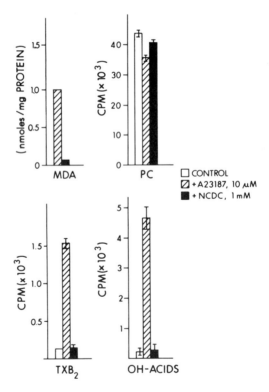

FIG. 4. Inhibition of A23187-induced release of phosphatidyl choline-arachidonate and its subsequent metabolism to MDA, TXB_2, and hydroxy acids (HETE + HHT) by NCDC.

tion may be necessary for the inhibitory action, we have no direct evidence for it, and the rapidity of the action of these compounds (within 1–5 min) may indicate that they may act over a short time scale as competitive reversible inhibitors of some platelet esterase or protease. We conclude therefore that the stimulus-induced mobilization of platelet arachidonate may require the activity of a serine-esterase (protease). This esterase could be one or more of the lipases involved in the breakdown of phospholipid or diglycerides, or a protease involved in their activation.

REFERENCES

1. Derksen, A., and Cohen, P. (1975): *J. Biol. Chem.,* 250:9342–9347.
2. Feinstein, M. B., Becker, E. L., and Fraser, C. (1977): *Prostaglandins,* 14:229–235.
3. Rittenhouse-Simmons, S. (1979): *J. Clin. Invest.,* 63:580–587.
4. Sun, G. Y., Su, K. L., Der, O. M., and Tang, W. (1979): *Lipids,* 14:229–235.
5. Vanderhoek, J. Y., and Feinstein, M. B. (1979): *Mol. Pharmacol.,* 16:171–180.

Advances in Prostaglandin and Thromboxane Research,
Vol. 6, edited by B. Samuelsson, P. W. Ramwell,
and R. Paoletti. Raven Press, New York © 1980.

Syntheses of New Prostacyclin Analogs

K. Shimoji, Y. Arai, H. Wakatsuka, and M. Hayashi

*Department of Chemistry, Research Institute, Ono Pharmaceutical Co., Ltd.,
Shimamoto-cho, Mishima-gun, Osaka 618, Japan*

It is well known that prostacyclin (PGI$_2$; Fig. 1, *1*) shows unique and very potent biological properties (4–7). Structurally, PGI$_2$ **1** possesses the enol-ether function, which is a clearly different moiety from those of the primary prostaglandins. Being interested in this moiety, we intended the syntheses of the two PGI$_2$ analogs **2** and **3** to know how the biological properties would be changed in comparison with the natural PGI$_2$. We wish to describe here the syntheses and biological properties of these PGI$_2$ analogs.

SYNTHESES

Preparation of Compounds 12 and 14

The Diels-Alder reaction of cyclopentadiene with chloroacrylonitrile gave compound **4** quantitatively (Fig. 2). Treatment of **4** with aqueous potassium hydroxide in dimethyl sulfoxide afforded the bicyclic ketone **5** quantitatively. The bicyclic ketone **5** was converted to the lactone iodohydrin **6** in 60% yield by Baeyer-Villiger oxidation, followed by the iodo-lactonization.

Epoxidation of the iodohydrin **6** to the epoxide **7** was carried out using potassium carbonate in isopropanol at 50°C and proceeded in 96% yield.

The epoxy-lactone **7** led to the acetal **8** and **9** by a method similar to that of Corey et al. (1).

The reaction of the epoxy-acetal **8** with the lithium salt of phenylallyl sulfide (2.0 eq) in dry tetrahydrofuran (THF) at −78°C gave a mixture of compounds **10** and **11** in 38 and 60% yield, respectively (Fig. 3).

Compound **10** was converted to the allylic alcohol **12** in three steps in 77% overall yield: (a) dihydropyran, *p*-toluenesulfonic acid in methylene chloride; (b) *m*-chloroperbenzoic acid (1.0 eq) in methylene chloride at −78°C; and (c) rearrangement of allylic sulfoxide with trimethyl phosphite in methanol (2).

The isomer **11** was also converted to the isomer **13** by the same method. Compound **14** is the enantiomeric isomer of the compound **13**.

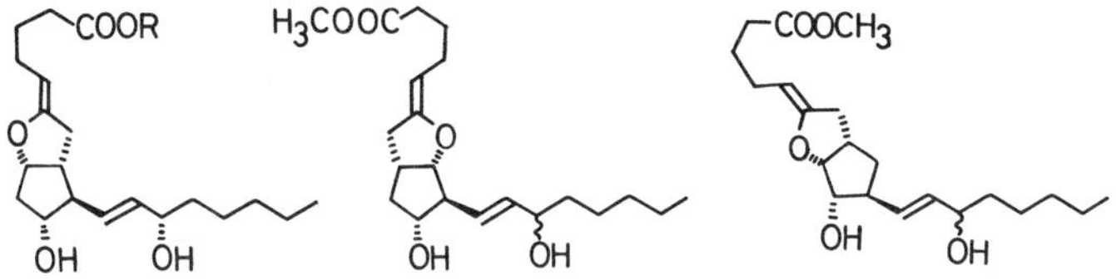

FIG. 1. Chemical structures of PGI₂ (**1**) and its analogs, **2** and **3**. R= H or methyl.

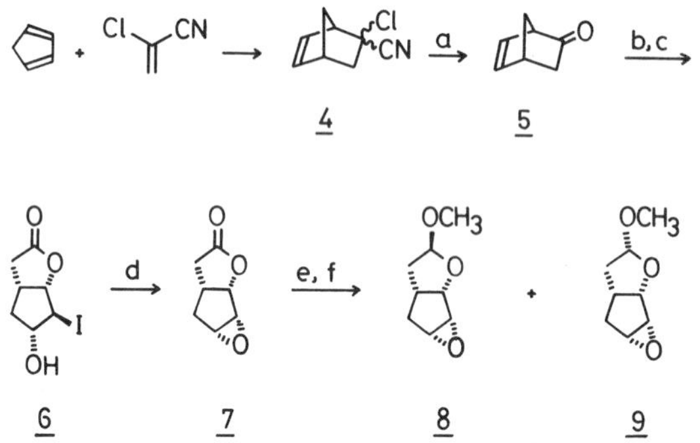

FIG. 2. Preparation of the epoxy-acetal **8**. a: KOH (aq. soln.) in dimethyl sulfoxide, **b:** H₂O₂ (aq. soln.) + NaOH (aq. soln.), c: KI₃ (aq. soln.), d: K₂CO₃ in isopropanol, e: diisobutylaluminum hydride in toluene at −78°C, f: borontrifluoride etherate in methanol at −20°.

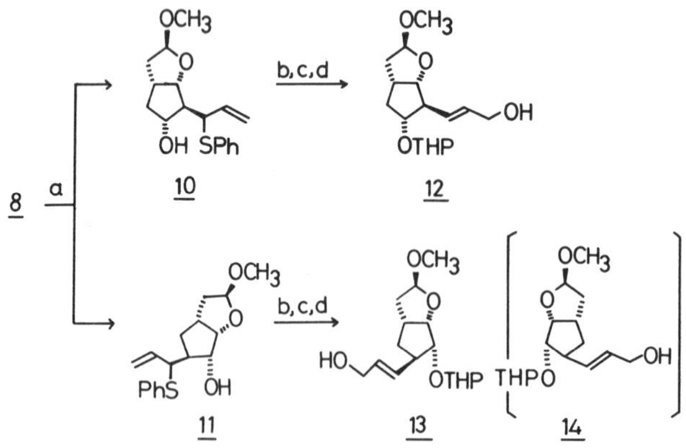

FIG. 3. Preparation of allylic alcohol **12** and **14**. a: PhSCHCH=CH₂ Li⁺ in tetrahydrofuran at −78°C, b: dihydropyran+ *p*-toluene-sulfonic acid in methylene chloride, c: *m*-chloroperbenzoic acid in methylene chloride at −78°C, d: trimethyl phosphite in methanol. THP = 2-tetrahydropyranyl; Ph = phenyl.

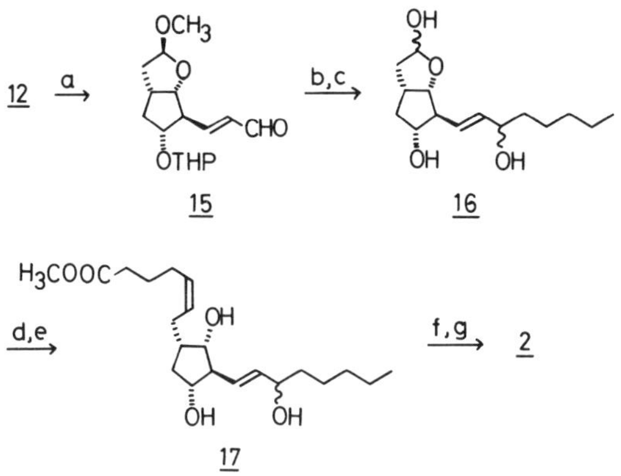

FIG. 4. Preparation of the PGI$_2$-analog **2**. a: Manganese dioxide in methylene chloride, b: n-C$_5$H$_{11}$MgBr in ether at $-20°$C, c: HC1 (aq. soln.) in methanol, d: Ph$_3$P=CH(CH$_2$)$_3$COONa in dimethyl sulfoxide, e: diazomethane in ether, f: I$_2$ + NaHCO$_3$ (aq. soln.) in methylene chloride, g: 1,8-diazabicyclo [5.4.0]-7-undecene. THP = 2-tetrahydropyranyl.

Preparation of Compound 2

The oxidation of the allylic alcohol **12** using manganese dioxide in methylene chloride gave the ene-aldehyde **15** in excellent yield. The reaction of the ene-aldehyde **15** with n-amyl magnesium bromide, followed by the acid hydrolysis of the acetal, afforded compound **16** (Fig. 4). The lactol **16** was converted to the PGF$_{2\alpha}$ analog **17** by the Wittig reaction, followed by methylation with diazomethane.

The PGI$_2$ analog **2** was prepared from compound **17** by the procedure of Johnson et al. (3).

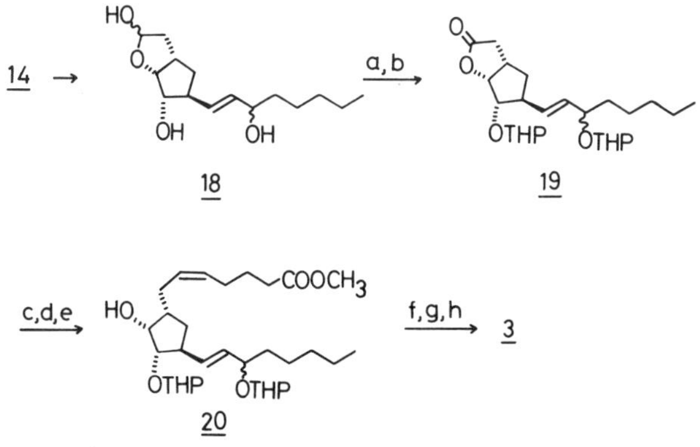

FIG. 5. Preparation of the PGI$_2$-analog **3**. a: Ag$_2$O + NaOH (aq. soln.), b: dihydropyran + p-toluenesulfonic acid in methylene chloride, c: diisobutylaluminum hydride in toluene at $-78°$C, d: Ph$_3$P=CH(CH$_2$)$_3$COONa in dimethyl sulfoxide, e: diazomethane in ether, f: N-bromosuccinimide in chloroform, g: acetic acid + water + tetrahydrofuran at $45°$C, h: 1,8-diazabicyclo[5.4.0]-7-undecene. THP = 2-tetrahydropyranyl.

Preparation of Compound 3

The allylic alcohol **14** was converted to the lactol **18** by the same method described above for compound **2**. The oxidation of the lactol **18** using silver oxide, followed by the tetrahydropyranylation, afforded the lactone **19**. And the lactone **19** was converted to the $PGF_{2\alpha}$ analog **20** in three steps: (a) diisobutyl-aluminum hydride in toluene at $-78°C$; (b) Wittig reaction; and (c) diazomethane in ether (Fig. 5).

The PGI_2 analog **3** was prepared from compound **20** in three steps: (a) N-bromosuccinimide in chloroform; (b) acid hydrolysis of the tetrahydropyranyl group by acetic acid-water-THF at $45°C$; and (c) dehydrohalogenation with 1,8-diazabicyclo[5.4.0]-17-undecene.

BIOLOGICAL PROPERTIES OF THE PGI_2 ANALOGS 2 AND 3

The two PGI_2 analogs **2** and **3** showed biological properties similar to those of the natural PGI_2.

For example, compound **2** possesses the inhibitory activity of adenosine mono-phosphate-induced platelet aggregation of the rat platelet-rich plasma. And compound **3** showed coronary vasodilatory activity in the isolated rabbit heart.

However, these activities were very low compared to those of natural PGI_2.

REFERENCES

1. Corey, E. J., Nicolaou, K. C., and Beames, D. J. (1974): *Tetrahedron Lett.,* 2439–2440.
2. Evans, D. A. (1974): *Acc. Chem. Res.,* 7:147–155.
3. Johnson, R. A., Lincoln, F. H., Nidy, E. G., Schneider, W. P., Thompson, J. L., and Axen, U. (1978): *J. Am. Chem. Soc.,* 100:7690–7705.
4. Moncada, S., Gryglewski, R. J., Bunting, S., and Vane, J. R. (1976): *Nature,* 263:663–665.
5. Moncada, S., Gryglewski, R. J., Bunting, S., Flower, R. J., and Vane, J. R. (1976): *Prostaglandins,* 12:685–713.
6. Moncada, S., Gryglewski, R. J., Bunting, S., and Vane, J. R. (1976): *Prostaglandins,* 12:715–737.
7. Moncada, S., Gryglewski, R. J., Bunting, S., and Vane, J. R. (1976): *Prostaglandins,* 12:897–913.

Advances in Prostaglandin and Thromboxane Research,
Vol. 6, edited by B. Samuelsson, P. W. Ramwell,
and R. Paoletti. Raven Press, New York © 1980.

Comparison of the Activities of Prostacyclin and Its Stable Analogs on the Platelet Aggregation and Cardiovascular Systems

Akiyoshi Kawasaki, Kenji Ishii, Korekiyo Wakitani, and Masami Tsuboshima

Department of Pharmacology, Research Institute, Ono Pharmaceutical Co., Ltd., 3-1-1 Sakurai, Shimamoto-cho, Mishima-gun, Osaka 618, Japan

Prostacyclin (PGI_2), the newly discovered unstable metabolite of arachidonic acid in vascular tissues, has potent antiplatelet aggregating and vasodilating properties. Whereas it has been hypothesized that PGI_2 plays an important physiological role in preventing platelet clumping on blood vessel walls, its study is very restricted because of its poor stability. Therefore, several investigators (1–3) have tried to synthesize more stable analogs retaining the potency of PGI_2. In an attempt to synthesize such analogs in aqueous solution, we found a few compounds which, although they are less potent than PGI_2, are 6 to 13 times more potent than prostaglandin E_1 (PGE_1). We now report the results of screenings carried out so far.

MATERIALS AND METHODS

The activity of PGI analogs as inhibitors of rat and human platelet aggregation was investigated. Blood was freshly collected into trisodium citrate (3.8%, w/v, 0.1 vol.) and centrifuged (400 x g for 10 min). Inhibition of platelet aggregation was determined in a Born-type aggregometer by incubating aliquots of the platelet-rich plasma (PRP) with PGI analogs for 2 min before the addition of sufficient adenosine diphosphate (ADP, 6–10 μg/ml). In three experiments, ID_{50} for analogs was compared with that of PGE_1 and expressed as relative to it. The hypotensive activity of PGI analogs was also determined after intravenous injection in dogs anesthetized with barbital sodium (250 mg/kg, i.p.). The hypotensive doses required to cause a fall of blood pressure of 20 to 40 mm Hg were compared with those of PGE_1 in three experiments. The hypotensive activity was determined after oral administration in fasting spontaneously hypertensive rats (SHR) using the tail-cuff method.

The stable PGI analogs used in experiments have the following basic structure: 5,6-dihydro-PGI_1, 6,9α-nitrilo-PGI_1, 6,9-methano-PGI_2, and 6,9-thio-PGI_2.

Furthermore, these basic analogs were modified by introduction of the methyl group at the C_{16} or C_{17} position, as well as being modified to the 16,18-methano- or 16,18-ethano- ring in the ω chain in order to increase the antiplatelet aggregating activity.

RESULTS AND DISCUSSION

Stability of PGI Analogs

The stability of PGI analogs was compared with those of the PGI_2 sodium salt and its methyl ester based on their hypotensive activity after intravenous injection in anesthetized dogs. Since the stability of the compound in solution depends on its concentration and the solvent used, PGI_2 sodium salt and its methyl ester were examined at 10 μg/ml in 20% ethanol–saline solution or under conditions of pH adjusted with glycine–sodium hydroxide buffer. While PGI_2 sodium salt and its methyl ester were not stable if the pH of solution was not adjusted either to 10 for the PGI_2 sodium salt or to 8.6 for its methyl ester (Fig. 1), the PGI analogs shown in Fig. 2 were stable in 20 to 50% ethanol–saline solution even 6 hr after solubilization compared with those freshly prepared, suggesting that PGI_1, nitrilo-, methano-, and thio- analogs are more stable than PGI_2 sodium salt and its methyl ester.

Biological Activities of Stable PGI Analogs

All PGI_1 analogs—including 16-S-methyl-, 17-S-methyl- and 16,18-methano-, and 16,18-ethano-ω-homo structures—were 1.0 to 2.3 times more potent than PGE_1 in antiaggregating activity in rat PRP. The hypotensive activities were less or almost equiactive to PGE_1 in anesthetized dogs. Among the nitrilo analogs, 17-S-methyl-ω-homo-6,9α-nitrilo-PGI_1 methyl ester 1 and 16,18-ethano-ω-homo-6,9α-nitrilo-PGI_1 methyl ester 3 were 11.4 and 10.1 times more active, respectively, than PGE_1 in antiplatelet activity in rat PRP, and their hypotensive potencies were more or less the same as PGE_1 (Table 1).

Of the methano- and thio- analogs, 17-S-methyl-ω-homo-methano-PGI_2 5 was 6.7 times more potent than PGE_1 in the antiaggregating activity and twice as active as PGE_1 in lowering blood pressure. Other analogs, except for 1, 3, and 5 described above, were almost equiactive to PGE_1 in both activities.

As shown in Table 1, since the antiaggregating activity of PGI_2 methyl ester was far less potent than PGI_2 sodium salt in human PRP compared with that in rat PRP, we studied analogs 2 and 4 having free carbonic acid instead of analogs 1 and 3 in human PRP. Analog 2 was 13.1 times more potent than PGE_1, with an ID_{50} of 2.6 ng/ml. Analogs 4 and 5 were about 6 times as active as PGE_1. On the other hand, comparing their hypotensive activity in SHR, analogs 1 and 2 were the most potent of all analogs at the doses tested.

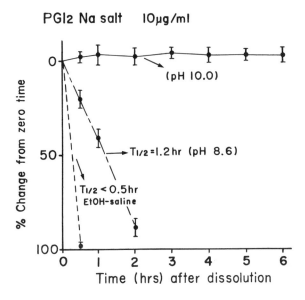

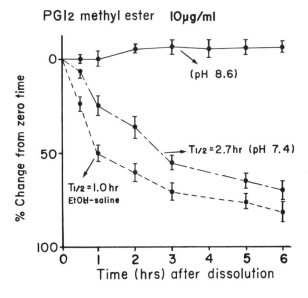

*estimated by their hypotensive activity after i.v. injection in anesthetized dogs

FIG. 1. Stability of PGI$_2$ sodium salt *(top)* and methyl ester *(bottom)* as estimated by bioassay of their hypotensive activities after intravenous injection in anesthetized dogs. They were stored at 10 μg/ml in 20% ethanol-saline solution either alone or adjusted to various pH by glycine-sodium hydroxide buffer at room temperature.

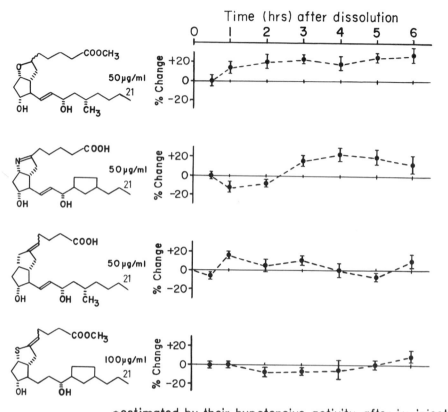

*estimated by their hypotensive activity after i.v. injection in anesthetized dogs

FIG. 2. The stability of PGI_1, nitrilo-, methano-, and thio- analogs stored at room temperature in 20–50% ethanol–saline solution as seen in Fig. 1.

This result may suggest that 17-S-methyl-ω-homo-6,9α-nitrilo- analogs are not so selective inhibitors of platelet aggregation as the analogs **3**, **4**, and **5**.

CONCLUSION

Comparing the antiaggregating activity of stable PGI analogs in aqueous solution with that of PGE_1, 17-S-methyl-ω-homo-6,9α-nitrilo-PGI_1, 16,18-ethano-ω-homo-6,9α-nitrilo-PGI_1, and 17-S-methyl-ω-homo-5EZ-6,9-methano-PGI_2 were 6 to 13 times more potent than PGE_1 in human PRP. In the light of the physiological importance of PGI_2 and its unstable nature, we consider that although they were 4 to 8 times less potent than PGI_2, such analogs are valuable in the system studied under conditions where stability is of importance.

TABLE 1. *Biological activities of stable and potent PGI analogs compared with those of PGI$_2$*

PGI$_2$ or analog	Inhibitory effect on ADP-induced platelet aggregation (relative to PGE$_1$ = 1.0)		Hypotensive activity	
	Rat	Human	Anesthetized dogs, i.v. (relative to PGE$_1$ = 1.0)	Minimum effective doses in SHR (mg/kg, p.o.)
PGI$_2$ sodium salt	48.8	46.9	10–20	>1
PGI$_2$ methyl ester	85.0	1.3	10–20	>1
17-S-Methyl-ω-homo-6,9α-nitrilo-PGI$_1$ methyl ester (1)	11.4	a	0.5	≧0.3
17-S-Methyl-ω-homo-6,9α-nitrilo-PGI$_1$ (2)	6.6	13.1	4.7	≧0.3
16,18-Ethano-ω-homo-6,9α-nitrilo-PGI$_1$ methyl ester (3)	10.1	a	1.5	>1
16,18-Ethano-ω-homo-6,9α-nitrilo-PGI$_1$ (4)	3.3	6.3	4.8	>1
17-S-Methyl-ω-homo-5EZ-6,9-methano-PGI$_2$ (5)	6.7	6.6	2.0	>3

a Not tested.

REFERENCES

1. Corey, E. J., Keck, G. E., and Szekély, I. (1977): *J. Am. Chem. Soc.,* 99:2006.
2. Fried, J., and Barton, J. (1977): *Proc. Natl. Acad. Sci. USA,* 74:2199.
3. Nicolaou, K. C., Barnette, W. E., Gasic, G. P., and Magolda, M. L. (1977): *J. Am. Chem. Soc.,* 99:7736.

Advances in Prostaglandin and Thromboxane Research,
Vol. 6, edited by B. Samuelsson, P. W. Ramwell,
and R. Paoletti. Raven Press, New York © 1980.

Syntheses and Biological Activities of Some Prostacyclin Analogs

S. Ohuchida, S. Hashimoto, H. Wakatsuka, Y. Arai, and M. Hayashi

Department of Chemistry, Research Institute, Ono Pharmaceutical Co., Ltd., 3-1-1 Sakurai, Shimamoto-cho, Mishima-gun, Osaka 618, Japan

In 1976, Moncada et al. (5) discovered a new prostaglandin, prostacyclin (PGI_2), and Johnson et al. (3) elucidated its chemical structure. Since PGI_2 is very unstable in spite of possessing high biological activities, the modification of the structure of PGI_2 is an important area of pharmacological study. We wish to describe a recent advance in the syntheses and biological activities of some PGI_2 analogs (Fig. 1).

SYNTHESES

The first analog **1** has a structure similar to that of thromboxane B_2. The preparation of this analog **1** was developed starting with thromboxane B_2 methyl ester **8** reported by Schneider and Morge (6). The compound **8** was converted with iodine and aqueous sodium bicarbonate into the iodoether, which by treatment with 1,8-diazabicycloundecene (DBU) provided the analog **1** in 70% yield.

Three analogs **2**, **3**, and **4**, described below, have the same carbon skeleton as that of PGI_2 and contain one extra methyl group in their α-chains. The synthesis of the analog **2** was realized starting with the ester **9**. Treatment of **9** with lithium diisopropylamide followed by methyl iodide gave α-methyl ester **10** in 80% yield. This compound **10** was reduced with diisobutylaluminum hydride to the corresponding alcohol, which was oxidized to the aldehyde quantitatively using the Collins reagent. The Wittig reaction of this aldehyde with the ylide derived from 5-triphenylphosphoniopentanoic acid and subsequent esterification led to the ester **11** in 63% yield. This ester **11** was transformed with 65% aqueous acetic acid to the triol, which was treated with N-bromosuccinimide (NBS) to give the bromoether in 87% yield. Exposure of the bromoether to DBU afforded the analog **2** in 39% yield, accompanied by the undesired Δ^4-compound in 40% yield.

The third analog **3** has a methyl group at C_5-position. The synthesis of this analog was achieved starting with the ester **12**. The 5,6-double bond in **12** was selectively oxidized with one equivalent of m-chloroperbenzoic acid into

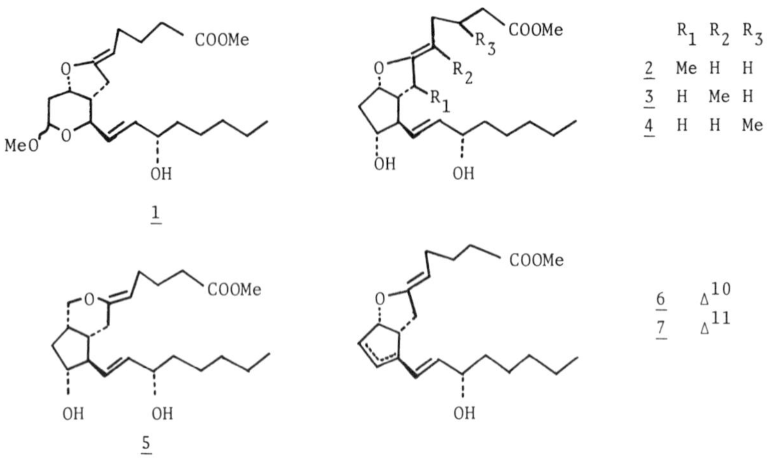

FIG. 1. Chemical structures of PGI analogs **1** and **7**.

5,6-epoxide, which was treated with potassium carbonate to furnish the cyclic ether **13** in 62% yield based on the compound **12**. Oxidation of **13** with anhydrous chromic acid and manganese sulfate followed by treatment with methylmagnesium iodide produced the compound **14** in 42% yield. The tetrahydropyranyl (THP) units in **14** were replaced with the acetyl groups in 64% yield, and then dehydration of the acetate with phosphoric chloride in pyridine afforded the desired Δ^5-compound **15** in 41% yield and the Δ^4-compound in 40% yield. Removal of the acetyl groups in **15** with potassium carbonate in methanol gave analog **3** in 62% yield.

The fourth analog **4** has a methyl group at the C_3-position. The starting material **12** was converted to the α,β-unsaturated ester in two steps: (a) phenylselenylation with diphenyldiselenide and (b) dephenylselenylacion with hydrogen peroxide in 54% overall yield. Reaction of the α,β-unsaturated ester with lithium dimethylcuprate produced compound **16** in 66% yield. The compound **16** was transformed into the desired analog **4** in 40% yield by the same method as described in the preparation of analog **2**.

The fifth analog **5** has a structure in which the unstable enolether moiety is not constructed in the five-membered ring but in the six-membered ring. In this synthesis we used compound **17** as a starting material, as reported by Bundy (1). Iodoetherification of **17** with iodine and aqueous sodium bicarbonate followed by treatment with DBU led to the analog **5** in 78% yield.

The sixth analog **6** is a PGA type and was prepared from compound **18** reported by Corey and Moinet (2) in 14% yield in three steps: (a) bromoetherification, (b) removal of the THP unit, and (c) dehydrohalogenation with DBU.

The last analog **7** is a PGC type and was obtained from the compound **19** reported by Kelly et al. (4) in the same way as described in the preparation of the analog **6** in 10% yield (Fig. 2).

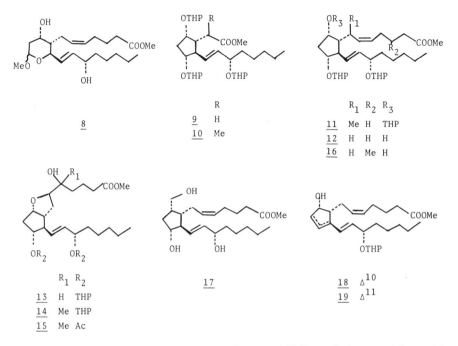

FIG. 2. Chemical structures of synthetic intermediates **8–19**. THP: tetrahydropyranyl; Ac: acetyl.

BIOLOGICAL ACTIVITIES

The biological activities of these analogs are summarized in Table 1. The two analogs **2** and **3** showed a stronger inhibitory effect on blood platelet aggregation than that of the natural PGE_1. Also, these analogs stimulated uterine contraction more strongly than the natural $PGE_{2\alpha}$. Additionally, they exerted more

TABLE 1. *Biological activities of PGI analogs*[a]

Analog	CVD ($PGE_1 = 1$)	IPA ($PGE_1 = 1$)	HA ($PGE_1 = 1$)	UCA ($PGF_{2\alpha} = 1$)
1	inactive	<0.003	pressor	<0.1
2		2.1	1.7	1
3	0.15	1.5	0.4	5
4	<0.1	0.14	<0.3	<0.1
5		0.003	inactive	<0.1
6	<0.1	0.023	pressor	<0.1
7	contraction	0.003	[b]	<0.1

[a] CVD, coronary vasodilating activity in rabbit isolated heart; IPA, inhibitory effect on rat platelet aggregation *in vitro* (adenosine diphosphate induced); HA, hypotensive activity in anesthetized dogs; UCA, uterine contractile activity in rats (to i.v. dose).
[b] Pressor followed by fall in blood pressure.

potent hypotensive activity than that of PGE_1 administered to dogs. The other analogs were hardly active or inactive altogether.

REFERENCES

1. Bundy, G. L. (1975): *Tetrahedron Lett.,* 1957.
2. Corey, E. J., and Moinet, G. (1973): *J. Am. Chem. Soc.,* 95:6831.
3. Johnson, R. A., Morton, D. R., Kinner, J. H., Gorman, R. R., McGuire, J. C., Sun, F. F., Whittaker, N., Bunting, S., Salmon, J., Moncada, S., and Vane, J. R. (1976): *Prostaglandins,* 12:915.
4. Kelley, R. C., Schletter, I., and Jones, R. L. (1973): *Prostaglandins,* 4:653.
5. Moncada, S., Gryglewski, R. J., Bunting, S., and Vane, J. R. (1976): *Nature,* 263:663.
6. Schneider, W. P., and Morge, R. A. (1976): *Tetrahedron Lett.,* 3283.

Advances in Prostaglandin and Thromboxane Research,
Vol. 6, edited by B. Samuelsson, P. W. Ramwell,
and R. Paoletti. Raven Press, New York © 1980.

Vasodilator and Antiplatelet Activities of Prostacyclins with Modified ω-Side Chain

B. A. Schölkens, W. Bartmann, G. Beck, U. Lerch, E. Konz, and
U. Weithmann

Hoechst AG, 6230 Frankfurt (Main) 80, Federal Republic of Germany

In consideration of the physiological importance of the natural prostacyclin (PGI), inhibition of platelet aggregation (10,14), relaxation of vascular smooth muscle (6), vasodepression in normotensive and hypertensive animals, as well as in man (1,7,13,14), various PGI analogs have been synthesized in search of therapeutically useful agents (12). Continuation of structure–activity studies in other PG series of analogs with modified ω-side chains (2,3,5) led to PGI analogs with residues attached to the 15-position, including cyclohexyl, 2-(2-furyl)ethyl, 2-(3-thienyl)ethyl, 3-thienyloxymethyl, and 1,1-dimethyloxaalkyl. To characterize the vasodepressor and antiaggregatory activities, the effects of these PGI analogs with modified ω-side chains were evaluated on systemic blood pressure (BP), isolated bovine coronary artery (BCA) and on arachidonic acid-induced platelet aggregation (PA).

METHODS AND MATERIAL

Vasodepressor Response in Anesthetized Rats

Arterial BP was recorded in pentobarbital-anesthetized Sprague-Dawley rats with a pressure transducer (Statham P 23 Db). PGI and its analogs were given as bolus injections into the jugular vein in doses of 0.1, 0.3, and 1 μg/kg or 0.1, 1, and 10 μg/kg. The vasodepressor response was expressed in terms of the dose causing a 25% decrease of the resting mean arterial BP (ED_{25}).

Relaxation of BCA Strips

Isolated strips of BCA were prepared according to the method of Dusting et al. (6) with minor modifications. The vasodilator action of the analogs was expressed as the dose of analog evoking 50% of the vasodilator action of 100 ng/ml PGI sodium salt (ED_{50}).

Inhibition of PA

Platelet-rich plasma was obtained from the blood of volunteers. PA was monitored by continuous recording of light transmission in a Born aggregometer

(4). Potency of PGI and its analogs was expressed as the concentration causing 50% inhibition of PA by 0.2 to 0.5 μM arachidonic acid per 0.25 ml platelet-rich plasma added after a 30-sec incubation (IC_{50}).

The PGI sodium salt and the methyl ester, as well as the PGI analogs, were synthesized according to Nicolaou et al. (11). The sodium salts were dissolved in phosphate buffer, while the PGI methyl ester and its analogs were dissolved in ethanol. Dilutions of stock solutions were made in phosphate buffer (pH 8.0). Appropriate controls were used for each type of vehicle. The data obtained were analyzed on a Univac computer system by a linear-regression program.

RESULTS

The sodium salt of PGI induced a dose-dependent decrease of BP with an ED_{25} of 0.23 μg/kg, i.v., a marked relaxation of BCA, and a strong inhibition

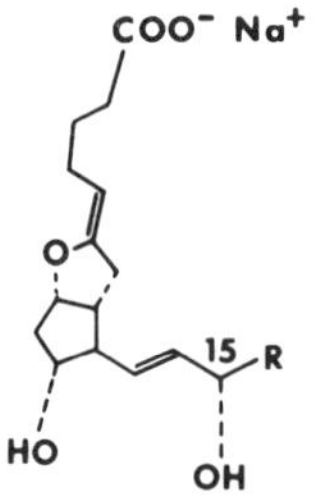

R	RAT BP ED_{25} [μg/kg i.v.]	RELAXATION OF BCA ED_{50} [ng/ml]	INHIBITION OF PA IC_{50} [M]
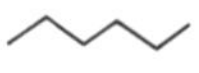	0.23	5.9	3×10^{-9}
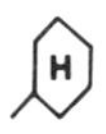	0.27	21.0	2×10^{-8}
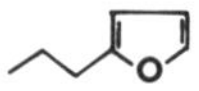	0.39	22.0	3×10^{-8}
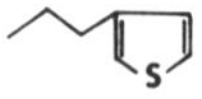	0.43	49.0	2×10^{-7}
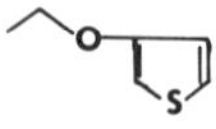	0.25	4.5	5×10^{-9}

FIG. 1. Biological effects of PGI sodium salt and its analogs with modified ω-side chains.

of PA with an IC_{50} of 3×10^{-9} M (Fig. 1). The PGI sodium salt in doses of
0.1, 0.3, and 1 μg/kg, i.v., induced a fall of mean arterial BP by 14, 27, and
45%, respectively. Substitution of the *n*-pentyl moiety of the sodium salt with
3-thienyloxymethyl or cyclohexyl resulted in analogs with comparable PGI vaso-

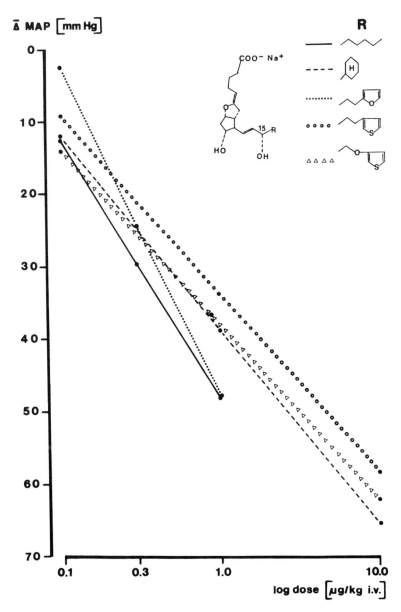

FIG. 2. Decrease of mean arterial blood pressure ($\bar{\Delta}$ MAP) by intravenous injection of PGI
sodium salt and analogs with modified ω-side chain in pentobarbital-anesthetized rats.

depressor activity; replacement by 2-(2-furyl)ethyl or 2-(3-thienyl)ethyl showed a slight diminished depressor activity, whereas substitution by 1,1-dimethyloxaalkyl was followed by a marked loss of activity, with an $ED_{25} > 10$ $\mu g/kg$ (Fig. 1). Regression lines relating the decrease in mean arterial BP to the dose of PGI sodium salt and analogs with modified ω-side chains demonstrate a good dose–response relationship for each analog (Fig. 2). The methyl ester of PGI also induced a decrease of BP with an ED_{25} of 0.55 $\mu g/kg$, i.v., a marked relaxation of BCA, and an inhibition of PA with an IC_{50} of 4×10^{-8} M. With respect to the analogs similar results were obtained as with analogs of the PGI sodium salt.

DISCUSSION

With respect to the broad spectrum of biological properties of PGI, an increasing body of evidence for possible therapeutic uses of its analogs emerges (12). These experiments have found that the potency estimates of the three independent test models used—rat BP, relaxation of BCA, and inhibition of PA—demonstrate that substitution of the *n*-pentyl moiety of the sodium salt or the methyl ester of PGI by cyclohexyl, 2-(2-furyl)ethyl, 2-(3-thienyl)ethyl, and especially 3-thienyloxymethyl resulted in analogs with comparable PGI activity, whereas 1,1-dimethyloxaalkyl and 2-cyclohexyl-1,1-dimethyl-2-oxaethyl residues were far less active. The order of potency among the analogs of the sodium salt and methyl ester of PGI was identical in all three test models used. The combined application of these three pharmacological methods, as well as similar pharmacological test combinations (8,9), seems to be a practical procedure of characterizing structurally modified PGI and identifying features of particular interest in structure–activity studies. Suitable modifications of the ω-side chain of PGI result in potent vasodilator and antiaggregatory agents.

REFERENCES

1. Armstrong, J. M., Lattimer, N., Moncada, S., and Vane, J. R. (1978): *Br. J. Pharmacol.,* 62:125–130.
2. Bartmann, W., Beck, G., and Lerch, U. (1974): *Tetrahedron Lett.,* 2441–2444.
3. Bartmann, W., Beck, G., Lerch, U., Teufel, H., and Schölkens, B. (1979): *Prostaglandins,* 17:301–311.
4. Born, G. V. R. (1968): *Nature,* 194:927–929.
5. Buendia, J., and Schalbar, J. (1977): *Tetrahedron Lett.,* 4499–4502.
6. Dusting, G. J., Moncada, S., and Vane, J. R. (1977): *Prostaglandins,* 13:3–15.
7. Fitzpatrick, T. M., Alter, I., Corey, E. J., Ramwell, P. W., Rose, I. C., and Kot, P. A. (1978): *Circ. Res.,* 42:192–194.
8. Gandolfi, C. A., and Gryglewski, R. J. (1978): *Pharmacol. Res. Commun.,* 10:885–896.
9. Gryglewski, R. J., and Nicolaou, K. C. (1978): *Experientia,* 34:1336–1338.
10. Moncada, S., Gryglewski, R. J., Bunting, S., and Vane, J. R. (1976): *Nature,* 263:663–665.
11. Nicolaou, K. C., Barnette, W. E., Gasic, G. P., Magolda, R. L., and Sipio, W. J. (1977): *J. Chem. Soc., Chem. Commun.,* 630–631.

12. Nicolaou, K. C., Gasic, G. P., and Barnette, W. E. (1978): *Angew. Chem., Int. Ed. Engl.,* 17:293–312.
13. Schölkens, B. A. (1978): *Prostaglandins Med.,* 1:359–372.
14. Szczeklik, A., Gryglewski, R. J., Nizankowski, R., Musial, J., Pieton, R., and Mruk, J. (1978): *Pharmacol. Res. Commun.,* 10:545–556.

Advances in Prostaglandin and Thromboxane Research,
Vol. 6, edited by B. Samuelsson, P. W. Ramwell,
and R. Paoletti. Raven Press, New York © 1980.

Pharmacological Evaluation of ONO 1206, a Prostaglandin E₁ Derivative, as Antianginal Agent

Toshimichi Tsuboi, Naonobu Hatano, Katsuyoshi Nakatsuji, Buichi Fujitani, Kouichi Yoshida, Masanao Shimizu, *Akiyoshi Kawasaki, *Moriyuki Sakata, and *Masami Tsuboshima

*Research Laboratories, Dainippon Pharmaceutical Co., Ltd., Enoki-cho, 33–94, Suita City, Osaka 564; and *Department of Pharmacology, Ono Pharmaceutical Co., Ltd., Mishima-gun, Osaka 618, Japan*

Angina pectoris is considered to be a state of imbalance between myocardial oxygen supply and demand that is often based on thrombotic and atherosclerotic lesions of the coronary artery. In this view, a compound having both an effect on coronary insufficiency and a suppressive effect on the thrombotic tendency seems to be valuable as an antianginal agent. We examined the effects of ONO 1206, 17-S-methyl-ω-homo-trans-Δ^2-prostaglandin E₁, on the cardiovascular system and platelet functions by oral administration in experimental animals.

METHODS

ST segment depression on an electrocardiogram (ECG) induced by vasopressin (0.2 IU/kg) in rats was performed by the method reported previously (4). Coronary blood flow was estimated by a flowmeter on a cannula bypassed from the coronary sinus to the external jugular vein. Resistance of the coronary vessel was estimated by the method of Winbury et al. (6). Platelet adhesiveness to a glass bead column was measured by the method reported previously (3). Platelet aggregation and bleeding time were measured by the methods of Born (2) and Arfores et al. (1), respectively. The intravenous infusion method using adenosine diphosphate (ADP) and collagen was reported previously (5).

RESULTS AND DISCUSSION

Cardiovascular System

As ST segment depression on ECG is commonly observed in patients with angina pectoris, ST segment depression induced by vasopressin in rats seems to be a suitable model of angina pectoris. ONO 1206 given per os (p.o.) at doses of more than 100 μg/kg showed the suppressive effect on ST segment depression induced by vasopressin in rats. The peak time of the effect was 0.5 to 1.0 hr after administration. Prostaglandin E_1 (PGE$_1$) showed a significant effect at the high dose of 10 mg/kg, p.o. Blood pressure of normotensive rats was decreased significantly, but temporarily, by ONO 1206 at 300 μg/kg, p.o. When ONO 1206 was injected in the coronary artery at doses from 1 to 100 ng/kg in anesthetized dogs, coronary blood flow increased markedly in a dose-related manner without any influence on heart rate, blood pressure, myocardial oxygen consumption, and redox potential. Resistance of the large coronary vessel of dogs decreased about 20% after intravenous injection at 1 and 3 μg/kg. The same effect was observed with nitroglycerin but not dipyridamole. Resistance of total coronary vessels also decreased about 30% at 1 and 3 μg/kg, and the effect lasted for more than 20 min, though the effect of nitroglycerin was temporary.

Platelet Function

ONO 1206 showed a significant inhibition of platelet adhesiveness to a glass bead column at 3 and 10 μg/kg, p.o., in guinea pigs and a peak inhibition time of 4 to 6 hr after administration. However, the inhibition disappeared at the higher doses of 30 and 100 μg/kg, p.o. This disappearance of the inhibition was not observed with *in vitro* experiments and in other *in vivo* methods testing platelet functions. PGE$_1$ showed a significant inhibition of platelet adhesiveness at the high dose of 10 mg/kg, p.o. Collagen-induced platelet aggregation in guinea pigs was inhibited in a dose-related manner at 30 to 300 μg/kg, p.o., 4 hr after administration, and ADP-induced aggregation was significantly inhibited at 300 μg/kg, p.o. Intravenous injection of ADP or collagen forms transient platelet aggregates in lung and other organs, and simultaneously causes a fall in the platelet count in circulating blood (5). This systemic injection of ADP or collagen seems to simulate the early thrombotic process. The fall of platelet count induced by ADP or collagen in guinea pigs was reversed 4 hr after 30 to 300 μg/kg, p.o., administration of ONO 1206. Bleeding time of the mesenteric artery in guinea pigs was prolonged 4 hr after ONO 1206 administration: primary bleeding time (time from cutting of artery to the first plug formation) was prolonged at doses of more than 30 μg/kg, p.o., and total bleeding time (total time of bleeding periods within 30 min after cutting of artery) was prolonged at doses more than 10 μg/kg, p.o.

Thus ONO 1206 seems to improve cardiac imbalance by its vasodilating action and to suppress thrombotic tendency by inhibiting platelet function.

REFERENCES

1. Arfores, K., and Bergquist, D. (1974): *Thromb. Res.*, 4:447–461.
2. Born, G. V. R. (1962): *Nature*, 194:927–929.

3. Fujitani, B., Tsuboi, T., Takeno, K., Yoshida, K., and Shimizu, M. (1976): *Thromb. Haemostas.,* 36:401–410.
4. Hatano, N., Nakatsuji, K., Nose, I., and Shimizu, M. (1977): *Folia Pharmacol. Jpn.,* 73:7p.
5. Tsuboi, T., Fujitani, B., Sasaki, J., Yoshida, K., and Shimizu, M. (1979): *Folia Pharmacol. Jpn.,* 75:17p.
6. Winbury, M. M., Howe, B. B., and Hefner, M. A. (1969): *J. Pharmacol. Exp. Ther.,* 168:70–95.

Advances in Prostaglandin and Thromboxane Research,
Vol. 6, edited by B. Samuelsson, P. W. Ramwell,
and R. Paoletti. Raven Press, New York © 1980.

The Influence of Sulprostone upon Platelet Function: *In Vitro* and *In Vivo* Studies

R. C. Briel and T. H. Lippert

Department of Obstetrics and Gynecology, 7400 Tübingen, W. Germany

Several investigators have demonstrated the influence of E prostaglandins, especially E_1 and E_2, on platelet function, whereas only a slight effect on blood coagulation and fibrinolysis has been found (1). This chapter deals with the effect of the new prostaglandin E_2 derivative sulprostone on platelet function both *in vivo* and *in vitro*.

MATERIALS AND METHODS

Sulprostone was given extraamniotically for induction of abortion (average dose 200 µg) in 10 patients, and intramuscularly (average dose 1,000 µg) in 6 patients, 3 for therapeutic abortion and 3 with missed abortion, in the 14th to 24th week of pregnancy. In the *in vitro* experiments, the blood was examined from 3 pregnant and from 4 nonpregnant women. ADP- and collagen-induced platelet aggregation were studied according to the method of Born and the spontaneous aggregation according to Breddin. Statistical evaluation was by the paired *t*-test.

RESULTS

One and 4 hr after extraamniotic sulprostone administration, the collagen-induced aggregation was enhanced to a small extent which was statistically significant; ADP-induced aggregation remained constant. The speed of aggregation showed a small increase, also statistically significant. The disaggregation phase did not show any change, nor did the spontaneous platelet aggregation (Table 1). When sulprostone was administered intramuscularly, similar results were obtained. The ADP- and collagen-induced platelet aggregation were only slightly increased and disaggregation was unchanged. The spontaneous platelet aggregation was not altered.

In the *in vitro* investigations, sulprostone produced an increasing effect on the spontaneous and induced aggregation which was concentration-dependent within the range of 0.005 to 0.5 µg/ml (Fig. 1).

TABLE 1. Parameters of platelet function (Born test) before and after administration of sulprostone—average values[a]

Route of administration / Number of patients	Time h	Maximal aggregation %			Speed of aggregation ctg$_{\alpha 1}$			Lag phase sec	Maximal disaggregation %		Speed of disaggregation ctg$_{\beta 1}$	
		2 μM ADP/ml	4 μM ADP/ml	20 μg Coll/ml	2 μM ADP/ml	4 μM ADP/ml	20 μg Coll/ml	20 μg Coll/ml	2 μM ADP/ml	4 μM ADP/ml	2 μM ADP/ml	4 μM ADP/ml
Extraamniotic 10	0	24	48	71	6.6	8.9	9.7	73	79	38	1.2	0.6
	1	22	49	77[a]	7.5[a]	9.7[a]	11.1[a]	69	78	45	1.6	0.8
	4	21	52	77[a]	7.2	9.7[a]	11.0[a]	69	78	36	1.6	0.5
	24	21	48	72	7.0	8.7	10.3	72	79	43	1.3	0.8
Intramuscular 6	0	45	54	80	8.2	10.1	12.1	79	48	42	1.4	0.6
	1	51[a]	70[a]	84	9.3[a]	10.6	12.1	71[a]	46	25	1.2	0.2
	24	38	62	75	7.8	9.8	11.0	75	50	26	1.1	0.2

[a] Significantly different from original values $p < 0.05$.

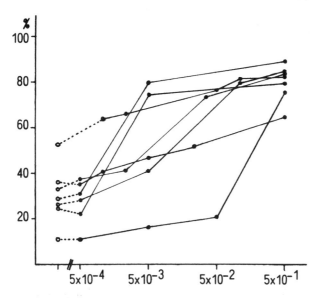

FIG. 1. ADP-induced platelet aggregation after addition of sulprostone and saline to platelet-rich plasma in seven cases. Ordinate: percentages of maximal aggregation. Abscissa: saline *(open circles)* and sulprostone concentrations in μg/ml *(full circles)*.

CONCLUSIONS

The present results demonstrate that the prostaglandin E_2 derivative sulprostone can enhance the aggregation of platelets *in vitro*. By extraamniotic and intramuscular administration, however, the changes are small. The slightly increased platelet aggregation may be partly due to the stress of labor and seems to be clinically unimportant. Blood coagulation and fibrinolysis were not altered significantly by sulprostone, as shown by other investigators (2,3). In summary, sulprostone appears to have no undesirable side effects regarding hemostasis when used for midtrimester abortion.

REFERENCES

1. Howie P. W. (1976): In: *Prostaglandins: Physiological, Pharmacological and Pathological Aspects,* edited by S. M. M. Karim, pp. 277–291. MTP Press, Lancaster, England.
2. Lechner K. (1978): In: International Sulprostone Symposium, Vienna. Pfizer, Inc., W. Germany. *(in press).*
3. Schander K., Budde U., and Bellmann, O. (1979): *Arch. Gynecol. (in press).*

Advances in Prostaglandin and Thromboxane Research,
Vol. 6, edited by B. Samuelsson, P. W. Ramwell,
and R. Paoletti. Raven Press, New York © 1980.

Synthesis and Biological Activity of 9-Deoxo-9-Methylene and Related Prostaglandins

G. L. Bundy, F. A. Kimball, A. Robert, J. W. Aiken,
K. M. Maxey, O. K. Sebek, N. A. Nelson, J. C. Sih, W. L. Miller,
and R. S. P. Hsi

The Upjohn Company, Kalamazoo, Michigan 49001

Prostaglandins (PGs) of the E type exhibit pharmacological profiles which suggest a number of potential clinical applications, e.g., as antifertility agents, gastric antisecretory agents, antithrombotic agents, antiasthma agents, and several others. However, the relative chemical instability of the β-hydroxyketone portion of the PGEs, with respect to dehydration to the PGAs and PGBs, has presented a continuing nuisance to the drug development of PGEs, particularly those which are not crystalline.

We describe the synthesis of a series of PG analogs in which the C-9 carbonyl group of several PGEs has been replaced by an exo-methylene group, thereby affording 9-deoxo-9-methylene-PGEs. Although a methylene group is less polar than the corresponding carbonyl group, the two functional groups require similar amounts of space as judged by molecular models. Furthermore, the sp_2 hybridization at C-9 in the exo-methylene analogs should provide the same flattening of the ring and constraint on side-chain conformation as that brought about by the carbonyl group of the PGEs. These 9-deoxo-9-methylene-PGEs constitute one of several possible solutions to the PGE stability problem, as they are chemically stable in aqueous media from pH 1 to 14. Most important, their biological properties are qualitatively very similar to those of the corresponding PGEs, and in some cases offer a significant improvement in biological specificity.

The novel 9-deoxo-9-methylene analogs described below and, in particular, 9-deoxo-16,16-dimethyl-9-methylene-PGE_2 have significant and useful activities for pregnancy termination. Clinical results to date suggest an important use both for termination of early pregnancy and for preoperative cervical dilatation in late first trimester abortion (2,3,4). 9-Deoxo-16,16-dimethyl-9-methylene-PGE_2, both by vaginal and oral administration, appears to be the best tolerated compound investigated thus far and is associated with a particularly low incidence of nausea and gastrointestinal side effects (2,3,4).

SYNTHESIS OF 9-DEOXO-9-METHYLENE-PGEs

The base instability of the PGEs renders several of the more common procedures for converting carbonyl groups to methylene groups inappropriate for

PG applications. For example, attempted Wittig olefination of PGE_2 methyl ester, 11,15-bis(trimethylsilyl ether), led only to mixtures of PGAs and PGBs. The necessary combination of increased nucleophilicity and decreased basicity was achieved in the anion of methylphenyl-N-methylsulfoximine, a reagent developed by Johnson et al. (8) for the methylenation of ketones. Addition of this reagent to PGE_2 methyl ester, 11,15-bis(trimethylsilyl ether), at $-78°C$ to avoid attack on the C-1 ester, afforded an intermediate β-hydroxysulfoximine mixture. Subsequent reductive elimination with aluminum amalgam in a mixture of acetic acid, water, and tetrahydrofuran (0°C, 30 min) then yielded the desired 9-deoxo-9-methylene-PGE_2 methyl ester.

Using the sulfoximine chemistry, or straightforward modifications thereof, the following 9-deoxo-9-methylene-PGEs were prepared from the corresponding C-9 ketones:

9-Deoxo-9-methylene-PGE_1 (**1**)

9-Deoxo-9-methylene-PGE_2 (**2**)

(15S)-9-Deoxo-15-methyl-9-methylene-PGE_2 (**3**)

9-Deoxo-9-methylene-16-phenoxy-17,18,19,20-tetranor-PGE_2 (**4**)

9-Deoxo-9-methylene-16-phenyl-17,18,19,20-tetranor-PGE_2 (**5**)

9-Deoxo-9-methylene-17-phenyl-18,19,20-trinor-PGE_2 (**6**)

9-Deoxo-16,16-dimethyl-9-methylene-PGE_2 (**7**)

9-Deoxo-16,16-dimethyl-9-methylene-cis-Δ^4-PGE_1 (**8**)

9-Deoxo-16,16-dimethyl-9-methylene-5-$trans$-PGE_2 (**9**)

9-Deoxo-16,16-dimethyl-9-methylene-PGE_1 (**10**)

9-Deoxo-16,16-dimethyl-9-methylene-$trans$-Δ^2-PGE_1 methyl ester (**11**)

9-Deoxo-16,16-dimethyl-9-methylene-PGE_2, N-methanesulfonamide (**12**)

In addition, in the case of **7**, several crystalline derivatives were synthesized by standard procedures to provide more easily handled solids and to offer a range of aqueous solubilities, e.g., the p-acetamidobenzamidophenyl ester (mp 195–197°C), the p-hydroxybenzaldehyde semicarbazone ester (mp 85–87°C), the sodium salt (mp 132–138°C), and the adamantanamine salt (mp 116–118°C).

Analogs **1** to **12** provide sufficient structural diversity to allow thorough biological evaluation of the 9-methylene modification, as they correspond to a number of metabolically stabilized PGs, several of which show clinical potential.

The preliminary biological screening results for 9-deoxo-9-methylene-PGE_1 and -PGE_2, summarized in Table 1, support the generalization that, qualitatively at least, the 9-deoxo-9-methylene analogs bear striking resemblance to their 9-keto congeners. Both 9-deoxo-9-methylene-PGE_1 and -PGE_2 are depressors of rat blood pressure and stimulators of gerbil colon. Both are weak antifertility agents in the hamster, and both are essentially equal to PGE_1 in their ability to inhibit human platelet aggregation. As summarized in Table 1, with the exception of the gastric antisecretory area, the two 9-methylene PGs (chemically stable entities) are apparently recognized by many biological systems as being PGE-like. Further demonstration that 9-methylene analogs can act as substitutes for their less stable 9-keto counterparts was provided by Fitzpatrick and Bundy

TABLE 1. *Biological activity of 9-deoxo-9-methylene-PGE$_1$ and -PGE$_2$*

Compound	Rat BP depressor (PGE$_1$ = 100)	Gerbil colon stimulation (PGE$_1$ = 100)	Hamster antifertility — No. nonpreg./no. treated	Dose (µg)	Human platelet aggreg. inhibition (rel. potency, PGE$_1$ = 1)	Primate uterine stimulation, i.v. (PGF$_{2\alpha}$ = 1)	15-PGDH substrate (PGE$_1$ = 100)	Rat gastric antisecretory (ED$_{50}$)	Rat gastric cytoprotection, p.o.
1	10–32	100–320	4/5 3/6	1,000 100	1	10	75–100	inactive (15 mg/kg)	100% (2 mg/kg)
PGE$_1$	100	100	6/6 0/6	200 100	1	10	75–100	2–5 mg/kg	100% (0.05 mg/kg)
2	10–32	320–1,000	6/6 0/6	1,000 100	1	10	> 100	inactive (15 mg/kg)	100% (2 mg/kg)
PGE$_2$	32–100	100–320	6/6 1/8	250 125	biphasic	10	> 100	2–5 mg/kg	81% (0.1 mg/kg) 65% (0.05 mg/kg)

TABLE 2. Biological activity of 9-deoxo-16,16-dimethyl-9-methylene-PGE analogs

Compound	Primate uterine stimulation, i.v. ($PGF_{2\alpha} = 1$)	Rat enteropooling, p.o. (ED_{50}, mg/kg)	Hamster antifertility		Gerbil colon stimulation ($PGE_1 = 100$)
			No. nonpreg./ no. treated	Dose (μg)	
7	100–150	0.15	6/6 3/6	1,000 50	109 (64–196)
8	100–150	0.15	toxic 2/6	1,000 50	212 (72–420)
9	75	0.6	1/6	1,000	223 (162–293)
10	50–80	0.09	1/5	1,000	102 (74–142)
18	5	0.4	5/6 0/6	1,000 30	257 (201–324)
19	10	0.1	1/6	1,000	103 (73–147)
23	100	0.01	toxic 4/6	1,000 30	140 (71–392)
11	10	0.12	4/6	1,000	6 (2–13)
12	20	1.2	1/6	1,000	112 (68–196)
34	100–150	0.0005	6/8 3/8	15 12	446 (168–765)

(6), who demonstrated that specific, high-affinity rabbit antibodies to 9-deoxo-9-methylene-PGE_2 cross-reacted quantitatively with PGE_2 itself and made possible the development of a useful PGE_2 radioimmunoassay procedure.

All of the 9-deoxo-9-methylene analogs **1** to **12** possessed biological activities reminiscent of the corresponding C-9 ketones. However, 9-deoxo-16,16-dimethyl-9-methylene-PGE_2 (**7**) and its crystalline derivatives exhibited particularly attractive biological profiles for fertility control agents (9,10). 9-Deoxo-16,16-dimethyl-9-methylene-PGE_2 was equipotent with 16,16-dimethyl-PGE_2 as a uterine stimulant (i.v., monkey), while being 300 times less enteropooling in rats (a measure of diarrhea potential) (Table 2). Additionally, Rhesus monkey core temperature measurements indicated that **7** was about 300 times less thermogenic than 16,16-dimethyl-PGE_2.

SYNTHESIS OF 9-DEOXO-9,16,16-TRIMETHYL- AND 9-DEOXO-16,16-DIMETHYL-PGE_2

In order to assess the importance of C-9 stereochemistry to the desired selective biological activity, the 9-deoxo-9α-methyl and 9-deoxo-9β-methyl analogs **18** and **19** were synthesized as outlined in Fig. 1. 16,16-Dimethyl lactone **13** (12) was reduced with lithium aluminum hydride, selectively silylated (5) on the primary hydroxyl, oxidized to the C-9 ketone **14** (Collins reagent), and converted to 9-deoxo-9-methylene intermediate **15** with sulfoximine chemistry (8). Hydroboration–oxidation of **15** yielded 9α-hydroxymethyl derivative **15a**, which was in turn transformed into the corresponding 9α-methyl intermediate (1. MsCl; 2. LiAlH$_4$) and, then following standard procedures, into 9-deoxo-9α-methyl analog **18**. The 9β-methyl **19** was obtained by oxidation of alcohol **15a** to aldehyde **16**, equilibration to the more stable 9β-aldehyde **17** (1,5-diazabicycloundecene, CH$_2$Cl$_2$), reduction to the 9β-methyl intermediate (1. NaBH$_4$; 2. MsCl; 3. LiAlH$_4$), and elaboration of carboxyl side chain (1. Bu$_4$NF; 2. Collins; 3. Wittig; 4. tetrahydropyranyl ether (THP) hydrolysis).

9-Deoxo-16,16-dimethyl-PGE_2 (**23**) was synthesized (Fig. 2) from 16,16-dimethyl-$PGF_2\alpha$, methyl ester, 11,15-bis(tetrahydropyranyl ether) **20** by conversion to 9β-bromide **22** (1. MsCl; 2. LiBr/HMPA), hydrolysis of the blocking groups, and reduction of the bromide with the ethylenediamine complex of chromous perchlorate (11).

BIOLOGY

Preliminary biological test results for 9-deoxo-16,16-dimethyl-9-methylene-PGE_2 **7** and closely related compounds **8** to **12**, **18**, **19**, and **23** are summarized in Table 2 (16,16-dimethyl-PGE_2 **34** is included for comparison purposes). In the pentobarbital-anesthetized, pentolinium-treated rat, **7** produced small and inconsistent pressor, depressor, or biphasic responses in the dose range of 0.01 to nearly 1.0 μg/kg. These responses were more like those produced by low

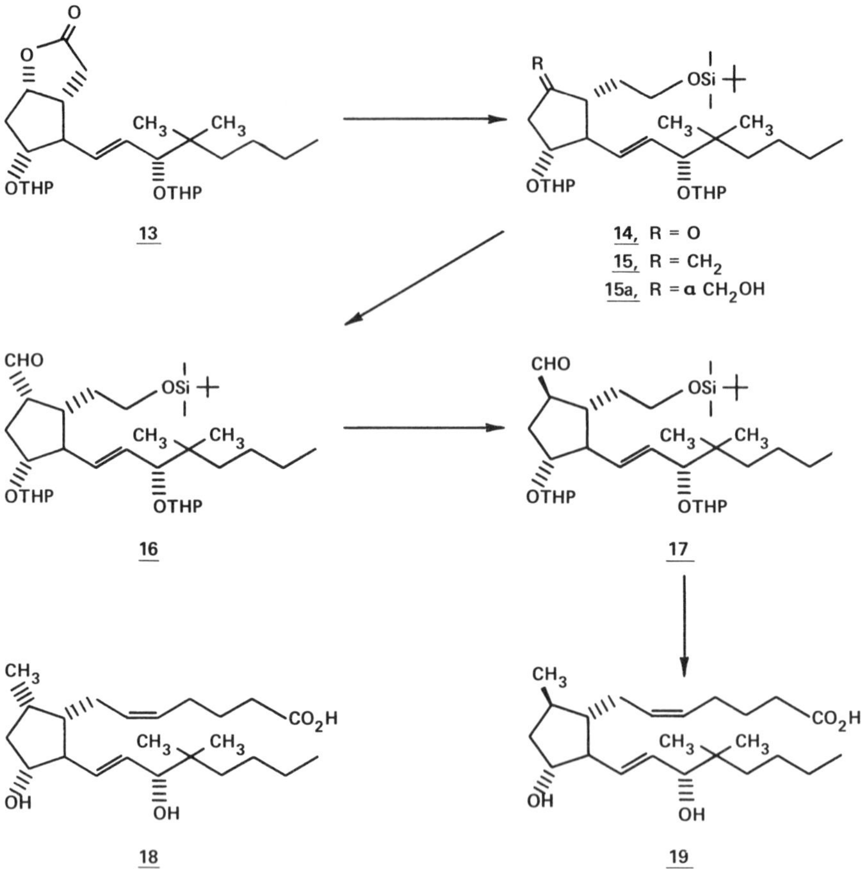

FIG. 1. Synthesis of 9-deoxo-9,16,16-trimethyl PGE$_2$.

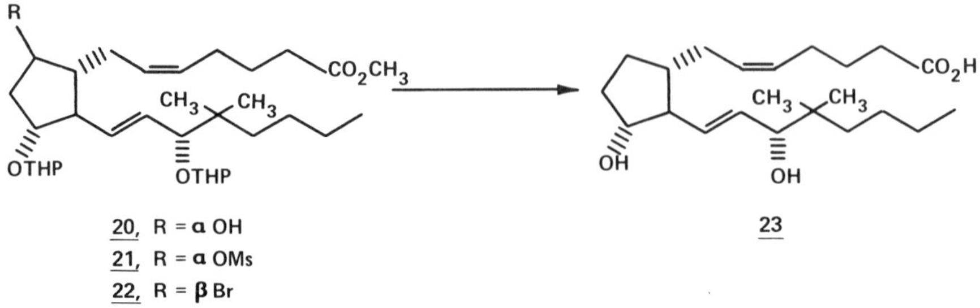

13

14, R = O
15, R = CH$_2$
15a, R = α CH$_2$OH

16

17

18

19

20, R = α OH
21, R = α OMs
22, R = β Br

23

FIG. 2. Synthesis of 9-deoxo-16,16-dimethyl PGE$_2$.

doses of PGF$_2\alpha$ (approximately 1 μg/kg) than like those produced by PGE$_1$. At 1 μg/kg and above, **7** was only depressor and was equipotent to PGE$_1$ in this activity. At higher doses, 100 μg/kg and above, tachyphylaxis was observed, which extended to both PGE$_1$ and PGF$_2\alpha$. Although several of the analogs in Table 2 are, like **7**, potent uterine stimulants (e.g., **8, 10, 23**), most are appreciably more enteropooling than analog **7**.

SYNTHESIS OF METABOLITES AND LABELED 7

3,3,4,4-Tetradeutero-9-deoxo-16,16-dimethyl-9-methylene-PGE$_2$, needed for development of a gas liquid chromatography–mass spectroscopy assay (1,7) for **7**, was obtained by conversion of the 9-methylene intermediate **15** into the corresponding C-6 aldehyde (1. Bu$_4$NF; 2. Collins), Wittig reaction with the appropriate tetradeuterated carboxybutylphosphorane (7) and deprotection of the hydroxyls.

Introduction of tritium into the metabolically stable C-11 position of **7** required a slightly more circuitous route (Fig. 3). The most polar of the sulfoximine adducts of 16,16-dimethyl-PGE$_2$ methyl ester, 11,15-bis(tetrahydropyranyl ether) (**24**), was deprotected, and then selectively silylated, affording diol **26** in high yield. A three-step sequence (1. dihydropyran; 2. Bu$_4$NF; 3. Jones reagent) gave ketone **27**, which on sodium borotritide reduction, aluminum amalgam reduction, and THP hydrolysis yielded [11β-^{3}H]**28** in high yield and purity. The reduction of ketone **27** gave a 11α-OH/11β-OH ratio of 10:1 with sodium

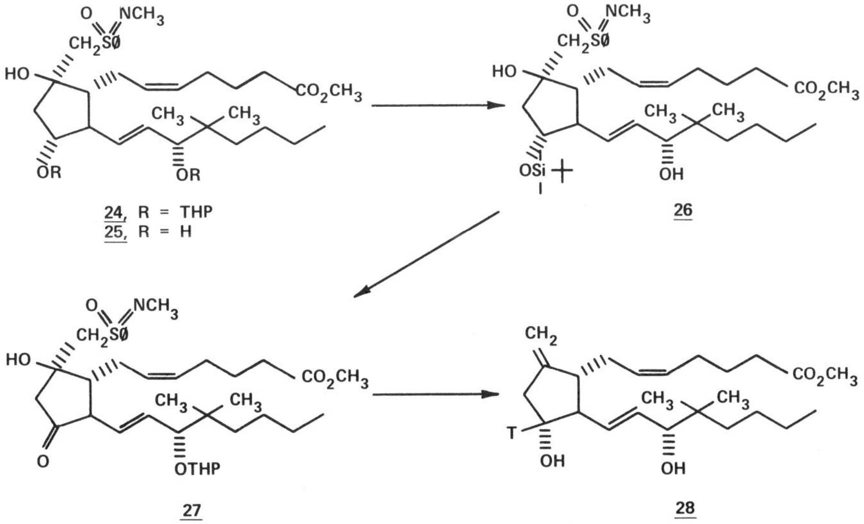

FIG. 3. Synthesis of tritium-labeled 9-deoxo-16,16-dimethyl-9-methylene PGE$_2$.

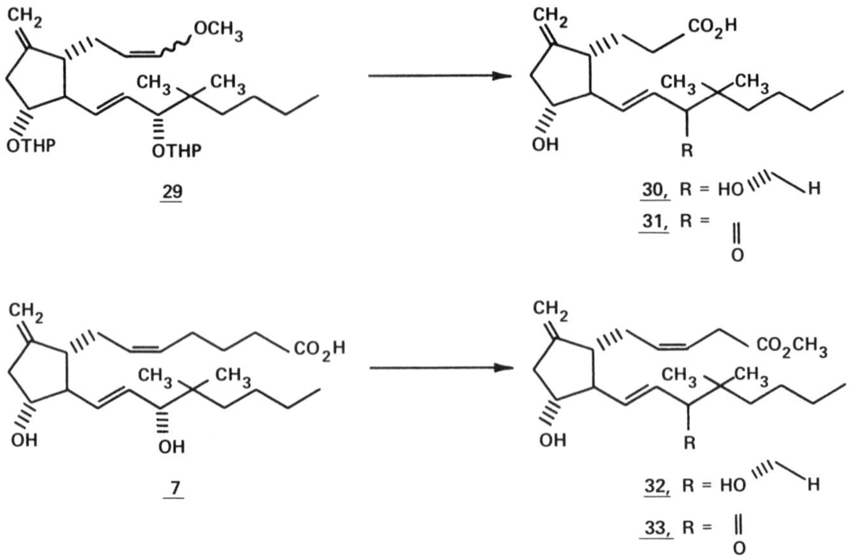

FIG. 4. Synthesis of metabolites of 9-deoxo-16,16-dimethyl-9-methylene PGE$_2$.

borohydride and about 4:1 with sodium borotritide. The specific activity of **28** was 6.16 mCi/mg.

Several metabolites of 9-deoxo-16,16-dimethyl-9-methylene-PGE$_2$ (14) were synthesized (Fig. 4). Treatment of the C-6 aldehyde (from **15**) with methoxymethylenetriphenylphosphorane yielded enol ether **29**, which on oxidation with pyridinium chlorochromate (13) followed by hydrolysis gave tetranor analog **30**. Low-temperature Jones oxidation afforded the corresponding 15-ketone **31**. The dinor metabolite **32** was obtained directly from **7** by microbiological β-oxidation with *Mycobacterium rhodochrous,* while the dinor 15-ketone **33** was, as above, the sole product of low-temperature Jones oxidation of **32**. (The 15-ketone corresponding to **7** was prepared in the same manner.)

The metabolites **30** to **33** and 15-keto-**7** all exhibited greatly diminished biological activity in the rat blood pressure, gerbil colon, and primate uterine stimulation assays (all < 1% of **7**).

SUMMARY

A number of PGE analogs have been synthesized in which the C-9 carbonyl group has been replaced by an exo-methylene group. These chemically stable 9-deoxo-9-methylene-PGEs exhibit biological profiles very similar to their less stable PGE relatives. 9-Deoxo-16,16-dimethyl-9-methylene-PGE$_2$ (7) retains the useful uterine-stimulating potency of 16,16-dimethyl-PGE$_2$ but is approximately 300 times less enteropooling in the rat. In preliminary clinical trials, **7** has shown efficacy for pregnancy termination by the oral and vaginal routes of administration, as well as relative freedom from gastrointestinal side effects.

ACKNOWLEDGMENTS

The authors gratefully acknowledge the skilled technical assistance of J. M. Baldwin, A. D. Forbes, M. J. Sutton, N. J. Crittenden, and V. R. Bockstanz. The authors also appreciate the efforts of E. E. Nishizawa in determining the effects of **1** and **2** on human platelets. In addition, we acknowledge the Prostaglandin Screening Laboratory of The Upjohn Company, under the direction of C. F. Lawson, for the preliminary gerbil colon and rat blood pressure results.

REFERENCES

1. Axen, U., Green, K., Horlin, D., and Samuelsson, B. (1971): *Biochem. Biophys. Res. Commun.,* 45:519–525.
2. Bergstrom, S. (1979): Presented at the *Fourth International Prostaglandin Conference,* Washington, D.C.
3. Bygdeman, M. (1979): *(this volume).*
4. Bygdeman, M., Green, K., Bergstrom, S., Bundy, G., and Kimball, F. A. (1979): *Lancet,* 1135.
5. Corey, E. J., and Venkateswarlu, A. (1972): *J. Am. Chem. Soc.,* 94:6190–6191.
6. Fitzpatrick, F. A., and Bundy, G. L. (1978): *Proc. Natl. Acad. Sci. USA,* 75:2689–2693.
7. Green, K., Granstrom, E., Samuelsson, B. and Axen, U. (1973): *Anal. Biochem.,* 54:434–453.
8. Johnson, C. R., Shanklin, J. R., and Kirchoff, R. A. (1973): *J. Am. Chem. Soc.,* 95:6462–6463.
9. Kimball, F. A. (1979): Presented at the *Fourth International Prostaglandin Conference,* Washington, D.C.
10. Kimball, F. A., Bundy, G. L., Robert, A., and Weeks, J. R. (1979): *Prostaglandins,* 17:657–666.
11. Kochi, J. K., and Singleton, D. M. (1968): *J. Org. Chem.,* 33:1027–1034.
12. Magerlein, B. J., Ducharme, D. W., Magee, W. E., Miller, W. L., Robert, A., and Weeks, J. R. (1973): *Prostaglandins,* 4:143–145.
13. Piancatelli, G., Scettri, A., and D.'Auria, M. (1977): *Tetrahedron Lett.,* 3483–3484.
14. Wickrema Sinha, A. J. (1979): Presented at the *Fourth International Prostaglandin Conference,* Washington, D.C.

Advances in Prostaglandin and Thromboxane Research,
Vol. 6, edited by B. Samuelsson, P. W. Ramwell,
and R. Paoletti. Raven Press, New York © 1980.

Comparative Luteolytic Effects of Prostaglandin $F_{2\alpha}$ and Its 13-Dehydro Analogs *In Vivo*

J. A. McCracken, M. E. Glew, S. S. Hull, Jr., L. Bovaird,
L. Underwood, and J. Fried

*Worcester Foundation for Experimental Biology, Shrewsbury, Massachusetts 01545; and
Department of Chemistry, University of Chicago, Chicago, Illinois 60637*

Prostaglandin (PG) $F_{2\alpha}$ was identified in the sheep as a uterine luteolytic hormone in 1972 (45), and evidence is accumulating that $PGF_{2\alpha}$ performs a similar physiologic function in several mammalian species including the guinea pig (53), the pig (14,19), the cow (33,48), and probably other species (27). However, in primates it seems clear that PGs of uterine origin are not essential for luteolysis. For example, hysterectomy is without effect on the life-span of the CL in women (4) and in monkeys (8). In addition, the primary metabolite of $PGF_{2\alpha}$ (15-keto-13:14-dihydro-$PGF_{2\alpha}$) is not elevated in the peripheral blood of women at the time of CL regression, as is observed in other species such as the sheep and cow (34,50). The possibility that luteolysis in the primate might be controlled by PGs generated locally within the ovary has been suggested by several authors (23,42,52). However, there is some disagreement as to whether $PGF_{2\alpha}$ levels rise in the human CL at the time of luteolysis (9,58,61). In any case, the extra luteal tissues of the ovary of the primate could be a significant source of PGs. In support of this possibility, it has recently been reported that estrogen treatment of cyclic female monkeys causes an increase in $PGF_{2\alpha}$ concentration in blood draining the ovary (2). Furthermore, the luteolytic effect of estrogen in monkeys is prevented by the administration of indomethacin (3).

Numerous attempts have been made to demonstrate a luteolytic effect of natural and synthetic PGs in both female monkeys and women. While there is good evidence that various PGs are luteolytic in monkeys (36,56,57), the evidence in the human female is less convincing (1,24,30,37,38). This may be due to the small amount of PG actually reaching the ovary as a result of rapid clearance by the PG-15-OH-dehydrogenase in lung (51) or perhaps to a relative lack of PG receptors in human luteal cells (52). In women, several PG analogs have been administered in an attempt to prolong the biologic activity of these substances. In many cases, the inherent smooth muscle activity of these analogs is also preserved, thus enhancing the powerful uterotonic action of some of these compounds. This latter property has been used by several research groups to effect the early termination of pregnancy in women (6,31,35,39,49,62). However, it is not yet clear whether this approach will be acceptable for routine clinical use in view of the side effects such as diarrhea and hypertension which are often associated with the use of this type of compound. In some cases, these compounds can produce uterine contractions which are so severe that uterine rupture has occurred during the first trimester of pregnancy (29).

The luteolytic 16-aryloxy derivatives of $PGF_{2\alpha}$ have been used with some success in domestic animals (5,10). However, in recent trials with this analog in monkeys (13,56) and women (11), side effects reached unacceptable levels. More recently, $PGF_{2\alpha}$ 1-15 lactone administered to cycling and early pregnant rhesus monkeys (60) appeared to cause a reduction in progesterone levels in both cases. However, there was evidence that smooth muscle activity was also potentiated in the case of this analog. Since it had been postulated that $PGF_{2\alpha}$ caused luteolysis by an effect on the vascular smooth muscle of the ovary or corpus luteum, it was not at all clear whether analogs with reduced smooth muscle activity would still cause luteolysis. However, we have shown that at the onset of $PGF_{2\alpha}$-induced luteolysis in the sheep, there is no change either in total blood flow through the ovary (41,43) or in capillary blood flow through the corpus luteum (46). However, 24 to 48 hr after functional luteolysis induced by $PGF_{2\alpha}$, total blood flow through the ovary eventually declines, presumably due to structural changes occurring within the corpus luteum. This eventual decline in blood flow through the ovary is also observed after naturally occurring luteolysis in the sheep (40).

Our own approach to the search for PG analogs with antifertility potential has been to selectively remove the smooth-muscle-stimulating properties of the molecule while still retaining luteolytic activity. We have been able to achieve this objective and have previously reported on the luteolytic activity of the 13-dehydro analogs of $PGF_{2\alpha}$ in both sheep and monkeys (16,46,47). This chapter summarizes these previous findings and also describes new results with these compounds in the early pregnant monkey model *(M. fascicularis)*.

RESULTS

Studies with Luteolytic 13-Dehydro PGs in Sheep

Attempts to control CL function in normal cycling sheep with the endogenous luteolysin $PGF_{2\alpha}$ produced somewhat variable results. It was observed that following the subcutaneous or intravaginal administration of 5 to 25 mg of $PGF_{2\alpha}$, only about ⅔ of these animals showed evidence of luteolysis (44). This was explained by the finding that after giving the above amounts of $PGF_{2\alpha}$, plasma levels of $PGF_{2\alpha}$ were elevated for less than 2 hr. This indicates that the sheep, like other species, appears to have a remarkable capacity to clear $PGF_{2\alpha}$ from the bloodstream. Because smooth muscle side effects were seen in these animals, it seemed logical to seek analogs that would have reduced smooth muscle activity but which would retain their luteolytic properties. Ideally, these analogs would also be resistant to metabolism by the PG-15-OH-dehydroge-nase which would prolong their biologic activity.

The first synthetic PGs which we examined were the 7-oxa-analogs of $PGF_{1\alpha}$ (18) in terms of luteolysis in the sheep ovarian autotransplant preparation. The latter model system (20,41) permits the determination of either direct luteolytic potency or resistance to metabolism *in vivo* by infusing the analogs respectively into either the arterial supply of the ovary or into the systemic circulation (i.v.). It was found that the replacement of the carbon atom in position 7 by an oxygen atom markedly diminished the luteolytic properties of these analogs compared to the parent compound, $PGF_{1\alpha}$ (7). We examined subsequently a number of acetylenic (13-dehydro) analogs of $PGF_{2\alpha}$ (17) examples of which are shown in Fig. 1. Several of the 13-dehydro analogs had luteolytic activity equal to or in some cases greater than the parent compound $PGF_{2\alpha}$ (16,46). The 16-fluoro derivative of 13-dehydro-$PGF_{2\alpha}$ was particularly potent in this respect, being about five times as luteolytic as $PGF_{2\alpha}$ in the ovarian transplant model when given intraarterially and 100 times when given i.v. The insertion of a fluorine atom in position 16—i.e., on the carbon α to the 15-hydroxyl group in the PG molecule (16)—was a direct analogy to previous work carried out with steroids (15) where the introduction of a halogen atom next to a hydroxyl group necessary for biologic activity resulted in a marked increase

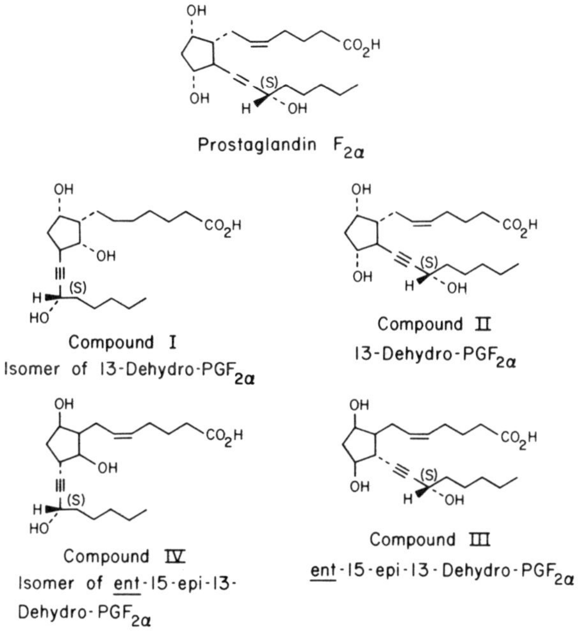

Prostaglandin $F_{2\alpha}$

Compound I
Isomer of 13-Dehydro-$PGF_{2\alpha}$

Compound II
13-Dehydro-$PGF_{2\alpha}$

Compound IV
Isomer of ent-15-epi-13-Dehydro-$PGF_{2\alpha}$

Compound III
ent-15-epi-13-Dehydro-$PGF_{2\alpha}$

FIG. 1. Examples of 13-dehydro (acetylenic) PG analogs. Further modifications included the addition of a fluorine atom in position 16 in compounds II and III.

TABLE 1. *Summary of luteolytic and smooth muscle activities of 13-dehydro analogs relative to PGF$_{2\alpha}$-sheep: Intraarterial administration* in vivo, *ovary and uterus*

	Potency (PGF$_{2\alpha}$ = 1)	
	Luteolysis	Smooth muscle
13-Dehydro-PGF$_{2\alpha}$	1.0	0.4
Ent-15-epi-13-dehydro-PGF$_{2\alpha}$	0.5	0.01
16-Fluoro-13-dehydro-PGF$_{2\alpha}$ (erythro)	5.0	0.2
16-Fluoro-13-dehydro-PGF$_{2\alpha}$ (threo)	0.25	0.2–0.4
Ent-15-epi-16-fluoro-13-dehydro-PGF$_{2\alpha}$ (erythro)	0.1	0.002

TABLE 2. *Comparative luteolytic effect in sheep with autotransplanted ovaries of PGF$_{2\alpha}$ and its 13-dehydro analogs: lowest effective dose given intraarterially into the ovary and the highest dose to date given systemically (i.v.)*

Dose/hr/6 hr (μg)	Route	% Decrease in progesterone secretion	Change in blood flow (↑↓)
PGF$_{2\alpha}$			
2.5 μg	i.a.	>95%	None
500.0 μg	i.v.	~25%	None
13-Dehydro-PGF$_{2\alpha}$			
2.5 μg	i.a.	>90%	None
50.0 μg	i.v.	~30%	None
Ent-15-epi-13-dehydro-PGF$_{2\alpha}$			
10.0 μg	i.a.	>90%	None
50.0 μg	i.v.	~30%	None
16-Fluoro-13-dehydro PGF$_{2\alpha}$ (erythro, mixture of 15,16 epimers)			
1.0 μg	i.a.	>80%[a]	None
25.0 μg	i.v.	>95%	None
16-Fluoro-13-dehydro-PGF$_{2\alpha}$ (threo, mixture of 15,16 epimers)			
10.0 μg	i.a.	>95%	None
50.0 μg	i.v.	~15%	None
Ent-15-epi-16-fluoro-13-dehydro-PGF$_{2\alpha}$ (erythro)			
40.0 μg	i.a.	>90%	None
300.0 μg	i.v.	>95%[b]	None

[a] Progesterone secretion was completely suppressed after 14 hr but rebounded to control values by 24 hr.

[b] Progesterone secretion was completely suppressed after 12 hr but rebounded to control values by 44 hr.

in potency of the steroid. The relative luteolytic activity of tne acetylenic analogs of $PGF_{2\alpha}$ is shown in Tables 1 and 2. All of these analogs also showed marked resistance to the PG-15-OH-dehydrogenase when infused intravenously, which is in agreement with previous findings *in vitro* (28). In the case of 16-fluoro-13-dehydro-$PGF_{2\alpha}$, the resistance to metabolism was very pronounced. It can be seen from Table 2 that as little as 25 μg (12.5 μg active epimer) of this analog infused i.v. caused complete luteal regression, whereas even 500 μg of the parent compound did not achieve this effect. Thus, by the systemic route 16-fluoro-13-dehydro-$PGF_{2\alpha}$ is about 100 times more active than the parent compound, $PGF_{2\alpha}$. We attribute this enhanced activity in part to the increased luteolytic potency of the molecule per se and in part to an increased resistance to metabolism in the circulation. Selected examples of the luteolytic effect of these analogs are shown in Figs. 2 and 3. With the *ent*-15-epi-16-fluoro-13-

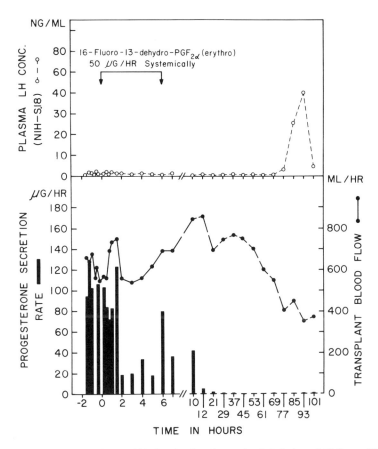

FIG. 2. Progesterone secretion and LH levels after the systemic infusion of 16-fluoro-13-dehydro-$PGE_{2\alpha}$ (mixture of 15,16 epimers, erythro) at 50 μg/hr for 6 hr in the ovarian transplanted sheep (from ref. 47).

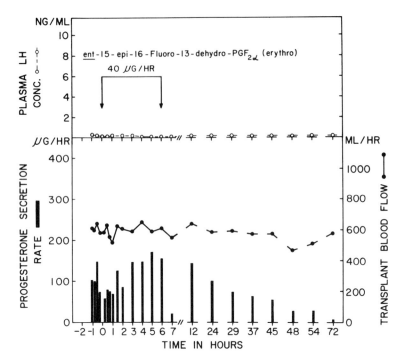

FIG. 3. Progesterone secretion and LH levels after the intraarterial infusion of *ent*-15-epi-16-fluoro-13-dehydro-PGF$_{2\alpha}$ (erythro) at 40 μg/hr for 6 hr into the ovarian transplant in the sheep (from ref. 47).

dehydro-PGF$_{2\alpha}$ analog, the fall in progesterone secretion occurred very slowly, a finding for which we as yet have no explanation.

Smooth muscle activity of the 13-dehydro-analogs was examined *in vivo* by infusing them into the arterial supply of the sheep uterus *in situ* on day 3 of the cycle using a method described previously (54). The results of these experiments are summarized in Table 1. An example of the smooth muscle activity of *ent*-15-epi-16-fluoro-13-dehydro-PGF$_{2\alpha}$ (erythro) is shown in Fig. 4. The fact that the 13-dehydro analogs show a diminished or complete absence of smooth muscle activity but are still luteolytic is compatible with our findings that PGF$_{2\alpha}$ does not initiate luteolysis via a vascular smooth muscle effect on the capillary bed of the CL (46). Furthermore, these results suggest that the receptors governing the luteolytic effect on the one hand, and the smooth muscle effect on the other, may possess different structural specificities.

Studies with 13-Dehydro Analogs in a Primate Model *(Macaca fascicularis)*

To determine the direct luteolytic effect of PGF$_{2\alpha}$ and its 13-dehydro analogs, a technique was devised to infuse these substances directly into the hilus of

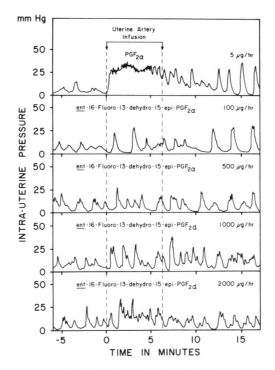

FIG. 4. Comparative effect of PGE$_{2\alpha}$ and *ent*-15-epi-16-fluoro-13-dehydro-PGF$_{2\alpha}$ (erythro) on uterine smooth muscle activity *in vivo* in the sheep (from ref. 47).

the ovary (46). Results using this technique are shown in Fig. 5 where it can be seen that both PGF$_{2\alpha}$ and its 13-dehydro analog at 5 μg/hr for 6 hr caused a fall in peripheral plasma progesterone concentration during the mid-luteal phase of the cycle. Control infusions of vehicle alone were without any immediate effect. It was also found that the 13-dehydro analog was active when given i.v. (100 μg/kg/hr for 6 hr), subcutaneously (1 mg/kg), or orally (2 mg/kg), again given during the mid-luteal phase (46). The steroid levels which we observed in the monkey model used *(Macaca fascicularis)* were comparable to those previously reported for this species (21).

The *ent*-15-epi-13-dehydro-PGF$_{2\alpha}$ analog also appeared to possess luteolytic activity during the mid-luteal phase of the cycle, but higher doses were required to effect luteolysis (46). The dose levels required were: i.v., 250 μg/kg/hr/6 hr; s.c., 1–2 mg/kg; and orally 3–4 mg/kg. The 16-fluoro derivative of 13-dehydro-PGF$_{2\alpha}$ was found to be the most active compound in the monkey model. The results are shown in Table 3 where it can be seen that the dose required by the various routes is less than with the other analogs listed above. This increase in potency of the 16-fluoro analog over its nonfluorinated counterpart is shown graphically in Fig. 6 where the 16-fluoro results are directly

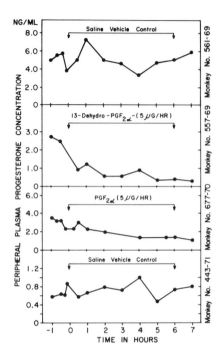

FIG. 5. Peripheral plasma progesterone levels in female monkeys (*Macaca fascicularis*) during the mid-luteal phase following the intraovarian infusion of 13-dehydro-PGF$_{2\alpha}$ or PGF$_{2\alpha}$, both at 5 µg/hr for 6 hr. (from ref. 47).

compared with PGF$_{2\alpha}$ and 13-dehydro-PGF$_{2\alpha}$, each given orally at a dose of 1 mg/kg. Experiments with the *ent*-15-epi-16-fluoro-13-dehydro compound are not yet complete, but preliminary results indicate that the potency of this analog is similar to its nonfluorinated equivalent. The administration of saline controls by these same routes was usually without any immediate effect on progesterone levels, although shortening of the cycle was observed in a few animals perhaps due to stress (63) or perhaps to a spontaneous short luteal phase (65).

Initial experiments in the monkey to determine the uterine smooth muscle effects *in vivo* of PGF$_{2\alpha}$ and its 13-dehydro analogs, using a similar approach to that described for the sheep, were unsuccessful because acute insertion of a

TABLE 3. *Summary of luteolytic effect of 16-fluoro-13-dehydro-PGF$_{2\alpha}$ in the monkey (Macaca fascicularis) during the mid-luteal phase of the cycle (day 21 to 22)*

Route	Dose	Luteolysis
I.O. Infusion	2.5 µg/hr/6 hr	Negative
Systemic infusion	50 µg/kg/hr/6 hr	Incomplete (65%)
	100 µg/kg/hr/6 hr	Incomplete (85%)
	150 µg/kg/hr/6 hr	Complete
	200 µg/kg/hr/6 hr	Complete
S.C. Injection	1.0 mg/kg	Positive
Per os	1.0 mg/kg	Positive
	2.0 mg/kg	Positive

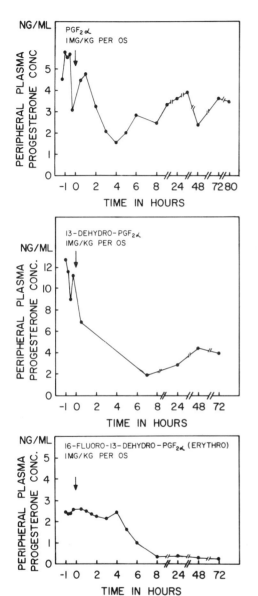

FIG. 6. Comparison of effect on peripheral plasma progesterone of $PGF_{2\alpha}$, 13-dehydro-$PGF_{2\alpha}$, and 16-fluoro-13-dehydro-$PGF_{2\alpha}$, each given orally at 1 mg/kg on day 21 to three different monkeys. (From ref. 47).

saline-filled balloon into the uterine lumen caused severe uterine hypertonus lasting many hours. The method described previously by Spilman and co-workers (32,59), which consisted of a small saline-filled silastic balloon chronically implanted in the myometrium, was used to determine smooth muscle activity *in vivo* in the primate model. The details of our use of this technique have been reported elsewhere (46). The results are summarized in Table 4. When the

TABLE 4. *Comparative effects of PGF$_{2\alpha}$ and its 13-dehydro analogs*
on uterine smooth muscle activity in vitro *in the primate*
(Macaca fascicularis)

Compound	Potency (PGF$_{2\alpha}$ = 1)
13-Dehydro-PGF$_{2\alpha}$	0.2
Ent-15-epi-13-dehydro-PGF$_{2\alpha}$	0.01
16-Fluoro-13-dehydro-PGF$_{2\alpha}$ (erythro)	0.5
16-Fluoro-13-dehydro-PGF$_{2\alpha}$ (threo)	0.25
Ent-15-epi-16-fluoro-13-dehydro-PGF$_{2\alpha}$ (erythro)	0.02

standard dose of PGF$_{2\alpha}$ was increased to 100 μg given as a single injection i.v., emesis or wretching was evoked in the test monkey, while doses of the analog, in some cases as high as 2,000 μg i.v., were without noticeable effect. These experiments performed with the 13-dehydro analogs in the monkey *in vivo* appear to closely parallel the results previously obtained in the sheep in terms of smooth muscle and luteolytic activity.

More recently, we have administered several of the 13-dehydro analogs to monkeys during early pregnancy (days 31 to 36 of the cycle during which the monkey conceived). Pregnancy was determined by the tube test for monkey urinary chorionic gonadotropin (26) which shows a positive result from about day 32 onwards. The conception rate based on controlled matings was surprisingly low. The results of our efforts to obtain early dated pregnancies are shown in Table 5, where it can be seen that only about 25% of the monkeys conceived following a 4-day exposure to a male at mid-cycle. This figure is remarkably close to a study in women where only 25% of 104 women who cohabitated at the expected time of ovulation actually conceived (55).

Our preliminary studies with the 13-dehydro analogs in early pregnant monkeys (days 31 to 36 of the pregnancy cycle) are shown in Table 6 (see also Fig. 7), where it can be seen that in the case of 13-dehydro-PGF$_{2\alpha}$, there was no effect on peripheral plasma progesterone in spite of the previous finding that this compound was active in the cyclic monkey. It therefore appears that

TABLE 5. *Conception rate in the monkey colony*
during the period January 1, 1978
to January 31, 1979

63 Monkeys mated in this period
12 Pregnancies
75% Ovulation rate[a]
63 × .75 = 47 Competent ovulations
$\frac{12 \text{ Pregnancies}}{47 \text{ Competent ovulations}}$ = 25.5% Conception rate

[a] Based on our previous determination from the same colony.

TABLE 6. *The effect of several 13-dehydro analogs of PGF$_{2\alpha}$ on peripheral plasma progesterone in the early pregnant monkey* (Macaca fascicularis) *following oral administration*

Expt #	Day of pregnancy	Dose (mg/kg)	% Fall in plasma prog.
13-Dehydro-PGF$_{2\alpha}$			
2 MG	36	4	No change
2 MK	36	6	No change
Ent-15-epi-13-dehydro-PGF$_{2\alpha}$			
2 MH	34	8	No change
2 MQ	34	24	30%
2 MX	34	36	50%
16-Fluoro-13-dehydro-PGF$_{2\alpha}$			
2 MB	31	2	85%
2 ML	35	3	60%

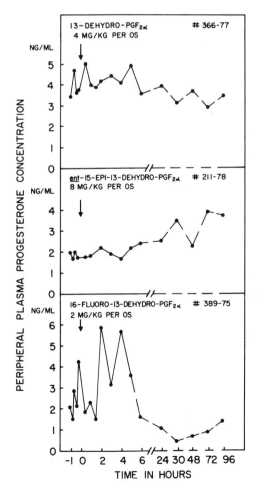

FIG. 7. Peripheral plasma progesterone levels following oral administration of three different 13-dehydro analogs of PGF$_{2\alpha}$ to monkeys during early pregnancy (days 31 to 36 of the cycle during which they conceived).

the corpus luteum of pregnancy is relatively resistant to PGs, possibly due to the presence of circulating levels of mCG. With the *ent*-epi analog, a dose of 8 mg/kg given orally—which was adequate in the cyclic monkey—was without effect in the pregnant monkey (Table 6 and Fig. 7). Because of the wide safety margin of this analog (lack of smooth muscle activity), we were able to give quite large doses (24 to 36 mg/kg) or this compound (Table 6). However, even these high doses only depressed progesterone by 30% to 50% (see Fig. 8). As in the cyclic monkey, we found 16-fluoro-13-dehydro $PGF_{2\alpha}$ to be the most active analog in the early pregnant monkey. However, although we obtained a substantial reduction in peripheral plasma progesterone concentration (60% to 85%), pregnancy was not terminated in either monkey (Table 6 and Fig. 7).

Recent luteectomy studies in the monkey have shown that even on day 29 of the pregnancy cycle, pregnancy was terminated in only 50% of the subjects in spite of the fact that peripheral plasma progesterone fell to low levels (22). The investigators in this latter study concluded that even at this early stage of pregnancy, the placenta in the monkey is able to produce enough progesterone

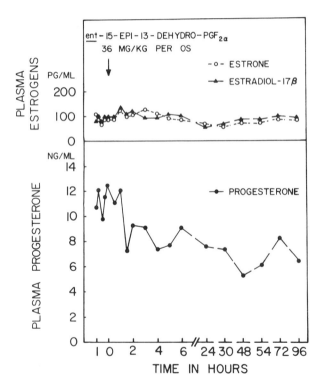

FIG. 8. Peripheral plasma progesterone and estrogen concentration following the oral administration of *ent*-15-epi-13-dehydro-$PGF_{2\alpha}$ (36 mg/kg) to a female monkey on day 34 of the cycle during which she conceived.

to support pregnancy locally but not enough to contribute significantly to peripheral blood levels. Thus, it would appear that—unlike the human female where the luteoplacental shift occurs around 6 to 8 weeks after conception (12)—the luteoplacental shift in the monkey occurs very early. The "window" during which a luteolytic drug will be able to terminate pregnancy in the monkey may be only a few days at best, whereas in women it is probably 4 weeks or more. It is interesting to note that while the 16-fluoro-13-dehydro analog was able to depress progesterone levels in the early pregnant monkey, there was no effect of this drug on peripheral plasma levels of mCG (see Fig. 9). This finding would suggest that these analogs have no direct embryotoxic effect on the conceptus per se. The fact that the corpus luteum of early pregnancy in the monkey is relatively resistant to the PG analogs suggests that mCG may have a protective effect on the CL. Indeed, it is even possible that one of the important physiological roles of mCG may be to protect the CL against endogenous PGs and hence prolong the life-span of the CL in early pregnancy. It

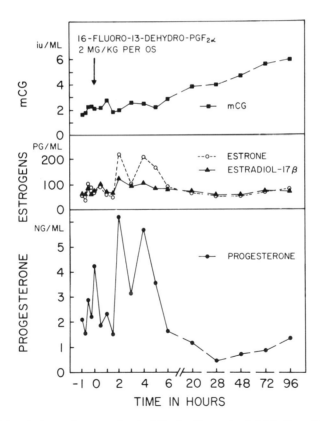

FIG. 9. Peripheral plasma hormone levels following the oral administration of 16-fluoro-13-dehydro-PGF$_{2\alpha}$ (2 mg/kg) to a female monkey on day 31 of the cycle during which she conceived.

would thus appear that the early pregnant monkey is really an essential model for our type of study since, to be of utility, these drugs must be able to depress progesterone levels in the presence of endogenous mCG. Alternatively, the hCG-treated monkey model (25,63,64) may prove to be a useful substitute for the early pregnant monkey model, especially since the latter are so time-consuming to obtain.

CONCLUSIONS

Several 13-dehydro analogs were shown to be luteolytic in both the cyclic sheep and cyclic primate models studied. The fact that these luteolytic analogs have diminished uterine smooth muscle activity suggests that the receptors governing the smooth muscle effect on the one hand, and the luteolytic effect on the other, may possess different structural specificities. In both species studied, the analogs showed marked resistance to the PG-15-OH-dehydrogenase *in vivo* as shown by their activity when infused intravenously. In the early pregnant monkey, the reduced luteolytic activity of the 13-dehydro analogs suggests that mCG may have a protective effect on the corpus luteum to PGs in general. Thus, the early pregnant monkey, or possibly the hCG-treated cyclic monkey, would appear to be "essential" models in the study of luteolytic agents in the primate. Finally, previous reports of termination of early pregnancy in monkeys with luteolytic PG analogs may have depended, at least in part, on their intrinsic smooth muscle activity on the uterus.

ACKNOWLEDGMENTS

The work at the Worcester Foundation was supported by contract No. HD-4-2801 (J.F.) and in part by NIH Grant No. HD 08129 (J.McC.). Thanks are due also to David Watson and his staff at the Herschel Lab for the analysis of steroids in primate samples. The studies involving primates were conducted at the New England Regional Primate Research Center, Southborough, Massachusetts which is supported by NIH Grant No. RR 00168 from the Division of Research Resources. Particular thanks are due to Dr. P. Sehgal and his staff for help with the primate study. The work at the University of Chicago was supported by NIH Grant AM 11499, Contract HD-4-2801 and RCA AM 21846. Acknowledgment is also made to NSF (GP 33116) and NIH (CA 14999) for funds to purchase nmr equipment used in the synthetic work.

REFERENCES

1. Arrata, W. S. M., and Chatterton, R. T. (1974): *Am. J. Obstet. Gynecol.,* 120:954–959.
2. Auletta, F. J., Agina, H., and Scommegna, A. (1978): *Endocrinology,* 103:1183–1189.
3. Auletta, F. J., Caldwell, B. V., and Speroff, L. (1976): *Prostaglandins,* 11:745–752.
4. Beavis, E. L. G., Brown, J. B., and Smith, M. A. (1969): *J. Obstet. Gynaec.,* 76:969–978.
5. Binder, D., Bowler, J., Brown, E. D., Crossley, N. S., Hutton, J., Senior, M., Slater, L., Wilkinson, P., and Wright, N. C. A. (1974): *Prostaglandins,* 6:87–90.

6. Bygdeman, M., Martin, J. N., Jr., Leader, A., Lundström, V., Ramadan, M., Eneroth, P., and Green, K. (1976): *Obstet. Gynecol.* 48:221.
7. Carlson, J. C., McCracken, J. A., and Fried, J. (1972): *Adv. Biosci. Suppl.,* 9:101.
8. Castracane, V. D., Moore, G. T., and Shaikh, A. A. (1979): *Biol. Reprod.,* 20:462–472.
9. Challis, J. R. G., Calder, A. A., Dilley, S., Foster, C. S., Hillier, K., Hunter, D. J. S., MacKenzie, I. Z., and Thorburn, G. D. (1976): *J. Endocrinol.,* 68:401–408.
10. Crossley, N. S. (1975): *Prostaglandins,* 10:5–18.
11. Csapo, A. I., and Mocsary, P. (1976): *Prostaglandins,* 11:155–162.
12. Csapo, A. I., and Pulkkinen, M. (1978): *Obstet. Gynecol. Survey,* 33:69–81.
13. Dukes, M., Russell, W., and Walpole, A. L. (1974): *Nature,* 250:330–331.
14. Eddy Moeljono, M. P., Bazer, F. W., and Thatcher, W. W. (1976): *Prostaglandins,* 11:737–743.
15. Fried, J., and Borman, A. (1958): *Vitamins and Hormones.* Academic Press, New York.
16. Fried, J., Lee, M-S., Gaede, B., Sih, J. C., Yoshikawa, Y., and McCracken, J. A. (1976): In: *Advances in Prostaglandin and Thromboxane Research,* Vol. 1, edited by B. Samuelsson and R. Paoletti, pp. 183–193. Raven Press, New York.
17. Fried, J., and Lin, C. H. (1973): *J. Med. Chem.,* 16:429–430.
18. Fried, J., Mehra, M. M., and Kao, W. L. (1971): *J. Am. Chem. Soc.,* 93:5594.
19. Gleeson, A. R., Thorburn, G. D., and Cox, R. I. (1974): *Prostaglandins,* 5:521–529.
20. Goding, J. R., McCracken, J. A., and Baird, D. T. (1967): *J. Endocrinol.,* 39:37–52.
21. Goodman, A. L., Descalzi, C. D., Johnson, D. K., and Hodgen, G. D. (1977): *Proc. Soc. Exp. Biol. Med.,* 155:479–481.
22. Goodman, A. L., and Hodgen, G. D. (1978): *Endocrinology,* 102:A368.
23. Henderson, K. M., and McNatty, K. P. (1975): *Prostaglandins,* 9:779–797.
24. Hillier, K., Dutton, A., Corker, C. S., Singer, A., and Embrey, M. P. (1972): *Br. Med. J.,* 4:333–336.
25. Hodgen, G. D. (1979): Personal communication.
26. Hodgen, G. D., and Ross, G. T. (1974): *J. Clin. Endocrinol. Metab.,* 38:927–930.
27. Horton, E. W., and Poyser, N. L. (1976): *Physiol. Rev.,* 56:595–651.
28. Jarabak, J., and Braithwaite, S. S. (1976): *Arch. Biochem. Biophys.,* 177:245.
29. Jerve, F., Fylling, P., and Stenby, S. (1979): *Prostaglandins,* 17:121–123.
30. Jones, G. S., and Wentz, A. C. (1972): *Am. J. Obstet. Gynecol,* 114:393–404.
31. Karim, S. M. M., and Ratnam, S. S. (1977): In: *Biochemical Aspects of Prostaglandins and Thromboxanes,* edited by N. Kharasch and J. Fried, pp. 115–132. Academic Press, New York.
32. Kimball, F. A., Kirton, K. T., Spilman, C. H., and Wyngarden, L. J. (1975): *Biol. Reprod.,* 13:482–489.
33. Kindahl, H., Edqvist, L.-E., Bane, A., and Granström,E. (1976): *Acta Endocrinol.,* 82:134–149.
34. Kindahl, H., Granstrom, E., Edqvist, L.-E., and Eneroth, P. (1976): In: *Advances in Prostaglandin and Thromboxane Research,* Vol. 2, edited by B. Samuelsson and R. Paoletti, pp. 667–671. Raven Press, New York.
35. Kinoshita, K., Eneroth, P., and Bygdeman, M. (1979): *Prostaglandins,* 17:469–481.
36. Kirton, K. T., Pharriss, B. B., and Forbes, A. D. (1970): *Proc. Soc. Exp. Biol. Med.,* 133:314–316.
37. Lehmann, F., Peters, F., Breckwoldt, M., and Bettendorf, G. (1972): *Prostaglandins,* 1:269–277.
38. Le Maire, W. J., and Shapiro, A. G. (1972): *Prostaglandins,* 1:259–267.
39. MacKenzie, I. Z., Embrey, M. P., Davies, A. J., and Guillebaud, J. (1978): *Lancet,* I:1223–1226.
40. Mattner, P. E., and Thorburn, G. D. (1969): *J. Reprod. Fertil.,* 19:547–549.
41. McCracken, J. A. (1971): *Annals NY Acad. Sci.,* 180:456–472.
42. McCracken, J. A. (1972): In: *Prostaglandins in Fertility Control,* Vol. 2, edited by S. Bergstrom, K. Green, and B. Samuelsson, p. 234. Karolinska Institute, Stockholm.
43. McCracken, J. A., Baird, D. T., and Goding, J. R. (1971): *Recent Prog. Horm. Res.,* 27:537–582.
44. McCracken, J. A., Barcikowski, B., Carlson, J. C., Green, K., and Samuelsson, B. (1973): *Adv. Biosci.,* 9:599–624.
45. McCracken, J. A., Carlson, J. C., Glew, M. E., Goding, J. R., Baird, D. T., Green, K., and Samuelsson, B. (1972): *Nature [New Biol.],* 238:129–134.

46. McCracken, J. A., Einer-Jensen, N., and Fried, J. (1979): In: *Ovarian Follicular and Corpus Luteum Function,* edited by C. P. Channing, J. Marsh, and W. A. Sadler, pp. 577–601. Plenum Press, New York.

47. McCracken, J. A., Fried, J., Lee, M.-S., Yoshikawa, Y., and Mammato, D.C. (1977): In: *Biochemical Aspects of Prostaglandins and Thromboxanes,* edited by N. Kharasch and J. Fried, pp. 215–242. Academic Press, New York.

48. Nancarrow, C. D., Buckmaster, J., Chamley, W., Cox, R. I., Cumming, I. A., Cummins, L., Drinan, J. P., Findlay, J. K., Goding, J. R., Restall, B. J., Schneider, W., and Thorburn, G. D. (1973): *J. Reprod. Fertil.,* 32:320.

49. Oshima, K., Matsumoto, K., Tsuda, T., Shibata, K., and Hayashi, M. (1978): *Prostaglandins,* 15:473–483.

50. Peterson, A. J., Tervit, H. R., Fairclough, R. J., Havik, P. G., and Smith, J. F. (1976): *Prostaglandins,* 12:551–558.

51. Piper, P. J., Vane, J. R., and Wyllie, J. H. (1970): *Nature,* 225:600–604.

52. Powell, W. S., Hammerström, S., Samuelsson, B., and Sjöberg, B. (1974): *Lancet,* I:1120.

53. Poyser, N. L. (1976): In: *Advances in Prostaglandin and Thromboxane Research,* Vol. 2, edited by B. Samuelsson and R. Paoletti, pp. 633–643. Raven Press, New York.

54. Roberts, J. S., and McCracken, J. A. (1976): *Biol. Reprod.,* 15:457–463.

55. Rock, J., and Hertig, A. T. (1948): *Am. J. Obstet. Gynecol.,* 55:6.

56. Russell, W. (1975): *Prostaglandins,* 10:163–183.

57. Shaikh, A. A., and Klaiber, E. L. (1974): *Prostaglandins,* 6:253–262.

58. Shutt, D. A., Shearman, R. P., Lyneham, R. C., Clarke, A. H., McMahon, G. R., and Goh, P. (1975): *Steroids,* 26:299–310.

59. Spilman, C. H. (1976): Personal communication.

60. Spilman, C. H., Beuving, D. C., Forbes, A. D., and Kimball, F. A. (1977): *Prostaglandins,* 14:477–488.

61. Swanston, I. A., McNatty, K. P., and Baird, D. T. (1977): *J. Endocrinol.,* 73:115–122.

62. Takagi, S., Sakata, H., Yoshida, T., Nakazawa, S., Fujii, K. T., Tominaga, Y., Iwasa, Y., Ninagawa, T., Hiroshima, T., Tomida, Y., Itoh, K., and Matsukawa, R. (1977): *Prostaglandins,* 14:791–798.

63. Wan, L. S., Khatamee, M., Niemann, W., Feller, C., and Bigelow, B. (1975): *Fertil. Steril.,* 26:111–120.

64. Wilks, J. W. (1979): In: *Ovarian Follicular and Corpus Luteum Function,* edited by C. P. Channing, J. Marsh, and W. A. Sadler, p. 757. Plenum Press, New York.

65. Wilks, J. W., Hodgen, G. D., and Ross, G. T. (1976): *J. Clin. Endocrinol. Metab.,* 43:1261–1267.

Advances in Prostaglandin and Thromboxane Research,
Vol. 6, edited by B. Samuelsson, P. W. Ramwell,
and R. Paoletti. Raven Press, New York © 1980.

Structure–Activity Relationships: A Look at the Structures of PG-Related Molecules

George T. DeTitta, David A. Langs, and Mary G. Erman

Medical Foundation of Buffalo, Inc., Buffalo, New York 14203

The model of the classical pharmacophore outlined by Kier (10) suggests that the study of molecular architecture is a fruitful avenue of research for those interested in structure–activity relationships. Here we wish to outline what various physical techniques tell us about the architecture of prostaglandins (PGs).

The overall shape of classical PGs has been characterized as "hairpin" in recognition of the U-shaped or approximately parallel arrangement of side chains first observed by Abrahamsson (1) in his diffraction study of a $PGF_{1\beta}$ derivative (Fig. 1A). Evidence for the "hairpin" motif comes from the lanthanide-induced shift nuclear magnetic resonance (NMR) studies of Leovey and Andersen (13), the surface tension–concentration studies of $PGF_{2\alpha}$ by Roseman and Yalkowsky (15) and the repeated observation of the "hairpin" in 11 diffraction studies of 14 PG molecules by crystallographic methods. The stability of the arrangement has been attributed to van der Waals attractive interactions between the parallel side chains by Rabinowitz et al. (14). The sole exception to the "hairpin" rule is PGB_1, which is L-shaped (4).

If the "hairpin" shape is the hallmark of a PG, then clearly more subtle conformational features must distinguish one PG from another. Loci of variability include ring conformations, ring–chain junction geometries, Δ^5- and Δ^{13}-double bond geometries, and the C_{15} hydroxyl region. The ring conformations of PGs are primarily governed by the C_8 and C_{12} substituents' needs to be diequatorial. Thus the range of observed ring conformations is restricted to approximately 30% of the pseudo rotation pathway of cyclopentane (Fig. 1B). Although the permissible range centers about a conformation midway between a C_8 β-envelope and a C_{10} half-chair, as in the monoclinic form of PGA_1 (5), the two most populous ring geometries are the C_9 α-envelope and the C_{12} α-envelope. The C_9 α-envelope conformation of $PGF_{2\alpha}$ is the only ring shape within the permissible range that brings the O_9 and O_{11} hydroxyls close enough together for the hydrogen bonding which was reportedly observed in the solution (CCl_4) infrared spectrum of $PGF_{1\alpha}$ by DeClercq et al. (3). Proton NMR spectroscopy of $PGF_{2\alpha}$ by Conover and Fried (2) first suggested the diequatorial orientation of $PGF_{2\alpha}$ side chains, subsequently observed by x-ray diffraction (11) (Fig. 1C).

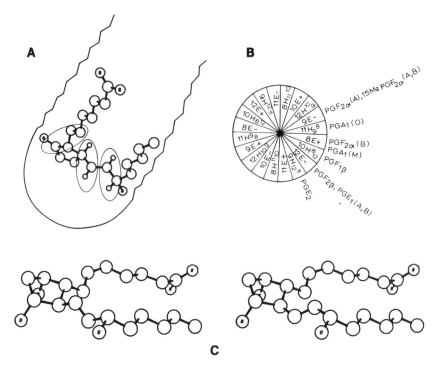

FIG. 1. A: The prototypical PG "hairpin" conformer, illustrated by PGA, and emphasized by the hairpin drawn around its periphery. **B:** The permissible "ideal" ring conformations of PGs, which range from a C_9 α-envelope (i.e., one with C_{10}–C_8 in a plane and C_9 below or α to the plane) to a C_9 half-chair (with C_{12} below and to the left and C_{11} above and to the right of the plane made by C_8–C_{10}). **C:** The major **(left)** and minor **(right)** Δ^{13}-conformers of $PGE_{2\alpha}$. The major form has H_{12} trans to H_{13} and H_{14} trans to H_{15}, while the minor form has H_{12} gauche to H_{13} and H_{14} gauche to H_{15}.

The C_8 junction geometries of the PG_1 series are predominantly *trans* to C_9 and gauche to C_{12}, while in the PG_2 series the opposite arrangement is found. The cis double bond at $C_6 = C_5$ kinks the α chain and the C_{12} *trans* junction geometry is probably necessary to keep the α and ω chains parallel. PG_{2} is an exception to the gauche-*trans* rule (7). Its C_8 junction geometry is –gauche to C_9 and +gauche to C_{12}. The normal PG_2 junction geometry is denied to PGE_2 by a close interaction between its keto O_9 and the C_6 hydrogen which would occur in that geometry (11).

The C_{12} junction geometry is much less variable. As predicted by the extended Hückel calculations of Hoyland and Kier (9), the observed geometry is predominantly H_{12} *trans* to H_{13}, placing the plane of the $C_{13} = C_{14}$ double bond approximately perpendicular to the ring and intersecting the C_9-C_{10} bond. Likewise, the C_{15} hydroxyl region *vis-à-vis* the double bond is well fixed, with H_{15} *trans* to H_{14} (i.e., C_{16} –anticlinal and O_{15} +anticlinal to C_{13}). Recent reanalysis of the diffraction study of $PGF_{2\alpha}$·Tris revealed that a minor conformer, in which the $C_{13} = C_{14}$ double bond has rotated such that H_{12} is $-$gauche to H_{13} and H_{14} is $+$gauche to H_{15}, is present in both crystallographically independent $PGF_{2\alpha}$ molecules. This unexpected retro conformer explains the media-dependent changes in the olefinic span of the circular dichroism spectrum of $PGF_{2\alpha}$ observed by Leovey and Andersen (13). Originally attributed to a conformational shift involving a reorientation of the Δ^5- and Δ^{13}-double bonds on going from less to more polar media, it is now more readily understood in a classical way as a shift of the Δ^{13}-chromophore relative to the asymmetric agent, in this case the 15-hydroxyl oxygen. Thus $PGF_{2\alpha}$ appears to be a PG which manifests not only two distinct ring conformations, but also two distinct Δ_{13}-conformations.

A rethinking of the body of physical data available for PGs suggests an unexpected, but gratifying, concordance—unexpected in view of the differing states in which PGs have been investigated (free molecule, solution, crystal) and gratifying in that this concordance leads to confidence that the observed shapes are of relevance in our understanding of PG activity. Since we are presently unable to examine the shapes of PGs *in situ* (at the receptor, in the enzyme, etc.) to check our results, we are forced to judge their relevance by their ability to explain and perhaps predict biological action. For example, the L-shape of PGB_1 has been put forward (6) as the reason PGB_1 is resistent to PGDH metabolism. Similarly, we now suggest that the enhanced antifertility activity of Grieco's 12-fluoro-$PGF_{2\alpha}$ (8) may be due to a locking of the Δ^{13}-double bond into the retro form, which in turn brings the H_{14} hydrogen gauche to H_{15}, thereby affording the molecule protection from metabolism by PGDH (8).

ACKNOWLEDGMENTS

We would like to thank our co-workers at the Medical Foundation for their support of this work and acknowledge support of the National Heart, Lung and Blood Institute, Department of Health, Education and Welfare, Grant HL-15378.

REFERENCES

1. Abrahamsson, S. (1963): *Acta Crystallogr.,* 16:409–418.
2. Conover, W. W., and Fried, J. (1974): *Proc. Natl. Acad. Sci.* USA, 71:2157–2161.
3. DeClercq, P., Samson, M., Tavernier, D., Van Haver, D., and Van de walle, M. (1977): *J. Org. Chem.,* 42:3140–3144.
4. DeTitta, G. T. (1976): *Science,* 191:1271–1272.
5. DeTitta, G. T., Edmonds, J. W., and Duax, W. L. (1975): *Prostaglandins,* 9:659–665.
6. DeTitta, G. T., Langs, D. A., and Edmonds, J. W. (1979): *Biochemistry,* 18:3387–3391.
7. Edmonds, J. W., and Duax, W. L. (1974): *Prostaglandins,* 5:275–281.
8. Grieco, P. A., Wang, C.-L. J., Owens, W., Williams, E., Sugahara, T., Yokoyama, Y., Okuniewicz, F. J., and Withers, G. P. (1979): In: *Chemistry, Biochemistry, and Pharmacological Activity of Prostanoids,* edited by S. M. Roberts and F. Scheinmann, pp. 87–99. Pergamon Press, New York.
9. Hoyland, J. R., and Kier, L. B. (1972): *J. Med. Chem.,* 15:84–86.
10. Kier, L. B. (1976): *Experentia (Suppl.)* 23; 151–160.

11. Langs, D. A., Erman, M., and DeTitta, G. T. (1977): *Science,* 197:1003–1005.
12. Leovey, E. M. K., and Andersen, N. H. (1975): *J. Am. Chem. Soc.,* 97:4148–4150.
13. Leovey, E. M. K., and Andersen, N. H. (1975): *Prostaglandins,* 10:789–794.
14. Rabinowitz, I., Ramwell, P., and Davison, P. (1971): *Nature* [*New Biol.*], 223:88–90.
15. Roseman, T. J., and Yalkowsky, S. H. (1973): *J. Pharm. Sci.,* 62:1680–1685.

Advances in Prostaglandin and Thromboxane Research,
Vol. 6, edited by B. Samuelsson, P. W. Ramwell,
and R. Paoletti. Raven Press, New York © 1980.

Evidence for Separate PGD_2 and $PGF_{2\alpha}$ Receptors in the Canine Mesenteric Vascular Bed

Larry Feigen and Barry Chapnick

Departments of Physiology and Pharmacology, Tulane University Medical Center,
New Orleans, Louisiana 70112

Studies on prostaglandin (PG) binding in various tissues suggest that there are receptors which are relatively specific for the PG family. These receptors are usually found not to be absolutely specific, however, since two or more PGs can usually compete for the same binding sites (3,5,6). Competitive antagonism among PGs has also been demonstrated in isolated organ studies involving the canine uterus (2) and rat mesenteric artery (4), suggesting that a sufficiently large dose of one PG can inhibit responses to other PGs. However, it is not clear whether these results indicate a nonspecific action of one PG on a number of receptors or rather that certain PGs share a common receptor.

We studied the question of whether there are separate, relatively specific receptors in the intact mesenteric vascular bed of anesthetized dogs, remembering that without specific antagonists, the term "receptor" must be used with caution.

METHODS AND MATERIALS

Using methods that have previously been reported (1), dogs were anesthetized with pentobarbital, and catheters were placed in the left ventricle (via a carotid artery), aorta, and inferior vena cava (via femoral vessels). The superior mesenteric artery was exposed through an incision high on the flank while the animal was suspended in the prone position from an overhead frame by subcutaneous wires. An electromagnetic flow probe was placed on the mesenteric artery, and a small needle cannula was inserted into the artery proximal to the probe. Interactions between PGs were studied by continuously infusing a PG systemically via the catheter in the left ventricle and concomitantly injecting substances into the mesenteric artery. Comparisons of the effect of injections before and during PG infusions were carried out. Because PGD_2 and $F_{2\alpha}$ are both potent mesenteric vasoconstrictors (1), we decided to examine whether one of these would inhibit responses to the other. A dose for ventricular infusion was chosen (100 ng/kg/min) that caused modest reductions in mesenteric blood flow, which was then reversed by direct infusions of nitroglycerine into the mesenteric artery. Under these conditions, relatively specific interactions between infused and injected PGs could be observed, and any influence of alterations in initial vascular resistance could be avoided.

RESULTS AND DISCUSSION

PGD_2 and $F_{2\alpha}$ produce dose-related decreases in mesenteric blood flow when injected into the superior mesenteric artery at doses of 10 to 100 ng and 0.1 to 1 μg, respectively. Figure 1 shows that during intraventricular infusion of prostaglandin $F_{2\alpha}$, responses to $PGF_{2\alpha}$ injections were reduced 60 to 70%. At this time, responses to PGD_2 were not affected in a consistent fashion. In contrast, when PGD_2 was infused, responses to bolus injections of PGD_2 were decreased 40 to 70%, but responses to $PGF_{2\alpha}$ were unaffected (Fig. 1). Mesenteric vascular responses to norepinephrine were not affected during infusion of either $PGF_{2\alpha}$ or PGD_2 (data not shown).

These data show that mesenteric vascular responses to close arterial injections of PGD_2 are reduced during systemic infusion of PGD_2 and that local responses to $PGF_{2\alpha}$ were reduced during systemic infusion of $PGF_{2\alpha}$. Since responses to PGD_2 were not affected by infusion of $PGF_{2\alpha}$ and vice versa, and since norepinephrine was not affected by either PG, these substances appear to act through noncompeting mechanisms. These results suggest that PGD_2 and $PGF_{2\alpha}$ act on different receptors in the mesenteric vascular bed.

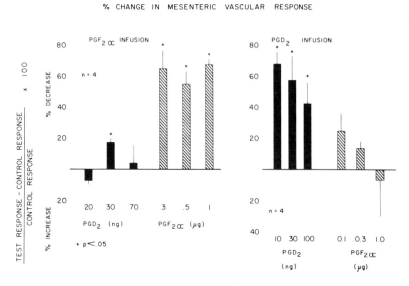

FIG. 1. Left. Effect of $PGF_{2\alpha}$ infusion on mesenteric vascular responses to injections of $PGF_{2\alpha}$ and D_2. Responses to $PGF_{2\alpha}$ injections were markedly reduced, but the effects of PGD_2 were not consistently changed. **Right:** Effect of PGD_2 infusion on responses to PGD_2 and $PGF_{2\alpha}$ injections. PGD_2 effects were significantly reduced, but responses to $PGF_{2\alpha}$ were not changed.

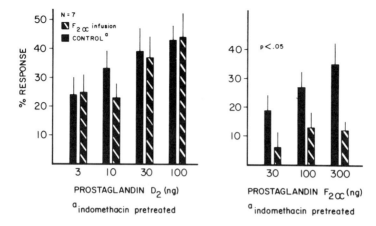

FIG. 2. Effect of PGF$_{2\alpha}$ infusion on mesenteric vascular responses to injections of PGF$_{2\alpha}$ and D$_2$ in dogs pretreated with indomethacin (2.5 mg/kg). Responses to PGF$_{2\alpha}$, but not PGD$_2$, injections were markedly reduced.

To assess the possibility that endogenous PG synthesis might complicate the interpretation of results obtained when vasoactive substances were administered, we repeated the infusion of PGF$_{2\alpha}$ in dogs treated with indomethacin (2.5 mg/ kg, i.v.). In these animals, mesenteric responses to arachidonic acid were reduced 70 to 90% by indomethacin treatment. Figure 2 shows that infusion of PGF$_{2\alpha}$ produced a 50 to 70% reduction in responses to PGF$_{2\alpha}$ injections, but that responses to PGD$_2$ were not reduced. These results support the previous data and strengthen the hypothesis that PGF$_{2\alpha}$ and PGD$_2$ produce mesenteric vaso-constriction by acting on separate receptors.

ACKNOWLEDGMENTS

We thank Dr. J. E. Pike of The Upjohn Company for the generous gifts of PGs. The work was supported in part by Grant 19997 and Contract 21882 of the National Heart, Lung and Blood Institute and by grants from the American and Louisiana Heart Associations.

REFERENCES

1. Chapnick, B. M., Feigen, L. P., Hyman, A. L., and Kadowitz, P. J. (1978): *Am. J. Physiol.,* 235:H326–H332.
2. Clark, K. E., and Brody, M. J. (1977): *Blood Vessels,* 14:204–211.
3. Lord, J. T., Ziboh, V. A., and Warren, S. (1976): In: *Advances in Prostglandin and Thromboxane Research,* Vol. 1, edited by B. Samuellson and R. Paoletti, pp. 291–296. Raven Press, New York.
4. Manku, M. S., Mtabaji, J. P., and Horribin, D. F. (1977): *Prostaglandins,* 13:701–709.
5. Rao, C. V. (1974): *J. Biol. Chem.,* 249:7203–7209.
6. Schillinger, E., and Prior, G. (1976): In: *Advances in Prostaglandin and Thromboxane Research,* Vol. 1, edited by B. Samuelsson and R. Paoletti, pp. 259–263. Raven Press, New York.

Advances in Prostaglandin and Thromboxane Research,
Vol. 6, edited by B. Samuelsson, P. W. Ramwell,
and R. Paoletti. Raven Press, New York © 1980.

Evaluation of Prostaglandin and Prostacyclin Antagonism at Platelet Receptors by Aggregometry

Thomas L. Eggerman, Lawrence A. Harker, Niels H. Andersen, and Cynthia H. Wilson

University of Washington, Seattle, Washington 98195

The multiplicity and individual specificities of platelet reactivity regulating receptors for prostanoids are key to our understanding of a wide variety of thrombotic diseases. Prostacyclin (PGI_2), prostaglandins (PGs) D_2, E_1, and E_2 all stimulate platelet adenylate cyclase (PAC); yet their actions on adenosine monophosphate-(ADP) induced human platelet-rich plasma aggregation are qualitatively and quantitatively distinct. We have used optical aggregometry in a study of synergistic and antagonistic interactions of these prostanoids (and a large selection of analogs). While our studies were in progress, others have presented data—species variation in relative potencies and selective inhibition (6), displacement of platelet-bound radiotracers (4,5), and cross-desensitization at PAC (1)—which support the notion that PGE_1 and PGI_2 share a PAC-related receptor, while PGD_2 acts at a distinct receptor coupled to the same PAC. However, the position of PGE_2 is far from clear. The radiotracer displacement data indicates minimal affinity for the E_1/I_2 receptor in contrast to Gorman's (1) cross-desensitization studies and the earlier suggestion by McDonald and Stuart (2) that the opposing effects of PGE_1 and PGE_2 on ADP-induced PRP aggregation is due to "competitive antagonism" by a partial agonist.

In our studies, ADP (8–10 μM) or collagen (2 μg/ml) was used to induce aggregation. The inhibiting agents [PGI_2, PGD_2, PGE_1, and exo-PGI_1—IC_{50} (nM) against ADP: 5, 45, 90, and 800; against collagen: 3, 15, 23, and 200] were added 60 sec prior to the aggregating stimulus. The antagonist (PGE_2) or partial agonist was either included in a 60-sec preincubation or added 120 sec after the stimulus. In runs employing preincubation, a full 6 to 8 point dose–response curve (DRC) for the inhibiting agent is obtained at each of several concentrations of the partial agonist or antagonist. The shifts in the inhibitor DRC resulting from preincubation with a partial agonist can, in principle, take three distinct forms as illustrated in Fig. 1, together with DRCs for PGI_2 alone and in the presence of PGD_2, PGE_1, and PGE_2. The three theoretical effects can be classified as synergism (potentiation), additivity, and antagonism. The

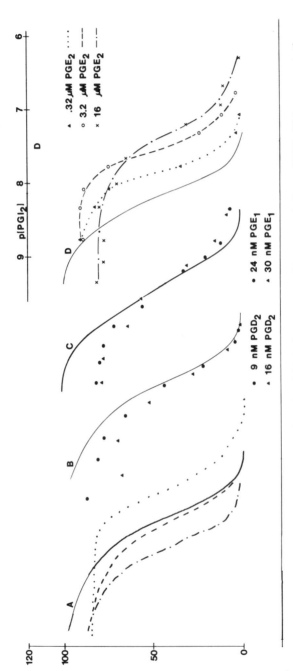

FIG. 1. DRCs. Percent of control aggregation vs. p[PGI$_2$] for PGI$_2$ in the presence of two concentrations of PGD$_2$ (B) two concentrations of PGE$_1$ (C), and three concentrations of PGE$_2$ (D). The p[PGI$_2$] scale is the same throughout and is included only for run D. The solid curve in each illustration is the control DRC of PGI$_2$ alone. A illustrates the expected DRCs for a partial agonist that is synergistic (- -), fully additive (---), or antagonistic (· · ·). The percent transmission change over 90 sec was used as the measure of aggregation.

additive response indicates either low-affinity but efficacious binding to the same receptor or binding to a distinct receptor. It is observed with PGD$_2$ (see Fig. 1), presumably due to the presence of two distinct receptors at the PAC, with exo-PGI$_1$ (see Fig. 2); and also with 18,18,20-trimethyl-PGE$_2$, 5-exo-PGI$_2$, and a variety of PGI$_2$ analogs (data not shown) of low potency (0.1–2% of PGI$_2$). The latter indicates that weak partial agonism at the PGI$_2$ receptor does not result in "competitive antagonism." PGE$_1$ does not show a fully additive action. Only PGE$_2$ displays antagonist activity.

PGE$_2$ is an equally effective antagonist of the inhibiting actions of PGE$_1$, exo-PGI$_1$ (date not shown), and even more effective in opposing the action of PGD$_2$. The efficacy of PGE$_2$ antagonism of PGI$_2$ and PGD$_2$ varies depending on which measure of aggregation is employed in constructing the DRCs Table 1.

The increase in [PG]$_{inhib}$ required to inhibit release (as measured by either net aggregation 90 sec after the stimulus or the maximal rate of change in percent transmission, which occurs during the release phase) is two to seven times that required to inhibit the initial response to ADP. Clearly, the major portion of the antagonism displayed by PGE$_2$ is the result of stimulated release which is observed with PGE$_2$ over a wide concentration range (0.01–5 μM), and also with PGE$_1$ at noninhibiting doses (2–15 nM), but not with any of the other partial inhibitors tested.

A further indication that the antagonism is not due to competitive binding can be seen in the absence of the expected antagonist concentration dependence. A 50-fold increase in [PGE$_2$] produces less than a 1.5-fold increase in the IC$_{50}$ of PGI$_2$ when aggregation is followed for 45 sec (see Fig. 2).

The potent antagonism (shown by PGE$_2$) of PGD$_2$, even when a major portion of the stimulated release is factored out by using initial aggregation rate data, is taken as a strong indication that the remaining antagonism is not due to competition for the E$_1$/I$_2$ receptor. Rather we must postulate another distinct PGE$_2$ receptor (presumably adenylate cyclase related). When this receptor is occupied, the efficacy of receptor bound PGI$_2$ (and particularly PGD$_2$) is greatly reduced. The effect at the physiological end point is the equivalent of displacement.

The aggregation-promoting actions of PGE$_2$ and PGE$_1$ are also evident when

TABLE 1. [PG] increase required for 50% inhibition of aggregation due to preincubation with PGE$_2$ (2–3.2 μM)

Inhibitor (%)		
PGI$_2$	PGD$_2$	Measure of aggregation
210	670	Initial rate [d (OD)/dt at 10–20 sec]
380	730	ΔOD (0–45 sec)
360	1,140	Net release (= OD at 90 sec)
520	3,500	Maximum aggregation rate [d (OD)/dt]$_{max}$

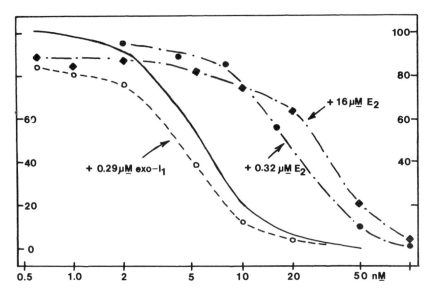

FIG. 2. DRCs for PGI₂. Aggregation to 45 sec after ADP (percent of uninhibited control) vs. concentration of PGI₂ (nM). The solid curve is for PGI₂ alone. The shifted DRCs are for preincubation PGs indicated.

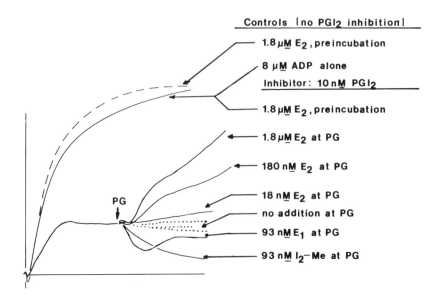

FIG. 3. The effect of PGs added 2 min after the ADP stimulus in aggregations partially inhibited by a 60-sec preincubation with 10 nM PGI₂. The aggregatory stimulus is 8 µM ADP throughout.

the agents are added after the ADP stimulus (see Fig. 3). PGE_2 addition produces a dose-dependent biphasic aggregation. PGE_1 produces an initial disaggregatory response followed by an increase in percent transmission associated with either stimulated release or displacement of PGI_2 from the receptor. PGD_2 and PGI_2 produce (data not shown) only a disaggregatory response. This assay also demonstrates the notable disaggregatory activity of the methyl ester of PGI_2 (ca. 10–15% that of PGI_2), which contrasts with the low intrinsic potency (0.4% of PGI_2) of the ester as an inhibitor of the initial aggregation observed on addition of ADP. Studies using preincubation periods from 10 to 210 sec demonstrate that these activities are not due to slow ester hydrolysis. PGI_2 esters may prove to be useful antithrombotic agents.

ACKNOWLEDGMENT

These studies were supported by contract NO1-HV-8-2933 from the National Heart, Lung and Blood Institute.

REFERENCES

1. Gorman, R. R. (1978): Presented at the *VIIth Winter Prostaglandin Conference,* Sarasota, Florida.
2. McDonald, J. W. D., and Stuart, R. K. (1974): *J. Lab. Clin. Med.,* 81:111.
3. Miller, O. V., and Gorman, R. R. (1979): *J. Pharmacol. Exp. Ther. (in press).*
4. Schafer, A. I., Cooper, B., and Hardin, R. I. (1978): *Clin. Res.,* 26:356A.
5. Siegl, A. M., Smith, J. B., Silver, M. J., Nicolaou, and Ahern, D. (1979): *J. Clin. Invest.,* 63:215. [See also (1978): *Fed. Proc.,* 37:260.]
6. Whittle, B. J. R., Moncada, S., and Vane, J. R. (1978): *Prostaglandins,* 16:373.

Advances in Prostaglandin and Thromboxane Research,
Vol. 6, edited by B. Samuelsson, P. W. Ramwell,
and R. Paoletti. Raven Press, New York © 1980.

^{3}H-PGD$_2$ Binding by Intact Human Platelets

A. M. Siegl, J. B. Smith, and M. J. Silver

*Cardeza Foundation and Department of Pharmacology, Thomas Jefferson University,
Philadelphia, Pennsylvania 19107*

Prostaglandins (PGs) E$_1$, D$_2$ and prostacyclin (PGI$_2$) are potent inhibitors of platelet aggregation (4) and stimulators of platelet adenyl cyclase (10). Previous studies with these three compounds have shown that the actions of PGI$_2$ and PGE$_1$ differ from those of PGD$_2$ in both species specificity (9) and dose–response characteristics (3). These differences, as well as differences in structure, led several workers to hypothesize that there are at least two types of PG receptors on human platelets: one which recognizes PGI$_2$ and PGE$_1$ and the other which recognizes PGD$_2$. We have previously reported on a specific PGI$_2$ binding site on platelets which recognizes PGI$_2$ and, to a lesser extent, PGE$_1$ but does not recognize PGD$_2$ (8). In order to confirm the hypothesis that there are separate receptors for PGI$_2$ and PGD$_2$, we have undertaken a series of receptor binding studies with ^{3}H-PGD$_2$.

MATERIALS AND METHODS

^{3}H-PGD$_2$ was biosynthesized from ^{3}H-arachidonic acid (New England Nuclear, Boston; specific activity, 61 Ci/mmole) using washed rabbit platelets, which had been preincubated with 2 mM imidazole to inhibit thromboxane A$_2$ (TX$_2$) synthetase, as the enzyme source (5). Fatty acid poor bovine serum albumin (4 mg/ml) was added after 3 min to accelerate the breakdown of endoperoxide and increase the yield of ^{3}H-PGD$_2$ (1). The incubation was terminated by acidification to pH 3.0 to 3.5, and the reaction mixture was extracted 3 times with 2 volumes of ethyl acetate. The ^{3}H-PGD$_2$ was purified by thin-layer chromatography using benzene/dioxane/acetic acid (50:25:2.5) as the solvent system. The ^{3}H-PGD$_2$ region, as determined by radiochromatography, was eluted with dry acetone and rechromatographed using the organic phase of the ethyl acetate/isooctane/acetic acid/water system (55:25:10:50) as the solvent system. The ^{3}H-PGD$_2$ was eluted, and its purity was confirmed by measuring the percent conversion to ^{3}H-PGF$_{2\alpha}$ in the presence of NaBH$_4$. (The final purity of all preparations was between 90 and 95%.) The yield of ^{3}H-PGD$_2$ by this method ranged from 2 to 12%. Binding experiments were performed as described previously (8). ^{3}H-PGD$_2$ was diluted to the appropriate specific activity by the addition of nonradioactive PGD$_2$. Nonradioactive PGs were a gift from Dr. John Pike, The Upjohn Co., Kalamazoo, Michigan.

RESULTS

The binding of 30 nM ^{3}H-PGD$_2$ was rapid, being essentially complete within 1 min and remaining at this level for at least the next 15 min (Table 1). This bound ^{3}H-PGD$_2$ could be rapidly and completely displaced by the addition of a 10 μM excess of nonradioactive PGD$_2$, indicating that the binding was reversible and not due to uptake by the platelet (Table 1). Concentration-dependent binding of ^{3}H-PGD$_2$ measured between 30 and 2,000 nM yielded a straight line on Scatchard analysis (7). This line represented a single binding site with a dissociation constant (K_D) of 4.13 ($\pm$ 1.76) $\times$ 10^{-7} M and a capacity of 760 ($\pm$ 120) sites per platelets. The specificity of this PGD$_2$ binding site was tested by measuring the ability of PGD$_2$, PGE$_1$, and PGF$_{2\alpha}$ to displace bound ^{3}H-PGD$_2$ (50 nM). The concentrations required for a 50% displacement of the bound ^{3}H-PGD$_2$ were 5 $\times$ 10^{-6} M, 1 $\times$ 10^{-3} M, $\gg$ 1 $\times$ 10^{-3} M, and $\gg$ 1 $\times$ 10^{-3} for PGD$_2$, PGE$_1$, PGI$_2$, and PGF$_{2\alpha}$, respectively, indicating that this site is specific for PGD$_2$. It is unlikely that the small degree (5%) of cross-reactivity of PGE$_1$ is physiologically significant because of the high concentrations involved.

DISCUSSION

To be relevant to the action of a hormone, data obtained in binding experiments should be consistent with respect to time and concentration with the time and concentration required for the hormone effects. The binding should exhibit struc-

TABLE 1. *Time course of binding of ^{3}H-PGD$_2$ by platelets and its displacement by nonradioactive PGD$_2$[a]*

Binding		Displacement	
Time (min)	Percent control	Time (min)	Percent control
0.5	55	0.5	37.4
1.0	92	1.0	19.4
2.0	91.5	2.0	16.5
4.0	100	4.0	0
8.0	103.5	8.0	0
16.0	124.5		

[a] Experiments were performed as described previously (8). Each point is the mean of four determinations on two subjects; 100% control is amount of ^{3}H-PGD$_2$ bound 4 min after the addition of 30 nM ^{3}H-PGD$_2$ to platelet-rich plasma (5.68 $\pm$ 0.23 fmoles/10^8 platelets). Displacement experiments were initiated by the addition of 10 μM nonradioactive PGD$_2$ at the 4 min (100% control) time point. Platelet counts were 5.43 $\pm$ 0.15 $\times$ 10^8/ml.

tural specificity also. The ^{3}H-PGD$_2$ binding site reported here fulfills these criteria. The rapid binding is consistent with the rapid inhibition of aggregation (9) and stimulation of adenyl cyclase (3) by PGD$_2$ reported by other investigators. The dissociation constant obtained, although somewhat higher than the concentrations required to inhibit aggregation, is consistent with the concentration for half-maximal stimulation of adenyl cyclase extrapolated from the report of Tateson et al. (10) and our own unpublished observations. Finally, the binding site exhibits structural specificity. PGD$_2$, but not PGE$_1$ and PGI$_2$, produced appreciable displacement of bound ^{3}H-PGD$_2$.

The physiologic significance of two PG binding sites on platelets with the same apparent function (to inhibit platelet aggregation) is a puzzle. A possible explanation may go as follows. PGI$_2$ produced at a constant low level by the vascular endothelium (2) may be responsible for the maintenance of platelets in a nonreactive state. With injury, however, especially one involving thrombin generation, the rapid production of PGD$_2$ by aggregating platelets (6) may act as a feedback inhibitor on other platelets to limit the uncontrolled growth of platelet thrombi. Subsequent production of PGI$_2$ by thrombin-stimulated endothelium (11) would then be additive with the PGD$_2$ effect (A. M. Siegl, J. B. Smith, *unpublished data*). The existence of platelet PGD$_2$ receptors, therefore, may represent a failsafe mechanism with considerable pathologic significance.

ACKNOWLEDGMENTS

This work supported by a grant from the Department of Health, Education and Welfare (HL 14890). A. M. S. was supported by an Advanced Predoctoral Grant from Pharmaceutical Manufacturers Association.

REFERENCES

1. Christ-Hazelhof, E., Nugteren, D. H., and Van Dorp, D. A. (1976): *Biochim. Biophys. Acta,* 450:450–461.
2. Gryglewski, R. S., Bunting, S., Moncada, S., Flower, R. J., and Vane, J. R. (1976): *Prostaglandins,* 12:685–713.
3. Mills, D. C. B., and Macfarlane, D. E. (1974): *Thromb. Res.,* 5:401–412.
4. Moncada, S., Vane, J. R., and Whittel, B. J. R. (1977): *J. Physiol. (Lond.),* 273:2P–4P.
5. Needleman, P., Raz, A., Ferrendelli, J. A., and Minkes, M. (1977): *Proc. Natl. Acad. Sci. USA,* 74:1716–1720.
6. Oelz, O., Oelz, R., Knapp, H. R., Sr., Sweetman, B. S., and Oates, J. A. (1977): *Prostaglandins,* 13:225–234.
7. Scatchard, G. (1950): *Ann. N.Y. Acad. Sci.,* 5:660–672.
8. Siegl, A. M., Smith, J. B., Silver, M. J., Nicolaou, K. C., and Ahern, D. (1979): *J. Clin. Invest.,* 63:215–220.
9. Smith, J. B., Silver, M. J., Ingerman, C. M., and Kocsis, J. J. (1974): *Thromb. Res.,* 5:291–299.
10. Tateson, J. E., Moncada, S., and Vane, J. R. (1977): *Prostaglandins,* 13:389–397.
11. Weksler, B. B., Lewy, C. W., and Jaffee, E. A. (1978): *J. Clin. Invest.,* 62:923–929.

Advances in Prostaglandin and Thromboxane Research,
Vol. 6, edited by B. Samuelsson, P. W. Ramwell,
and R. Paoletti. Raven Press, New York © 1980.

PGI₂ or PGE₂ Selectively Antagonize Responses to Excitatory PGs in Human Isolated Myometrium

G. J. Sanger and A. Bennett

Department of Surgery, King's College Hospital Medical School, Denmark Hill, London SE5 8RX, United Kingdom

The human myometrium can form various prostanoids and products of lipoxygenase (E. A. Willman and W. P. Collins, *personal communication;* C. N. Hensby, G. J. Sanger, I. F. Stamford, and A. Bennett, *unpublished*). Prostaglandins (PGs) D_2, E_2, or prostacyclin (PGI_2) may cause relaxation of the isolated myometrium, and PGI_2 can in addition antagonize contractions to $PGF_{2\alpha}$ without greatly affecting those to $BaCl_2$ (1,4; and A. Bennett and G. J. Sanger, *unpublished*). We have therefore studied the effects of PGE_2 and PGI_2 on contractions of the human isolated myometrium to acetylcholine (ACh), $PGF_{2\alpha}$ or U-46619, the $(15\text{-}S)$-hydroxy-$9\alpha,11\alpha$-(epoxymethano)prosta-5Z,13E-dienoic acid analog of PGH_2.

METHODS

Uterus was obtained from patients hysterectomized 1 to 11 days after the start of their last menstrual cycle for menorrhagia or fibroids. Myometrial strips, approximately $4 \times 4 \times 50$ mm were cut parallel to the uterine axis and used immediately or after overnight storage at 4°C in Krebs solution (NaCl, 7.1; $CaCl_2 \cdot 6H_2O$, 0.55; KH_2PO_4, 0.16; KCl, 0.35; $MgSO_4 \cdot 7H_2O$, 0.29, $NaHCO_3$, 2–1; dextrose, 1.0 g/liter) equilibrated with 5% CO_2 in O_2. Each strip was suspended under a load of 1 g in a 10-ml tissue bath containing normal Krebs solution or low-calcium Krebs solution to inhibit spontaneous muscle contractions ($CaCl_2 \cdot 6H_2O$, 0.02–0.11 g/liter; 37°C; 5% CO_2 in O_2). All drug concentrations are expressed as free acid or salt.

In each experiment, consistent, submaximal contractions to one PG ($PGF_{2\alpha}$, 20–500 ng/ml; U-46619, 5–300 ng/ml) were compared with approximately equal submaximal contractions to ACh (0.1–1.5 µg/ml), using 30-sec contact times and at least 5-min cycle times. Consistent responses to these doses were then obtained in the presence of PGE_2 or PGI_2. The results for seven experiments with each PG are expressed as medians and semiquartile ranges and analyzed using the Wilcoxon matched-pairs test.

RESULTS

In normal Krebs solution, PGI_2, 100 ng/ml to 10 μg/ml, inhibited spontaneous activity (3 tissues). The low-calcium concentration inhibited muscle activity and made relaxations difficult to detect, but sodium PGI_2, 1 μg/ml, either slightly reduced muscle tone or had no effect. PGE_2, 1 μg/ml, acted similarly, except that 3 out of 10 specimens initially contracted.

In low-calcium Krebs solution, sodium PGI_2, 1 μg/ml, resulted in mean reduced contractions to $PGF_{2\alpha}$ and U-46619 of 78 and 89%, respectively ($P = 0.05$; ranges: 7–95 and 57–100%, respectively), but no significant effect on those to ACh was observed (6% reduction; range, 21 to -11%). PGE_2 1 μg/ ml reduced contractions to $PGF_{2\alpha}$, U-46619, and ACh by 83, 89, and 50%, respectively (ranges: 76–97, 72–95, and 17–65%, respectively). The greater effect of PGE_2 on the agonist PGs compared with ACh was statistically significant ($p < 0.05$).

DISCUSSION

There have been many demonstrations that PGs can modulate the response to other substances, but there is little previous evidence that they can modulate the responses to each other. In rat isolated mesentery, PGE_1 reduced contractions to PGE_2 (2), but selectivity was not demonstrated. In the longitudinal muscle of human isolated stomach, PGI_2, 1 μg/ml, caused relaxation and reduced contractions to PGE_2 without greatly affecting those to ACh or U-46619 (A. Bennett and G. J. Sanger, *unpublished*).

Our results suggest that an imbalance of the types of PG formed might cause deranged uterine function. However, it may not be possible to predict this accurately from studies *in vitro,* as the effects of PGI_2 or PGE_2 on the human isolated myometrium may not always reflect their action *in vivo;* in normal nonpregnant women the uterus may relax to PGE_2 only during menses (3).

ACKNOWLEDGMENT

We thank the Medical Research Council (England) for support and The Wellcome Laboratories and The Upjohn Company Ltd. for PGs.

REFERENCES

1. Bygdeman, M. (1964): *Acta Physiol. Scand. (Suppl.* 242), 63:1–78.
2. Manku, M. S., Mtabayi, J. P., and Horrobin, D. F. (1977): *Prostaglandins,* 13:701–709.
3. Martin, J. N., Jr., Bygdeman, M., and Eneroth, P. (1978): *Acta Obstet. Gynecol. Scand.,* 57:141–147.
4. Omini, C., Pasargiklian, R., Foko, G. C., Fano, M., and Berti, F. (1978): *Prostaglandins,* 15:1045–1054.

Advances in Prostaglandin and Thromboxane Research,
Vol. 6, edited by B. Samuelsson, P. W. Ramwell,
and R. Paoletti. Raven Press, New York © 1980.

Prostaglandin-Specific Binding to Several Microsomal Fractions from Bovine Myometrium

Mary E. Carsten and *Jordan D. Miller

*Departments of Obstetrics and Gynecology and *Anesthesiology, School of Medicine,
University of California, Los Angeles, California 90024*

The first step in the action of prostaglandins (PGs) on the cellular level must be the binding of PGs to cellular components. Although PG binding to myometrial homogenates has been well documented (4), it is not known which cellular components are involved. The most likely sites are the cell membrane (CM) and the sarcoplasmic reticulum (SR). The latter is an intracellular calcium sink, which supplies at least part of the calcium for myometrial contraction. The remainder of the activator calcium enters the cell from outside.

To define the specific uterine binding site, a microsomal pellet was obtained from bovine uterine homogenates by differential centrifugation between 15,000 and 40,000 $\times$ g (1). Centrifugation on a discontinuous sucrose gradient of 24, 28, 33, and 45% sucrose in Spinco 27.1 rotor for 3 hr yielded protein bands at the interfaces as seen in Fig. 1. The protein homogenates were withdrawn with a syringe. Our data suggest that the 24 to 28% layer is largely SR, whereas the 28 to 33% and 33 to 45% layers exhibit CM properties. Characterization was by adenosine triphosphate (ATP)-dependent calcium accumulation and enzyme assays. ATP-dependent calcium binding is defined as the difference in calcium accumulation in the presence and absence of ATP from an incubation medium in 8 min at 37°C. Calcium is measured after centrifugation by atomic absorption spectroscopy (1). 5'-Nucleotidase served as a marker for CM (3). Table 1 shows that ATP-dependent calcium binding is highest in the 24 to 28% layer, whereas 5'-nucleotidase is highest in the 28 to 33% and 33 to 45% sucrose layers. For the purpose of this presentation the 24 to 28% layer will be called SR and the 28 to 33% and 33 to 45% layers will be called CM. Further documentation will be presented elsewhere.

To see which cell components would bind PGE_2 specifically, ^3H-PGE_2 was added to the 40,000 $\times$ g pellet in the absence and presence of unlabeled PGE_2 and allowed to equilibrate for 1 hr at room temperature. After centrifugation on a sucrose density gradient, radioactivity was counted in the protein layers. Since PGE_2 is equilibrated with the protein placed on the sucrose gradient and only a small fraction of the counts are expected to be bound, the free counts will diminish going down the gradient. The use of unlabeled ligand

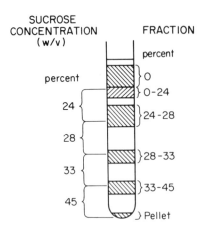

SUCROSE
CONCENTRATION
(w/v)

FRACTION

percent

percent
24
28
33
45

0
0–24
24–28
28–33
33–45
Pellet

FIG. 1. Diagram of discontinuous sucrose density gradient. **Left:** Original sucrose concentration. **Right:** Protein layers withdrawn at interfaces.

TABLE 1. *Characterization of layers from bovine myometrium[a]*

Layer (sucrose concentration, %)	ATP-dependent Ca binding (nmol Ca/mg protein/8 min)	5′-Nucleotidase (μmol P_i/mg protein/hr)
Initial	+10.5 ± 0.9	3.34 ± 0.91
0	—	0.87 ± 0.42
0–24	+8.3 ± 1.5	3.29 ± 0.81
24–28	+12.9 ± 0.4[b]	6.09 ± 1.02[b]
28–33	+7.4 ± 0.9[c]	13.92 ± 3.02[c]
33–45	+3.0 ± 1.1	16.24 ± 3.44
Pellet	+5.8 ± 5.9	5.82 ± 0.97

[a] Values shown are means ± SEM.
[b] $p < 0.001$.
[c] $p < 0.01$.

controls this phenomenon. Specific binding is therefore defined as the decrease in counts in the presence of excess unlabeled ligand. Table 2 shows that specific PGE_2 binding occurred almost uniformly in the 24 to 28%, the 28 to 33%, and the 33 to 45% layers, suggesting that both SR and CM bind PGE_2. However, only the SR exhibited statistically significant specific binding ($p < 0.05$).

Figure 2 illustrates PGE_2 binding to the SR fraction. Binding of ^3H-PGE_2 is carried out in the absence of unlabeled PGE_2 (total binding) and in the presence of unlabeled PGE_2 (nonspecific binding). The excess unlabeled PGE_2 (10 times highest ^3H-PGE_2) will saturate the high-affinity binding component, so that the remaining binding of labeled ligand is nonspecific (2). The difference in counts between total and nonspecific binding is proportional to the specific binding. This is based on the finding that nonspecific binding is not saturable, whereas specific binding reaches a limiting value, clearly demonstrated in Fig. 2.

TABLE 2. *Specific PGE$_2$ binding in sucrose density gradient layers, average of 7 experiments*

	PGE$_2$ concentration			
	1×10^{-10} M	5×10^{-9} M	Δ	Percent
Initial value	692[a]	668[a]	−24[a]	−3.3
Sucrose concentration (%)				
0	1,659	1,894	+235	+14.2
0–24	810	754	−56	−7.0
24–28 (SR)	259[b]	129[b]	−130	−50.5
28–33 ⎫ (CM)	271	96	−175	−64.6
33–45 ⎭	208	59	−149	−71.8
Pellet	125	49	−76	−61.0

[a] cpm/mg protein (bound and free).
[b] $p < 0.05$, by paired comparison.

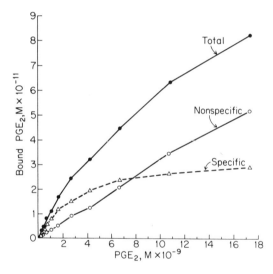

FIG. 2. ^{3}H-PGE$_2$ binding to SR fraction from bovine myometrium.

To futher explore specific PGE$_2$ binding, experiments were carried out with the starting material (15–40,000 $\times$ g pellet), the SR and CM fractions, combining the 28 to 33% and 33 to 45% fractions. Figure 3 presents the data in form of Scatchard plots for a representative experiment. The dissociation constant for SR is 3.57×10^{-9} M, and the number of binding sites is 3.65×10^{-11} mol/g protein. CM showed very similar results, i.e., $K_d = 3.96 \times 10^{-9}$ M and 2.9×10^{-11} mol/g binding sites. The initial protein again had a similar K_d but fewer binding sites per gram protein. Table 3 shows the dissociation constants and number

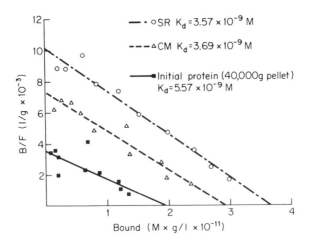

FIG. 3. Scatchard plots of specific PGE_2 binding: B, concentration of ^3H-PGE_2 bound; F, concentration of ^3H-PGE_2 free.

TABLE 3. *Dissociation constants and binding sites for PGE_2 specific binding[a]*

	K_d (M)	Number of binding sites (m/g)	Number of experiments
40,000 × g pellet	$3.07 \pm 1.11 \times 10^{-9}$	$1.69 \pm 0.35 \times 10^{-11}$	3
SR	$2.62 \pm 0.37 \times 10^{-9}$	$3.55 \pm 0.10 \times 10^{-11}$	4
CM	$2.60 \pm 0.49 \times 10^{-9}$	$4.15 \pm 0.85 \times 10^{-11}$	4

[a] Values shown are means $\pm$ S.E.M.

of binding sites, averaged for several experiments. The similarity of the dissociation constants suggests that the PGE_2 receptor in the SR, the CM, and the initial protein (40,000 × g pellet) are the same. However, the increase in the number of binding sites from the initial protein to CM and SR indicates purification of the receptor.

CONCLUSIONS

Specific PGE_2 binding was demonstrated in a sucrose density gradient, which produced separation of SR and CM. The affinity of PGE_2 binding was the same in the SR and CM layers. A more detailed study of the isolated SR and CM layers confirmed these results. The initial protein and the SR and CM preparations had the same K_d, which means that a single receptor is present in both SR and CM fractions. A comparable number of binding sites were observed in SR and CM preparations. Whether PG receptors are present inherently in both SR and CM cannot be ascertained until determination of the purity of the fractions and specific binding studies are done in the same experiment. This is necessitated by the variable purity of the fractions from experiment to experiment. The increase in the number of binding sites over the initial protein is due to purification of the PGE_2 receptor.

ACKNOWLEDGMENTS

This investigation was supported by Grant HD-00010, NICHD. The authors are indebted to Stephen Strann for assistance and to The Upjohn Company for the generous supply of PGs.

REFERENCES

1. Carsten, M. E., and Miller, J. D. (1977): *J. Biol. Chem.*, 252:1576–1581.
2. Chamness, G. C., and McGuire, W. L. (1975): *Steroids*, 26:538–542.
3. Chang, K. J., Bennet, V., and Cuatrecasas, P. (1975): *J. Biol. Chem.*, 250:488–500.
4. Kimball, F. A., Kirton, K. T., Spilman, C. H., and Wyngarden, L. J. (1975): *Biol. Reprod.*, 13:482–489.

Advances in Prostaglandin and Thromboxane Research,
Vol. 6, edited by B. Samuelsson, P. W. Ramwell,
and R. Paoletti. Raven Press, New York © 1980.

Prostaglandin Receptor: Induction of Density Changes in Rat Liver Plasma Membrane

Maureen G. Rice, *John R. McRae, and R. Paul Robertson

Division of Clinical Pharmacology, University of Washington, and *Veterans Administration
Medical Center, Seattle, Washington 98108

Prostaglandins (PGs) of the E series have been reported to increase hepatic glucose production (3) and circulating glucose levels (2). It has been reported that PGE binds to liver plasma membranes (5) and stimulates adenylate cyclase (1). An important consideration in studies of hormone action is determining whether alterations in the level of endogenous ligand result in reciprocal changes in the density of binding sites. The purpose of this study was to investigate the relationship between endogenous PGE *in vivo* and regulation of PGE binding sites on rat liver plasma membranes.

METHODS

All studies were performed on littermate pairs of male Sprague-Dawley rats. Plasma membranes were isolated from liver using sucrose density gradients as previously described (5). Identification of the membrane fraction was confirmed by electron microscopy, 5'-nucleotidase, and adenylate cyclase activity. All binding studies were performed using 500 μg of membrane protein. ^{3}H-PGE$_1$ (4,000 dpm; 87 Ci/mM) and various concentrations of cold PGE$_2$ were incubated for 30 min at 37°C. Nonspecific binding was defined as the amount of bound ^{3}H-PGE$_1$ not displaced by excess unlabeled ligand.

In order to study down-regulation, rats were treated with PGE$_2$; however, since native PGE is rapidly degraded *in vivo*, the 16,16-dimethyl-PGE$_2$ (DiM) analog, which has been shown not to be a substrate for the 15-OH-dehydrogenase, was used. This analog competes for PGE binding sites identically with PGE$_1$ and PGE$_2$ and has essentially the same dissociation constant. In order to study up-regulation, rats were treated with the PG synthesis inhibitors, aspirin, or indomethacin for 4 days. To determine whether these inhibitors were effective in lowering endogenous PG levels, plasma concentrations of 13,14-dihydroxy-15-keto-PGE$_2$ (DHK-PGE$_2$) were measured in treated rats.

RESULTS AND DISCUSSION

Plasma membranes in this system have binding sites which are specific for PGEs. PGE_1 and PGE_2, as well as DiM, compete identically for binding sites, all having K_D of approximately 5×10^{-9} M. Other PGs tested, including PGA_1, PGB_1, and $PGF_{2\alpha}$, did not compete effectively at the concentrations examined. Although prostacyclin has been reported to share binding sites with PGE on platelets, it did not compete effectively for PGE binding sites in liver. When the binding data were analyzed by the method of Scatchard (4), which examines the relationship between the PGE specifically bound and the bound to free ratio, a straight line was generated. The linearity of this plot ($r = 0.97$) indicates a single class of binding sites.

Since the intercept from a Scatchard plot represents binding site density, this value can be used to determine whether alterations in available PG *in vivo* will result in compensatory changes in binding site density. In order to increase available PGE, pairs of rats were treated *in vivo* with either 50 μg of its DiM analog or the diluent. The rats were sacrificed and the plasma membranes isolated. When the binding data for control and experimental rats were examined, it was found that membranes from control rats ($n = 4$) initially bound 33 $\pm$ 2%, while membranes from experimental rats ($n = 4$) bound only 21 $\pm$ 2% of the available ^{3}H-PGE_1. Control membranes bound more PG than experimental membranes at all concentrations of cold PG up to 1,000 pg; however, nonspecific binding was identical for both groups. When the data were analyzed by the Scatchard method, the binding data for control and experimental rats generated two parallel lines. Since the slopes were identical, treatment with DiM did not change the affinity for PGE (control $K_A = 5.1 \times 10^8$ M; experimental $K_A = 4.7 \times 10^8$ M). In contrast, the DiM treatment resulted in a 37% decrease in the number of binding sites compared to control. It appears, therefore, that increased levels of available PGE *in vivo* result in decreased numbers, or down-regulation, of PGE binding sites.

The opposite hypothesis, i.e., that decreased endogenous PGE would result in increased numbers of PGE binding sites (up-regulation), was also examined. The efficiency of aspirin or indomethacin in lowering endogenous PGE levels was examined in rats with chronically implanted jugular catheters. Plasma levels of DHK-PGE_2 were obtained before and during 4 days of treatment so that each rat served as its own control. Both drugs lowered DHK-PGE_2 levels to 50% of control by day 2 and levels remained low throughout the study.

Membranes from treated rats and their paired controls were subjected to binding studies and Scatchard analysis. Aspirin treatment resulted in a 38% increase in the number of binding sites compared to control. Additionally, plasma membranes from aspirin-treated rats had a larger K_A than control. These changes were not observed if plasma membranes were treated with aspirin *in vitro*. Membranes from indomethacin-treated rats also showed a 40% increased density of PGE binding sites when compared to their paired controls. In contrast to aspirin treatment, indomethacin treatment resulted in a decreased affinity constant. As with aspirin, indomethacin *in vitro* did not change the characteristics of the binding.

In conclusion, changes in available PG *in vivo* result in compensatory and reciprocal changes in the density of PG binding sites. The alterations in affinity induced by aspirin and indomethacin may be unrelated to the decrement in endogenous PGE but rather separate non-PG effects of the drugs.

REFERENCES

1. Okamura, N., and Terayama, H. (1977): *Biochim. Biophys. Acta,* 465:54–67.
2. Robertson, R. P., and Chen, M. (1977): *J. Clin. Invest.,* 60:747–753.
3. Sacca, L., Perez, G., Rengo, F., and Condorelli, M. (1974): *Diabetes,* 23:532–535.
4. Scatchard, G. (1949): *Ann. N.Y. Acad. Sci.,* 51:660–672.
5. Smigel, M., and Fleischer, S. (1974): *Biochim. Biophys. Acta,* 332:358–373.

Advances in Prostaglandin and Thromboxane Research,
Vol. 6, edited by B. Samuelsson, P. W. Ramwell,
and R. Paoletti. Raven Press, New York © 1980.

Fenalcomine Hydrochloride Inhibits the Action of PG on the Smooth Muscle but Stimulates That of TXA₂

Pham Huu Chanh, A. Pham Huu Chanh, and M. Nguyen van Thoai, and In Sokan

E.R. 164 C.N.R.S. Institut de Physiologie, F- 31400 Toulouse, France

It has been demonstrated that the metabolism of arachidonic acid results not only in prostaglandins (PGs), but also in thromboxanes (TXs) and prostacyclin (PGI_2). These products present different, often opposing, pharmacological properties. These compounds are very active, and not always beneficially so; indeed, they are sometimes harmful. For these reasons, much research has been carried out in order to find the antagonists and stimulants of their biosynthesis and their effects on their receptors. The most well-known discoveries were those of Vane on the antiinflammatory agents (8).

In the field of the research on the inhibitors of the biosynthesis and of the receptors of PGs and derivatives, we have demonstrated that fenalcomine hydrochloride (FH), 2[N-[β-(4-(α-hydroxypropyl)phenoxy)ethyl]amino]1-phenylpropane, antagonized the effects of PGE_2 and $PGF_{2\alpha}$ on the smooth muscle.

The present study was undertaken to reassess the effects of FH on the biosynthesis of PGs and TXA_2, as well as on their activities on smooth muscle.

MATERIALS AND METHODS

Biosynthesis of PGs, PG endoperoxides, and TXA_2 was achieved using two methods. In the first, rabbit lung extract was incubated with Na arachidonate (5). In the second bovine seminal vesicle microsomes (BSVM, 200–300 μg protein) were incubated without cofactors with sodium arachidonate (AA, 5 μg) at room temperature (22°C) for 3 min. This resulted in products that behaved like PGs, contracting rat stomach strips (RSS) and rat colon (RC), and PG endoperoxides (PGG_2, PGH_2), which were measured by the contractile responses of thoracic aorta strips. Further incubation of PG endoperoxides with horse platelet microsomes (200–250 μg protein) for 30 sec at 0°C yielded a TXA_2-like product (3): its contractile effects on rabbit thoracic aorta strips were more powerful than those of PG endoperoxides (5).

Biological characterization of PGs, PG endoperoxides, and TXA_2 was carried out by the cascade method (7) using RC, RSS, and spiral strips of rabbit thoracic aorta (RbAo) continuously superfused at 10 ml/min with oxygenated Krebs solution (5% CO_2, 95% O_2) at 37°C.

The Krebs solution contained a mixture of pharmacological antagonists (mepyramine maleate, 1×10^{-7} g/ml; hyoscine bromide, 1×10^{-7} g/ml; propranolol hydrochloride, 2×10^{-6} g/ml; phenoxybenzamine hydrochloride, 1×10^{-7} g/ml; and methylsergide bimaleate, 2×10^{-7} g/ml) to make the assay specific for PGs. Indomethacin (1 μg/ml) was also added to the superfusion medium to prevent PG biosynthesis by the assay tissues (8).

The lung extract was prepared according to Svensson et al. (5): 2 g of rabbit lung was chopped and homogenized in 5 ml of ice-cold 0.1 M potassium phosphate buffer, pH 7.4, and centrifuged for 12 min at 8,000 × g; the supernatant contained mainly microsomal and soluble fractions.

BSVM were prepared as described by Takeguchi et al. (6): 80 g of bovine seminal vesicles were trimmed of their adjacent tissues, chopped, and homogenized in 150 ml of ice-cold 0.1 M phosphate buffer pH 8.0. The homogenate was centrifuged for 10 min at 12,000 × g. The supernatant was filtered through a cheesecloth and centrifuged for 1 hr at 105,000 × g. The pellet was resuspended in phosphate buffer (5 mM, pH 7.5–8.0), redistributed in small tubes, lyophilized, and stored in a freezer.

Horse platelet-rich plasma was centrifuged for 15 min at 2,000 × g. The pellet containing platelets were resuspended in ice-cold saline (0.9% NaCl) solution and subjected to shell freezing and thawing (5 times) and again centrifuged for 15 min at 8,000 × g to remove cell debris. The supernatant was centrifuged for 45 min at 100,000 × g. The pellet was resuspended in 5 ml phosphate buffer, lyophilized, and stored in a freezer (1).

The protein from each sample of BSVM and of horse platelet microsomes (HPM) was determined by the method of Lowry et al. (2).

RESULTS

Incubation of BSVM with FH in concentrations ranging from 1×10^{-8} to 1×10^{-4} M before addition of sodium arachidonate did not provoke any change in the quantities of PG- and endoperoxide-like products. On the contrary, indomethacin (1 μg/ml) totally inhibited the formation of these compounds. Neither FH nor indomethacin, added to HPM before incubation with PG endoperoxides, significantly changed the quantities of PGs and TXA₂ formed, however. The same results were obtained from incubation of lung extract with AA.

When infused over the assay tissues for 10 min prior to testing the effects of preformed TXA₂ and PGs, FH greatly modified the action of these compounds on their receptors: this action varied according to the product under consideration (Fig. 1). In fact, FH inhibited the action of PGs on the smooth muscle, as was previously demonstrated (4): it was more active against PGF₂α than PGE₂. The concentration of FH necessary to inhibit 50% of the effect of PGF₂α

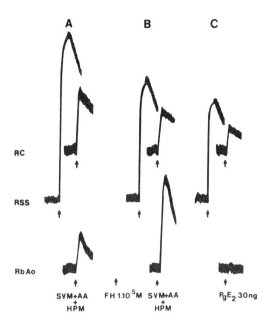

FIG. 1. Effects of FH, infused over the assay tissues, on the action of preformed PGs and TXA$_2$ on the smooth muscle. SVM (250 μg protein) were incubated in 500 μl of phosphate buffer (50 mM, pH 8.0) with 5 μg of AA at room temperature for 3 min; then HPM were added, and the mixture was tested on the cascade: PG- and TXA$_2$-like activities were measured by the contractile response of the tissue. FH at 1×10^{-5} M stimulated the TXA$_2$-like activity and inhibited the PG-like activity. PGE$_2$ at 30 ng contracted RSS but had no action on RbAo.

is 2.21×10^{-4} M and that necessary to inhibit 25% of the effect of PGE$_2$ is 2.58×10^{-4} M. In contrast, FH stimulated the effects of TXA$_2$ on RbAo: the concentration necessary to enhance the action of TXA$_2$ by 50% is 9.75×10^{-5} M (Fig. 2).

These effects were cencentration dependent. The correlation coefficient was 0.99 ($p \le 0.01$) for PGF$_{2\alpha}$, PGE$_2$, and TXA$_2$.

CONCLUSION

In the experimental conditions adopted, it therefore appeared that FH, in the concentrations studied, manifested no action on PG, nor on PG endoperoxide synthetase, in contrast to indomethacin. Furthermore, FH had no effect on TX synthetase.

The present experiments have confirmed the results previously obtained. In fact, it has been demonstrated that with synthetic PGs, FH antagonized the contractile effect of PGE$_2$ and PGF$_{2\alpha}$ on the smooth muscle: FH was more effective on the action of PGF$_{2\alpha}$ than on that of PGE$_2$. But only the antagonism between FH and PGE$_2$ was competitive. Moreover, the replacement of its second-

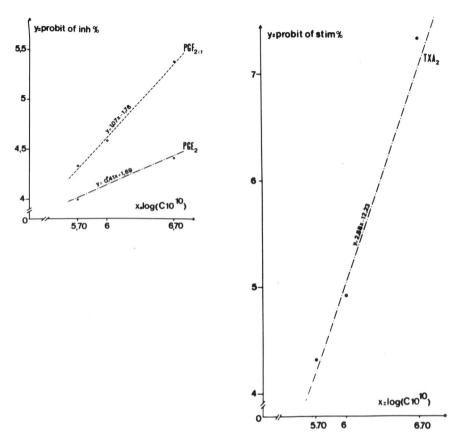

FIG. 2. Effects of FH, infused over the assay tissues, on the action of preformed PGF$_{2\alpha}$ and PGE$_2$ **(left, inhibition)** and of TXA$_2$ **(right, stimulation)** on smooth muscle. Ordinates: Probit of inhibition percentages of PG-like effects **(left)** or of stimulation percentages of TXA$_2$-like effects **(right)** on smooth muscle. Abscissas: concentrations of FH. (Number of experiments for each concentration of FH = 5.)

ary alcoholic function by a ketonic function suppressed the competitive anti-PGE$_2$ activity of FH and reinforced its antispasmodic action (4).

In contrast, FH has been shown to stimulate the TXA$_2$-like effects on the smooth muscle; this activity was powerful and concentration dependent.

At this stage of our research, it is not possible for us to draw conclusions either on the action mechanism of FH or on the relationship between these actions and the pharmacological properties of FH.

However, due to its particular properties, FH could be used in the future as a pharmacological tool which may reveal some new activities of PGs and TX in physiology and pathophysiology. It could be for us a new way to determine the mechanism of action of drugs.

ACKNOWLEDGMENT

This work was supported by grants from Dēlégation Générale pour la Recherche Scientifique et Technique and Fondation pour la Recherche Médicale. We are grateful to Mrs. M. Laroche, PDG of Laboratories Laroche-Navarron, Paris; Dr. John E. Pike of The Upjohn Co., Kalamazoo, Michigan; and to Dr. J. C. Le Douarec of Merck, Sharp & Dohm Laboratories, Clermont-Ferrand, for the generous gifts of respectively FH, PGs, and indomethacin.

REFERENCES

1. Eakins, K. E., and Kulkarni, P. S. (1977): *Br. J. Pharmacol.,* 60:135–140.
2. Lowry, O. H., Rosebrough, N. J., Farr, A. L., and Randall, R. J. (1951): *J. Biol. Chem.,* 193:265–275.
3. Moncada, S., Needleman, P., Bunting, S., and Vane, J. R. (1976): *Prostaglandins,* 12:323–335.
4. Pham Huu Chanh, and Pham Huu Chanh, A. (1979): *IRCS Med. Sci.,* 7:103.
5. Svensson, J., Hamberg, M., and Samuelsson, B. (1975): *Acta Physiol. Scand.,* 94:222–228.
6. Takeguchi, C., Kohno, E., and Sih, C. J. (1971): *Biochemistry,* 10:2372–2376.
7. Vane, J. R. (1964): *Br. J. Pharmacol.,* 23:360–373.
8. Vane, J. R. (1971): *Nature* [*New Biol.*], 231:232–235.

Advances in Prostaglandin and Thromboxane Research,
Vol. 6, edited by B. Samuelsson, P. W. Ramwell,
and R. Paoletti. Raven Press, New York © 1980.

Biochemical and Pharmacological Evaluation of Thromboxane Synthetase Inhibitors

Robert R. Gorman

Experimental Biology Research, The Upjohn Company, Kalamazoo, Michigan 49001

Since the discovery by Hamberg et al. (7) that human platelets convert the prostaglandin endoperoxide (PGG_2) into a labile ($t_{1/2} = 32$ sec) proaggregatory molecule thromboxane A_2 (TXA_2), researchers have sought compounds that could selectively inhibit the biological activity of TXA_2. This end may be achieved in two different ways: (a) the synthesis of TXA_2 can be blocked by inhibiting the TXA_2 synthetase, or (b) a compound could be a receptor-level antagonist of TXA_2. It is impossible to predict which molecule would be more useful as a biological probe, but as a therapeutic agent, a case can be made that favors the development of a TXA_2 synthetase inhibitor. The rationale for this is outlined in Fig. 1. The human platelet can synthesize only the proaggregatory and vaso-constrictive TXA_2, while the vessel wall can synthesize only the vasodilator and antiaggregatory PGI_2. Under normal circumstances, the balance between these two PGs controls human platelet aggregation through the "reciprocal regulation" of platelet cyclic adenosine monophosphate (cAMP) levels (3). In certain pathological states, PGI_2 synthesis could be impaired, and TXA_2 would become the dominating force, inducing both thrombotic episodes and vasocon-striction. A TXA_2 synthetase inhibitor would allow PGH_2 to accumulate, escape the platelet, and be converted to PGI_2 by the vessel wall. Although this model employs platelet–blood vessel interactions, the same mechanism could be useful in other circumstances as well. A typical example is the human lung. TXA_2 is a potent constrictor of airways, while PGI_2 dilates airways. During respiratory distress, a TXA_2 synthetase inhibitor would be useful by diverting PGH_2 from TXA_2 toward PGI_2 synthesis.

A number of molecules have been reported to be TXA_2 synthetase inhibitors (2,5,10), one a receptor-level antagonist of TXA_2 (1) and another seeming to have a mixed activity that includes both enzyme inhibition and receptor-level antagonism (12). Unfortunately, of all the reported compounds, few have been properly evaluated. In this chapter I will describe methods by which a compound can be evaluated as a potential TXA_2 synthetase inhibitor or antagonist and attempt to establish criteria which should be met before a compound is admitted to the literature. If these criteria are rigorously followed, the literature will not become unnecessarily confused with erroneous reports of TXA_2 synthetase

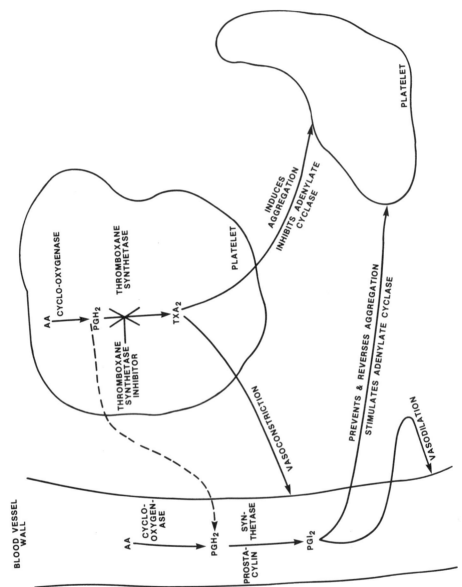

FIG. 1. Regulation of human platelet aggregation by PGI_2 and TXA_2.

inhibitors or antagonists which are really cyclooxygenase inhibitors or stimulators of cyclic AMP accumulation.

EVALUATION OF TXA$_2$ SYNTHETASE INHIBITORS AND RECEPTOR-LEVEL ANTAGONISTS

The most complete method of evaluating whether or not a compound is a potential TXA$_2$ synthetase inhibitor and/or a TXA$_2$ receptor-level antagonist is through the use of a combination of analytical and bioassay techniques.

The most direct analytical assessment of a potential inhibitor is by radioimmunoassay of *both* TXB$_2$ and PGE$_2$ during arachidonic acid-induced human platelet aggregation in platelet-rich plasma (PRP). Radiographic thin-layer chromatography of the products formed from [1-^{14}C]arachidonate (AA) is also acceptable. TXA$_2$ synthetase inhibitors that do not influence the cyclooxygenase give a characteristic pattern in platelets aggregated with AA. As TXA$_2$ synthesis is inhibited, the production of PGE$_2$ increases (Table 1). Any agent that suppresses both PGE$_2$ and TXB$_2$ synthesis from AA should be suspected as a possible cyclooxygenase inhibitor. These techniques in intact platelets have two marked advantages over experiments done in microsomes or purified enzyme preparations. Only those compounds that actually penetrate the cell membrane will be active, and cyclooxygenase inhibitors can be eliminated.

When a compound has been found that inhibits TXB$_2$ synthesis but elevates PGE$_2$ production, one can be almost certain that it is a TXA$_2$ synthetase inhibitor. A final check is done using the endoperoxides (PGH$_2$ or PGG$_2$) to induce human platelet aggregation in PRP. There are now several easily reproduced methods for endoperoxide synthesis (4,6,11).

A typical final analysis using PGH$_2$ is shown in Fig. 2. PGH$_2$ induces a

TABLE 1. *Influence of TXA$_2$ synthetase inhibitors and TXA$_2$ receptor-level antagonists on TXB$_2$ and PGE$_2$ synthesis from AA[a]*

Time (sec)	Control (ng/ml)		Azo analog I (ng/ml)		9,11 E.I.P. (ng/ml)	
	PGE$_2$	TXB$_2$	PGE$_2$	TXB$_2$	PGE$_2$	TXB$_2$
30	3	14	3	3	3	13
60	3	22	8	8	5	25
90	5	140	23	8	5	146
120	8	213	35	26	9	212
150	10	275	58	41	12	278
180	12	282	63	54	12	288
210	13	284	77	62	14	290
240	15	288	74	77	16	286

[a] Human PRP was incubated for 2 min at 37°C with either 5.6 µM azo analog I, or 5.6 µM 9,11 E.I.P. The platelets were then exposed to 1.3 mM AA and 50-µl samples removed every 30 sec for TXB$_2$ and PGE$_2$ analysis by radioimmunoassay. Control response corresponds to platelets that received only AA.

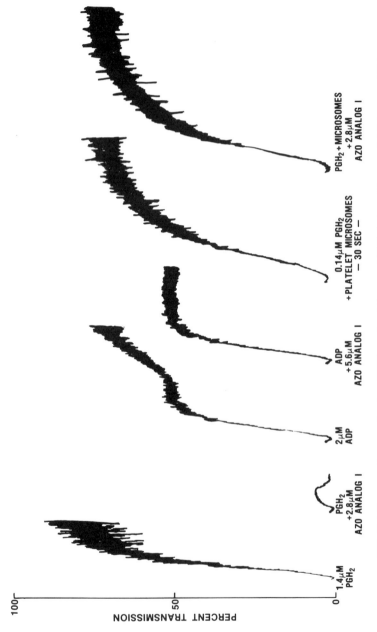

FIG. 2. Influence of azo analog I on PGH₂-, epinephrine-, and TXA₂-induced human platelet aggregation.

PGH₂+MICROSOMES
+2.8μM
AZO ANALOG I

0.14μM PGH₂
+PLATELET MICROSOMES
— 30 SEC —

ADP
+5.6μM
AZO ANALOG I

2μM
ADP

PGH₂
+2.8μM
AZO ANALOG I

1.4μM
PGH₂

100

50

0

PERCENT TRANSMISSION

marked aggregation, and preincubation of platelets with 9,11-azoprosta-5,13-dienoic acid (azo analog I) blocks the PGH_2 response. This is suggestive of a useful inhibitor. However, it is possible that the compound could elevate cyclic AMP, and any agent that elevates cyclic AMP blocks PGH_2-induced aggregation (8).

An easy way to evaluate for cyclic AMP elevation is to use either epinephrine or adenosine diphosphate (ADP) to aggregate platelets. These two agonists induce distinctive first and second waves of aggregation. An agent that elevates cyclic AMP blocks *both* the first and second wave of epinephrine- or ADP-induced aggregation. PGI_2 is an example of this class of compound. A molecule that selectively blocks TXA_2 synthesis will inhibit *only* the second wave of aggregation, and not antagonize aggregation induced by exogenously added TXA_2 (Fig. 2). When a compound blocks both PGH_2-induced aggregation and the second wave of ADP or epinephrine and does not antagonize exogenous TXA_2, there is unequivocal evidence that the compound is a TXA_2 synthetase inhibitor.

If desired, the TXA_2 synthetase inhibitor can also be used to block the synthesis of rabbit aorta contracting activity (RCS). Using the technique of Needleman et al. (9), incubation of human platelet microsomes (HPM) with PGH_2 results in the formation of a potent labile RCS (Fig. 3). Incubation of HPM with the TXA_2 synthetase inhibitor blocks the RCS formed from PGH_2 + HPM. In summation, the profile of activities of a selective TXA_2 synthetase inhibitor are as follows:

1. attenuates AA-induced aggregation and blocks TXA_2 synthesis but elevates PGE_2 levels;
2. blocks PGH_2-induced aggregation;
3. selectively blocks the second wave of ADP- or epinephrine-induced aggregation;
4. does not block aggregation induced by exogenously added TXA_2; and
5. blocks the synthesis of RCS activity from PGH_2 + HPM.

Using the same protocol that we followed with the TXA_2 synthetase inhibitor (azo analog I), we will evaluate a second compound 9,11-epoxyimino-5,13-dienoic acid (9,11 E.I.P). This compound will clearly demonstrate the necessity of evaluating a potential inhibitor in several different systems. Analytical evaluation of an AA-induced aggregation in the presence of increasing concentrations of 9,11 E.I.P. shows that although AA-induced aggregation is attenuated by 9,11 E.I.P., there is no inhibition of either PGE_2 or TXB_2 synthesis (Table 1). These data show that 9,11 E.I.P. is not a cyclooxygenase inhibitor or a TXA_2 synthetase inhibitor, but does influence aggregation of human platelets. These data suggest 9,11 E.I.P. either is a receptor-level antagonist of TXA_2 or increases platelet cyclic AMP levels.

Bioassay of 9,11 E.I.P. in human platelets gives the following profile of actives. PGH_2-induced aggregation is blocked by 9,11 E.I.P. as is the second wave of epinephrine- and ADP-induced aggregation (eliminates cyclic AMP) (Fig. 4). The use of exogenously generated TXA_2 is also antagonized by 9,11 E.I.P.,

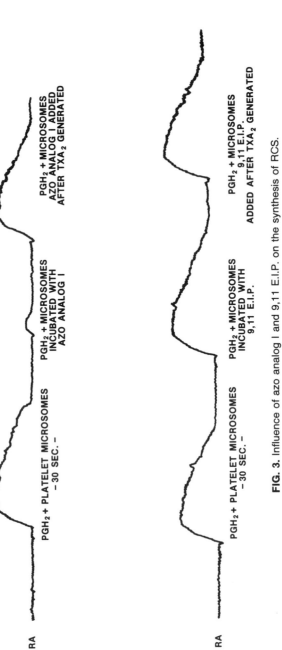

RA

PGH₂ + PLATELET MICROSOMES — 30 SEC. —

PGH₂ + MICROSOMES INCUBATED WITH AZO ANALOG I

PGH₂ + MICROSOMES AZO ANALOG I ADDED AFTER TXA₂ GENERATED

RA

PGH₂ + PLATELET MICROSOMES — 30 SEC. —

PGH₂ + MICROSOMES INCUBATED WITH 9,11 E.I.P.

PGH₂ + MICROSOMES 9,11 E.I.P. ADDED AFTER TXA₂ GENERATED

FIG. 3. Influence of azo analog I and 9,11 E.I.P. on the synthesis of RCS.

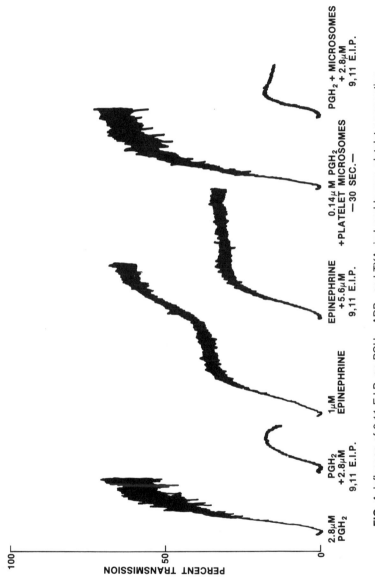

PERCENT TRANSMISSION

2.8μM PGH₂

PGH₂ +2.8μM 9,11 E.I.P.

1μM EPINEPHRINE

EPINEPHRINE +5.6μM 9,11 E.I.P.

EPINEPHRINE 0.14μM PGH₂ +PLATELET MICROSOMES —30 SEC.—

PGH₂ + MICROSOMES +2.8μM 9,11 E.I.P.

FIG. 4. Influence of 9,11 E.I.P. on PGH₂-, ADP-, and TXA₂-induced human platelet aggregation.

finishing a series of biological responses that would be consistent with TXA_2 receptor-level antagonism. RCS synthesis is not blocked by 9,11 E.I.P., and this is also consistent with receptor-level antagonism of TXA_2 and inconsistent with either cyclooxygenase or TXA_2 synthetase inhibition.

The profile of activities for a selective TXA_2 receptor-level antagonist are as follows:

1. attenuates AA-induced aggregation but does not influence either TXB_2 or PGE_2 synthesis in human PRP;
2. blocks PGH_2-induced aggregation;
3. blocks selectively the second wave of epinephrine- and ADP-induced aggregation;
4. blocks aggregation induced by exogenously added TXA_2; and
5. *does not* block the synthesis of RCS activity from PGH_2 + HPM.

DISCUSSION

Through a combination of bioassay and biochemical measurements in intact cells compounds can be easily evaluated as possible TXA_2 synthetase inhibitors and/or as TXA_2 receptor-level antagonists. The use of only part of the evaluation scheme is not sufficient. The minimum standards which should be met are summarized in Table 2.

There are, of course, several other refinements which can be evaluated. Does the compound block PGI_2 synthesis and antagonize the effect of TXA_2 on isolated arteries. And there is the question of whether TXA_2 synthetase inhibitors block PGH_2-induced aggregation, still a controversial issue. However, in our hands, we have never found a TXA_2 synthetase inhibitor that is devoid of intrinsic agonist activity that does not block PGH_2-induced aggregation. Irrespective of minor disagreements, if the above criteria are rigorously followed, few mistakes in data interpretation will be made, and this entire field of research will be put on a more solid scientific basis.

TABLE 2. *Minimum standards that TXA₂ synthetase inhibitors should meet*

Action	TXA_2 synthetase inhibitor	TXA_2 receptor-level antagonist
Blocks TXB_2 synthesis from AA	+	−
Does not inhibit PGE_2 synthesis from AA	+	+
Attenuates both PGH_2- and AA-induced aggregation	+	+
Blocks RCS synthesis from PGH_2 + HPM	+	−
Blocks aggregation by exogenously added TXA_2	−	+

REFERENCES

1. Fitzpatrick, F. A., Bundy, G. L., Gorman, R. R., and Honohan, T. (1978): *Nature,* 275:4230–4231.
2. Gorman, R. R., Bundy, G. L., Peterson, D. C., Sun, F. F., Miller, O. V., and Fitzpatrick, F. A. (1977): *Proc. Natl. Acad. Sci. USA,* 74:4007–4011.
3. Gorman, R. R., Fitzpatrick, F. A., and Miller, O. V. (1978): *Advances in Cyclic Nucleotide Research,* Vol. 9, edited by W. J. George and L. J. Iguarro, pp. 597–609. Raven Press, New York.
4. Gorman, R. R., Sun, F. F., Miller, O. V., and Johnson, R. A. (1977): *Prostaglandins,* 13:1043–1053.
5. Gryglewski, R., Zmuda, A., Korbut, R., Kverioch, E., and Beiron, K. (1978): *Nature,* 267:627–628.
6. Hamberg, M., and Samuelsson, B. (1973): *Proc. Natl. Acad. Sci. USA,* 70:899–903.
7. Hamberg, M., Svensson, J., and Samuelsson, B. (1975): *Proc. Natl. Acad. Sci. USA,* 72:2994–2998.
8. Miller, O. V., and Gorman, R. R. (1976): *J. Cyclic Nucleotide Res.,* 2:79–87.
9. Needleman, P., Moncada, S., Bunting, S., Vane, J. R., Hamberg, M., and Samuelsson, B. (1976): *Nature,* 261:558–560.
10. Needleman, P., Raz, A., Ferrendelli, J., and Minkes, M. (1977): *Proc. Natl. Acad. Sci. USA,* 74:1716–1720.
11. Nugteren, D. H., and Hazelhof, E. (1973): *Biochim. Biophys. Acta,* 326:448–461.
12. Venton, D. L., Enke, S., and LeBreton, G. C. (1979): *J. Med. Chem. (in press).*

Advances in Prostaglandin and Thromboxane Research,
Vol. 6, edited by B. Samuelsson, P. W. Ramwell,
and R. Paoletti. Raven Press, New York © 1980.

Synthesis and Biological Properties of Selective Inhibitors of the Prostaglandin Cascade

Josef Fried, J. Barton, S. Kittisopikul, Philip Needleman, and
A. Wyche

*Department of Chemistry, University of Chicago, Chicago, Illinois 60637; and Department
of Pharmacology, Washington University, St. Louis, Missouri 63110*

Selective inhibitors of the individual enzymes involved in the prostaglandin (PG) cascade have been of considerable interest because of their potential value both as probes to answer questions of mechanism and as potential therapeutic agents. Our own interest in this subject, which dates back several years (2), has been rekindled following the discovery of prostacyclin (PGI_2) and thromboxane A_2 (TXA_2), as well as of the enzymes responsible for their formation, PGI_2 synthetase and PG endoperoxide TX isomerase. Of particular interest are inhibitors of the latter enzyme, and a number of interesting inhibitors of that enzyme have recently been reported (3,4).

SYNTHESIS

Two approaches to the problem are described, one involving stable carbocyclic analogs of TXA_2 and the second involving 8,12-seco-PGs, which may be viewed as straight-chain fatty acid derivatives possessing PG-like functionality at appropriate positions. Others have reported on the synthesis and PG-like properties of 11,12-seco-PGs (1).

The synthesis of the first class of substances is shown in Figs. 1 and 2. Starting materials are the readily available naturally occurring monoterpenes (+) α-pinene and (−) β-pinene. These are ideally suited to produce the target products in chiral form of the absolute configuration present in the natural PGs. The choice of the oxygen-containing lower side chain was predicated on our earlier findings that the presence of such simple side chains favored inhibitory over agonist properties (2).

The synthesis of the straight-chain 8,12-seco-PG analogs is shown in Figs. 3 and 4. The target compounds include both those in which the fully developed eight-carbon side chain has been incorporated (Fig. 3) and others possessing simpler alkyl substituents (Fig. 4). The synthetic routes are clearly evident from these charts.

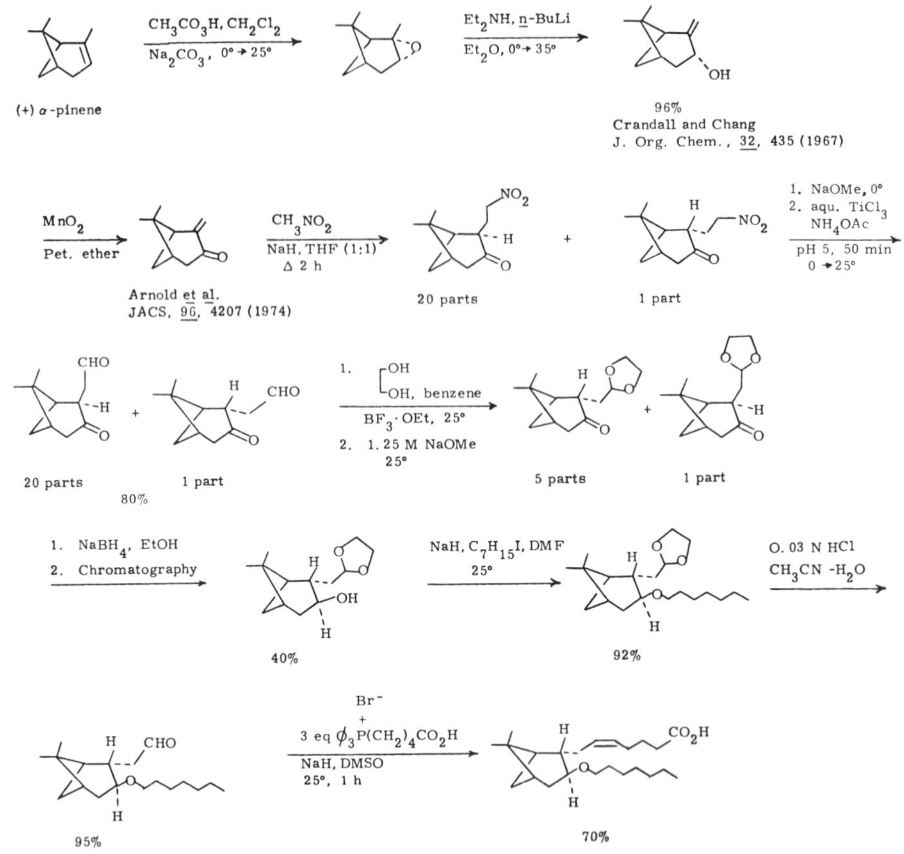

FIG. 1. Synthesis of TXA₂ analog A.

ASSAY PROCEDURES

Endoperoxide–TX Isomerase Assay

$$WP + [^{14}C]PGH_2 \xrightarrow{30°C} [^{14}C]TXB_2$$

Incubation Conditions

Washed platelets (400 μl) were incubated with $[^{14}C]PGH_2$ (20,000 cpm) for 10 min at 37°C. The $[^{14}C]TXB_2$ was acidified, extracted with ethyl acetate, and chromatographed on silica gel plates in benzene/dioxane/acetic acid (60:30:3). The plates were scanned and the peaks eluted and counted. Control TXB_2 was taken to be 100% and compared with the effect of preincubation of the test compounds for 10 min at room temperature with the washed platelets.

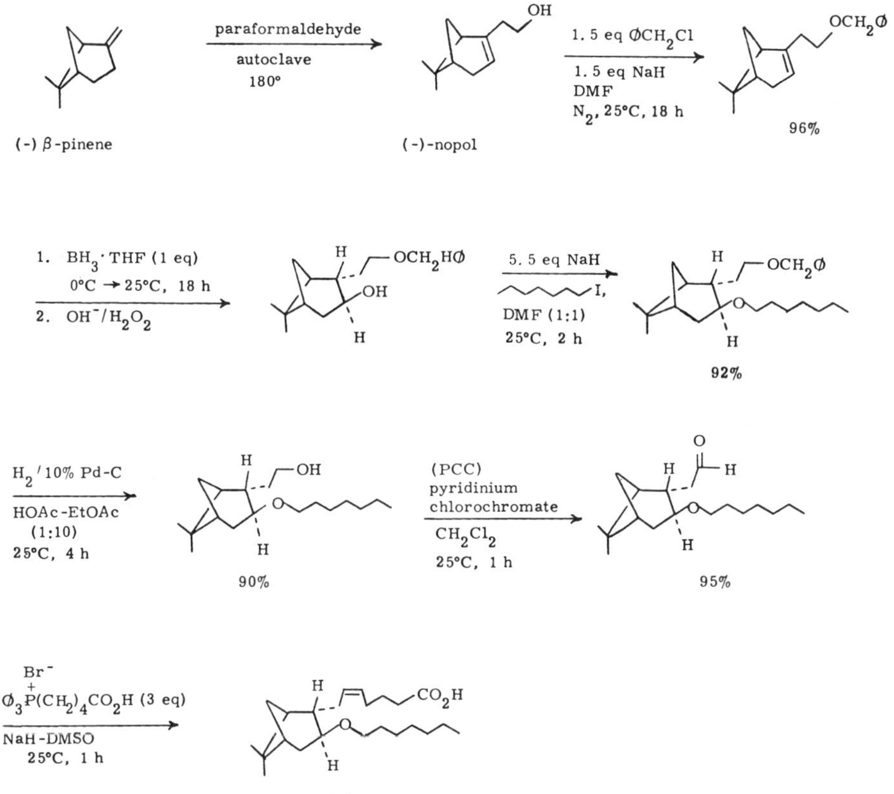

FIG. 2. Synthesis of carboxylic TXA₂ analog B.

Cyclooxygenase and Endoperoxide–TX Isomerase Assay

$$\text{WP} + [^{14}\text{C}]\text{arachidonate} \xrightarrow{15°\text{C}} [^{14}\text{C-PGH}_2] \rightarrow [^{14}\text{C}]\text{TXB}_2$$
$$(1\ \mu\text{g},\ 300{,}000\ \text{cpm}) \qquad\qquad\qquad (100\%)$$

PGI₂ Synthetase Assay

$$\text{Blood vessel microsomes} + [^{14}\text{C}]\text{PGH}_2 \rightarrow [^{14}\text{C}]\text{6-Keto-PGF}_{1\alpha}$$
$$100\ \mu\text{l} \qquad\qquad 30{,}000\ \text{cpm} \qquad\qquad (100\%)$$

Control: 15-hydroperoxy-arachidonic acid (AA) at 2 μg/ml produced a 93% inhibition of the vascular PGI₂ synthetase.

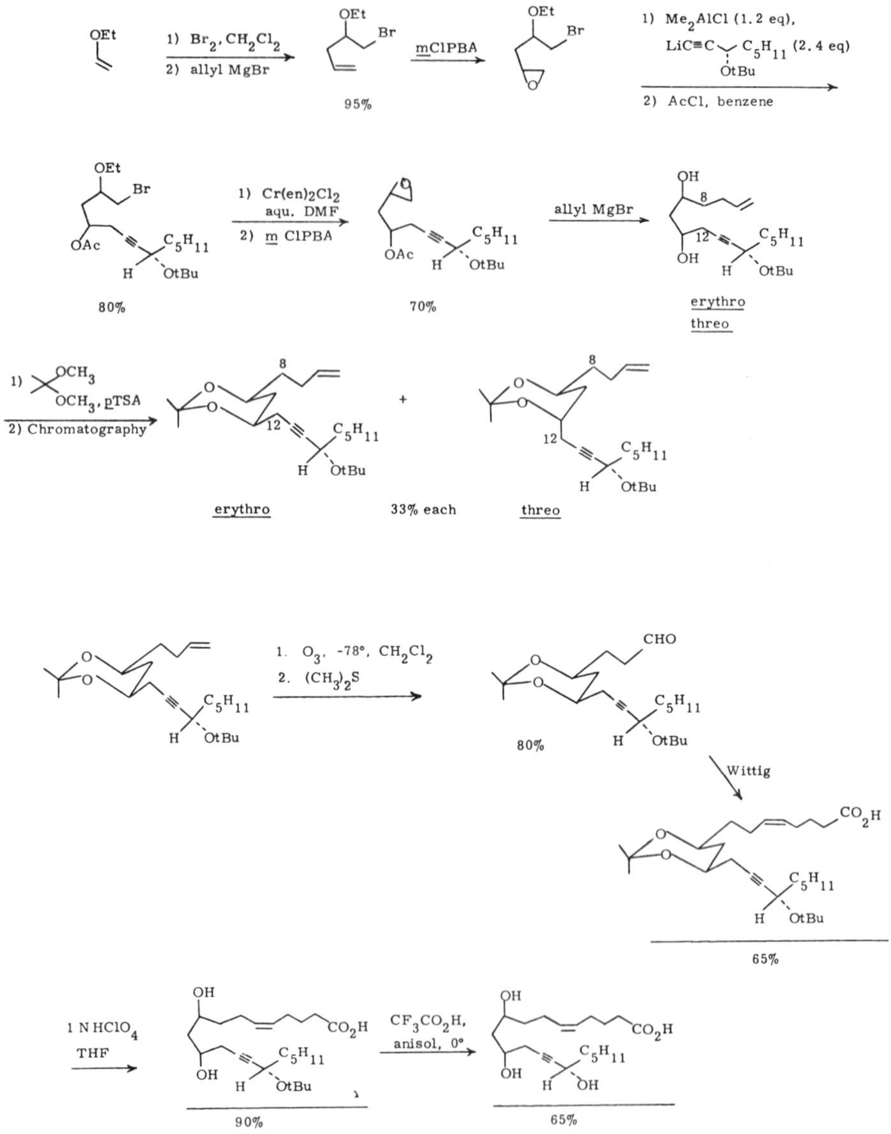

FIG. 3. Synthesis of 8,12-seco-13-dehydro-PGs.

RESULTS AND DISCUSSION

The results are shown in Tables 1 to 3. The first columns of the tables show the inhibition of TXB_2 formation from AA in washed rabbit platelets as the composite of inhibition of both cyclooxygenase and TXA_2 synthetase, while

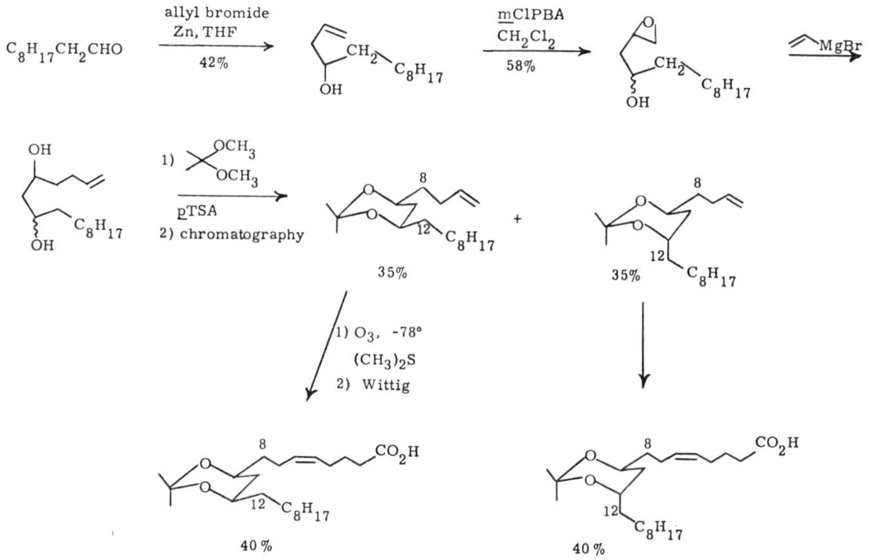

FIG. 4. Synthesis of 8, 12-13, 14-dihydro-PGs.

the second column shows the inhibition of the latter enzyme alone. The third column shows inhibition of PGI_2 synthetase as indicated by measurement of 6-keto-$PGF_{1\alpha}$ using bovine arterial microsomes. The fourth column in Table 1 shows the percent inhibition of platelet aggregation induced by both arachidonate and collagen in human platelet-rich plasma (HPRP) and human washed platelets (HWP). No inhibition was observed with HPRP even at levels of 300 μg of the inhibitor. On the other hand, the first entry in column 4 of Table 1 shows complete inhibition with HWP at 20 μg. The compounds listed in Tables 2 and 3 were likewise tested for inhibition of aggregation in HPRP but showed no effect even at the 300-μg level.

It is clear from inspection of all the tables that most of the substances showed no inhibition of prostacyclin synthetase. Only the last two entries in Table 3 show substantial inhibition of that enzyme. Achieving specificity of inhibition of thromboxane synthetase was more difficult. The substances shown in Table 2 possess only cyclooxygenase inhibition, which is abolished when the lower side chain is shortened by one methylene group. Several of the seco acids shown in Table 3 possess TXA_2 synthetase inhibition, with minimal effect on cyclooxygenase. These data do not exclude pure TXA_2 synthetase inhibition for some of the substances, and further work is clearly indicated. None of the compounds showed contraction of bovine artery, rabbit aorta, or chick rectum at the 300-μg/ml level.

TABLE 1. Inhibition of cyclooxygenase and TXA$_2$ and PGI$_2$ synthetase by carbocyclic analogs of TXA$_2$

	Percent inhibition										
	WRP + ^{14}CAA (TXB$_2$)			WRP + ^{14}CPGH$_2$ (TXB$_2$)			BAM + ^{14}CPGH$_2$ (6-Keto PGF$_{1\alpha}$)			Aggregation of HPRP HWP	
	2 µg	10 µg	50 µg	10 µg	50 µg	100 µg	10 µg	100 µg	300 µg	5 µg	20 µg
	11	50	90	0	15	75	0	0	0	75	100
	—	—	—	—	—	—	—	—	0	0	Slight delay at 50 µg

TABLE 2. Inhibition of cyclooxygenase and TXA_2 and PGI_2 synthetase by 8,12-seco-15-deoxy-prostaglandins

	Percent inhibition								
	WRP + ^{14}CAA (TXB_2)			WRP + ^{14}CPGH$_2$ (TXB_2)			BAM + ^{14}CPGH$_2$ (6-Keto $F_{1\alpha}$)		
	10 µg	50 µg	100 µg	10 µg	50 µg	100 µg	10 µg	50 µg	100 µg
	0	22	36	—	—	0	—	—	0
	0	40	45	—	—	0	—	—	0
	—	0	—	—	0	—	—	0	—

TABLE 3. Inhibition of cyclooxygenase, TXA$_2$ and PGI$_2$ synthetase by 15-oxygenated 8,12-seco-PGs

	Percent inhibition								
	WRP + ^{14}CAA (TXB$_2$)			WRP + ^{14}CPGH$_2$ (TXB$_2$)			BAM + ^{14}CPGH$_2$ (6-Keto F$_{1\alpha}$)		
Structure	10 µg	50 µg	100 µg	10 µg	50 µg	100 µg	10 µg	50 µg	100 µg
	0	50	60	0	25	50	0	—	0
	6	—	69	14	36	64	0	—	0
	6	—	81	7	7	43	5	—	8
	11	75	85	0	45	65	0	—	0

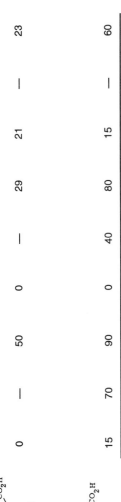

0	—	50	0	—	29	21	23
15	70	90	0	40	80	15	60

ACKNOWLEDGMENTS

Supported by Public Health Service contract HV-72945 research grant AM 11499, and Diabetes Research Training Center AM 20595, NMR facility by CA.

REFERENCES

1. Bicking, J. B., Robb, C. M., Smith, R. L., and Cragoe, E. J., Jr. (1977): *J. Med. Chem.,* 20:35–43.
2. Fried, J. C., Lin, C, Mehra, M., Kao, W., and Dalven, P. (1971): *Ann. N.Y. Acad. Sci.,* 180:38–63.
3. Gorman, R. R., Bundy, G. L., Peterson, D. C., Sun, F. F., Miller, O. V., and Fitzpatrick, F. A. (1977): *Proc. Natl. Acad. Sci. USA,* 74:4007–4011.
4. Yoshimoto, T. S., Yamamoto, S., and Hayaishi, O. (1978): *Prostaglandins,* 16:529–540.

Advances in Prostaglandin and Thromboxane Research,
Vol. 6, edited by B. Samuelsson, P. W. Ramwell,
and R. Paoletti. Raven Press, New York © 1980.

Effect of SQ 80,338 (1-(3-Phenyl-2-Propenyl)-1H-Imidazole) on Thromboxane Synthetase Activity and Arachidonic Acid-Induced Platelet Aggregation and Bronchoconstriction

D. N. Harris, R. Greenberg, M. B. Phillips, G. H. Osman, Jr.,
and M. J. Antonaccio

*Department of Pharmacology, The Squibb Institute for Medical Research,
Princeton, New Jersey 08540*

The role of blood platelets in hemostasis and thrombosis has been greatly clarified in recent years. Two major breakthroughs have helped in elucidating the role of prostaglandins (PGs) in platelet function. First, there was the discovery of thromboxane A_2 (TXA_2), the major PG product in platelets—a potent platelet aggregator, bronchoconstrictor, and vasoconstrictor (6). Second, prostacyclin (PGI_2), formed from arachidonic acid (AA) by endothelial cells of blood vessels, was found to have biological actions opposing those of TXA_2 (9). Normally there is a homeostatic balance maintained between TXA_2 and PGI_2. In some pathological conditions, the blood vessels become denuded, resulting in less endothelium to synthesize PGI_2. Thus the normal balance is upset, allowing the mainly detrimental properties of the now predominant TXA_2 to persist. Selective inhibition of TX synthetase therefore appears to be a means of restoring the homeostatic balance between TXA_2 and PGI_2. Imidazole has been shown to be a specific inhibitor of TX synthetase (8). Experiments were therefore done to determine the effect of SQ 80,338 (1-(3-phenyl-2-propenyl)-1H-imidazole) on TX synthetase activity, AA-induced platelet aggregation, and bronchoconstriction in the guinea pig.

METHODS

TX synthetase was prepared from fresh platelet-rich plasma (PRP) according to the procedure of Nijkamp et al. (11). Briefly, a platelet pellet was washed in physiological saline and then lysed by a combination of freeze–thaw cycles and homogenization. This platelet lysate was divided into small aliquots and stored at $-70°C$ until used.

TX synthetase activity was determined by radiochromatographic assay. Human platelet TX synthetase preparations were incubated with ^{14}C-AA for 3 to 5 min to generate TXB_2. Then TXB_2, PGE_2, $PGF_{2\alpha}$, and AA were isolated by thin-layer chromatography and radioactivity determined by liquid scintillation spectrometry.

Platelet aggregation of PRP was studied photometrically using a Chronolog aggregometer connected to a linear recorder (2). SQ 80,338 was preincubated with PRP for 2.5 min at 37°C before AA, adenosine monophosphate (ADP), epinephrine, or collagen were added and the optical transmission recorded for at least 3 min. The rate of increase in optical transmission, which is a measure of the initial velocity of aggregation, was measured by determining the slope of the steepest part of the curve.

Male guinea pigs weighing 480 to 520 g were anesthetized with urethane (1.5 g/kg, i.p.). Spontaneous respiration was arrested with succinylcholine (1.5 mg/kg, i.p.). The guinea pigs were artificially ventilated with a Palmer pump through a tracheal cannula at a rate of 72 strokes/min and a stroke volume of 3 ml. Pulmonary resistance (R) and dynamic compliance (C) were measured as previously described (5).

RESULTS

TX synthetase activity was linearly related to protein concentration. The formation of TXB_2 increased over fourfold at enzyme concentrations between 0.1 and 0.9 $\mu g/\mu l$. At this same enzyme concentration range, the formation of PGE_2 and $PGF_{2\alpha}$ increased only about 30%. SQ 80,338 inhibited the increase in TXB_2 formation 50% at a concentration of approximately 30 μM (Fig. 1). On the other hand, the formation of PGE_2 and $PGF_{2\alpha}$ were both maximally

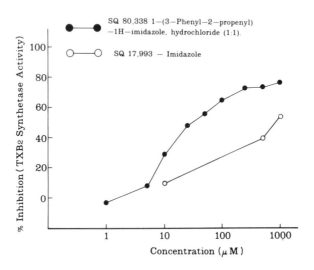

FIG. 1. Effect of SQ 80,338 and imidazole on TXB_2 synthetase activity of human blood platelets. Each point is the mean of at least two determinations.

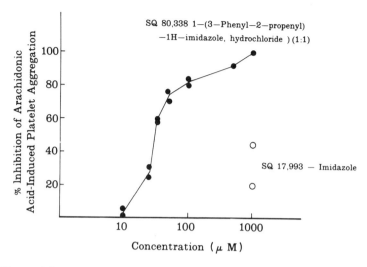

FIG. 2. Effect of SQ 80,338 and imidazole on arachidonic acid-(700 μM) induced aggregation of human blood platelets. Each point is the mean of at least two determinations.

increased 10-fold at 250 μM (data not shown). By comparison, imidazole inhibited TX synthetase activity 50% at 800 μM.

SQ 80,338 inhibited platelet aggregation induced by AA 50% at 30 μM (Fig. 2). SQ 80,338 also inhibited the secondary phase of epinephrine-induced platelet aggregation with an ID_{50} value of 48 μM and inhibited collagen-induced aggregation of 10% at 100 μM but had no effect on the primary phase of ADP- or epinephrine-induced aggregation (data not shown). Imidazole at 1 mM caused less than 50% inhibition of AA-induced aggregation (Fig. 2).

AA (0.25 mg/kg, i.v.) was administered to groups of 4 to 8 guinea pigs 15 min before and 3 and 10 min after the administration of SQ 80,338 (0.1, 0.3, and 1.0 mg/kg, i.v.) or saline. The AA caused large increases in R and decreases in C which were significantly antagonized by SQ 80,338 but not by saline (Fig. 3). The inhibitory effect lasted for less than 10 min in 5 guinea pigs. Imidazole (10 mg/kg, i.v.) caused a slight inhibition of the AA-induced bronchoconstriction. In four similar experiments SQ 80,338 (1.0 mg/kg, i.v.) did not alter the bronchoconstrictor response to histamine (5.0 μg/kg, i.v.).

DISCUSSION

The results of these experiments show that SQ 80,338 selectively inhibits platelet TX synthetase activity while increasing the formation of PGE_2 and $PGF_{2\alpha}$, probably by shunting the endoperoxides to the "stable" PGs. These results confirm those of others, who also showed that imidazole and its derivatives substituted at the 1-position are selective inhibitors of this enzyme and therefore are inhibitors of AA-induced platelet aggregation (1,3,10,14,17). The selectivity

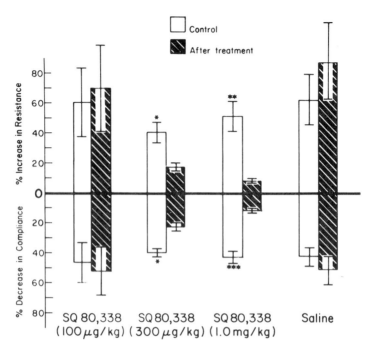

FIG. 3. Effect of SQ 80,338 on bronchoconstrictor response to AA (0.25 mg/kg, i.v.) in the anesthetized guinea pig. Each bar represents the mean ± S.E. of the response in 4 to 8 experiments. Significance of the difference from controls (*t*-test for paired data): *$p < 0.05$, **$p < 0.01$, ***$p < 0.001$.

of inhibition by SQ 80,338 was further shown by its inhibition of the secondary phase of epinephrine- and collagen-induced platelet aggregation, which are also caused by TXA_2 (4,13,15), while having no effect on the first phase of epinephrine- or ADP-induced platelet aggregation.

In the anesthetized guinea pig, SQ 80,338 effectively inhibited AA-induced bronchoconstriction without having an effect on histamine-induced bronchoconstriction. It is well established that AA-induced bronchoconstriction is mediated by PGs (7,12). It has also been shown that AA causes the release of PGs and TXA_2 from isolated guinea pig lung (16).

The results presented here therefore indicate that the inhibition of AA-induced platelet aggregation and bronchoconstriction is due to inhibition of TXA_2 synthesis.

ACKNOWLEDGMENTS

The authors are indebted to Mrs. Susan M. Smith and Mrs. Helen Stofko for invaluable secretarial assistance. SQ 80,338 was synthesized by Dr. H. Höhn of Chemische Fabrik von Heyden, Regensburg, Germany.

REFERENCES

1. Blackwell, G. J., Flower, R. J., Russell-Smith, N., Salmon, J. A., Thorogood, P. B., and Vane, J. R. (1978): *Br. J. Pharmacol.,* 64:435P.
2. Born, G. V. R. (1962): *Nature,* 194:927–929.
3. Fitzpatrick, F. A., and Gorman, R. R. (1978): *Biochim. Biophys. Acta,* 539:162–172.
4. Gorman, R. R. (1979): *Fed. Proc.,* 38:83–88.
5. Greenberg, R., Smorong, K., and Bagli, J. F. (1976): *Prostaglandins,* 11:961–980.
6. Hamberg, M., and Samuelsson, B. (1973): *Proc. Natl. Acad. Sci. USA,* 70:899–903.
7. Lefort, J., and Vargaftig, B. B. (1978): *Br. J. Pharmacol.,* 63:35–42.
8. Moncada, S., Bunting, S., Mullane, K., Thorogood, P., Vane, J. R., Raz, A., and Needleman, P. (1977): *Prostaglandins,* 13:611–618.
9. Moncada, S. Gryglewski, R., Bunting, S., and Vane, J. R. (1976): *Nature,* 263:663–665.
10. Needleman, P., Raz, A., Ferrendelli, J. A., and Minkes, M. (1977): *Proc. Natl. Acad. Sci. USA,* 74:1716–1720.
11. Nijkamp, F. P., Moncada, S., White, H. L., and Vane, J. R. (1977): *Eur. J. Pharmacol.,* 44:179–186.
12. Saeed, S. A., McDonald-Gibson, W. J., Cuthbert, J., Copas, J. L., Schneider, C., Gardiner, P. J., Butt, N. M., and Collier, H. O. J. (1977): *Nature,* 270:32–36.
13. Smith, J. B., Ingerman, C., Kocsis, J. J., and Silver, M. J. (1974): *J. Clin. Invest.,* 53:1468–1472.
14. Tai, H. H., and Yuan, B. (1978): *Biochem. Biophys. Res. Commun.,* 80:236–242.
15. Vapaatalo, H., and Parantainen, J. (1978): *Med. Biol.,* 56:163–183.
16. Vargaftig, B. B., and Dao Hai, N. (1973): *Eur. J. Pharmacol.,* 24:283–288.
17. Yoshimoto, T., Yamamoto, S., and Hayaishi, O. (1978): *Prostaglandins,* 16:529–540.

Advances in Prostaglandin and Thromboxane Research,
Vol. 6, edited by B. Samuelsson, P. W. Ramwell,
and R. Paoletti. Raven Press, New York © 1980.

Selective Inhibitor of Thromboxane Synthetase: Pyridine and Its Derivatives

Tsumoru Miyamoto, Ken Taniguchi, Tadao Tanouchi, and
Fumio Hirata

*Department of Biochemistry, Research Institute, Ono Pharmaceutical Co., Ltd., 3-1-1
Sakurai, Shimamoto-cho, Mishima-gun, Osaka 618, Japan*

Since thromboxane A_2 (TXA$_2$) is considered to play an important role in platelets and arteries, attempts to develop selective inhibitors of TX synthetase are being made. Several inhibitors of TX synthetase have been reported so far; namely, imidazole and its derivatives (6,9,10), prostaglandin (PG) endoperoxide analog (8), L-8027 (3), N-0164 (4), and dipyridamole (1). In order to develop a new class of TX synthetase inhibitors, we examined the inhibitory effects of various heterocyclic compounds and found that TX synthetase was inhibited by pyridine and its derivatives.

MATERIALS AND METHODS

[1-^{14}C]Arachidonic acid was purchased from New England Nuclear. Sheep vesicular gland microsomes were obtained from Ran Biochemicals (Tel Aviv, Israel). [1-^{14}C]PGH$_2$ was prepared by the method of Yoshimoto et al. (10).

Fresh citrated rabbit or human blood was centrifuged at $200 \times g$ for 10 min. The platelet-rich plasma was removed and recentrifuged at $2,000 \times g$ for 20 min. The pellets were suspended in a cold 0.1 M Tris-HCl, pH 8.0 (4×10^9/ml, washed platelets). Prostacyclin (PGI$_2$) synthetase from bovine aorta was obtained by a slight modification of the method of Gryglewski et al. (2). PG endoperoxide synthetase from bovine vesicular gland was prepared by the methods previously described (5).

For the formation of TXB$_2$ (TX synthetase assays), the washed platelets (4×10^7) were incubated with 50 μM [1-^{14}C]PGH$_2$ (5×10^4 cpm) at 24°C for 1 min in 0.1 M potassium phosphate, pH 7.4 (0.1 ml). PGI$_2$ synthetase assays were performed with the same reaction mixture described above except that the washed platelets were replaced with bovine aorta microsomes. In all cases, termination of the reaction and extraction of the radioactive materials were performed by previously described methods (5). Thin-layer chromatography was carried out in chloroform/ethyl acetate/methanol/acetic acid/water (70:30:8:1:0.5). The radioactive zones were located by autoradiography and quantitated by a standard liquid scintillation counting procedure. PG endoperoxide synthetase assays were performed according to the previously described methods (5).

RESULTS AND DISCUSSION

We screened the inhibitory effects of TX synthetase using commercially available heterocyclic compounds, and found that pyridine inhibited TX synthetase. The ID_{50} value of pyridine (60 μM) was similar to that of imidazole (50 μM). No significant inhibition of PG endoperoxide synthetase or PGI_2 synthetase was observed at the concentrations tested. Thus pyridine was a selective inhibitor of TX synthetase. We further examined the methyl derivatives of pyridine and found that substitution at β- or γ-position retained the inhibitory action of pyridine, while substitution at other positions caused decreases in activity.

Based on these findings, a number of pyridine derivatives substituted at β- or γ-position were synthesized and tested for their inhibitory potencies. Among the synthetic pyridine derivatives examined, β-[4-(2-carboxy-1-propenyl)benzyl]pyridine hydrochloride (OKY-1555, Fig. 1) was the most potent inhibitor of TX synthetase. Figure 2 shows the inhibition of TXB_2 formation from PGH_2 at nM concentrations. The ID_{50} values of OKY-1555 for TX synthetase from rabbit platelet and from human platelet were 2 and 3 nM, respectively. It should be noted that OKY-1555 affected neither PG endoperoxide synthetase nor PGI_2

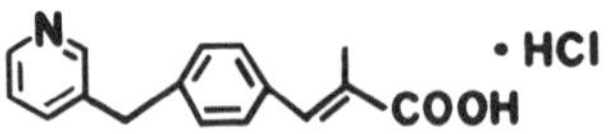

FIG. 1. Chemical structure of β-[4-(2-carboxy-1-propenyl)benzyl]pyridine hydrochloride (OKY-1555).

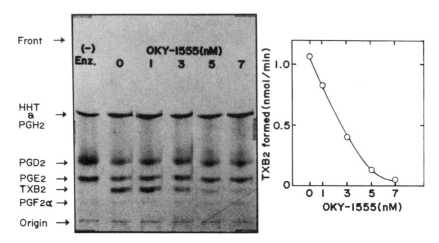

FIG. 2. Inhibitory effects of OKY-1555 on the formation of TXB_2 from PGH_2 of washed rabbit platelets. Reactions were carried out in the presence of OKY-1555 at various concentrations as described in the text. Thin-layer chromatography was performed at room temperature.

synthetase at the concentration of 1 mM. Furthermore, when [1-^{14}C]arachidonic acid was incubated with the washed platelets in the presence of 0.1 μM OKY-1555, the TXB_2 formation was greatly reduced, whereas PGH_2 was markedly accumulated. These findings indicate that OKY-1555 is a very potent and highly selective inhibitor of TX synthetase in platelet enzymes. The kinetic analysis of the inhibition of TX synthetase by OKY-1555 indicated that it was a noncompetitive inhibitor ($K_i = 2$ nM).

OKY-1555 also blocked the rabbit platelet aggregation induced by arachidonate in the dose-dependent manner ($ID_{50} = 0.3$ μM), though it did not affect the platelet aggregation induced by ADP or thrombin *in vitro*. We further investigated the effects of OKY-1555 *in vivo* on experimental thrombosis induced by the methods of Silver et al. (7). When arachidonate (4 mg/kg) was administered intravenously to rabbits, all animals died within 1 to 3 min. Under these conditions, the arachidonate-induced sudden death in rabbits was prevented by the pretreatment with OKY-1555. The complete effective dose of OKY-1555 was 1 mg/kg, i.v., and 30 mg/kg, p.o. These results suggest that TX formation may be an essential factor in the lethal effects of arachidonate in rabbits, because OKY-1555 inhibited neither PG endoperoxide synthetase nor PGI_2 synthetase, only TX synthetase. The properties of OKY-1555 described in this report suggest that it may contribute in elucidating the mode of action of TXA_2 in other biological systems.

REFERENCES

1. Greenwald, J. E., Wong, L. K., Rao, M., Bianchine, J. R., and Panganamala, R. V. (1978): *Biochem. Biophys. Res. Commun.*, 84:1112–1118.
2. Gryglewski, R. J., Bunting, S., Moncada, S., Flower, R. J., and Vane, J. R. (1976): *Prostaglandins*, 12:685–713.
3. Gryglewski, R. J., Zmuda, A., Korbut, R., Krecioch, E., and Bieron, K. (1977): *Nature*, 267:627–628.
4. Kulkarni, P. S., and Eakins, K. E. (1976): *Prostaglandins*, 12:465–469.
5. Miyamoto, T., Ogino, N., Yamamoto, S., and Hayaishi, O. (1976): *J. Biol. Chem.*, 251:2629–2636.
6. Moncada, S., Bunting, S., Mullane, K., Thorogood, P., and Vane, J. R. (1977): *Prostaglandins*, 13:611–618.
7. Silver, M. J., Hoch, W., Kocsis, J. J., Ingerman, C. M., and Smith, J. B. (1974): *Science*, 183:1085–1087.
8. Sun, F. F. (1977): *Biochem. Biophys. Res. Commun.*, 74:1432–1440.
9. Tai, H. H., and Yuan, B. (1978): *Biochem. Biophys. Res. Commun.*, 80:236–242.
10. Yoshimoto, T., Yamamoto, S., and Hayaishi, O. (1978): *Prostaglandins*, 16:529–540.

Advances in Prostaglandin and Thromboxane Research,
Vol. 6, edited by B. Samuelsson, P. W. Ramwell,
and R. Paoletti. Raven Press, New York © 1980.

Inhibition of Thromboxane Synthesis and Platelet Aggregation by Pyridine and Its Derivatives

Hsin-Hsiung Tai, Nancy Lee, and Chen L. Tai

Department of Biochemistry, North Texas State University Health Sciences Center/Texas College of Osteopathic Medicine, Fort Worth, Texas 76107

Thromboxane A_2 (TXA$_2$) and prostacyclin (PGI$_2$) are two novel prostaglandin (PG)-like substances which are derived from arachidonic acid via PG endoperoxides (PGG$_2$ and PGH$_2$). TXA$_2$ is a potent labile platelet aggregator and vascular constrictor (4), whereas PGI$_2$ is a potent labile antithrombotic compound and vasodilator (1). Factors that may specifically affect the enzyme activities catalyzing the synthesis of these two biologically potent substances are of great interest in controlling the balance of these two opposing actions.

Among a number of inhibitors of TX synthetase discovered so far, imidazole has been found to be the most selective inhibitor (6,7). We and others have shown that the inhibitory potency of imidazole can be greatly altered by introducing substituents at different positions of the heterocyclic ring (11,14). In this chapter, we shall describe another selective inhibitor of TX synthetase, pyridine, and the structure–activity relationship of pyridine derivatives. In addition, the effect of these inhibitors on human platelet aggregation will also be reported.

MATERIALS AND METHODS

Pyridine derivatives were obtained from the Aldrich Chemical Company. Methyl and hexyl nicotinates were obtained from the Sigma Chemical Company. Ethyl and butyl nicotinates were synthesized according to Levine and Sneed (5). [1-^{14}C]Arachidonic acid was purchased from Applied Science. PG standards were kindly supplied by The Upjohn Company. PG endoperoxide, PGH$_2$, was prepared according to Hamberg and Samuelsson (3). Microsomal fractions from human platelets and swine lung were prepared as described previously (12,13). TX synthetase was assayed by following the formation of TXB$_2$ immunoreactivity from PGH$_2$ using a specific radioimmunoassay for TXB$_2$ (10). Platelet aggregation experiments were done with fresh platelet-rich plasma (PRP) in a Chrono-Log model 330 platelet aggregometer.

RESULTS AND DISCUSSION

Pyridine inhibited TX synthetase from both human platelet and swine lung microsomes in a concentration-dependent manner. The concentrations which gave 50% inhibition (IC_{50}) was found to be 270 μM for platelet enzyme (Table 1). The inhibitory potency of pyridine appeared to increase if an alkyl or an aryl substituent was introduced at the 3- or 4-position. Substitution at the 3-position yielded more potent inhibitors, as shown in Table 1. However, substitution at the 2-position apparently abolished the inhibitory power of pyridine or its 3-substituted derivatives. The substituent needs to be of hydrophobic nature for higher inhibitory potency. This is best demonstrated by the fact that nicotinic acid (pyridine-3-carboxylic acid) is a poorer inhibitor than pyridine (Table 1). However, the inhibitory potency was dramatically increased after forming methyl ester of nicotinic acid. The inhibitory power of nicotinic acid ester increased as the alkyl chain was extended.

The specificity of inhibition by pyridine and its active derivatives was also investigated. The microsomal fraction of mammalian lung has been shown to exhibit appreciable TX, PGE, and PGI_2 synthetase activities. This provides a unique system to test the effect of inhibitors on various enzyme systems. Figure 1 shows that inhibition of TX synthesis by both pyridine (10 mM) and 3-ethyl pyridine (1 mM) was accompanied by the concurrent increase in PGE_2 and 6-keto-$PGF_{1\alpha}$ synthesis using [1-^{14}C]arachidonic acid as substrate. The total amount of products formed was not decreased in the presence of inhibitors. These results suggest that enzymes other than TX synthetase in the arachidonic acid cascade are not inhibited.

TABLE 1. *Inhibitory potency of pyridine and its derivatives on TX synthetase of human platelet microsomes[a]*

Inhibitors	IC_{50} (μM)
Pyridine	270
2-Ethyl pyridine	>1,000
3-Ethyl pyridine	16
4-Ethyl pyridine	60
5-Ethyl-2-methyl pyridine	>1,000
Nicotinic acid (pyridine-3-carboxylic acid)	>1,000
Methyl nicotinate	173
Ethyl nicotinate	33
Butyl nicotinate	18
Hexyl nicotinate	10

[a] The assay was carried out using PGH_2 as substrate in the manner described previously (12). Six different concentrations of each inhibitor were employed to determine the IC_{50}. The amount of microsomal protein used per assay was 75 μg.

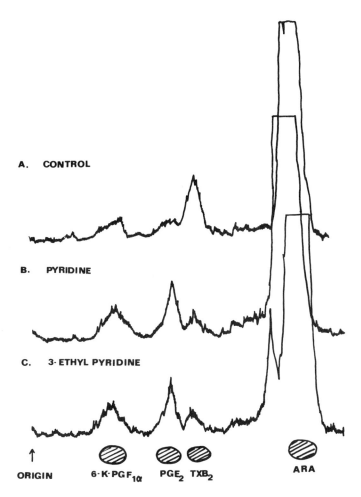

FIG. 1. Effect of pyridine and 3-ethyl pyridine on the biosynthesis of 6-keto-PGF$_{1\alpha}$, TXB$_2$, and PGE$_2$ by swine lung microsomes. The assay mixture contained: [1-^{14}C]arachidonic acid (16 nmol, 60,000 cpm), DL-isoproterenol (1 μmol), swine lung microsomes (2.5 mg protein), and inhibitor in 1 ml 0.05 M Tris-HCl buffer, pH 7.5. Pyridine and 3-ethyl pyridine were added at the concentrations of 10 and 1 mM, respectively. Incubation, extraction, and chromatography were carried out as described previously (13). Thin-layer plates were then scanned for radioactivity using a Berthold thin-layer scanner.

The effects of pyridine and their positional derivatives on human platelet aggregation in PRP were also examined. As shown in Fig. 2, 1.5 mM pyridine inhibited platelet aggregation induced either by 0.37 mM arachidonic acid or 10 μM adenosine triphosphate (ADP). Pyridine also inhibited the second phase of platelet aggregation induced by ADP, indicating the blockade of the release reaction. Three different ethyl derivatives of pyridine were also evaluated for their effects on platelet aggregation induced by either arachidonic acid or ADP

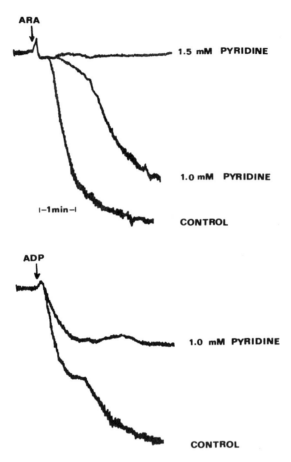

FIG. 2. Inhibition of arachidonic acid- or ADP-induced platelet aggregation by pyridine. Platelet aggregation in human PRP was induced by 0.37 mM arachidonic acid **(top)** or by 10 μM ADP **(bottom).** Pyridine at the indicated concentrations was preincubated with PRP for 5 min before addition of arachidonic acid or ADP.

(Fig. 3). 3-Ethyl pyridine, 0.25 mM, completely inhibited platelet aggregation induced by arachidonic acid and ADP, while the same concentrations of 4-ethyl pyridine and 2-ethyl pyridine resulted in only partial inhibition or none at all, respectively. The relative potency of three ethyl pyridines in inhibiting platelet aggregation is consistent with their power as TX synthetase inhibitors. This observation supports the contention that PGH_2 must be converted to TXA_2 in the induction of human platelet aggregation (2).

Our finding that 3-substituted pyridines are inhibitors of TX synthetase has interesting implications. Nicotinic acid, various nicotinates, and 3-pyridyl-*N,N*-disubstituted cyanoguanidines—which are 3-substituted pyridines—have been shown to possess vasodilatory and hypotensive activities (8,9). It is possible

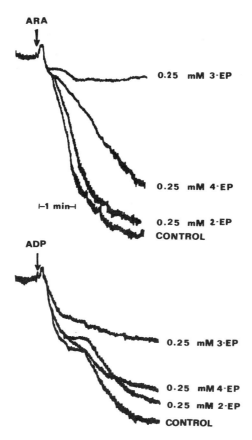

FIG. 3. Inhibition of arachidonic acid- or ADP-induced platelet aggregation by three different ethyl pyridines (EPs). Platelet aggregation in human PRP was induced by 0.5 mM arachidonic acid **(top)** or by 10 μM ADP **(bottom)**. Three different EPs at a concentration of 0.25 mM were incubated with PRP for 5 min before the addition of arachidonic acid or ADP.

that these drugs inhibit TX synthesis and concurrently stimulate PGI_2 synthesis *in vivo* in a manner similar to that found in *in vitro* (Fig. 1), since suppressed synthesis of TX may direct PG endoperoxide to increased formation of PGI_2— a potent vasodilator. This provides new insight to the elucidation of the mechanism of action of certain vasodilators and antihypotensive agents. Further studies on the synthesis and testing of various pyridine derivatives may yield some valuable vasodilatory, antihypertensive, and antithrombotic drugs.

SUMMARY

Pyridine inhibited the conversion of PG endoperoxide to TXA_2 catalyzed by TX synthetase from human platelet and swine lung microsomes. The inhibitory potency of pyridine is abolished by derivatizing pyridine at the 2-position but is increased by introducing hydrophobic substituents at 3- or 4-positions, with 3-substituted pyridines being the most potent inhibitors. Inhibition by pyridine and its derivatives was also selective, since other enzymes in the arachidonic acid cascade were not significantly affected. Pyridine and the active derivatives also inhibited human platelet aggregation induced by arachidonic acid or ADP.

ACKNOWLEDGMENT

This work was supported by grants from the U.S. Public Health Service (GM-25247) and from the American Heart Association (78–865).

REFERENCES

1. Bunting, S., Gryglewski, R., Moncada, S., and Vane, J. R. (1976): *Prostaglandins,* 12:897–913.
2. Gorman, R. R., Bundy, G. L., Peterson, D. C., Sun, F. F., Miller, O. V., and Fitzpatrick, F. A. (1977): *Proc. Natl. Acad. Sci. USA,* 74:4007–4011.
3. Hamberg, M., and Samuelsson, B. (1973): *Proc. Natl. Acad. Sci. USA,* 70:899–903.
4. Hamberg, M., Svensson, J., and Samuelsson, B. (1975): *Proc. Natl. Acad. Sci. USA,* 72:2994–2998.
5. Levine, R., and Sneed, J. K. (1951): *J. Am. Chem. Soc.,* 73:5614–5616.
6. Moncada, S., Bunting, S., Mullane, K., Thorogood, P., Vane, J. R., Raz, A., and Needleman, P. (1977): *Prostaglandins,* 13:611–618.
7. Needleman, P., Raz, A., Ferrendelli, J. A., and Minkes, M. (1977): *Proc. Natl. Acad. Sci. USA,* 74:1716–1720.
8. Oelkers, H. A. (1965): *Arzneim. Forsch.,* 12:1416.
9. Petersen, H. J., Nielsen, C. D., and Arrigoni-Mortelli, E. (1978): *J. Med. Chem.,* 21:773–781.
10. Tai, H. H., and Yuan, B. (1978): *Anal. Biochem.,* 87:343–349.
11. Tai, H. H., and Yuan, B. (1978): *Biochem. Biophys. Res. Commun.,* 80:236–242.
12. Tai, H. H., and Yuan, B. (1978): *Biochim. Biophys. Acta,* 531:286–294.
13. Tai, H. H., Yuan, B., and Wu, A. T. (1978): *Biochem. J.,* 170:441–444.
14. Yoshimoto, T., Yamamoto, S., and Hayaishi, O. (1979): *Prostaglandins,* 16:529–540.

Advances in Prostaglandin and Thromboxane Research,
Vol. 6, edited by B. Samuelsson, P. W. Ramwell,
and R. Paoletti. Raven Press, New York © 1980.

Inhibition of Arachidonate Metabolism by Selected Compounds *In Vitro* with Particular Emphasis on the Thromboxane A$_2$ Synthase Pathway

L. D. Tobias and J. G. Hamilton

Roche Research Center, Hoffmann-La Roche Inc., Nutley, New Jersey 07110

Imidazole and a number of its substituted analogs were first tested and found to be inhibitors of thromboxane A$_2$ (TXA$_2$) synthase by Moncada et al. (8). Tai and Yuan (10) later investigated a series of imidazoles and found that 1-nonyl-imidazole and 1-(2-isopropyl phenyl)-imidazole were potent, selective, inhibitors of TXA$_2$ synthase. The inhibition was found to be competitive with respect to prostaglandin endoperoxide (PGH$_2$) substrate. This work has been extended further by Yoshimoto et al. (12) who quantified the inhibition of TXA$_2$ synthase by 1-carboxyalkylimidazoles.

Besides 1-substituted imidazoles, a number of other compounds have been reported to inhibit TXA$_2$ synthase. These include *p*-benzyl-4-[1-oxo-2-(4-chloro-benzyl)-3-phenylpropyl] phenyl phosphonate (N0164) (3), 2-isopropyl-3-nicotinyl indole (L8027) (6), and several endoperoxide analogs (1,2,4,5,9).

This report describes a compilation of the results obtained in our laboratory concerning the inhibition of arachidonate metabolism by various compounds with particular emphasis on selective inhibition of the TXA$_2$ pathway.

MATERIALS AND METHODS

PG synthase activity was monitored via an oxygen electrode using sheep seminal vesicular gland microsomes (SSVM) as the enzyme source (11). Bovine aortic microsomes (BAM) (Ran Biochemicals, Tel Aviv, Israel) were used as the source of prostacyclin (PGI$_2$) synthase. Either human platelet microsomes (HPM) (Ran Biochemicals) or guinea pig lung microsomes (GPLM) were used as the source of TXA$_2$ synthase.

Inhibition of PGI$_2$ or TXA$_2$ synthase was monitored as follows:

To a 12 × 75-mm tube containing [1-^{14}C]PGH$_2$ (0.5 µg, 0.01 µCi) and potential inhibitor (typically 100 µM or 1 mM final conc. in 10 µl of ethanol) in 200 µl of phosphate buffer (0.1 M, pH 7.5) was added an aliquot of microsomal suspension (typically 50 μl, containing either BAM, 500 μg of protein; HPM, 150 μg protein; or GPLM, 400 μg protein, respectively).

After a 2-min incubation at 22°C, ether (2 ml) and HCl (25 μmoles) were added with vigorous agitation. The aqueous phase was frozen at −78°C, and products were identified as described previously (7). Quantitation was accomplished via cutting out the thin-layer chromatography region corresponding to the peak area in question and determining the cpm using a suitable fluor.

RESULTS AND DISCUSSION

The assay conditions were adjusted such that 5 to 10% of the [1-^{14}C]PGH$_2$ remained unconverted. When boiled microsomes were substituted in the assay procedure, approximately 10 to 15% of the added [1-^{14}C]PGH$_2$ was converted nonenzymatically to products which consisted of mainly PGD$_2$ and PGE$_2$.

The effect of various compounds on TXA$_2$ synthase is noted in Table 1.

TABLE 1. *Effect of various compounds on TXA$_2$ synthase from GPLM and HPM*

Compound	Concentration (mM)	Enzyme source	Effect
Acetylsalicylic acid	1	GPLM	−
Ascorbic acid	1	GPLM	−
Azathioprine	1	GPLM	−
Benzydamine	1	GPLM	−
Bromazepam	1	GPLM	−
Butaclamol	1	GPLM	−
Chlorodiazepoxide	1	GPLM	−
Clonazepam	1	GPLM	+
Cromolyn	1	GPLM	−
Diazepam	1	GPLM, HPM	+, +
Flunitrazepam	1	GPLM	+
Flurazepam	1	GPLM	−
Haloperidol	1	GPLM	−
1-Histidine	1	GPLM	−
Hydralazine	1	GPLM	−
Imidazole	1	GPLM, HPM	+, +
2-Imidazoline	1	GPLM	−
Indomethacin	1	HPM	+
L8027	1	GPLM, HPM	+, +
Levamisole	1	GPLM	−
Metaxolone	1	GPLM	−
Methocarbamol	1	GPLM	−
Minoxidil	1	GPLM	−
Molindone	1	GPLM	−
Nicotine	0.1	HPM	−
Nicotinic acid	1	GPLM	−
4-Nitroimidazole	1	GPLM, HPM	+, +
N0164	1	GPLM, HPM	+, +
Papaverine	1	GPLM	−
Phenidone	1	GPLM	−
Salicylic acid	1	GPLM	−
Theophylline	1	GPLM	−

TABLE 2. *Effect of selected compounds on TXA$_2$ synthase from GPLM and HPM on PGI$_2$ Synthase from BAM and on the cyclooxygenase enzyme from SSVM*

	IC$_{50}$			
Compound	GPLM TXA$_2$ synthase (μM)	HPM TXA$_2$ synthase (μM)	BAM PGI$_2$ synthase (mM)	SSVM cyclooxygenase (mM)
Imidazole	600	600	>1	>1
L8027	900	2	0.1–1	0.002
N0164	104	10	0.1–1	0.105
Diazepam	800	nd[a]	>1	~1

[a] nd, not determined.

The 50% inhibition concentrations (IC$_{50}$) of selected compounds for TXA$_2$ synthase and PGI$_2$ synthase were calculated on the basis of the percent PGH$_2$ remaining and are summarized in Table 2.

In summary, imidazole was found to be a weak inhibitor (IC$_{50}$ = 600 μM) of TX formation from PGH$_2$ but had no effect (IC$_{50}$ > 1 mM) on either PG formation from arachidonate or PGI$_2$ formation from PGH$_2$. Diazepam was found to have an inhibitory profile equivalent to imidazole, while chlorodiazepoxide hydrochloride was without effect. L8027 and N0164 were more potent inhibitors of TX formation using HPM (IC$_{50}$ = 2.0 and 9.0 μM, respectively) as compared to TXA$_2$ formation using GPLM (IC$_{50}$ = 630 and 104 μM, respectively). Both imidazole and diazepam were equipotent inhibitors of TXA$_2$ formation from either HPM or GPLM. L8027 and N0164 inhibited PG formation (IC$_{50}$ = 2.0 and 105 μM, respectively), and both were rather weak inhibitors of PGI$_2$ formation (100 μM < IC$_{50}$ > 1 μM). Of the other benzodiazepines tested, flunitrazepam and clonazepam were weak inhibitors of TX formation from GPLM, while bromazepam and flurazepam were inactive. Other representative skeletal muscle relaxants (methocarbamol and metaxolone) and tranquilizers (butaclamol, haloperidol, and molindone) had no effect on TX formation from GPLM.

ACKNOWLEDGMENTS

The authors wish to note the invaluable technical assistance of Lynn A. Bevere and Robin L. Schwier and also thank Sue Ann Bremner for her excellent assistance in the preparation of the manuscript.

REFERENCES

1. Bundy, G. L., and Peterson, D. C. (1978): *Tetrahedron Lett.,* 1:41–44.
2. Corey, E. J., Niwa, H., Bloom, M., and Ramwell, P. W. (1979): *Tetradedron Lett.,* 8:671–674.
3. Eakins, K. E., and Kulkarni, P. S. (1977): *Br. J. Pharmacol.,* 60:135–140.
4. Fitzpatrick, F. A., and Gorman, R. R. (1978): *Biochim. Biophys. Acta,* 539:162–172.

5. Gorman, R. R., Bundy, G. L., Peterson, D. C., Sun, F. F., Miller, O. V., and Fitzpatrick, F. A. (1977): *Proc. Natl. Acad. Sci. USA,* 74:4007–4011.
6. Gryglewski, R. J., Zmuda, A., Korbut, R., Krecioch, E., and Bieron, K. (1977): *Nature,* 267:627–628.
7. Hamilton, J. G., and Tobias, L. D. (1977): *Prostaglandins,* 13:1019.
8. Moncada, S., Bunting, S., Mullane, K., Thorogood, P., Vane, J. R., Raz, A., and Needleman, P. (1977): *Prostaglandins,* 13:611–618.
9. Needleman, P., Bryan, B., Wyche, A., Bronson, S. D., Eakins, K., Ferrendelli, J. A., and Minkes, M. (1977): *Prostaglandins,* 14:897–907.
10. Tai, H.-H., and Yuan, B. (1978): *Biochim. Biophys. Acta,* 80:236–242.
11. Wallach, D. P., and Daniels, E. G. (1971): *Biochim. Biophys. Acta,* 231:445–447.
12. Yoshimoto, Y., Yamamoto, S., and Hayaishi, O. (1978): *Prostaglandins,* 16:529–540.

Advances in Prostaglandin and Thromboxane Research,
Vol. 6, edited by B. Samuelsson, P. W. Ramwell,
and R. Paoletti. Raven Press, New York © 1980.

Inhibition of Dog Platelet Reactivity Following 1-Benzylimidazole Administration

R. H. Harris, T. Fitzpatrick, J. Schmeling, R. Ryan, P. Kot, and
P. W. Ramwell

*Department of Physiology and Biophysics, Georgetown University Medical Center,
Washington, D.C. 20007*

Thromboxane A_2 (TXA_2) is recognized as the primary metabolite mediating the actions of arachidonate in platelets (1). These include the induction of platelet aggregation, the stimulation of dense granule release, and a potentiation of the effects of other platelet stimuli (2). Thus, TXA_2 joins with the other intracellular mediators, ADP and serotonin, as messengers to stimulate surrounding platelets and to recruit them in the formation of a developing thrombus.

Because of the pivotal role of TXA_2 in platelet activation, a thromboxane synthetase inhibitor, which would block the conversion of the intermediate endoperoxides into TXA_2, may be expected to have therapeutic potential for preventing mural thrombi formation in atherosclerotic and chronically obstructed vessels. Several thromboxane synthetase inhibitors have already been reported (3–8). Most of these, which inhibit arachidonate or endoperoxide metabolism to thromboxanes in cellular and subcellular preparations, also inhibit arachidonate-induced platelet aggregation in platelet-rich plasma (PRP). However, very little has been reported about their antiplatelet or pharmacologic activity in the intact animal. Therefore, we have studied in the dog 1-benzylimidazole (1-BI), a known inhibitor of human thromboxane synthetase (8).

Dog platelets differ from human platelets in their response to an arachidonate challenge (9). In general, arachidonate does not induce aggregation, even though following metabolism to TXA_2 it induces a shape change and potentiates the effects of other aggregation stimuli (9,10). Since these two activities are dependent on thromboxane synthesis, an inhibitor would be expected to alter these two parameters in addition to thromboxane synthesis.

MATERIALS AND METHODS

Dog PRP was prepared from citrated (3.8%; 1:9, v/v) blood, and physical measurements were made in an aggregometer. For metabolic studies, platelets were washed and incubated with ^{14}C-arachidonate. The products were extracted and subsequently separated and quantitated by TLC.

RESULTS

In this system, 1-BI inhibited the production of radiolabeled TXB_2 from arachidonate. However, the I_{50} (100 μM) contrasts with the value (0.25 μM) reported using human platelet microsomes as enzyme source (8). This decreased activity may result from poor intracellular penetration by the compound, or from extensive nonspecific binding in the more complex cell system, or because of species differences in enzyme sensitivity to 1-BI.

In vitro platelet function was also altered by 1-BI. Concentrations of 1–10 μM inhibited the arachidonate-induced shape change and potentiation of ADP aggregation, when marginally active concentrations of arachidonate were used. However greater than 100 μM 1-BI was sometimes required to inhibit higher arachidonate concentrations. The finding that both processes were affected by similar arachidonate and 1-BI concentrations is consistent with their being thromboxane-mediated effects. The dependence of 1-BI potency on substrate concentration may also explain why higher 1-BI concentrations were needed in our metabolic study, which utilized excess arachidonate.

The compound was subsequently tested for *in vivo* activity. Mongrel dogs, anesthetized with nembutal, were surgically prepared by cannulation of the femoral artery and vein. Systemic pressure was monitored throughout the study. Arterial blood samples were removed prior to the intravenous injection of 1-BI (10 mg/kg) and at selected times afterward. The PRP was prepared and tested as soon as possible after sampling.

Thirty minutes after 1-BI administration, the platelets were less sensitive to arachidonate-induced shape change (Fig. 1). The concentration of arachidonate

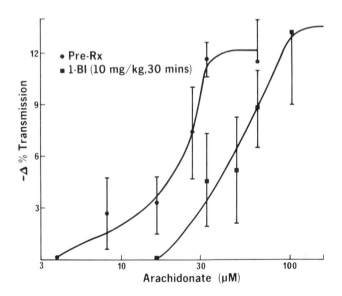

FIG. 1. Dose response of arachidonate-induced platelet shape change in PRP from dogs prior to (●) or 30 min after 1-benzylimidazole administration (■).

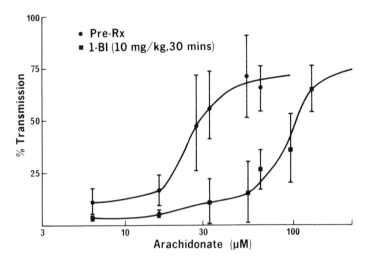

FIG. 2. Dose response of arachidonate-induced potentiation of ADP aggregation. Arachidonate was added 1 min prior to a suprathreshold ADP challenge. PRP was obtained from dogs prior to (●) or 30 min after 1-benzylimidazole (■).

necessary to produce a half-maximal change in shape (EC_{50}) had increased from 26 to 54 μM. Similarly, the EC_{50} for the potentiation of ADP aggregation was shifted from 32 to 66 μM (Fig. 2), while primary aggregation to ADP was unaffected. Indomethacin (2.5 mg/kg) proved more effective than 1-BI. It completely blocked both effects induced by arachidonate up to 330 μM. In addition, two dogs whose platelets aggregated irreversibly to arachidonate were included in this study. In both cases, higher arachidonate concentrations were required to induce aggregation after 1-BI administration.

The alterations in platelet sensitivity appeared very rapidly and persisted for up to 4 hr (Table 1). The extent of inhibition was very similar for both the shape change and potentiation responses. Marked increases in systemic pressure

TABLE 1. *Time course of 1-benzylimidazole activity*

Posttreatment (min)	% Δ baseline			EC_{50} arachidonate (μM)	
	SAP	Platelet	Hematocrit	Shape change	Potentiation
2	42.7 ± 7.4[a]	5 ± 6	7.7 ± 4.5	66 ± 9[a]	63 ± 13[a]
10	20.3 ± 8.5[a]	37 ± 16[a]	11.6 ± 4.5[a]	53 ± 7[a]	63 ± 12[a]
30	2.8 ± 3.3	37 ± 12[a]	17.6 ± 6.1[a]	54 ± 10[a]	66 ± 17[a]
120	−9.2 ± 11.5	72 ± 30[a]	18.1 ± 6.1[a]	65 ± 13[a]	62 ± 17[a]
240	−0.1 ± 7.3	20 ± 10	18.9 ± 5.3[a]	53 ± 13[a]	53 ± 13[a]
Pretreatment levels	127 ± 5 (mm Hg)	120 ± 30 (×10³/μl)	31 ± 2	26 ± 6 (μM)	32 ± 9 (μM)

[a] Significantly different from pretreatment values ($p < .05$).
SAP is systemic arterial pressure.

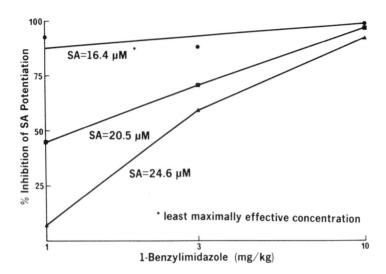

FIG. 3. Effectiveness of 1-benzylimidazole as an inhibitor of arachidonate potentiation. PRP from dogs pretreated with 1-benzylimidazole (30 min) was stimulated with increasing arachidonate concentrations. Inhibition was relative to a pretreated control sample.

also occurred almost immediately but generally normalized by one-half hour. Increases in platelet counts and hematocrit were noted; the former started to decline during the study but the latter remained elevated.

This increase in platelets may have arisen from the breakdown of circulating platelet aggregates or their release from vessel walls, two thromboxane-regulated processes. But the accompanying rise in hematocrit and systemic pressure favors the more likely explanation that splenic contraction leading to the expulsion of sequestered platelets and red cells may be responsible. It is known that splenic sequestration of these blood elements occurs during anesthesia. Such a state would be favorable to this proposed action for 1-BI.

Attempts to separate the cardiovascular effects from the antiplatelet activity were unsuccessful. Oral administration of 1-BI (20–25 mg/kg) produced pressure changes comparable to the intravenous route. Doses of 1 and 3 mg/kg i.v. produced smaller elevations in pressure, but also less effectively inhibited platelet function (Fig. 3). Activity for 1 mg/kg 1-BI could be demonstrated when a minimally effective arachidonate challenge was used, but activity rapidly fell off as the arachidonate challenge was increased.

CONCLUSIONS

1-Benzylimidazole inhibits the actions of arachidonate in canine platelets by blocking thromboxane synthesis. Platelets from dogs treated with 1-BI are similarly desensitized. However, the undesirable pressor effects—which could not be separated from the platelet activity—preclude the use of 1-benzylimidazole as an antithrombotic agent. Despite this, the search for a suitable thromboxane synthetase inhibitor remains attractive. Aspirin, which inhibits the cyclooxygenase, has received considerable attention as a therapy in thrombosis-sensitive diseases. A thromboxane synthetase inhibitor may be even more beneficial in this regard. Unlike aspirin, it would not affect nonplatelet production of prostacyclin. The normal production of this natural antiplatelet metabolite of arachidonate then would complement the antithrombotic actions of a thromboxane synthetase inhibitor.

ACKNOWLEDGMENTS

This work was supported by grants from American Heart Association, Washington Chapter 1V1-4G-0011280, and from NIH HL-18718.

REFERENCES

1. Hamberg, M., Svensson, J., and Samuelsson, B. (1975): *Proc. Natl. Acad. Sci. USA,* 72:2994–2998.
2. Silver, M. J., Smith, J. B., Ingerman, C. M., and Kocsis, J. J. (1973): *Prostaglandins,* 4:863–875.
3. Moncada, S., Bunting, S., Vane, J. R., Mullane, K., Thorogood, P., Raz, A., and Needleman, P. (1977): *Prostaglandins,* 13:611–618.
4. Alusy, V. D., and Hammarstrom, S. (1977): *FEBS Lett.,* 82:107–110.
5. Gryglewski, R. G., Zmuda, A., Dembinska-Kiec, A., and Krecioch, E. (1977): *Pharmacol. Res. Comm.,* 9:109–116.
6. Kulkarni, P. S., and Eakins, K. E. (1976): *Prostaglandins,* 12:465–469.
7. Fitzpatrick, F. A., and Gorman, R. R. (1978): *Biochim. Biophys. Acta,* 539:162–172.
8. Tai, H. H., and Yuan, B. (1978): *Biochem. Biophys. Res. Commun.,* 80:236–242.
9. Chignard, M., and Vergaftig, B. B. (1976): *Eur. J. Pharmacol.,* 38:7–18.
10. Chignard, M., and Vergaftig, B. B. (1976): *Prostaglandins,* 14:222–240.

Advances in Prostaglandin and Thromboxane Research,
Vol. 6, edited by B. Samuelsson, P. W. Ramwell,
and R. Paoletti. Raven Press, New York © 1980.

Effect of an Inhibitor of TXA$_2$ Synthesis and of PGE$_2$ on the Formation of 12-L-Hydroxy-5,8,10-Heptadecatrienoic Acid in Human Platelets

J. E. Vincent, F. J. Zijlstra, and *H. van Vliet

*Departments of Pharmacology and *Haematology, Medical Faculty, Erasmus University, 3000 DR Rotterdam, The Netherlands*

In platelets, arachidonic acid (AA) is transformed during aggregation into thromboxane A$_2$ (TXA$_2$), 12-L-hydroxy-5,8,10-heptadecatrienoic acid (HHT), 12-L-hydroxy-5,8,10,14-eicosatetraenoic acid (HETE), and small amounts of prostaglandins (PGs) E$_2$, F$_{2\alpha}$, and D$_2$ (3,4). Several substances have been described which inhibit the formation of TXA$_2$ from the endoperoxide PGH$_2$, which is an intermediate in this reaction (2,5,6,7,10,11). This inhibition leads to an increased formation of PGE$_2$, PGF$_{2\alpha}$, and PGD$_2$ (7,9,11).

It is not yet clear whether TXA$_2$ or PGH$_2$ is the precursor of HHT. It was also proposed that TXA$_2$ and HHT are formed from a common precursor (1). In a number of experiments in which the formation of TXB$_2$ from AA and PGH$_2$ was compared, we found that more HHT than TXB$_2$ was formed from AA, whereas equal amounts were formed from PGH$_2$. This was further investigated by measuring the effect of the inhibition of the synthesis of TXA$_2$ on the formation of TXB$_2$ and HHT. The effect of the addition of PGE$_2$ on the formation of the above-mentioned substances was also investigated.

MATERIALS AND METHODS

Citrated blood was collected from male volunteers who had not taken aspirin or other antiinflammatory drugs for at least a week. The blood was centrifuged for 5 min at 300 × g; the supernatant (PRP) was collected and to 2 ml PRP was added 0.4 ml of a 3.3% acid citrate dextrose solution and 0.2 ml of a 1% (w/v) ethylenediaminetetraacetic acid solution. Platelets were centrifuged for 15 min at 1400 × g and resuspended in Tris buffer (pH 6.2; ca. 1 ml/20 ml PRP). To this suspension was added Ca^{2+}-free Krebs-Henseleit buffer to a final concentration of 300 × 10^6 platelets/ml. Platelet aggregation was induced by collagen and measured as previously described (12).

The labeling of the resuspended platelets with [1-^{14}C]AA, the extraction, separation, and the determination of the PGs, TXB$_2$, and HHT by thin-layer chromatography (TLC) were performed as previously described for rat platelets

(11). The thin-layer chromatograms were developed using the following systems: First direction: $CHCl_3/MeOH/HAc/H_2O = 90:8:1:0.8$.

Second direction: diethyl ether/methanol/acetic acid (90:1:2) was used in the separation of PGs and TXB_2. The organic phase of ethyl acetate/*iso*-octane/ acetic acid/water (55:25:10:50) was used in the separation of HHT, HETE, and AA. TLC plates were scanned with a two-dimensional Berthold Dünnschicht scanner, using a dot printer. Dots were scratched off and counted in a Packard scintillation counter.

[1-^{14}C]AA (specific activity, 60.2 mCi/mmole) was obtained from the Radiochemical Center, Amersham. [1-^{14}C]PGH$_2$ (specific activity, 0.4 mCi/mmole) was a gift of E. Christ-Hazelhof, Unilever ResearchVlaardingen, The Netherlands. PGD_2 was a gift of Dr. Pike, The Upjohn Co. PGE_2, $PGF_{2\alpha}$, F_2, and PGA_2 were obtained from Sigma Chemical Co. All chemicals used were analytical grade from Merck, Darmstadt, West Germany.

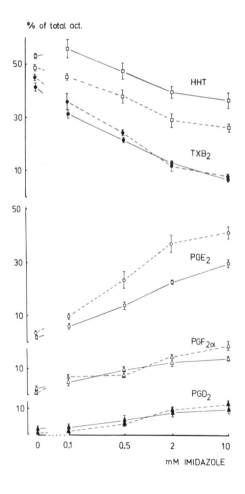

FIG. 1. Metabolites formed from AA in resuspended human platelets. The values shown express the percentage of the total amount of radioactivity of TXB_2, PGE_2, $PGF_{2\alpha}$, PGD_2, and HHT. Incubations: imidazole for 1 min, followed by [1-^{14}C]AA for 3 min and collagen, 40 μg/ ml, for 2 min. Imidazole (—) and PGE_2, 5 μg, + imidazole (---). $N = 4$.

TABLE 1. *Metabolites formed from PGH_2 in resuspended human platelets*[a]

	$PGF_{2\alpha}$	TXB_2	PGE_2	PGD_2	HHT	N
PRS	4.08 ± 0.30	21.08 ± 1.13	36.12 ± 1.18	15.48 ± 0.94	23.28 ± 1.21[b]	5
PRS + imidazole	8.13 ± 0.70	4.83 ± 0.23	59.83 ± 1.94	19.77 ± 0.94	7.50 ± 1.48	3
PRS + PGE_2	3.63 ± 0.40	20.68 ± 0.88	40.30 ± 1.45	16.93 ± 0.48	18.48 ± 1.61[b]	4
PRS + PGE_2 + imidazole	7.03 ± 0.26	4.58 ± 0.24	57.78 ± 1.40	22.80 ± 1.00	7.83 ± 0.99	4
Krebs	6.03 ± 0.69	4.50 ± 0.97	55.88 ± 1.20	21.09 ± 2.37	12.43 ± 1.33	7

[a] The values shown express the percentage of the total amount of radioactivity of TXB_2, PGE_2, $PGF_{2\alpha}$, PGD_2, and HHT. Incubations: imidazole 10 mM and PGE_2, 5 µg for 1 min, followed by $[1 - {}^{14}C]$ PGH_2 for 3 min and collagen, 40 µg/ml, for 2 min. PRS = platelet-rich suspension.
[b] The difference is statistically significant ($p < 0.05$).

RESULTS AND DISCUSSION

The products formed from AA in platelets during aggregation have been determined. The amount of HHT formed is higher than that of TXB_2. Formation of small quantities of PGE_2, $PGF_{2\alpha}$, and PGD_2 also takes place. When imidazole is added, the formation of both TXB_2 and HHT is inhibited and that of the PGs increased. The synthesis of TXB_2 is inhibited to a greater extent than that of HHT (Fig. 1). The addition of PGE_2 leads to a decrease in the formation of HHT. There is no effect on the synthesis of TXB_2, whereas the formation of PGE_2 is increased.

The substances formed from PGH_2 in platelets after aggregation were also determined (Table 1). These included TXB_2, HHT, PGE_2, $PGF_{2\alpha}$, and PGD_2 with the amounts of TXB_2 and HHT formed being equal. The addition of imidazole leads to the inhibition of the formation of both TXB_2 and HHT. The inhibitory effect is greater on the synthesis of TXB_2, which may be ascribed to the formation of larger amounts of HHT from PGH_2 in buffer.

These results may be explained by assuming the existence of two pathways in the formation of HHT. In the first one, this substance is formed from TXA_2 and in the second from an intermediate which is situated before the formation of PGH_2. The last one could be PGG_2. It is supposed that only the first pathway is inhibited by imidazole. The addition of PGE_2 leads to a decreased amount of HHT formed from AA. This could be due to the inhibition of the second pathway of HHT formation. The effect of PGE_2 shows that interrelationships exist between the substances formed from AA, and this may form part of a feedback mechanism.

REFERENCES

1. Diczfalusy, U., Falardeau, P., and Hammarström, S. (1977): *FEBS Lett.,* 84:271–274.
2. Eakins, K. E., and Kulkarni, P. S. (1977): *Br. J. Pharmacol.,* 60:135–140.

3. Hamberg, M., Svensson, J., and Samuelsson, B. (1974): *Proc. Natl. Acad. Sci. USA*, 71:3824–3828.
4. Hamberg, M., Svensson, J., and Samuelsson, B. (1975): *Proc. Natl. Acad. Sci. USA*, 72:2994–2998.
5. Kulkarni, P. S., and Eakins, K. E. (1976): *Prostaglandins*, 12:465–469.
6. Moncada, S., Bunting, S., Mullane, K., Thorogood, P., and Vane, J. R. (1977): *Prostaglandins*, 13:611–618.
7. Needleman, P., Bryan, B., Wyche, A., Bronson, S. D., Eakins, K., Ferrendelli, J. A., and Minkes, M. (1977): *Prostaglandins*, 14:897–907.
8. Needleman, P., Raz, A., Ferrendelli, J. A., and Minkes, M. (1977): *Proc. Natl. Acad. Sci. USA*, 74:1716–1720.
9. Nijkamp, F. P., Moncada, S., White, H. L., and Vane, J. R. (1977): *Eur. J. Pharmacol.*, 44:179–186.
10. Raz, A., Aharony, D., and Kenig-Wakshal, R. (1978): *Eur. J. Biochem.*, 86:447–454.
11. Vincent, J. E., and Zijlstra, F. J. (1978): *Prostaglandins*, 15:629–636.
12. Vincent, J. E., Zijlstra, F. J., and Bonta, I. L. (1975): *Prostaglandins*, 10:899–911.

Advances in Prostaglandin and Thromboxane Research,
Vol. 6, edited by B. Samuelsson, P. W. Ramwell,
and R. Paoletti. Raven Press, New York © 1980.

Partial Agonism of Prostaglandin H_2 Analogs and 11-Deoxy-Prostaglandin $F_{2\alpha}$ to Thromboxane-Sensitive Preparations

R. L. Jones and N. H. Wilson

Department of Pharmacology, University of Edinburgh, Edinburgh EH8 9JZ, Scotland

One method of searching for antagonists of a particular receptor is to rigorously examine possible compounds for evidence of partial agonism. If these investigations are fruitful, then chemical modification of the partial agonist may eventually lead to selective antagonists of high potency. We have investigated a large number of prostaglandin analogs with the object of detecting partial agonist activity at thromboxane (TX) receptor sites. Two typical TXA_2 actions, the contraction of isolated vascular smooth muscle (7) and the aggregation of human blood platelets *in vitro* (1), have been monitored. The chemical instability of the natural agonist, TXA_2 ($t_{1/2}$ at 37°C in water, 30–40 sec) (2), poses a problem in this type of experiment. Our policy has been to use a stable compound with TX-like actions as the standard agonist in initial studies and then to perform similar experiments with biologically generated TXA_2.

METHODS

Platelet Aggregation

Human blood (100 ml) obtained by venipuncture was added to citrate anticoagulant (20 ml of a solution containing 2 g disodium hydrogen citrate and 3 g dextrose in 120 ml water). After centrifugation (200 × g for 15 min), the platelet-rich plasma (PRP) was removed. Aggregation of the platelets was measured by the optical method. The cuvette contents—1.0 ml of PRP, 1.0 ml of Krebs–Henseleit solution, and 0.4 ml of 0.9% (w/v) NaCl solution—were stirred with a polished steel rod at about 1000 rpm and maintained at 37°C. After a 2-min equilibration period, compounds were added to the cuvette, dissolved in 0.10 ml of 0.9% (w/v) NaCl solution, and the aggregation process recorded. The response was taken as the maximum decrease in light absorption occurring during the first 100 sec after addition of the drug. In some of the inhibition studies the potential inhibitor was added 2 min before the addition of the aggregatory agent.

Rat blood was obtained from male rats (250–350 g) under ether anesthesia by needle puncture of the abdominal aorta. Citrated PRP was prepared as described above.

Isolated Vascular Preparations

Thoracic aortas from young male rabbits were removed immediately after they had been killed. Lateral saphenous veins were obtained from pentobarbital-anesthetized dogs of either sex within 30 min of induction of anesthesia. Spiral strips of vessel, 3 mm wide, were cut and suspended in Krebs–Henseleit solution (NaCl, 118; KCl, 5.4; $MgSO_4$, 1.0; $CaCl_2$, 2.5; NaH_2PO_4, 1.2; $NaHCO_3$, 25; dextrose, 10 mmoles/liter) gassed with 95% O_2 and 5% CO_2 and maintained at 37°C. The organ bath volume was 8 ml. Tension changes were recorded with a Grass FTO3 force displacement transducer linked to a Grass polygraph.

Compounds

The following compounds were gifts from The Upjohn Company, (U.S.): $PGF_{2\alpha}$, 15-*S*-15-methyl-$PGF_{2\alpha}$, 16,16-dimethyl $PGF_{2\alpha}$, PGE_2, 15-*S*-15-methyl PGE_2, 16,16-dimethyl PGE_2, PGD_2, 15-*S*-hydroxy-11α,9α-(epoxy-methano)-prosta-5Z,13E-dienoic acid (U 46619), 15-S-hydroxy-9α,11α-azoprosta-5Z,13E-dienoic acid (U 51093). The following compounds (all racemic) were donated by ICI Pharmaceuticals Division (U.K.): the 16-*p*-fluorophenoxy (ICI 79939) and 16-*p*-chlorophenoxy (ICI 79492) derivatives of 17,18,19,20-tetranor-$PGF_{2\alpha}$; 16-*p*-chlorophenoxy-17,18,19,20-tetranor-PGE_2 (ICI 80205), 15-δ-hydroxy-9α,11α-etheno-prosta-5*Z*,13*E*-dienoic acid (ICI 86841). PGI_2 sodium salt was donated by Schering AG, Berlin. 11-Deoxy-$PGF_{2\alpha}$ analogs were prepared in this laboratory by sodium borohydride reduction of the corresponding PGA_2 compounds. The following racemic compounds were also synthesized; 15-*S*-hydroxy-9α,11α-ethano-prosta-5Z,13E-dienoic acid and its 15-S-15-methyl analog; and 15-*S*-hydroxy-9α,11α-etheno-16-*p*-fluorophenoxy-17,18,19,20-tetranorprosta-5Z,13E-dienoic acid (EP 011), its 9α,11α-ethano derivative (EP 031), its 9α,11α-ethano-16-*p*-chlorophenoxy derivative (EP 032), and its 16-*p*-chlorobenzyl derivative (EP 016) (all racemic).

RESULTS

Vascular Smooth Muscle Preparations

In terms of TX-like action on "slow" preparations such as the rabbit aorta and the dog saphenous vein, the only practical method of obtaining complete concentration–effect relationships is by *cumulative* addition of suitable doses to the organ bath. Our initial experiments were preformed on the rabbit aorta with the 11,9-epoxymethano-PGH_2 analog as the standard agonist. However, on many preparations the rate of decay of either a maximum or near-maximum response following washout of the organ bath was tediously slow. We therefore decided to obtain comprehensive data using the dog saphenous vein preparation and 16-*p*-fluorophenoxy-17,18,19,20-tetranor-PGF$_{2\alpha}$ (ICI 79939) as the standard agonist, this combination giving the fastest return to resting tension on washout. We have recently shown that ICI 79939 has potent TX-like actions on several preparations (3).

Full Agonists

All the 16,16-dimethyl, 16-*p*-fluorophenoxy, and 16-p-chlorophenoxy analogs tested were found to be full agonists on the saphenous vein preparation. Equipotent molar ratios (11,9-epoxymethano-PGH$_2$ = 1.0) are given in Table 1. In addition, 9,11-azo PGH$_2$ and the 15-*S*-15-methyl derivatives of PGF$_{2\alpha}$ and 11-deoxy PGF$_{2\alpha}$ were full agonists with concentration–effect curves parallel to that of ICI 79939. There are considerable variations in potency among these compounds, the 16-*p*-fluorophenoxy derivatives of 9,11-etheno and 9,11-ethano-PGH$_2$ combining high potency with a remarkably persistent duration of contractile action following washout (4).

Partial Agonists

Six compounds gave maxima lower than ICI 79939 (= 100%). They were PGF$_{2\alpha}$ (50–70%), 11-deoxy-PGF$_{2\alpha}$ (50–75), 9,11-etheno-PGH$_2$ (70–80%) and its 16-*p*-chlorobenzyl analog (15–55%), and 9,11-ethano-PGH$_2$ (70–80%) and its 15-methyl analog (75–85%). Marked antagonism of ICI 79939 was observed with the higher concentrations of these compounds, whereas the contractile action of epinephrine was not opposed. A typical tracing showing the action

TABLE 1. *Potencies of compounds acting as full agonists on the dog saphenous vein preparation[a]*

Ring system	Side chain	Equipotent molar ratios (11,9-epoxymethano-PGH$_2$ = 1.0)				
	Natural[b]	15-Me	16,16-diMe	16-O-ϕ-F	16-O-ϕ-Cl
F$_\alpha$	PA[c]	360	15	4.0	4.8
E	↓	↓	55	5.0	8.5
D	↓			16.5	
11-deoxy-F$_\alpha$	PA	6.9	0.80		0.60
9,11-azo-H	1.2				
9,11-etheno-H	PA			0.52	
9,11-ethano-H	PA	PA		0.90	3.2

[a] All compounds have the *cis*-Δ-5,6 side chain.
[b] ↓ Indicates that these compounds relax saphenous vein preparations partially contracted with 11,9-epoxymethano-PGH$_2$, ICI 79939, or norepinephrine.
[c] PA, partial agonist.

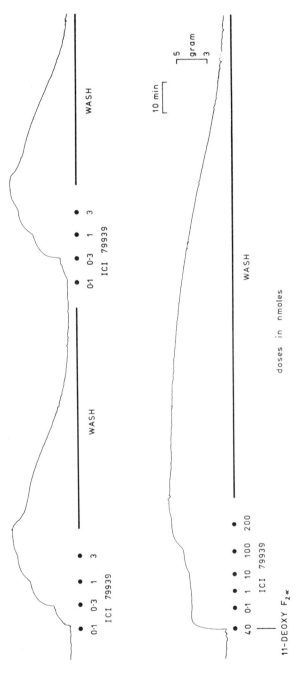

FIG. 1. Partial agonism exhibited by 11-deoxy PGF$_{2\alpha}$ in the dog saphenous vein *in vitro*.

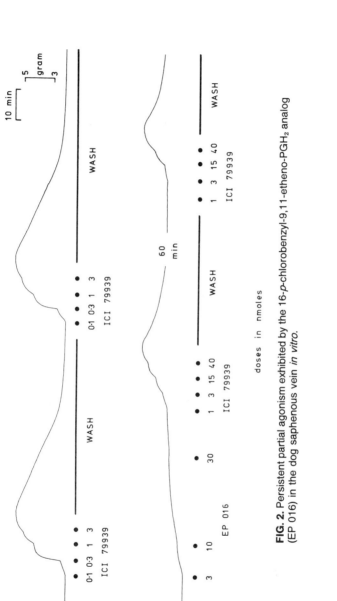

10 min

5
gram
3

WASH

ICI 79939
0·1 0·3 1   3

WASH

ICI 79939
0·1 0·3 1   3

60
min

WASH

ICI 79939
1   3 15 40

WASH

ICI 79939
1   3 15 40

30

EP 016

10

3

doses in nmoles

FIG. 2. Persistent partial agonism exhibited by the 16-*p*-chlorobenzyl-9,11-etheno-PGH₂ analog (EP 016) in the dog saphenous vein *in vitro*.

of 11-deoxy $PGF_{2\alpha}$ is shown in Fig. 1. With the bicycloheptane/ene compounds, particularly the 16-p-chlorobenzyl analog (EP 016), both the contractile action and the antagonism of ICI 79939 persisted after washout (Fig. 2).

Platelet Aggregation

The 11,9-epoxymethano-PGH₂ analog and adenosinediphosphate (ADP) were used as the standard aggregatory agents.

Inhibitors of Aggregation

We observed that PGI_2, PGE_1, and PGD_2 were more effective inhibitors of the aggregation induced by the PGH₂ analog than of aggregation produced by ADP (2–4-fold difference in concentration). PGI_2 (threshold concentration, $0.5-1 \times 10^{-9}$ M) was 10 to 20 times more potent than PGE_1 and PGD_2.

Compounds Producing Irreversible Platelet Aggregation

All the compounds which were full agonists on the dog saphenous vein (given in equipotent molar ratios, Table 1) elicited irreversible aggregation of human platelets. With the exception of the PGE analogs, the characteristics of the responses were identical; with increasing concentration, these responses consisted of a shape change, a primary reversible aggregation wave, occasionally a primary wave merging into a secondary irreversible wave, and a rapid and smooth irreversible wave. The magnitude of the primary aggregation induced by each agent was unaffected by the presence of indomethacin (10^{-5}M) in the cuvette.

Substances Producing Only Platelet Shape Change and/or Reversible Aggregation

We shall now consider the six compounds that exhibited partial agonist activity on the dog saphenous vein. $PGF_{2\alpha}$ had no effect on human platelets, either stimulatory or inhibitory, at concentrations up to 10^{-4}M. The 15-methyl-9,11-ethano-PGH₂ analog produced irreversible aggregation and was estimated to be 5 times less active than 11,9-epoxymethano-PGH₂. 9,11-Etheno- and 9,11-ethano-PGH₂ produced primary reversible aggregation waves over the concentration range 5×10^{-6} to 1×10^{-4}M. Simultaneous addition of either one of these analogs and the 11,9-epoxymethano-PGH₂ analog resulted in significantly smaller responses than predicted from the addition of their separate effects (Fig. 3). Similar experiments in which one of the analogs and ADP were added simultaneously to the platelet suspension resulted in a synergistic action on platelet aggregation. Combinations of ICI 79939 and ADP and 11,9-epoxymethano-PGH₂ and ADP were also synergistic.

The 16-p-chlorobenzyl-PGH₂ analog elicited a concentration-dependent shape

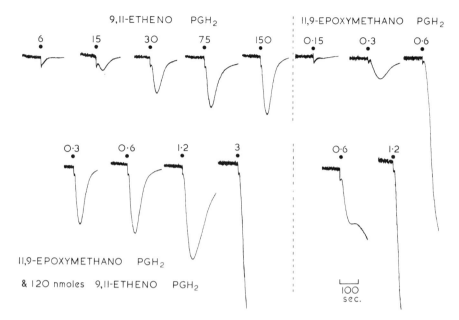

FIG. 3. Aggregation responses (measured by a change in light absorbance of the suspension) to 11,9-epoxymethano PGH₂ and 9,11-etheno PGH₂ in human platelets *in vitro.* Doses expressed in nmoles; final volume, 2.5 ml. Upper and lower traces are consecutive in time.

change but never a wave of aggregation (highest concentration tested, 10^{-4}M) (Fig. 4). Simultaneous addition of this analog and the 11,9-epoxymethano-PGH₂ analog resulted in antagonism of the aggregatory action of the latter compound. This profile of activity was essentially unaltered in the presence of indomethacin (10^{-5}M). The aggregatory activity of arachidonic acid was also markedly reduced, whereas that of ADP was slightly potentiated.

11-Deoxy-PGF$_{2\alpha}$ produced a unique profile of activity on human platelets. A platelet shape change was observed with concentrations of 5×10^{-7} to 3×10^{-6}M; higher concentrations (up to 10^{-4}M) produced a *small* reversible wave of aggregation of rapid onset and reversal. This effect could be mimicked by simultaneously adding the 11,9-epoxymethano-PGH₂ analog and either PGE₁ or PGD₂ to the cuvette.

11-Deoxy-PGF$_{2\alpha}$, 0.5 to 1×10^{-5}M, inhibited the aggregatory action of the 11,9-epoxymethano analog added 2 min later; ADP action was unaffected. Higher concentrations ($3-6 \times 10^{-5}$M) of 11-deoxy-PGF$_{2\alpha}$ inhibited ADP. On rat PRP, both PGI₂ and PGE₁ inhibited ADP at low concentrations, whereas PGD₂ was without effect. 11,9-Epoxymethano-PGH₂ elicited the platelet shape change over the concentration range 3×10^{-7} to 3×10^{-6}M. 11-Deoxy-PGF$_{2\alpha}$ (up to 5×10^{-5}M) showed no inhibitory action on the aggregation induced by ADP. On cat PRP, PGI₂ and PGE₁ were again inhibitory to ADP at low concentrations (2×10^{-9} and 10^{-7}M, respectively), whereas much higher doses

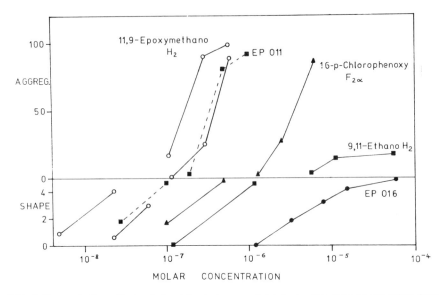

FIG. 4. Concentration–effect relationships in human platelets *in vitro*. Results are taken from two experiments: the 11,9-epoxymethano-PGH₂ curve to the left corresponds to the EP 016 curve; the one to the right to the remaining compounds. The response units correspond to 0.1-inch divisions on the pen recorder.

of PGD₂ were required ($>10^{-5}$M). 11,9-Epoxymethano-PGH₂ caused irreversible aggregation at concentrations of 2 to 5 × 10^{-7}M; 11-deoxy-PGF₂α produced an identical pattern of response at concentrations some 20-fold higher.

CONCLUSIONS

1. For compounds which show no inhibition of ADP-induced aggregation on human platelets, there is a good correlation between their full agonist/partial agonist properties on the dog saphenous vein and on human platelets. The persistent partial agonism of the bicycloheptane/ene analogs is of particular interest. Investigations of their interaction with TXA₂ are in progress.

2. 11-Deoxy-PGF₂α is also a partial agonist on the dog saphenous vein but, unlike the other compounds, blocks ADP-induced aggregation of human platelets at high concentrations. This effect may be due to a weak PGD₂-like action. It has no inhibitory action on cat and rat platelets, which are insensitive to PGD₂ but sensitive to PGE₁ and PGI₂ (5,6). It is therefore not possible to ascertain the nature of the direct interaction of 11-deoxy-PGF₂α with the TX receptor of human platelets.

ACKNOWLEDGMENTS

The gifts of PGS from ICI Pharmaceuticals Division, U.K.; The Upjohn Company, U.S.; and Schering AG, Berlin, are gratefully acknowledged. We wish to record our appreciation of the support and encouragement of Professor E. W. Horton during these studies.

REFERENCES

1. Hamberg, M., Svensson, J., and Samuelsson, B. (1975): *Proc. Natl. Acad. Sci. USA,* 72:2994–2998.
2. Hamberg, M., Svensson, J., and Samuelsson, B. (1976): *Advances in Prostaglandin and Thromboxane Research,* Vol. 1, edited by B. Samuelsson and R. Paoletti, pp. 19–27. Raven Press, New York.
3. Jones, R. L., and Marr, C. G. (1977): *Br. J. Pharmacol.,* 61:694–696.
4. Jones, R. L., and Wilson, N. H. (1978): *Br. J. Pharmacol.,* 63:372P.
5. Mills, D. C. B., and MacFarlane, D. E. (1977): In: *Prostaglandins in Hematology,* edited by M. J. Silver, J. B. Smith, and J. J. Kocsis, pp. 219–233. Spectrum Publications, New York.
6. Moncada, S., Vane, J. R., and Whittle, B. J. R. (1977): *J. Physiol.,* 273:2P–4P.
7. Needleman, P., Moncada, S., Bunting, S., Vane, J. R., Hamberg, M., and Samuelsson, B. (1976): *Nature,* 261:558–560.

Advances in Prostaglandin and Thromboxane Research,
Vol. 6, edited by B. Samuelsson, P. W. Ramwell,
and R. Paoletti. Raven Press, New York © 1980.

Thromboxane Molecules Are Not Hairpin Conformers

D. A. Langs, G. T. DeTitta, M. G. Erman, and S. Fortier

Medical Foundation of Buffalo, Inc., Buffalo, New York 14203

The book jacket of this series, as well as the cover illustration of the journal *Prostaglandins,* displays a conformational model of a prostaglandin (PG) molecule. For many years we have been subject to this subliminal suggestion of the importance of conformation to PG biochemistry, yet none of us is foolish enough to believe that these molecules do not bend. But although these hormones may appear to be nearly infinitely flexible and conformationally nondescript, the chemical evidence strongly suggests that the more probable conformations are severely restricted to what have been characterized as hairpin forms (1).

Diffraction methods have been used to explore the range of hairpin flexibility of various PG hormones, and it will be interesting to further investigate whether the details of the conformational dissimilarities of these hormones will prove useful in formulating tentative structure–activity relationships and encourage the testing of hormone analogs which might be designed to stress certain conformational characteristics thought important.

At present the structure–activity relationships inferred for thromboxane (TX) hormones and analogs are based on chemical rather than conformational differentiation (5,8). Although the short half-lives (6) of these interesting compounds discourage direct conformational investigation, no one has suggested that the conformational patterns of the TX hormones would be significantly different from the hairpin forms observed for PGs.

THROMBOXANE CONFORMATION

We have recently examined the crystalline conformation of TXB_2, which we suggest may be a good model for TXA_2 with regard to ring junction geometry and side chain conformations. TXB_2 was found to crystallize with two conformationally distinct molecules in the unit cell, neither of which could be described as a hairpin form. These two conformers offer interesting possibilities for reexamining the duality of physiological activity exhibited by TXs in arterial vasoconstriction (9) and blood platelet aggregation (6). An unusual conformational similarity between the ω-chains of the two TXB_2 molecules may in part explain

477

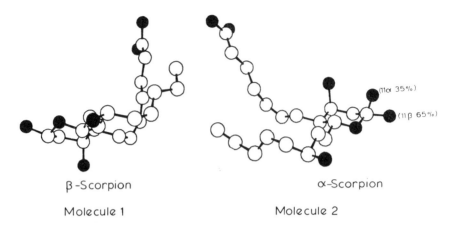

β -Scorpion   α-Scorpion

Molecule 1   Molecule 2

FIG. 1. Molecular models of the α- and β-tail scorpion conformers of TXB₂. The equilibrium percentages for the anomeric disorder of the O11 hydroxyl group of the α-tail scorpion conformer are given.

the resistance of these compounds to degradation by 15-hydroxy-PG dehydrogenase (PGDH) (7,10).

Unlike hairpin conformers, which require fully extended side chains, the side chains of TXB₂ are folded back on one another to give the molecules a decidedly bowed appearance. This is particularly noted in the torsional angles which flank the *cis*-C5=C6 double bond. These angles in PG2-series compounds are both generally in the range of +145 to +180°, imparting a shallow S-curve normal to the direction of the chain as it extends through the double-bond region. The flanking *cis*-C5=C6 torsional angles for TXB₂ have opposite signs, indicating that the α-chains fold back on themselves rather than extend. In one TXB₂ conformer, the carboxylic acid chain turns up through a right angle in the direction of the β-face of the molecule; in the other conformer, this side chain turns down through a right angle in the direction of the α-face of the molecule. It may be convenient to refer to these two distinct conformational types as either the β- or α-tail "scorpion" conformation as is illustrated in Fig. 1. The ω-chains of these two molecules are somewhat unusual in that the C16–C17 torsion angles are both (+)syn-clinal rather than trans-planar, as has been noted for all PG hairpin conformers. This unusual kink has the effect of foreshortening the ω-chain and allowing its end to fold in close to the double-bond region of the α-chain. The α-tail scorpion conformer exists as a statistically disordered 2:1 mixture of β- versus α-11-hydroxy anomers in the crystal; the β-tail conformer was found ordered in the β-11-hydroxy configuration.

ACTIVITY OF TXA₂ ANALOGS

The activity data which can logically be inferred for TX compounds from the work of Needleman et al. (8) in blood platelet aggregation and arterial vasoconstriction is worth enumerating. Whereas TXA₂ was known to be potent for both platelet aggregation and vasoconstriction, TXA_1 exhibited neither of these activities. TXA_3 constricted arteries but did not affect aggregation, while nor-2-TXA_2 aggregated platelets but did not affect arterial contractions. These data suggested that a *cis*-Δ^5 unsaturation was a necessary, if not sufficient, *chemical* condition for activity by either assay. The observed TXB_2 conformers suggest a *structural* rather than a chemical role for the *cis*-C5=C6 bond, i.e., the ability to drastically bend the α-chain away from a trans-planar geometry. Molecular models suggest that TXA_1 is inactive because it is a hairpin conformer possessing the α-chain with a trans-planar C8–C12 ring junction geometry.

DISCUSSION

It is not clear why TXA_3 and nor-2-TXA_2 should express only the mutually exclusive activities of TXA_2 unless the recognition sites encoding platelet aggregation and vasoconstriction required different conformational presentations of the hormone. If this duality of activity for TXA_2 is indicative of its ability to equilibrate between two drastically different conformations, could the two antipodal conformers seen for TXB_2 be relevant or might the relevant conformers escape the chosen accident of crystallization. If one should believe that the α- and β-tail scorpion conformers encode one or the other of the two activities, then TXA_3 and nor-2-TXA_2 must be expected to adopt opposing conformations. Although it seems reasonable to associate nor-2-TXA_2 with the α-tail conformer, which would produce an intramolecular hydrogen bond between the carboxyl group and O9, it is far more difficult to envision how a *cis*-Δ^{17} unsaturation might effect the conformational equilibrium in a unidirectional way.

The (+)gauche twist in the ω-chains of both TXB_2 conformers correlates well with the resistance (7,10) of TXB_2 to PGDH metabolism. The mechanism of action of the enzyme is understood to require NAD+ abstraction of H15 from the β-facial side of the substrate molecule (3,4). If the nicotinamide group of NAD+ is positioned directly above H15 in the active site of PGDH, it should be fairly clear that a (+)gauche twist would block access to H15 by turning the end of the ω-chain in that direction. The observation that significant amounts of TXB_2 were degraded to the 15-keto metabolite by PGDH in an antigen-challenged isolated perfusion system provided by sensitized guinea pig lung tissue (2) is not at variance with the previously noted TXB_2 resistance to PGDH metabolism under normal physiological conditions. This observation does suggest, however, that the conformational preference for the (+)gauche twist is not sufficient to prevent less probable, but conformationally more agreeable, forms of the substrate from reacting with the enzyme over prolonged exposure periods.

ACKNOWLEDGMENTS

We wish to express our thanks to Drs. J. Pike and G. Bundy of The Upjohn Company for offering the TXB_2 used in this study. Dr. S. Hannessian made useful suggestions regarding crystallization procedures and Dr. D. C. Rohrer supervised the diffractometry. This work was supported in part by Grant HL-15378 awarded by the National Heart, Lung and Blood Institute, Department of Health, Education and Welfare.

REFERENCES

1. Andersen, N. H., Ramwell, P. W., Leovey, E. M. K., and Johnson, M. (1976): In: *Advances in Prostaglandin and Thromboxane Research,* Vol. 1., edited by B. Samuelsson and R. Paoletti, pp. 271–289. Raven Press, New York.
2. Dawson, W., Boot, J. R., Cockerill, A. F., Mallen, D. N. B., and Osborne, D. J. (1976): *Nature,* 699–702.
3. DeTitta, G. T. (1976): *Science,* 191:1271–1272.
4. Eventoff, W., Rossmann, M. G., Taylor, S. S., Torff, H.-J., Meyer, H., Keil, W., and Kiltz, H.-H. (1977): *Proc. Natl. Acad. Sci. USA,* 74:2677–2681.
5. Falardeau, P., Hamberg, M., and Samuelsson, B. (1976): *Biochim. Biophys. Acta,* 441:193–200.
6. Hamberg, M., Svensson, J., and Samuelsson, B. (1975): *Proc. Natl. Acad. Sci. USA,* 72:2994–2998.
7. Kindahl, H. (1977): *Prostaglandins,* 13:619–629.
8. Needleman, P., Minkes, M., and Raz, A. (1976): *Science,* 193:163–165.
9. Piper, P. J., and Vane, J. R. (1969): *Nature,* 223:29–35.
10. Roberts, J. L., Sweetman, B. J., Morgan, J. L., Payne, N. A., and Oates, J. A. (1977): *Prostaglandins,* 13:631–648.

Advances in Prostaglandin and Thromboxane Research.
Vol. 6, edited by B. Samuelsson, P. W. Ramwell,
and R. Paoletti. Raven Press, New York © 1980.

Synthesis of Thromboxane A₂ Analogs

K. C. Nicolaou, R. L. Magolda, and D. A. Claremon

Department of Chemistry, University of Pennsylvania, Philadelphia, Pennsylvania 19104

In 1975 Hamberg et al. (2) described the presence of an unstable molecule ($t_{1/2} \simeq 30$ sec at pH 7.4 and 37°C) in blood platelets with potent aggregating and smooth muscle contracting properties. This substance was termed thromboxane A₂ (TXA₂) and was assigned the structure shown in Fig. 1 on the basis of chemical evidence (2). The isolation or chemical synthesis of this important biomolecule member of the arachidonic acid cascade (3) remains elusive. Furthermore, no structural analogs of this architecturally unusual compound have been reported to date. On the other hand, although prostacyclin (PGI₂) (Fig. 1) was disclosed later (1976) by Vane and his group (4), its chemical synthesis has been achieved and a plethora of analogs have emerged (3). We now wish to report the synthesis of the first structural analogs of TXA₂, namely, pinane TXA₂ (PTXA₂, **8a**) (5) and carbocyclic TXA₂, (CTXA₂, **10**).

The construction of the PTXA₂ analog **8a** was achieved from (−)-myrtenol (**1**) as shown in Fig. 2. (−)-Myrtenol was oxidized to the α,β-unsaturated aldehyde **2** (MnO₂, CH₂Cl₂, 25°C, 48 hr) in 95% yield. 1,4-Addition of the mixed cuprate derived from (±)-*trans*-lithio-1-octen-3-ol-*tert*-butyldimethylsilyl ether and 1-pentynylcopper hexamethylphosphorous triamide complex with the aldehyde **2** proceeded smoothly to furnish the adduct **3** (80%). Reaction of **3** with methoxymethylenetriphenylphosphorane in toluene–tetrahydrofuran solution yielded the enol ether **4** in 94% yield as a mixture of geometrical isomers. Treatment of **4** with Hg(OAc)₂–KI in aqueous tetrahydrofuran liberated the aldehyde **5** quantitatively. The upper side chain was attached by a Wittig reaction of **5** with the sodium salt of 4-carboxybutyltriphenylphosphorane in dimethylsulfoxide, furnishing, after exposure to diazomethane, the methyl ester of the protected TXA₂ analog **6** (mixture of epimers at the oxygen-bound carbon) in 80% yield. Removal of the silyl ether (acetic acid/water/tetrahydrofuran, 3:2:2, 45°C) afforded the methyl esters **7a** and **7b** (1:1,100%), which were separated chromatographically (silica, ether/petroleum ether, 1:1; **7a**, $R_f = 0.53$; **7b**, $R_f = 0.59$). Basic hydrolysis (LiOH in aqueous tetrahydrofuran) of the more polar compound furnished the PTXA₂ analog **8a** in quantitative yield, whereas similar treatment of the less polar methyl ester **7b** produced the epimeric PTXA₂ analog **8b**. The ¹³C-nuclear magnetic resonance (NMR) spectra of **7a** and **7b** were of crucial importance in assigning the stereochemistry of these compounds. In

COOH
O
O
OH
PGH2
PGI2 synthetase
TA2 synthetase
COOH
O
HO
OH
PGI2
COOH
O
O
OH
TA2
O
COOH
HO
HO
OH
6-Keto-PGF1α
OH
COOH
HO
O
OH
TB2

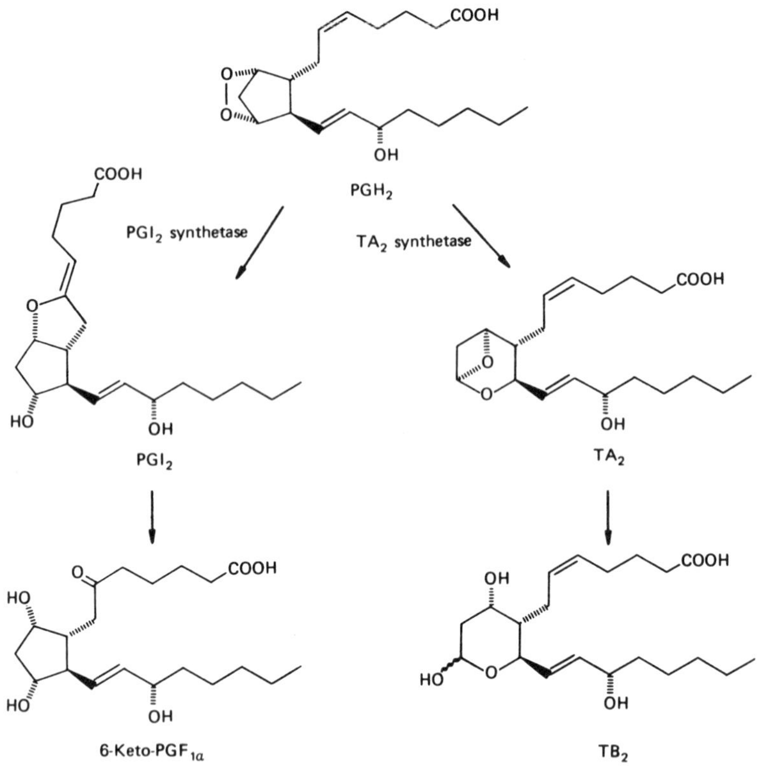

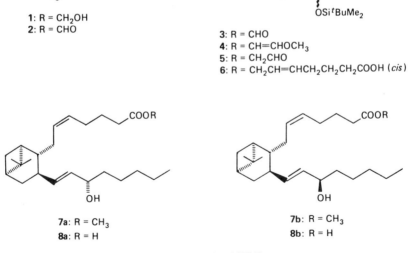

FIG. 1. Biosynthesis and degradation of TXA_2 and PGI_2.

R
1: R = CH2OH
2: R = CHO
R
OSitBuMe2
3: R = CHO
4: R = CH=CHOCH3
5: R = CH2CHO
6: R = CH2CH=CHCH2CH2CH2COOH (cis)
COOR
OH
7a: R = CH3
8a: R = H
COOR
OH
7b: R = CH3
8b: R = H

FIG. 2. Synthesis of $PTXA_2$.

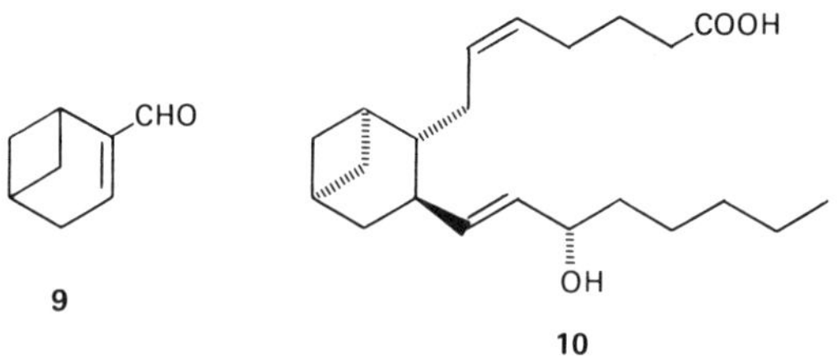

FIG. 3. CTA₂.

particular, the relatively low chemical shift for the C-10 (PG numbering) in the ^{13}C-NMR spectra of both **7a** and **7b** ($\delta = 33.3 \pm 2$) revealed the relative stereochemistry of the upper side chain by analogy to the corresponding model epimeric compounds from the pinane family, which exhibit this carbon at $\delta = 33.2$ (C trans to the side chain) and 24.2 (C cis to the side chain) (1). The PTXA₂ is indefinitely stable at 25°C in solution or neat.

Following similar methodology as for the synthesis of PTXA₂ (**8a**) and starting from the α,β-unsaturated aldehyde **9** (prepared from 1,4-cyclohexanedione or bicyclo[2.2.1]hexan-2-one in several steps), the CTXA₂ analog **10** was also synthesized efficiently.

REFERENCES

1. Bohlmann, F., Zeisberg, R., and Klein, E. (1975): *Org. Magn. Reson.,* 7:426–432.
2. Hamberg, M., Svensson, J., and Samuelsson, B. (1975): *Proc. Natl. Acad. Sci. USA,* 72:2994–2998.
3. Moncada, S., Gryglewski, R., Bunting, S., and Vane, J. R. (1976): *Nature,* 263:663–665.
4. Nicolaou, K. C., Gasic, G. P., and Barnette, W. E. (1978): *Angew. Chem., Int. Ed. Engl.,* 17:293–312.
5. Nicolaou, K. C., Magolda, R. L., Smith, J. B., Aharony, D., Smith, E. F., and Lefer, A. M. (1979): *Proc. Natl. Acad. Sci. USA (in press).*

*Advances in Prostaglandin and Thromboxane Research,
Vol. 6*, edited by B. Samuelsson, P. W. Ramwell,
and R. Paoletti. Raven Press, New York © 1980.

A Structural Analog of Thromboxane A₂

*M. F. Ansell, M. P. L. Caton, M. N. Palfreyman, K. A. J. Stuttle,
D. Tuffin, and J. L. Walker

*May and Baker Ltd., Dagenham, Essex, RM10 7XS; and *Queen Mary College, University
of London, London, E1 4NS*

Although the structure of thromboxane A₂ (TXA₂) was assigned several years ago (3), so far as we are aware, no synthetic work in this area has been published. We here report the synthesis and biological evaluation of stable analogs (Fig. 1, I) of TXA₂ in which the ether oxygens are replaced by carbon groupings.

Hydroboration with 9-BBN of the THP ether of 2[(1*R*, 5*S*)-6,6-dimethylbicyclo *[3.1.1.]* hept-2-en-2-yl] ethanol (Nopol) (Fig. 2, IIb) and carbonylation with carbon monoxide afforded the aldehyde (IVa), the stereochemistry of which was assigned by analogy with the known stereospecific hydroboration of α-pinene (IIa) to the borane (IIIa) (1) and the fact that carbonylation of boranes is known to occur with retention of configuration (2).

Wittig-Horner reaction of (IVa) with dimethyl-(2-oxoheptyl)-phosphonate gave the enone (IVb), which on hydrolysis with acetic acid in aqueous tetrahydrofuran (THF) and then oxidation with chromium trioxide and sulfuric acid in dimethylformamide afforded the carboxylic acid (Fig. 3, Va). Reduction of the latter with lithium tri-*s*-butylborohydride (L-Selectride®) in THF gave a mixture of alcohols (Vb and Vc), which were separated by thin-layer chromatography (TLC) on silica (ether/ethyl acetate/*n*-hexane, 3:1:1) and each taken forward by the sequence of esterification (diazomethane), THP ether formation, and lithium aluminium hydride reduction to the primary alcohols (VIa and VIb).

The latter were then oxidized with pyridinium chlorochromate in dichloromethane to the corresponding aldehydes, which afforded the two diastereomeric TXA₂ analogs (I) on Wittig elaboration with the phosphorane generated *in*

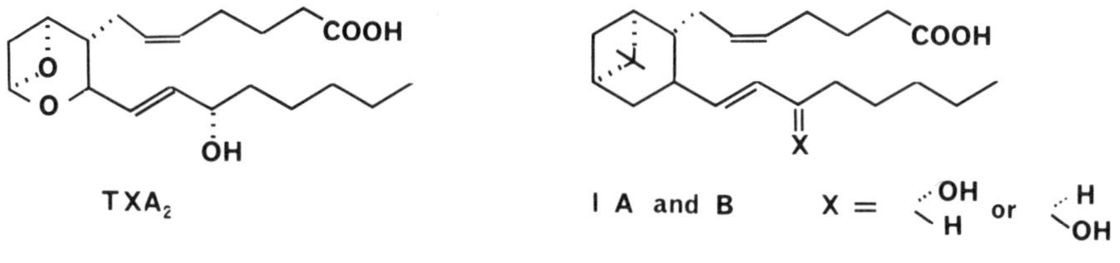

TXA₂   I A and B   X = OH or H
                                           H   OH

FIG. 1.

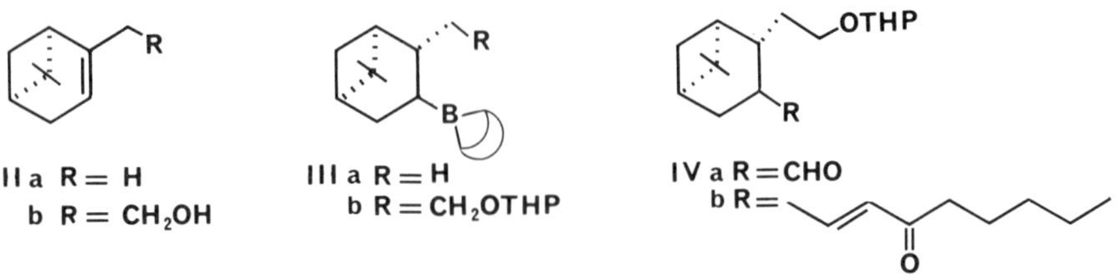

II a R = H
   b R = CH_2OH

III a R = H
    b R = CH_2OTHP

IV a R = CHO
   b R =

FIG. 2.

V a X = O
   b X = H, OH
   c X = OH, H

VI a X = OTHP, H
    b X = H, OTHP

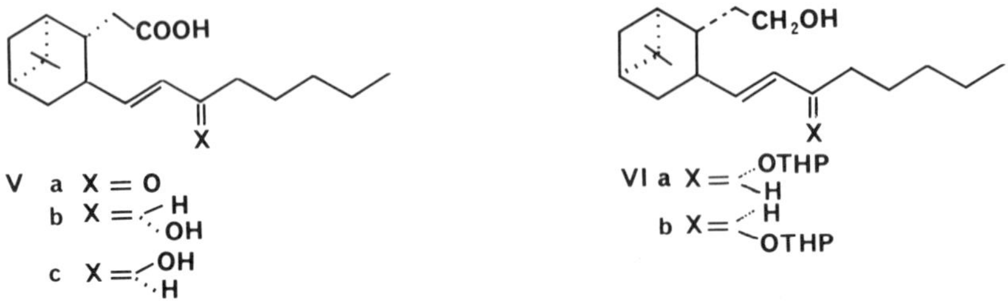

FIG. 3.

situ from (4-carboxybutyl)triphenyl phosphonium bromide by potassium-*t*-butoxide in THF and then acid hydrolysis. These two diastereomers are distinguishable by TLC on silica (ethyl acetate/cyclohexane/formic acid, 40:40:1), the faster-moving isomer being designated isomer A and the slower isomer B.

Compounds A and B have undergone preliminary testing *in vitro* for TXA_2-like activity and for antagonism of TXA_2 action. The tests used to detect TXA_2-like activity were (a) spasmogenic action on strips of arterial tissue [rabbit aorta (RbA), rabbit mesenteric artery (RbM), and pig coronary artery] and (b) aggregation of human platelets in platelet-rich plasma. Antagonism of TXA_2 action was determined by (a) inhibition of the spasmogenic activity of TXA_2, generated from arachidonic acid-perfused guinea pig lungs and assayed on RbA and RbM, and (b) inhibition of collagen-induced aggregation of human platelets.

Preliminary tests indicate that both compounds A and B may have slight agonist activity on RbA and RbM at 1.0 μg/ml. Isomer B appeared more potent than isomer A. In concentrations up to 1.0 μg/ml, both isomers also appeared to antagonize slightly the action of TXA_2 on RbA and RbM. No proaggregatory activity on human platelets was found with either compound in concentrations up to 50 μg/ml. Isomer A partially inhibited collagen-induced aggregation of human platelets at 50 μg/ml (one experiment).

ACKNOWLEDGMENTS

We acknowledge the skilled technical assistance of Mr. A. Stuttle and Miss J. Lang.

REFERENCES

1. Brown, H. C. (1975): In: *Organic Syntheses via Boranes.* Wiley & Sons, New York, p. 15–35.
2. Brown, H. C., Rogié, M. M., Rathke, M. W., and Kabalka, G. W. (1969): *J. Am. Chem. Soc.,* 91:2150–2152.
3. Hamberg, M., Svensson, J., and Samuelsson, B. (1975): Proc. Natl. Acad. Sci. USA, 72:2994–2998.

Advances in Prostaglandin and Thromboxane Research,
Vol. 6, edited by B. Samuelsson, P. W. Ramwell,
and R. Paoletti. Raven Press, New York © 1980.

Pinane Thromboxane A_2: A TXA_2 Antagonist with Antithrombotic Properties

D. Aharony, J. B. Smith, E. F. Smith, *A. M. Lefer, R. L. Magolda, and †K. D. Nicolaou

Cardeza Foundation and Departments of Pharmacology and Physiology, Thomas Jefferson University, Philadelphia 19107; and Department of Chemistry, University of Pennsylvania, Philadelphia, Pennsylvania 19104

Since thromboxane A_2 (TXA_2) can cause platelet aggregation and constriction of coronary arteries, it may be involved in myocardial infarction and be the cause of the angina associated with arterial thrombosis (4). Stable prostaglandin (PG) analogs have been reported which block the formation of TXA_2 or its effects on platelet aggregation, but they do not inhibit the constriction of the vessel wall induced by TXA_2 (1,2). The synthesis of TXA_2 analog pinane TXA_2 (PTA_2) (Fig. 1) was performed on the assumption that it would antagonize all of the biological effects of TXA_2 and thus might be a useful antithrombotic compound (3).

METHODS

The inhibitory effect of PTA_2 on vasoconstriction induced by PGH_2 analogs was determined using cat coronary arteries perfused constantly with Krebs–Hanseleit buffer. For platelet aggregation studies, human platelet-rich plasma was preincubated for 1 min with various concentrations of PTA_2 in an aggregometer cuvette (0.5 ml, 37°C) and adenosine diphosphate (ADP), sodium arachidonate, epinephrine, 9,11-azo-PGH_2, 9,11-methanoepoxy-PGH_2 (U46619), or 9,11-epoxymethano-PGH_2 (U44069) as added. TX synthesis was assayed using washed rabbit platelets preincubated with up to 100 μM PTA_2 (5 min at 37°C)

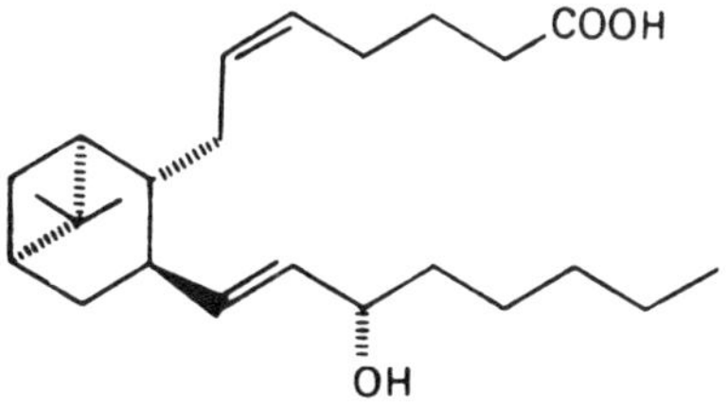

FIG. 1. Structure of PTA_2.

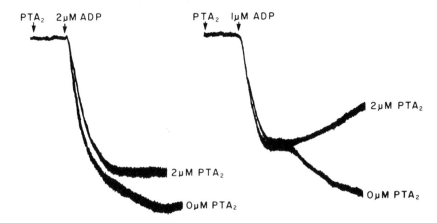

FIG. 2. Inhibition of ADP-induced second wave of aggregation by PTA₂.

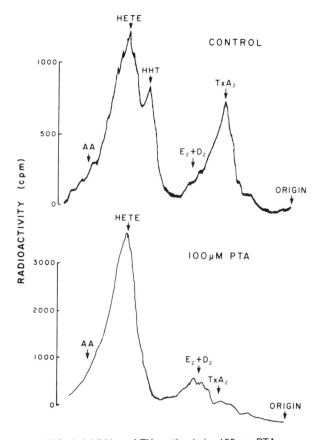

FIG. 3. Inhibition of TX synthesis by 100 μM PTA₂.

TABLE 1. *Lack of effect of PTA₂ on PGI₂ synthesis*

Dose (μM)	Total cpm	6-Keto-PGF$_{1\alpha}$	
		cpm	Percent
—	22,840	14,198	62.2
—	24,508	15,212	62.1
10	23,094	14,521	62.9
25	23,151	15,622	67.5
100	21,296	13,215	62.1
100	24,811	15,983	64.4

before addition of 0.5 μCi [1-¹⁴C]arachidonic acid. 6-keto-PGF$_{1\alpha}$ synthesis was assayed using ram seminal vesicle microsomes preincubated with up to 100 μM PTXA₂ before addition of 0.02 μCi [1-¹⁴C]arachidonic acid. In both latter assays, products were extracted and subjected to thin-layer chromatography and appropriate zones were scraped and counted for radioactivity.

RESULTS

At 0.1 μM, PTXA₂ inhibited the constriction of coronary arteries induced by 30 nM 9,11-azo-PGH₂ by 50%, and 1 μM PTA₂ completely abolished this constriction. At 2 μM, PTA₂ abolished aggregation induced by arachidonic acid, inhibited the second wave of aggregation induced by 50 μM epinephrine or 2 μM ADP, and also reversed the aggregation induced by 1 μM of ADP (Fig. 2). The same concentration of PTA₂ caused 50% inhibition of aggregation induced by the endoperoxide analogs 9,11-azo-PGH₂ (0.3–0.6 μM), 9,11-methanoepoxy-PGH₂ (0.3–0.6 μM), or 9,11-epoxy-methano-PGH₂ (1–3 μM) (3). PTA₂ did not antagonize the inhibitory effect of PGI₂ or PGD₂ on platelet aggregation. At 100 μM, PTA₂ inhibited TXB₂ synthesis by 83% (Fig. 3) but had no effect on 6-keto-PGF$_{1\alpha}$ (Table 1).

DISCUSSION

PTA₂ is potent and selective antagonist of the vasoconstriction and platelet aggregation activities of PG endoperoxide analogs. At concentrations of two orders of magnitude higher than required to abolish vasoconstriction, it inhibits TX synthesis. Unlike cyclooxygenase inhibitors which may prevent the formation of PGI₂, PTA₂ had no effect at all on PGI₂ formation. These differences in PTA₂ effects and potencies are very suitable for a potent antithrombotic drug that selectively antagonizes TXA₂ but does not impair PGI₂ synthesis or effects.

REFERENCES

1. Fitzpatrick, F. A., Bundy, G. L., Gorman, R. R., and Honohan, T. (1978): *Nature*, 275:764–766.

2. Gorman, R. R., Bundy, G. L., Peterson, D. C., Sun, F. F., Miller, O. V., and Fitzpatrick, F. A. (1977): *Proc. Natl. Acad. Sci. USA,* 74:4007–4011.
3. Nicolaou, K. C., Magolda, R. L., Smith, J. B., Aharony, D., Smith, E. F., and Lefer, A. M. (1979): *Proc. Natl. Acad. Sci. USA (in press).*
4. Shimamoto, T., Kobayashi, M., Takahashi, T., Motomiya, T., Numano, F., and Morooka, S. (1977): *Proc. Jpn. Acad., Ser. B,* 53:38–42.

*Advances in Prostaglandin and Thromboxane Research,
Vol. 6,* edited by B. Samuelsson, P. W. Ramwell,
and R. Paoletti. Raven Press, New York © 1980.

Stereocontrolled Synthesis of 7-Oxabicyclo (2.2.1) Heptane Prostaglandin Analogs as Thromboxane A₂ Antagonists

P. W. Sprague, J. E. Heikes, *D. N. Harris, and *R. Greenberg

*Departments of Chemistry and *Pharmacology, The Squibb Institute for Medical Research,
Princeton, New Jersey 08540*

The 7-oxabicyclo[2.2.1]heptane ring system bears a resemblance to the bicyclic portion of either prostaglandin H_2 (PGH₂) or thromboxane A_2 (TXA₂) (Fig. 1) depending on how the oxa and dimethylene bridges are viewed in relation to the natural products. We hypothesized that attachment of PG-like side chains to this ring system might lead to compounds with TXA₂ synthetase inhibitory or TXA₂ antagonistic activity. To test this concept we have synthesized eight diastereomers 1a to 1h (Fig. 2) which include all possible permutations of side chain stereochemistry about the bicyclic nucleus.

CHEMISTRY

These syntheses have been accomplished, as depicted in Fig. 3, with complete stereocontrol by strategic manipulation of the readily available Diels-Alder adducts 2 and 3. Adduct 2 (2) was reduced in two steps to *endo*-hemiacetal 4, a key intermediate leading to six of the eight isomers of 1. Homologation of 4 to *endo*-hemiacetal 5 and attachment of the PG acid side chain yields 6. This

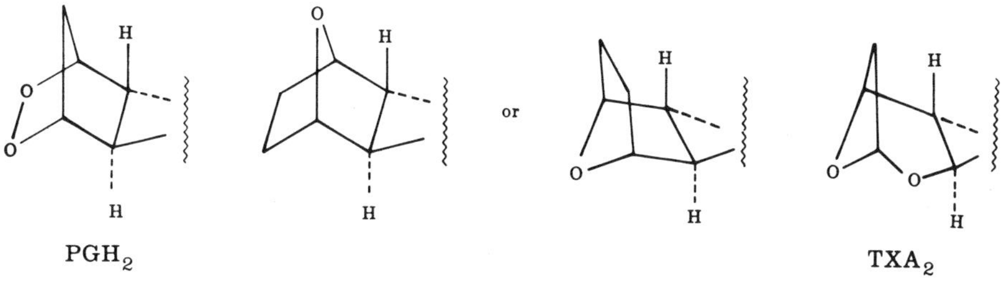

FIG. 1.

493

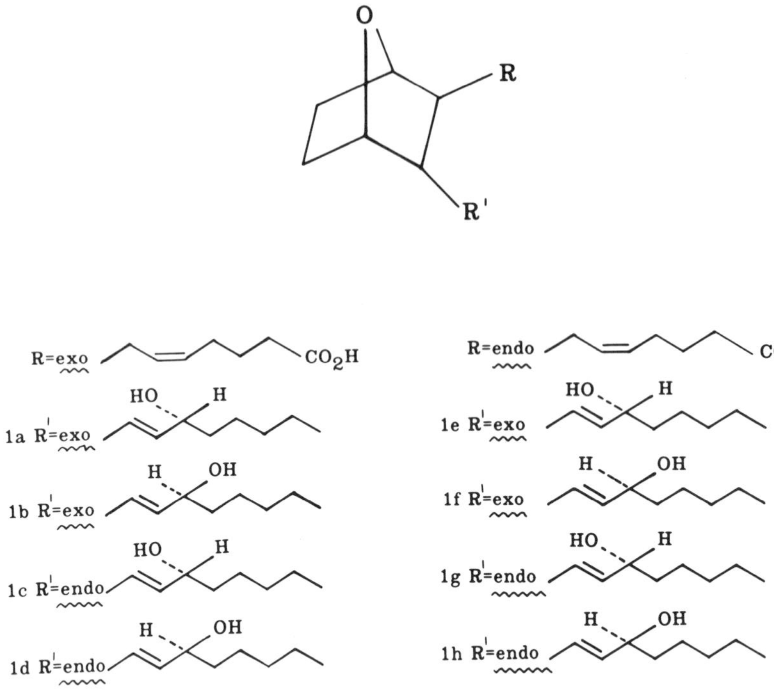

FIG. 2.

substance could be carried on to all-*endo* isomers **1g** and **1h** or epimerized first to *exo*-aldehyde **7** and then converted to *trans* isomers **1e** and **1f**. The synthesis of the alternate *trans* isomers **1c** and **1d** required that we reverse our sequence of side chain attachment. Hemiacetal **4** was trapped as its ring-opened aldehyde tautomer (as acetate **9**) via *endo*-hydrazone **8**, then transformed to *exo*-aldehyde **10**. The *trans* compounds **1c** and **1d** followed from **10** by straight-forward methods. The remaining *exo-cis* side chain pattern in **1a** and **1b** was readily accessible from the well-known Diels-Alder adduct **3** (5) through the application of similar chemistry.

BIOLOGICAL ACTIVITY

Acids **1a** to **1c** and **1e** to **1g** were evaluated in arachidonic acid (AA)-induced platelet aggregation (1) and TXA₂ synthetase inhibition (3) tests. The results (Table 1) suggest that these compounds function as TXA₂ antagonists. Compounds **1a** and **1e** have also been shown to inhibit AA-induced bronchoconstriction (4) in guinea pigs.

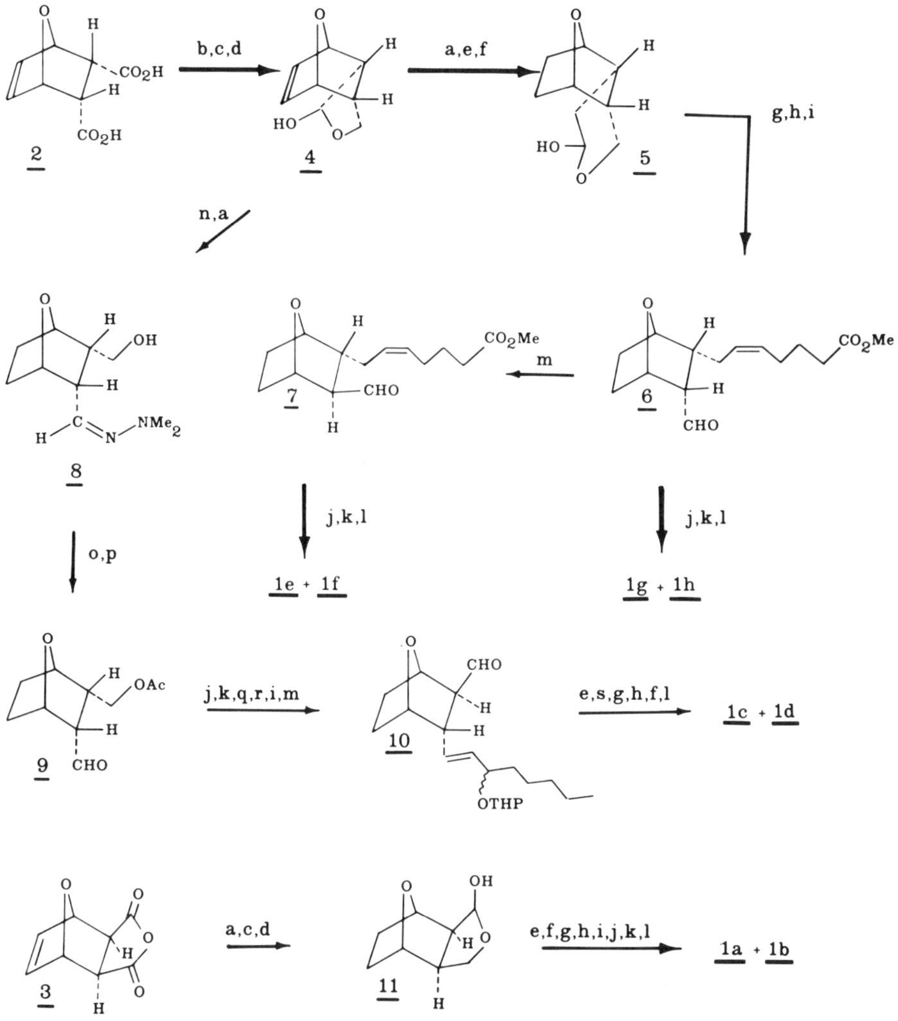

FIG. 3. The synthesis of the PG analogs involved the following reactions: a. H_2, Pd/C; b. trifluoroacetic anhydride (TFA); c. $NaBH_4$, tetrahydrofuran (THF); d. diisobutylatuminum hydride, (DIBAL); e. $\varnothing_3P = CHOCH_3$; f. TFA, H_2O; g. $\varnothing_3P = CH(CH_2)_3CO_2{\ominus}Na{\oplus}$, dimethyl sulfoxide; h. CH_2N_2, ether; i. CrO_3, pyridine, CH_2Cl_2; j. $(MeO)_2$ P—CH—C—C_5H_{11}, dimethoxyethane;

k. $NaBH_4$, $CeCl_3$, MeOH; l. LiOH, THF, H_2O; m. NaOMe, MeOH; n. H_2N—NMe₂; o. Ac₂O; p. CuCl₂, phosphate buffer (pH 7); q. dihydropyrane (DHP), tosic acid, benzene; r. Na₂CO₃, MeOH; s. Hg(OAc)₂, KI.

TABLE 1. *Activity of 7-oxabicyclo[2.2.1]heptane PG analogs as inhibitors of TXA synthetase and arachidonic acid-induced platelet aggregation*

Compound	AA-induced platelet aggregation inhibition, ID_{50} (μM)	TXA synthetase inhibition at 1,000 μM (%)
1a	68	40–60
1b	stimulates aggregation	40–60
1c	27	not tested
1e	0.82	48
1f	54	34
1g	15	45
PGI_2	0.0006	
Imidazole	42% inhibition at 1,000 μM	72

REFERENCES

1. Born, G. V. R. (1962): *Nature,* 194:927–929.
2. Eggelte, T. A., DeKoning, H., and Huisman, H. O. (1973): *Tetrahedron,* 29:2491–2493.
3. Nijkamp, F. P., Moncada, S., White, H. L., and Vane, J. R. (1977): *Eur. J. Pharmacol.,* 44:179–186.
4. Saeed, S. A., McDonald-Gibson, W. J., Cuthbert, J., Copas, J. S., Schneider, C., Gardiner, P. J., Butt, N. M., and Collier, H. O. J. (1977): *Nature,* 270:32–36.
5. Woodward, R. B., and Baer, H. (1948): *J. Am. Chem. Soc.,* 70:1161.

*Advances in Prostaglandin and Thromboxane Research,
Vol. 6,* edited by B. Samuelsson, P. W. Ramwell,
and R. Paoletti. Raven Press, New York © 1980.

Thromboxane A₂ Receptor Antagonism Selectively Reverses Platelet Aggregation

*G. C. Le Breton and †D. L. Venton

*Department of Pharmacology, College of Medicine, and †Department of Medicinal
Chemistry, College of Pharmacy, University of Illinois, Chicago, Illinois 60680

Recent evidence has suggested that prostaglandin H_2 (PGH_2) and/or thromboxane A_2 (TXA_2) is capable of directly stimulating platelet aggregation. In this connection it was demonstrated that platelets deficient in releasable adenosine diphosphate (ADP) will aggregate in response to arachidonic acid (AA) (2,7,9). Furthermore, it was also demonstrated that addition of low concentrations of endoperoxide to platelet-rich plasma (PRP) will induce reversible aggregation in the absence of measurable secretion (1). Since, however, this study also indicated that aggregation induced by AA was always accompanied by ADP secretion, it has not been possible to assess whether endogenously elaborated PGH_2 or TXA_2 plays a significant role in directly initiating the aggregation of normal platelets in response to moderate doses of AA.

In the present study we examined this question through use of a direct TXA_2 antagonist. We recently provided evidence that 13-azaprostanoic acid (13-APA) (8) specifically inhibits AA-induced aggregation through inhibition of the platelet TXA_2/PGH_2 receptor (3). Subsequent experiments have demonstrated that in addition to preventing AA-induced aggregation, 13-APA will also reverse aggregation once the process has been initiated.

RESULTS

It can be seen in Fig. 1 that addition of 13-APA (100 μM) 15 sec subsequent to AA (350 μM) results in platelet deaggregation. This thrombolytic effect is also apparent when 13-APA is added at 30 or 45 sec following AA addition. It can also be seen that the ability of 13-APA to reverse aggregation decreases with time. Consequently, at 50 sec 13-APA produces only partial reversal; and at 60 sec 13-APA is without effect (not shown). The time at which 13-APA is added to the plasma is therefore crucial relative to its ability to cause deaggregation. It should be pointed out that the onset of irreversibility appears to depend on the individual platelet donor. Some platelets underwent deaggregation well beyond 45 sec, whereas others would only deaggregate at a maximum of 35

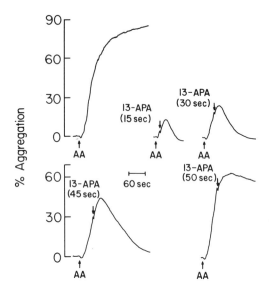

FIG. 1. Reversal of AA-induced aggregation by 13-APA. Citrated, human PRP was aggregated by 350 μM AA; 100 μM 13-APA was added to the plasma at 15, 30, or 45 sec subsequent to AA.

sec. The values reported here, therefore, represent the median response between these extremes.

In order to determine whether this thrombolytic property is specific for AA-induced platelet aggregation, 13-APA reversal of ADP or epinephrine-induced aggregation was also evaluated (Fig. 2). In these experiments aggregation was induced by either 5μM ADP or epinephrine. 13-APA (100 μM) was then added to the plasma at 15, 30, or 45 sec after the aggregating agent. It is apparent from the aggregation traces that 13-APA is completely without effect in altering the normal ADP or epinephrine response at each time examined.

These findings therefore suggest that the ability of 13-APA to deaggregate platelets is specific for PGH₂- or TXA₂-mediated functional change. This specificity is in marked contrast to the thrombolytic properties of prostacyclin (PGI₂). Moncada et al. (5) have demonstrated that PGI₂ will also reverse platelet aggregation. Since, however, its mechanism of action is presumably mediated through stimulation of adenylate cyclase, PGI₂ will not selectively reverse aggregation induced by AA (Fig. 3). Thus the addition of 3 ng/ml PGI₂ not only deaggregates AA-stimulated (350 μM) platelets at 15, 30, and 45 sec, but also reverses aggregation induced by 10 μM ADP or epinephrine.

It is possible that the ability of 13-APA to specifically deaggregate AA-stimulated platelets is related to an alteration in the rate of metabolism of AA to PGH₂ or TXA₂. This possibility, however, was excluded on the basis that neither indomethacin nor imidazole produced a similar thrombolytic effect even at the earliest time tested, i.e., 15 sec (Fig. 4). The preincubation traces illustrate that

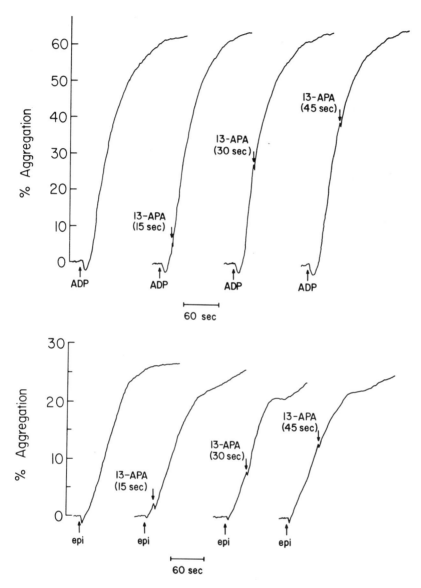

FIG. 2. Effect of 13-APA on the process of aggregation induced by ADP or epinephrine. Citrated, human PRP was pretreated with 20 μM indomethacin to inhibit the production of TXA₂ from endogenous AA. Platelet aggregation was induced by either 5 μM ADP or epinephrine. Following addition of aggregating agent, 100 μM 13-APA was added at 15, 30, or 45 sec.

addition of 20 μM indomethacin or 300 μg/ml imidazole 5 sec prior to AA will almost completely block the aggregation process. This result demonstrates that both agents act quite rapidly in inhibiting cyclooxygenase or TX synthetase activity. Nevertheless, neither compound produced deaggregation. On the other

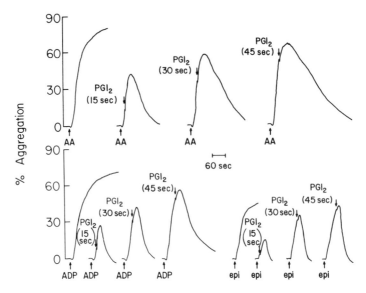

FIG 3. Reversal of aggregation by PGI₂. Citrated human PRP was aggregated with either 350 μM AA, 10 μM ADP, or 10 μM epinephrine; 3 ng/ml PGI₂ was added to the plasma at 15, 30, or 45 sec subsequent to aggregating agent.

hand, it is apparent that the extent of aggregation progressively decreases as indomethacin or imidazole is added at shorter time intervals subsequent to AA. This finding is presumably associated with decreased TXA₂ production,

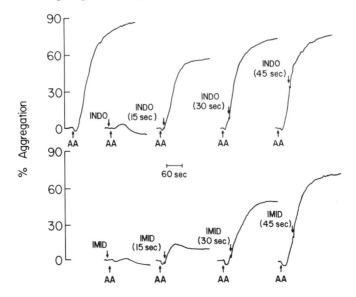

FIG. 4. Effect of indomethacin or imidazole on the process of aggregation induced by AA. Indomethacin (20 μM) or imidazole (300 μg/ml) was added to citrated human PRP 5 sec prior to AA (350 μM) or 15, 30, or 45 sec subsequent to AA (350 μM).

which would serve to limit the aggregation response. The suppression of aggregation in the absence of reversal therefore suggests that partial reduction of PGH_2 and/or TXA_2 synthesis is not itself sufficient to cause platelet deaggregation, but rather once reactive AA metabolites are formed, receptor antagonism is required to specifically reverse the aggregation process.

This concept is supported by the observation that 13-APA will also cause reversal of aggregation induced by the stable endoperoxide analog U46619 (Fig.

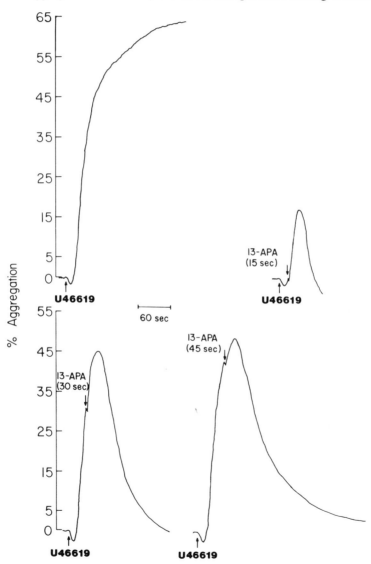

FIG. 5. Reversal of U46619-induced aggregation by 13-APA. Citrated human PRP was aggregated by 0.75 μM U46619; 100 μM 13-APA was added to the plasma at 15, 30, or 45 sec subsequent to U46619.

5). It can be seen that 100 μM 13-APA will completely deaggregate platelets at 15, 30, and 45 sec subsequent to the addition of 0.75 μM U44619, which in the absence of 13-APA caused irreversible aggregation.

CONCLUSIONS

If irreversible aggregation induced by AA were exclusively mediated through secretion of ADP (4,6), 13-APA would not be expected to reverse the aggregation process. Since, however, deaggregation was observed for up to 45 sec subsequent to the addition of AA, we propose that in normal platelets, endogenously elaborated PGH₂ and/or TXA₂ plays a major role in directly stimulating the development of platelet adhesiveness. Thus 13-APA was found to completely reverse AA-induced aggregation when the process was approximately 50% complete and 13-APA deaggregated U46619-stimulated platelets even though 80% of the control aggregation had developed. Based on these findings, it appears that during the early stages of AA-induced aggregation, continued TXA₂ receptor occupation is required for the maintenance of platelet adhesiveness. Consequently, during this phase of aggregation, secreted ADP is not itself sufficient to sustain the aggregation response.

Although the relative contribution of TXA₂ and ADP to the aggregation process is presently unclear, it is possible that as secretion continues the requirement for PGH₂ and/or TXA₂ is reduced. Thus with time continued platelet adhesiveness becomes solely an ADP-dependent process. This suggestion would be consistent with our finding that specific TXA₂ antagonism will only reverse aggregation within a limited period subsequent to the addition of AA.

Experiments are currently in progress to measure secretion during both the 13-APA reversible and irreversible phases of aggregation in order to establish the temporal relationship between reversibility and secretion of platelet ADP.

ACKNOWLEDGMENTS

U46619 and PGI₂ were kindly provided by Dr. J. Pike, The Upjohn Company. The authors wish to thank Bruce Robin for expert technical assistance. This work was supported in part by grants from the Chicago Heart Association and the University of Illinois.

REFERENCES

1. Charo, I. F., Feinman, R. D., Detwiler, T. C., Smith, J. B., Ingerman, C. M., and Silver, M. J. (1977): *Nature*, 269:66–69.
2. Kinlough-Rathbone, R. L., Reimers, H. J., Mustard, J. F., and Packham, M. A. (1976): *Science*, 192:1011–1012.
3. Le Breton, G. C., Venton, D. L., Enke, S. E., and Halushka, P. V. (1979): *Proc. Natl. Acad. Sci. USA*, 76:4097–4101.
4. Malmsten, C., Hamberg, M., Svensson, J., and Samuelsson, B. (1975): *Proc. Natl. Acad. Sci. USA*, 72:1446–1450.

5. Moncada, S., Gryglewski, R. J., Bunting, S., and Vane, J. R. (1976): *Prostaglandins,* 12:715–737.
6. Samuelsson, B., Hamberg, M., Malmsten, C., and Svensson, J. (1976): In: *Advances in Prostaglandin and Thromboxane Research,* Vol. 2, edited by B. Samuelsson, and R. Paoletti, pp. 737–746. Raven Press, New York.
7. Smith, J. B., Ingerman, C. M., and Silver, M. J. (1976): In: *Advances in Prostaglandin and Thromboxane Research,* Vol. 2, edited by B. Samuelsson, and R. Paoletti, pp. 747–753. Raven Press, New York.
8. Venton, D. L., Enke, S. E., and Le Breton, G. C. (1979): *J. Med. Chem.,* 22:824–830.
9. Weiss, H. J., Willis, A. L., Kuhn, D., and Brand, H. (1976): *Br. J. Haematol.,* 32:257–272.

Advances in Prostaglandin and Thromboxane Research,
Vol. 6, edited by B. Samuelsson, P. W. Ramwell,
and R. Paoletti. Raven Press, New York © 1980.

Vasopressin Stimulates Thromboxane Synthesis in the Toad Urinary Bladder: Effects of Thromboxane Synthesis Inhibition

*Ronald M. Burch, *Daniel R. Knapp, and *†Perry V. Halushka

*Departments of *Pharmacology and †Medicine, Medical University of South Carolina,
Charleston, South Carolina 29403*

In the toad urinary bladder, vasopressin increases water permeability (3) and activates phospholipase A_2 (14) to release free arachidonic acid. Arachidonic acid is then transformed into prostaglandin E_2 (PGE_2) (15), which acts as a negative modulator to reduce the vasopressin induced increase in water permeability (1,7,11). In a preliminary report (12), imidazole—a selective inhibitor of thromboxane synthetase (8,9)—was shown to decrease vasopressin-stimulated water flow in the urinary bladder of the toad, *Bufo bufo.* The purpose of this study was to determine (a) if vasopressin stimulates thromboxane as well as PG synthesis and (b) the effects of imidazole on the action of vasopressin in the isolated toad urinary bladder.

MATERIALS AND METHODS

Synthesis of Immunoreactive PGE

Hemibladders were removed from Mexican toads *(Bufo marinus)* and incubated at 25°C in a Ringer's solution with the following composition (mM): NaCl, 90; KCl, 3.0; $NaHCO_3$, 25; $MgSO_4$, 3.9; KH_2PO_4, 0.5; $CaCl_2$, 1.0; and glucose, 6.0. Control and experimental hemibladders were obtained from the same toad. After incubation, media were acidified with formic acid to pH 3.5 and extracted twice with ethyl acetate, and dried under nitrogen. The dried extract was reconstituted and chromatographed on a silicic acid column (13). The PGE fraction was isolated (13) and converted to PGB, assayed by radioimmunoassay (2), expressed as immunoreactive PGE (iPGE).

Gas Chromatography–Mass Spectrometric Confirmation of Thromboxane Synthesis

Bladder incubation media (2.2 liters, Ringer's) were acidified to pH 3.5 with formic acid and extracted twice with 3 volumes of ether. [³H]Thromboxane

B$_2$ (TXB$_2$; 10,000 cpm) was added to the residue to serve as a marker. The extract was subjected to silicic acid column chromatography (4), then to silicic acid thin-layer chromatography (8). The TX methyl ester was formed with ethereal diazomethane and subjected to thin-layer chromatography as above. The methoxime tri-trimethylsilyl (TTMS) derivative was formed (6) and subjected to combined gas chromatography–mass spectrometry. A blank was prepared of [^{3}H]TXB$_2$ (10,000 cpm) and treated as above. The blank was below the limits of detectability of the mass spectrometer.

iTXB$_2$ Synthesis

Following extraction and silicic acid column chromatography, the samples were assayed for TXB$_2$ using a previously described radioimmunoassay (5) with an antibody provided by Dr. J. B. Smith, Cardeza Foundation, Philadelphia.

Vasopressin-Stimulated Water Flow

Osmotic water flow was measured gravimetrically by the method of Bentley (3).

RESULTS AND DISCUSSION

Since previous studies on the metabolism of arachidonic acid by the isolated toad urinary bladder have not demonstrated TXB$_2$ synthesis, we chose first to establish the presence or absence of the TX pathway. A methyl ester methoxime TTMS derivative was formed from the partially purified extract of toad bladder bathing media. A single peak corresponding in retention time to a sample of authentic derivatized TXB$_2$ was eluted, and its mass spectrum was identical to that produced by authentic derivatized TXB$_2$ (Fig. 1). Thus the toad urinary bladder is capable of synthesizing TXB$_2$ from endogenous precursors.

It has been previously shown in several tissues that imidazole, by inhibiting TX biosynthesis, shunts PG endoperoxide intermediates to other PGs (9,10). In the isolated toad urinary bladder, imidazole, at concentrations of 0.1 to 1.0 mM, produced a dose-related increase in iPGE synthesis (Fig. 2) from a basal level of 0.22 ± 0.01 pmole/min/hemibladder, reaching a maximum of 0.34 ± 0.04 pmoles/min/hemibladder.

To determine the effect of imidazole on vasopressin-stimulated water flow, hemibladders were incubated with 1 mM imidazole in Bentley chambers. Although basal water flow was not affected by imidazole, vasopressin-stimulated water flow was significantly less ($p < 0.05$) in the imidazole-treated hemibladders (Fig. 3). Vasopressin significantly ($p < 0.05$) increased TX synthesis, and this increase was significantly ($p < 0.05$) inhibited by imidazole. Imidazole did not affect basal iTXB$_2$ synthesis. Imidazole significantly increased basal ($p < 0.05$) and vasopressin-stimulated iPGE synthesis ($p < 0.01$) (Fig. 3). Thus inhibition

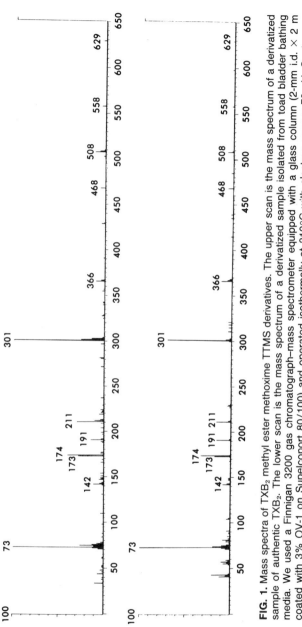

FIG. 1. Mass spectra of TXB_2 methyl ester methoxime TTMS derivatives. The upper scan is the mass spectrum of a derivatized sample of authentic TXB_2. The lower scan is the mass spectrum of a derivatized sample isolated from toad bladder bathing media. We used a Finnigan 3200 gas chromatograph–mass spectrometer equipped with a glass column (2-mm i.d. × 2 m coated with 3% OV-1 on Supelcoport 80/100) and operated isothermally at 210°C with electron energy 70 eV. Carrier gas was helium flowing at a rate of 25 ml/min. (From ref. 5, with permission.)

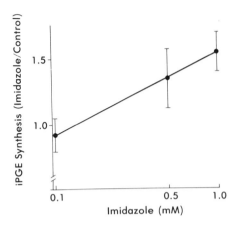

FIG. 2. Effects of imidazole on i-PGE synthesis. Hemibladders were removed and incubated in Ringer's solution. i-PGE synthesis was measured from 0 to 15 min after the addition of imidazole and is presented as the ratio of synthesis in the imidazole-treated hemibladders to synthesis in their paired controls at the same time ($n = 6$ at each concentration, $r = 0.89$, $p < 0.05$). (From ref. 5 with permission.)

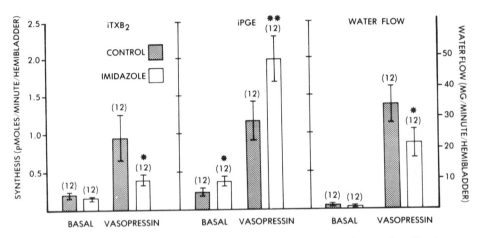

FIG. 3. Effects of imidazole (1 mM) on i-TXB$_2$ and i-PGE synthesis and water flow. Numbers of hemibladders in each group are shown in the parentheses ($*p < 0.05$, $**p < 0.01$).

of water flow associated with increased iPGE synthesis is consistent with the hypothesis that PGE acts as a negative modulator of vasopressin-stimulated water flow.

Another TX synthetase inhibitor, 7-(1-imidazolyl)-heptanoic acid (71-HA) was tested on the toad bladders, and it also blocked vasopressin-stimulated water flow and iTXB$_2$ synthesis but did not alter iPGE synthesis at the concentration tested (data not shown). Thus the hypothesis that TXA$_2$ may act as a positive modulator of vasopressin-stimulated water flow is suggested, and future investigations of the relation between vasopressin, arachidonic acid metabolism, and the mechanism of action of this peptide hormone must consider TX synthesis.

ACKNOWLEDGMENTS

We wish to acknowledge Drs. J. Pike and U. Axen, The Upjohn Company, Kalamazoo, Michigan, for the PGs. We are grateful to Ms. Brenda Garner, Ms. Shirley Kratz, and Ms. Betsy Powell for their expert technical assistance, and Ms. Marie Truesdell for typing the manuscript. Research was supported in part by Grants GM20387 and GM07404.

REFERENCES

1. Albert, W. C., and Handler, J. G. (1974): *Am. J. Physiol.,* 226:1382–1386.
2. Alexander, R. W., Kent, K. M., Pisano, J. J., Keiser, H. R., and Cooper, T. (1975): *J. Clin. Invest.,* 55:1174–1181.
3. Bentley, P. J. (1958): *Endocrinol.,* 17:201–209.
4. Bills, T. K., Smith, J. B., and Silver, M. J. (1976): *Biochim. Biophys. Acta,* 424:303–314.
5. Burch, R. M., Knapp, D. R., and Halushka, P. V. (1979): *J. Pharmacol. Exp. Ther.,* 210:344–348.
6. Fitzpatrick, F. A. (1977): *Anal. Chem.,* 50:47–52.
7. Flores, A. G. A., and Sharp, G. W. G. (1972): *Am. J. Physiol.,* 233:1392–1397.
8. Moncada, S., Bunting, S., Mullane, K., Thorogood, P., Vane, R. J., Raz, A., and Needleman, P. (1977): *Prostaglandins,* 13:611–618.
9. Needleman, P., Raz, A., Ferrendelli, J. A., and Minkes, M. (1977): *Proc. Natl. Acad. Sci. USA,* 74:1716–1720.
10. Nijkamp, F. P., Moncada, S. D., White, H. L., and Vane, J. R. (1977): *Eur. J. Pharmacol.,* 44:179–186.
11. Ozer, A., and Sharp, G. W. G. (1972): *Am. J. Physiol.,* 222:674–680.
12. Puig Muset, P., Puig Parellada, P., and Martin-Esteve, J. (1972): *Biochemical and Pharmacological Aspects of Imidazole,* pp. 99–101, published by the authors, Barcelona, Spain.
13. Webb, J. G., Saelens, D. A., and Halushka, P. V. (1978): *J. Neurochem.,* 31:13–19.
14. Zusman, R. M., and Keiser, H. R. (1977): *J. Biol. Chem.,* 252:2069–2071.
15. Zusman, R. M., Keiser, H. R., and Handler, J. S. (1977): *J. Clin. Invest.,* 60:1339–1347.

Advances in Prostaglandin and Thromboxane Research,
Vol. 6, edited by B. Samuelsson, P. W. Ramwell,
and R. Paoletti. Raven Press, New York © 1980.

Use of Inhibitors of Prostaglandin Synthesis in Patients with Breast Cancer

*T. J. Powles, *P. J. Dady, †Judith Williams, †G. C. Easty,
and †R. C. Coombes

*Chester Beatty Institute for Cancer Research and † Unit of Human Cancer Biology,
Ludwig Institute for Cancer Research, Royal Marsden Hospital,
Sutton, Surrey, United Kingdom

Prostaglandin (PG) synthesis has been implicated in many physiological, pathological, and biological processes that might influence the progress of the tumor in patients with breast cancer. This chapter is concerned particularly with the spread to and development of metastases in bone.

We have previously shown that some human breast tumors release osteolytic substances which cause breakdown of bone. These may be detected in vitro by use of an organ culture system and may, in part, be inhibited by anti-inflammatory agents like aspirin and indomethacin. Patients with active tumors are more likely to develop bone metastases (4,6) and development of osteolytic bone tumors in rats can be prevented by antiinflammatory drugs like aspirin and indomethacin. We have also previously shown that tumor osteolysis depends, in part, on PG synthesis by tumor and/or bone (1,2,5), and we have therefore, examined for possible effects of antiinflammatory and antiosteolytic agents in patients with breast cancer.

We have found that Benoral, an aspirin–paracetamol conjugate was as effective as aspirin at preventing bone metastases in rats (Table 1). We therefore set up a double-blind clinical trial to examine for possible effects of Benoral on 160 patients with primary poor-risk cancer.

From January, 1975, all patients who had stage II or anaplastic primary breast carcinoma underwent primary treatment, including mastectomy and radiotherapy where appropriate. They were stratified according to prognostic criteria and then randomized to Benoral [10 ml (4 g) twice a day] or placebo, which was continued for 18 months. All patients were fully staged before primary treatment and have been serially staged and clinically followed since.

There were no differences for overall relapse or development of bone metastases between the two groups (Figs. 1 and 2). At the present time there is no overall difference in survival between the two groups (Fig. 3).

In collaboration with Dr. Lawrence Levine at Brandeis University, Boston, the plasma levels of thromboxane B_2 (TXB_2) in some patients were measured

TABLE 1. *Effect of aspirin, Benoral, or paracetamol on development of bone and soft tissue metastases in rats after intra-aortic injection of 10⁴ Walker 265 tumor cells*

Drug	Dose per animal (mg/kg/day)	Change in tumor (%)	
		Soft tissue	Bone
Aspirin	176	+ 6	− 16
	440	−33	−100
	480	+52	−100
Benoral	140	+24	− 35
	240	+90	− 40
	845	−18	−100
Paracetamol	140	+ 5	+ 18
	540	−41	+ 18

by radioimmunoassay. Patients on treatment had significantly lower levels than control patients (Fig. 4).

The disparity between the rat and human experiments is disappointing. It is possible that medication, although sufficient to reduce the plasma TXB_2 levels was not enough to inhibit local tumor PG synthesis. Alternatively, the time course or mechanisms in the rat tumor may be different from that in human breast cancer.

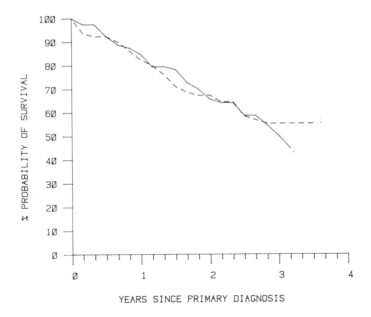

FIG. 1. Probability of developing any metastases in 160 patients with breast cancer given Benoral, 10 ml twice daily (—), or placebo (- - - - -).

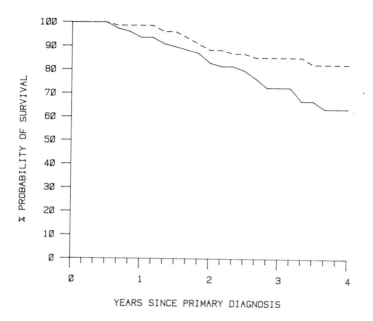

FIG. 2. Probability of survival of 160 patients with primary breast cancer given Benoral, 10 ml twice daily (—), or placebo (- - - - -).

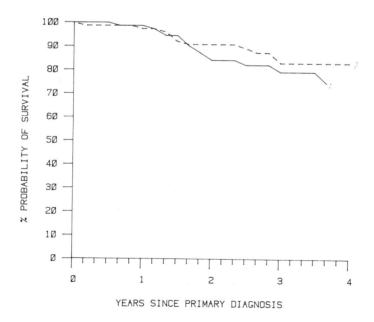

FIG. 3. Probability of developing bone metastases in 160 patients with primary breast cancer given Benoral, 10 ml twice daily (—), or placebo (- - - - -).

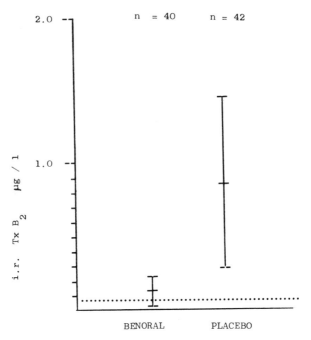

FIG. 4. Plasma levels of immunoreactive TXB₂ in patients with primary breast cancer given Benoral or placebo.

Although drugs like aspirin and indomethacin will prevent development of tumor deposits in bone (3,4) once osteolytic deposits are established, these agents have no effect on subsequent development (3). We have therefore used bone in organ culture to test other agents for antiosteolytic properties. We have shown that indomethacin, flurbiprofen, calcitonin, and mithramycin are all inhibitors of *in vitro* osteolysis (Table 2). We have therefore examined these agents for possible antiosteolytic properties in patients with breast cancer and bone metastases.

Osteolytic metastases cause breakdown of the collagen matrix and complexed calcium phosphate apatite crystals which constitute bone, causing release of calcium and hydroxyproline into the circulation. This is associated with bone pain, hypercalcaemia, and hydroxyprolinuria. Evidence of antiosteolytic activity may be reflected by changes in any or all of these features. Twenty-two patients with histologically proven breast cancer and radiological evidence of widespread osteolytic bone metastases were studied on 34 separate occasions for periods ranging from 5 to 70 days according to response. Patients were given daily aspirin, 2,700 mg, and indomethacin, 300 mg (9 patients), or calcitonin, 1 mg, s.c. (7 patients), or flurbiprofen, 300 mg (9 patients) or twice weekly mithramycin, 1 mg, i.v. (8 patients). Sequential radiological, isotopic scan, and pain assessment were carried out and urinary hydroxyproline and serum calcium were estimated.

TABLE 2. *Effect of mithramycin, human calcitonin, and indomethacin on* in vitro *resorption of ^{45}Ca-labelled neonatal mouse calvaria stimulated by PGE$_2$, bovine parathyroid hormone (PTH), and trypsin*[a]

Experiment	^{45}Ca release at 65 hr (%)		
	PGE$_2$ (1 μg/ml)	PTH (1 IV/ml)	Trypsin (1 μg/ml)
Control	1.95 ± 0.43	2.53 ± 0.47	1.74 ± 0.4
Mithramycin (50 ng/ml)	1.25 ± 0.22	0.91 ± 0.15	1.19 ± 0.11
Control	1.56 ± 0.15	1.66 ± 0.16	
Calcitonin (10 ng/ml)	1.05 ± 0.11	0.95 ± 0.05	
Control			2.57 ± 0.44
Indomethacin (1 μg/ml)			1.26 ± 0.18

[a] Assays performed in Biggers medium + 0.5% bovine plasma albumin. Results expressed as a ratio of percent total ^{45}Ca release from stimulated and control bones ± SEM.

The results are summarized in Table 3. Apart from relief of pain, aspirin and indomethacin failed to show any evidence of antiosteolytic activity. Pain relief also occurred with flurbiprofen administration but was associated with reduction of hypercalcaemia and hydroxyproline excretion in two patients. Calcitonin therapy was associated with pain relief (2/7) and reduction of serum calcium (1/1).

Mithramycin, an agent which we have previously reported to relieve hypercalcaemia in breast cancer (7) was also effective at relieving pain (3/8) and one patient showed good evidence of resclerosis of bone metastases.

These results indicate that although these agents show some evidence of antiosteolysis in some patients with bone metastases, in terms of cancer therapy they

TABLE 3. *Effects of aspirin, indomethacin, calcitonin, flurbiprofen, and mithramycin on osteolysis in patients with osteolytic bone metastases and breast cancer*

	Aspirin + indomethacin	Flurbiprofen	Calcitonin	Mithramycin
Number of patients	10	9	7	8
Number with hypercalcaemia	4	4	1	4
Duration of treatment (days)	5–8	21–28	21	28–70
Reduction in bone pain	2/10	2/9	2/7	3/8
Reduction in serum calcium	0/4	2/4	1/1	2/4
Reduction in hydroxyproline excretion	0/10	2/8	0/6	2/8
Radiological sclerosis	—	0/7	0/7	1/8

are trivial. Although these results are disappointing, the experimental work strongly indicates the need for further experimental and clinical investigation.

ACKNOWLEDGMENTS

We would like to thank the Boots Company Limited, United Kingdom, for supplying flurbiprofen and the Medical Research Council for supporting Dr. Judith Williams on a training fellowship.

REFERENCES

1. Dowsett et al. (1976): *Nature,* 263:72.
2. Dowsett et al. (1976): *Prostaglandins,* 2:447.
3. Galasko, C. S. B., and Bennett, A. (1976): *Nature,* 263:508.
4. Powles et al. (1973): *Br. J. Cancer,* 28:316.
5. Powles et al. (1973): *Nature* [*New Biol.*], 245:83.
6. Powles et al. (1976): *Lancet,* 1:608.
7. Smith, I. E., and Powles, T. J. (1975): *Br. Med. J.,* 1:268.

Advances in Prostaglandin and Thromboxane Research,
Vol. 6, edited by B. Samuelsson, P. W. Ramwell,
and R. Paoletti. Raven Press, New York © 1980.

Prostaglandin Enhancement of Skin Tumor Initiation and Promotion

Susan M. Fischer, Greta L. Gleason, Jeffrey S. Bohrman, and Thomas J. Slaga

Biology Division, Oak Ridge National Laboratory, and the University of Tennessee—Oak Ridge Graduate School of Biomedical Sciences, Oak Ridge, Tennessee 37830

Skin tumors on mice can be induced by a two-step procedure defined as initiation and promotion. The second step, promotion, is characterized by hyperplasia and inflammation (7). Prostaglandin (PG) involvement is suggested not only because of its direct function in inflammation, but also because of its structural similarities with the phorbol ester tumor promoters (5) and the stimulation of PG production in some cell types by such promoters (2). PGs have been used in conjunction with phorbol ester promoters but only in a limited study in which idiosyncratic behavior was reported (1). In addition, a report has appeared on the enhancement of complete skin carcinogenesis by PGs (3). It has also been demonstrated that PG synthetase can contribute to the metabolic activation of polycyclic aromatic hydrocarbons (4,6). These reports suggested that PGs may influence both tumor initiation and tumor promotion, although by different mechanisms.

METHODS AND MATERIALS

Seven-week-old Sencar mice, bred at the Oak Ridge National Laboratory, were shaved 2 days prior to the first treatment, and only those mice in the resting phase of the hair cycle were used in the tumor experiments. Groups of 30 mice, housed 10 per cage and fed *ad libitum,* were used, and the incidence of papillomas was recorded weekly. In the promotion experiments, the various PGs (Sigma Chemical Co.) or indomethacin (Merck, Sharp & Dohme) were applied topically at the same time as the topical application of the tumor promoter 12-O-tetradecanoylphorbol-13-acetate (TPA). In the initiation experiments, the PGs were applied topically at prescribed times before, during, and after the application of the carcinogen 7,12-dimethylbenz[a]anthracene (DMBA).

RESULTS AND DISCUSSION

Promotion

The involvement of the PGs in skin tumor promotion by TPA was studied by comparing the 2-series (PGE_2 and $PGF_{2\alpha}$) with the 1-series (PGE_1), as well as looking at the effect of the precursor arachidonic acid and the PG synthesis inhibitor indomethacin. As shown in Figs. 1 and 2, PGE_2 and $PGF_{2\alpha}$ increased the number of papillomas produced when applied simultaneously with TPA over the number seen with TPA alone. None of the PGs by themselves produced tumors in initiated mice. $PGF_{2\alpha}$ is slightly more potent than PGE_2 insofar as doses of 1 and 5 μg were nearly as effective as 10 μg. Only the 10-μg dose of PGE_2 produced a comparable 50% increase in tumor number.

PGE_1, however, has repeatedly produced an inhibition, even at a dose as low as 1 μg (Fig. 3). This would suggest that the differences between the 1- and 2-series of PGs may be more important with respect to tumor promotion than the differences within a series.

Arachidonic acid, precursor of the 2-series, produced an unexpected dose–response inhibition of promotion (Fig. 4). An 80% inhibition was observed with the highest dose employed (500 μg). The percentage of arachidonate converted to either PGE_2 or $PGF_{2\alpha}$ in this system is unknown. It is probable that other PG metabolites are responsible for the inhibition seen.

Indomethacin has been reported to inhibit TPA promotion (7). In this study,

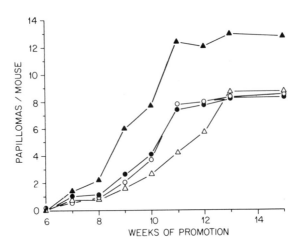

FIG. 1. Enhancement of tumor promotion by simultaneous treatment with TPA plus PGE_2. Each group consisted of 30 mice and all mice were initiated with 100 nmoles (25.6 μg) DMBA and promoted with 1 μg TPA twice weekly starting 1 week after initiation. Data expressed as average number of papillomas per mouse as a function of weeks of promotion. Symbols used: ○, control (TPA alone); ●, TPA plus 1 μg PGE_2; △, TPA plus 5 μg PGE_2; and ▲, TPA plus 10 μg PGE_2.

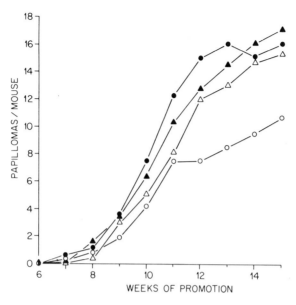

FIG. 2. Enhancement of tumor promotion by simultaneous treatment with TPA plus $PGF_{2\alpha}$. Each group consisted of 30 mice and all mice were initiated with 100 nmoles (25.6 μg) DMBA and promoted with 1 μg TPA twice weekly starting 1 week after initiation. Data expressed as average number of papillomas per mouse as a function of weeks of promotion. Symbols used: ○. control (TPA alone); ●, TPA plus 1 μg $PGF_{2\alpha}$; △, TPA plus 5 μg $PGF_{2\alpha}$; and ▲, TPA plus 10 μg $PGF_{2\alpha}$.

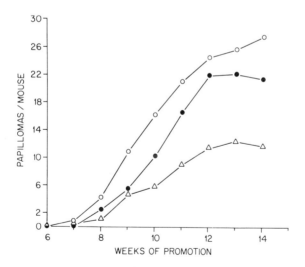

FIG. 3. Inhibition of tumor promotion by simultaneous treatment with TPA plus PGE_1. Each group consisted of 30 mice and all mice were initiated with 100 nmoles (25.6 μg) DMBA and promoted with 1 μg TPA twice weekly starting 1 week after initiation. Data expressed as average number of papillomas per mouse as a function of weeks of promotion. Symbols used: ○, control (TPA alone); ●, TPA plus 1 μg PGE_1; △, TPA plus 5 μg PGE_1.

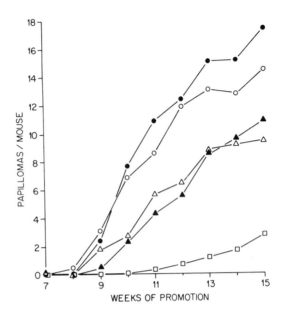

FIG. 4. Inhibition of tumor promotion by simultaneous treatment with TPA plus arachidonic acid. Each group consisted of 30 mice and all mice were initiated with 100 nmoles (25.6 μg) DMBA and promoted with 1 μg TPA twice weekly starting 1 week after initiation. Data expressed as average number of papillomas per mouse as a function of weeks of promotion. Symbols used: ○, control (TPA alone); ●, TPA plus 1 μg arachidonic acid; △, TPA plus 10 μg arachidonic acid; ▲, TPA plus 100 μg arachidonic acid; and □, TPA plus 500 μg arachidonic acid.

however, a lower range of doses was used, which resulted in an enhanced tumor yield (Fig. 5). Since it is known that indomethacin blocks PG synthesis at the level of the cyclooxygenase and also that it inhibits the TPA induction of ornithine decarboxylase in a manner that is reversible with the addition of PGE_1 or PGE_2 (8), the mechanism by which low doses of indomethacin augments tumorigenesis is unknown.

Initiation

The ability of PG synthetase to oxidize benzo[*a*]pyrene to reactive electrophilic metabolites (6) suggested that PGs may enhance the initiation stage of skin carcinogenesis. As shown in Fig. 6, the application of either PGE_1, PGE_2, $PGF_{2\alpha}$, or arachidonic acid increased the tumor yield. In considering time of application with respect to the carcinogen, arachidonic acid gave the greatest enhancement (60%) when applied 8 hr before DMBA, but the PGs had a greater effect when given at the same time as or slightly after DMBA. The time differences may be explained by the time required for the metabolism of arachidonic acid to the PGs. Further studies are being conducted to better delineate this phenomena.

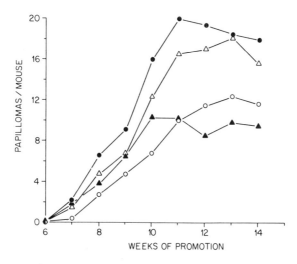

FIG. 5. Enhancement of tumor promotion by simultaneous treatment with TPA plus indometha-cin. Each group consisted of 30 mice and all mice were initiated with 100 nmoles (25.6 μg) DMBA and promoted with 2 μg TPA twice weekly starting 1 week after initiation. Data expressed as average number of papillomas per mouse as a function of weeks of promotion. Symbols used: ○, control (TPA alone); ●, TPA plus 25 μg indomethacin; △, TPA plus 50 μg indomethacin; and ▲, TPA plus 100 μg indomethacin.

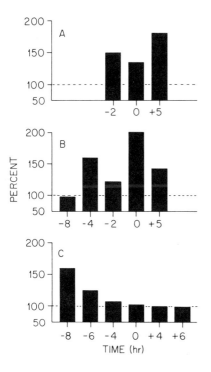

FIG. 6. Enhancement of DMBA tumor initia-tion by treatment with either PGE_1, $PGF_{2\alpha}$, or arachidonate. Each group consisted of 30 mice and all mice were initiated with 100 nmoles (25.6 μg) DMBA and promoted with 1 μg TPA twice weekly starting 1 week after initiation. PGs or arachidonate were applied as single doses at given times before or after DMBA. Data expressed as percentage of control of average number of papillomas per mouse as a function of time in hours before or after initiation. **A**: 10 μg PGE_1; **B**: 10 μg $PGF_{2\alpha}$; and **C**: 100 μg arachidonic acid.

In summary, TPA tumor promotion can be enhanced by PGE_2, $PGF_{2\alpha}$, or indomethacin but is inhibited by PGE_1 or arachidonic acid. Initiation with DMBA is enhanced by all the PGs tested, although to various extents. The mechanism operative in each of these stages is believed to be different.

ACKNOWLEDGMENTS

This research was sponsored jointly by the National Cancer Institute under Interagency Agreement Y01-CP-70227 and the Office of Health and Environmental Research, U.S. Department of Energy, under contract W-7405-eng-26 with the Union Carbide Corporation. J.S.B. is a postdoctoral investigator supported by Carcinogenesis Training Grant CA 05296 from the National Cancer Institute.

REFERENCES

1. Bellman, S., and Troll, W. (1978): *Carcinogenesis, Vol. 2. Mechanisms of Tumor Promotion and Cocarcinogenesis,* edited by T. J. Slaga, A. Sivak, and R. K. Boutwell, pp. 117–134. Raven Press, New York.
2. Levine, L., and Ohuchi, K. (1978): *Cancer Res.,* 38:4142–4146.
3. Lupulescu, A. (1978): *J. Natl. Cancer Inst.,* 61:97–106.
4. Marnett, L. J., Reed, G. A., and Johnson, J. T. (1977): *Biochem. Biophys. Res. Commun.,* 79:569–575.
5. Rohrschneider, L. R., and Boutwell, R. K. (1973): *Nature,* 243:212–213.
6. Sivarajah, K., Anderson, M. W., and Eling, T. E. (1978): *Life Sci.,* 23:2571–2578.
7. Slaga, T. J., Fischer, S. M., Viaje, A., Berry, D. L., Bracken, W. M., LeClerc, S., and Miller, D. R. (1978): In: *Carcinogenesis, Vol. 2. Mechanisms of Tumor Promotion and Cocarcinogenesis,* edited by T. J. Slaga, A. Sivak, and R. K. Boutwell, pp. 173–195. Raven Press, New York.
8. Verma, A. K., Rice, H. M., and Boutwell, R. K. (1977): *Biochem. Biophys. Res. Commun.,* 79:1160–1166.

Advances in Prostaglandin and Thromboxane Research,
Vol. 6, edited by B. Samuelsson, P. W. Ramwell,
and R. Paoletti. Raven Press, New York © 1980.

Effects of Diazepam on Tumor Growth and Plasma Prostaglandin E_2 in Rats

R. A. Karmali, A. Volkman, *P. Muse, *T. M. Louis

Department of Pathology and Laboratory Medicine and *Department of Anatomy, School
of Medicine, East Carolina University, Greenville, North Carolina 27834

Prostaglandins (PGs) have been shown to be present at high levels in a large number of human and experimental tumors (2,4,6). Such increased PG synthesis suggests loss of inhibitory regulation of the PG pathway. It has been suggested that thromboxane A_2 (TXA_2), a product which is rapidly inactivated, may provide this regulatory control (3). When diazepam was employed as a TXA_2 antagonist (1) in rats bearing the R3230AC mammary carcinoma, increased tumor growth was observed (5). Present data show increased growth of yet another tumor—Walker 256—following diazepam treatment. This phenomenon and the concomitant elevation in plasma PGE_2 levels were dose related.

MATERIALS AND METHODS

Male (Lewis $\times$ BN) F_1 hybrid rats (300 g) were obtained from the Trudeau Institute, Saranac Lake, New York. Groups of 7 animals were treated daily with 0.25-ml injections containing 0.9% saline, diazepam at 500 μg (1.7 mg/kg) and at 1,250 μg (4.2 mg/kg). The treatments were started 2 days before 5×10^5 Walker 256 tumor cells in single-cell suspension were transplanted under the left kidney capsule in each animal. After 14 days, rats were anesthetized with ether, and individual blood samples were drawn from the left and right renal veins. Five-ml chilled hypodermic syringes (23-gauge needle) containing heparin and 50 μg indomethacin were used. Lymph from the cannulated abdominal portion of the thoracic duct was collected in similar conditions. PGE_2 measurements in plasma and thoracic duct lymph were made by specific radioimmunoassay.

RESULTS AND DISCUSSION

The data in Table 1 summarize the effects of the treatments on tumor growth and PGE_2 in thoracic duct lymph. By 14 days after grafting, tumor growth increased significantly ($p < 0.01$) in rats treated with 500 μg diazepam but not with 1,250 μg. PGE_2 levels in the thoracic duct lymph were not significantly

TABLE 1. *Tumor growth and PGE$_2$ levels in thoracic duct lymph in rats bearing Walker 256 tumor (means ± SEM)*

	Control	Diazepam	
		500 µg/day	1,250 µg/day
Tumor growth[a]	1.025 ± 0.0200	1.133 ± 0.0298	1.090 ± 0.240
		($p < 0.01$)	($p < 0.01$)
PGE$_2$ (pg/ml)	306 ± 36.2	217 ± 60.0	270 ± 32.4

[a] Expressed as weight of left kidney/weight of right control kidney.

TABLE 2. *Plasma PGE$_2$ (pg/ml) in rats bearing Walker 256 tumor in the left kidney (means ± SEM)*

Control		Diazepam, 500 µg/day		Diazepam, 1,250 µg/day	
Left	Right	Left	Right	Left	Right
615 ± 36.8	502 ± 56.0	1,445 ± 318.6[a]	1,038 ± 222.0	717 ± 134.6	623 ± 103.6

[a] Diazepam 500 µg/day vs. control: ($p < 0.02$).
Analysis of variance ($p < 0.02$).

altered by 500 µg diazepam treatment. PGE$_2$ from the left tumor-bearing renal vein plasma was generally higher than that in the right control renal vein plasma in each group. This difference in levels was significant in the saline-treated group ($p < 0.02$) (Table 2). When PGE$_2$ levels in plasma from the tumor-bearing kidneys were compared, they were significantly higher after 500 µg than after 1,250 µg and in controls.

In conclusion, the data show dose-related increases in intrarenal tumor growth and renal vein PGE$_2$ levels in diazepam-treated rats. In unpublished experiments we have found that diazepam has no effect on plasma PGE$_2$ levels in rats bearing no tumors. The relationship of diazepam to the changes in tumor growth and PGE$_2$ levels in the present experiments remains to be elucidated.

REFERENCES

1. Ally, A. I., Manku, M. S., Horrobin, D. F., Karmali, R. A., Morgan, R. O., and Karmazyn, M. (1978): *Neurosci. Lett.,* 7:31–34.
2. Bennett, A., Charlier, E. M., McDonald, A. M., Simpson, J. S., Stanford, I. F., and Zebro, T. (1977): *Lancet,* 2:624–626.
3. Horrobin, D. F., Karmali, R. A., Manku, M. S., Ally, A. I., Karmazyn, M., Morgan, R. O., Swift, A., and Zinner, H. (1977): *IRCS J. Med. Sci.,* 5:547–549.
4. Jaffe, B. M. (1974): *Prostaglandins,* 6:453–461.
5. Karmali, R. A., Horrobin, D. F., Ghayur, T., Manku, M. S., Cunnane, S. C., Morgan, R. O., Ally, A. I., Karmazyn, M., and Oka, M. (1978): *Cancer Lett.,* 5:205–208.
6. Tashjian, A. H., Voelkel, E. F., and Levine, L. (1977): *Prostaglandins,* 14:309–317.

Advances in Prostaglandin and Thromboxane Research,
Vol. 6, edited by B. Samuelsson, P. W. Ramwell,
and R. Paoletti. Raven Press, New York © 1980.

The VX-2 Carcinoma: Humoral Effects and Arachidonic Acid Metabolism

*W. C. Hubbard, †A. Hough, *A. R. Brash, *R. M. Johnson,
and *‡J. A. Oates

*Departments of *Pharmacology, †Pathology, and *‡Medicine, Vanderbilt University,
Nashville, Tennessee 37232*

The VX-2 carcinoma-bearing rabbit has been employed as an animal model for study of humorally mediated hypercalcemia of malignant disease (4,8,10, 11,12). Rabbits receiving implants of VX-2 carcinoma tissue intramuscularly (i.m.) in the hind limb develop significant hypercalcemia within 10 to 21 days. The elevation in the serum calcium levels is preceded by increased prostaglandin E_2 (PGE_2) production (8,10). Concomitant with the hypercalcemia are osseous changes that are consistent with systemic bone resorption. The administration of agents to hypercalcemic tumor-bearing animals that inhibit PGE_2 biosynthesis lower, or in some instances normalize, the serum calcium levels. Since PGE_2 is a potent osteoclastic stimulator *in vitro* (2,5) and is produced in relatively large quantities by rabbits bearing the VX-2 carcinoma i.m., it has been postulated that the hypercalcemic syndrome in this tumor-bearing animal model and perhaps certain types of malignancy in man (9) may be due to the secretion and release of PGE_2, which in turn leads to increased systemic bone resorption.

In addition to becoming hypercalcemic, rabbits bearing the VX-2 carcinoma i.m. also develop a myelocytic leukemoid syndrome characterized by granulocytosis and severe bone marrow hyperplasia (4). Granulocytosis is observed concomitant with or shortly after the onset of hypercalcemia. Thus a relationship between PGE_2 production and the onset of granulocytosis similar to that observed in the development of hypercalcemia can be established. The effect of inhibitors of PGE_2 biosynthesis on the granulocytic leukemoid syndrome has not been determined.

The humoral effects of the VX-2 carcinoma vary significantly in relation to the site of implantation of neoplastic tissue. Rabbits receiving implants of tumor tissue intra-abdominally (i.a.) fail to develop hypercalcemia (12) and the myelocytic leukemoid syndrome (W. C. Hubbard and A. Hough, *unpublished observations*) even in the presence of an extensive neoplastic burden. We have evaluated these differences in the humoral effects of the neoplasm in relation to PGE_2 production *in vivo* and to the metabolism of arachidonic acid (AA) by VX-2 carcinoma tissue *in vitro.*

Comparisons of the serum calcium levels, white blood cell (WBC) counts and plasma levels of the 15-keto-13,14-dihydro-metabolite of PGE_2 ($15K-H_2-PGE_2$) in normal and in tumor-bearing rabbits are summarized in Table 1. The data summarized in Table 1 suggest that the differences in the humoral effects of the VX-2 carcinoma subsequent to i.m. and i.a. implantation are not related to differences in PGE_2 production *in vivo* or to differences in the circulating level of $15K-H_2-PGE_2$.

In subsequent studies of the metabolic profile of AA, the fatty acid precursor of PGE_2, by VX-2 carcinoma tissue *in vitro,* we observed no differences in tumor tissue harvested from the two different implant sites. During these studies we observed that in addition to being a precursor of PGE_2, AA is converted to 11-hydroxy-eicosatetraenoic acid (11-HETE) and 15-hydroxy-eicosatetraenoic acid (15-HETE). More significantly, we observed that linoleic acid is also oxygenated by tumor homogenates to 9-hydroxyoctadecadienoic acid (9-HODD) and 13-hydroxy-octadecadienoic acid (13-HODD). The conversion of linoleic acid (LA) to 9-HODD and 13-HODD appears to be the only pathway in the metabolism of the polyenoic fatty acid. Indirect measurements of 9-HODD and 13-HODD produced by VX-2 carcinoma tissue *in vitro* indicate that the quantities of these compounds produced by the tumor approximate that of PGE_2 biosynthesis. The oxygenation of AA to 11-HETE and 15-HETE and LA to 9-HODD and 13-HODD is inhibited by indomethacin.

Our data indicate that the humoral effects of the VX-2 carcinoma produced subsequent to i.m. and i.a. implantation may be due to more complete presystemic inactivation or removal of the humoral agent(s) released from i.a. implants by metabolism sequentially in the liver and the lung than by the lung alone when the implants are i.m. Since PGE_2 is rapidly inactivated by both the lung and liver (1,3,6,7), the differences in the humoral effects of the VX-2 carcinoma may be related to differences in the ability of the liver and lung to convert monohydroxy-polyenoic fatty acids (HPFA) to inactive compounds or to remove them from the circulation. The possibility that the differences in the humoral effects of the VX-2 carcinoma may be related to differences in the ability of the lung and liver to remove or to inactivate HPFA produced by the tumor and evaluation of the role of these compounds in the production of the myelocytic

TABLE 1. *Serum calcium levels, WBC counts, and plasma levels of 15K-H_2-PGE$_2$ in normal and in tumor-bearing rabbits*[a]

Site of implant	Serum Ca²⁺ (mg/dl)	WBC/mm (× 10³)	15K-H₂-PGE₂ (ng/ml)
None (control)	14.9 ± 0.3	7.1 ± 1.5	0.05 ± 0.02
IA	13.9 ± 0.5	8.6 ± 1.8	11.1 ± 6.0[b]
IM	17.9 ± 0.5[a]	21.2 ± 3.1[a]	15.2 ± 3.8[b]

[a] Samples for evaluation taken 4 weeks after tumor implantation.
[b] $p < 0.001$.

leukemoid syndrome and hypercalcemia in the VX-2 carcinoma-bearing rabbit warrants further investigation.

ACKNOWLEDGMENTS

This work was supported by NIH Grant GM 15431.

REFERENCES

1. Bakhle, Y. S., and Vane, J. R. (1974): *Physiol. Rev.,* 54:1007–1045.
2. Dietrich, J. W., Goodson, J. M., and Raisz, L. G. (1975): *Prostaglandins,* 10:231–240.
3. Hamberg, M., and Samuelsson, B. (1971): *J. Biol. Chem.,* 246:1073–1077.
4. Hough, A., Jr., Seyberth, H. W., Oates, J. A., and Hartmann, W. (1977): *Am. J. Pathol.,* 87:537–552.
5. Klein, D. C., and Raisz, L. G. (1970): *Endocrinology,* 86:1436–1440.
6. Samuelsson, B., Goldyne, M., Granström, E., Hamberg, M., Hammarström, S., and Malmsten, C. (1978): *Ann. Rev. Biochem.,* 47:997–1029.
7. Samuelsson, B., Granström, E., Green, K., Hamberg, M., and Hammarström, S. (1975): *Ann. Rev. Biochem.,* 44:669–695.
8. Seyberth, H. W., Hubbard, W. C., Oelz, O., Sweetman, B. J., Watson, J. T., and Oates, J. A. (1977): *Prostaglandins,* 14:319–331.
9. Seyberth, H. W., Segre, G. V., Morgan, J. L., Sweetman, B. J., Potts, J. T., Jr., and Oates, J. A. (1975): *N. Engl. J. Med.,* 293:1278–1283.
10. Tashjian, A. H., Jr., Voelkel, E. F., and Levine, L. (1977): *Prostaglandins,* 14:309–317.
11. Voelkel, E. F., Tashjian, A. H., Jr., Franklin, R., Wasserman, E., and Levine, L. (1975): *Metabolism,* 24:973–986.
12. Young, D. V., Fioravanti, J. L., Prieur, D. J., and Ward, J. M. (1976): *Lab. Invest.,* 35:30–46.

Advances in Prostaglandin and Thromboxane Research,
Vol. 6, edited by B. Samuelsson, P. W. Ramwell,
and R. Paoletti. Raven Press, New York © 1980.

Increased Prostaglandin Synthesis in Hodgkin's Disease: A Lymphocyte–Monocyte Interaction

P. L. Amlot, A. Chivers, D. Heinzelmann, and L. J. F. Youlten

Department of Medicine and Pharmacology, Guy's Hospital Medical School, London Bridge, SE1 9RT London, United Kingdom

An immunoregulatory role for prostaglandins (PGs) has been suggested from the inhibitory effect of exogenous PGE_2 on lymphocyte function *in vitro* and the augmentation of lymphocyte responses by indomethacin and other PG synthetase inhibitors *in vitro* (3,5). It has also been claimed that an adherent suppressor cell (presumably a monocyte) synthesizing increased quantities of PG is the cause of the depressed lymphocyte function commonly seen in Hodgkin's disease (3). This claim is examined in the present study.

Paired controls and untreated patients with Hodgkin's disease (HD) were studied using established microculture lymphocyte transformation techniques (4) and responses were evaluated at 48 hr by ^{3}H-thymidine (^{3}HTdR) uptake. The effect of indomethacin at 1 μg/ml on mitogen-induced lymphocyte proliferation is shown in Fig. 1. Significant increases in ^{3}HTdR uptake by mitogen-stimulated cultures in the presence of indomethacin were seen in both controls and HD patients. ^{3}HTdR uptake was augmented in unstimulated control cultures by the presence of indomethacin but not in unstimulated HD cultures. Indomethacin did not restore the optimum phytohemagglutinin (PHA) dose response observed in HD cultures to normal control values. HD patients show normal lymphocyte responsiveness to pokeweed mitogen (PWM) and the effect of indomethacin is the same in both HD and controls.

PGE_2 and $PGF_{2\alpha}$ synthesized *in vitro* over 48 hr by unstimulated peripheral blood mononuclear cells (PBMCs) were measured by radioimmunoassay using specific antisera obtained from the Institut Pasteur. Because of the important contribution by monocytes to PG synthesis, May Grunewald Giemsa and nonspecific esterase staining were used to estimate the percentage of monocytes in cell preparations. Ficoll-Triosil separation of whole blood (1) yielded PBMC preparations with a significantly greater percentage of monocytes in HD than in controls (Table 1). Virtually all the remaining cells were lymphocytes. The relatively lymphoctye-enriching procedures of plastic adherence and phagocyte depletion using polycarbonyl iron yielded approximately equal monocyte contamination of these lymphocyte preparations in both HD and controls.

If monocyte numbers were ignored, PGE_2 and $PGF_{2\alpha}$ synthesis by HD PBMC

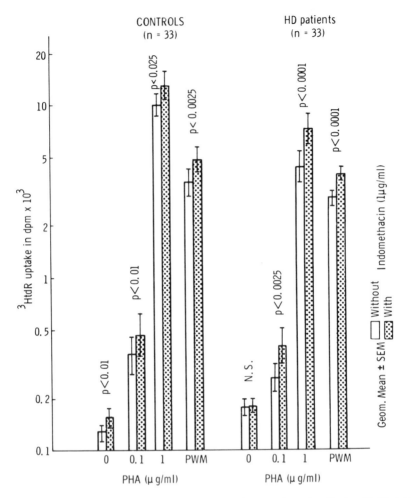

FIG. 1. Effect of indomethacin on mitogen response in controls and patients with Hodgkin's disease. Indomethacin was added at 1 μg/ml.

in vitro was considerably greater than from control PBMC (Table 2). When PG production was standardized to ng/10^6 monocytes/48 hr, no difference was seen between HD and controls when isolated adherent cell cultures of 80 to 90% monocytes were examined. However, a significantly higher PGE_2 synthesis by PBMC from HD persisted; this was not seen with $PGF_{2\alpha}$ (Table 3). That the excess PG production in HD PBMC cultures did not derive from lymphocytes is shown in Table 4, where much lower levels of PGE_2 and $PGF_{2\alpha}$ were found in phagocyte-depleted cultures. Indeed, nearly all of the PG production in these cultures could be attributed to residual monoctye contamination.

No significant correlation between PG synthesis and lymphocyte mitogen

TABLE 1. *Percent monocytes in PBMCs in HD and control subjects*

	Controls ($n = 77$)	HD patients ($n = 54$)
PBMC	22.7 ± 1.1^a	36.4 ± 2^b
Plastic nonadherent	6.6 ± 1.2	5.3 ± 0.5
Phagocyte depleted	0.6 ± 0.1	0.7 ± 0.1

[a] Mean $\pm$ SEM.
[b] $p < 0.001$.

TABLE 2. *PG production in the total cell culture*

	Controls ($n = 19$)	HD patients ($n = 19$)
PGE_2	18.6 ± 3.1^a	74.9 ± 17.1^b
$PGF_{2\alpha}$	12.4 ± 1.5	27.8 ± 6.2^c

[a] Mean $\pm$ SEM (ng/10^6 PBMC/48 hr).
[b] $p < 0.0025$.
[c] $p < 0.01$.

TABLE 3. *Standardized PG production*

	Controls ($n = 19$)	HD patients ($n = 19$)
All PBMC		
PGE_2	71.9 ± 8.9^a	187.7 ± 52^b
$PGF_{2\alpha}$	61.3 ± 8.7	78.3 ± 21.1
Adherent cells		
PGE_2	110.5 ± 13	136.4 ± 23.9
$PGF_{2\alpha}$	85.1 ± 15.2	75.3 ± 11.1

[a] Mean $\pm$ SEM (ng/10^6 monocytes/48 hr).
[b] $p < 0.01$.

TABLE 4. *PG production by phagocyte-depleted cells*

	Controls ($n = 12$)	HD patients ($n = 12$)
PGE_2	1.6 ± 0.8^a	0.8 ± 0.5
$PGF_{2\alpha}$	0.32 ± 0.15	0.31 ± 0.14

[a] Mean $\pm$ SEM (ng/10^6 cells/48 hr).

TABLE 5. ^{3}HTdR uptake by unstimulated cell cultures

	Control ($n = 34$)	HD patients ($n = 34$)
All PBMC	123 ± 12^a	170 ± 20^b
Adherent cells	56 ± 8	69 ± 10
Phagocyte depleted	89 ± 12	78 ± 9

[a] Mean $\pm$ SEM (dpm counts).
[b] $p < 0.005$.

response measured in ^{3}HTdR uptake or with the change in response induced by indomethacin was found.

These results suggest that a lymphocyte–monocyte interaction in HD induces increased PGE$_2$ production by monocytes. It is noteworthy, therefore, that the same appears true for the increased uptake of ^{3}HTdR by unstimulated PBMC cultures frequently reported in HD (2) (Table 5).

We draw the following conclusions:

a. most of the increased PG production by HD PBMC is due to the greater number of monocytes present therein;

b. a lymphocyte–monocyte interaction augments the production of PGE$_2$ by monocytes in HD; and

c. the indomethacin effect does not seem explicable on the simple basis of cumulative PG production *in vitro* suppressing mitogen response.

REFERENCES

1. Böyum, A. (1968): *Scand. J. Clin. Lab. Invest. (Suppl. 21)*, 97:77.
2. Crowther, D., Fairley, G. H., and Sewell, R. L. (1969): *Br. Med. J.*, 2:473.
3. Goodwin, J. S., Messner, R. P., Bankhurst, A. D., Peake, G. T., Saiki, J. H., and Williams, R. C., Jr. (1977): *N. Engl. J. Med.*, 279:963.
4. Janossy, G., and Greaves, M. S. (1972): *Clin. Exp. Immunol.*, 10:525.
5. Webb, D. R., (1977): *Cell Immunol.*, 33:1.

Advances in Prostaglandin and Thromboxane Research,
Vol. 6, edited by B. Samuelsson, P. W. Ramwell,
and R. Paoletti. Raven Press, New York © 1980.

Prostaglandin and Thromboxane Production by Fibroblasts and Vascular Endothelial Cells

A. E. Ali, J. C. Barrett, and T. E. Eling

*National Institute of Environmental Health Sciences, Research Triangle Park,
North Carolina 27709*

Prostaglandin I_2 (PGI$_2$, prostacyclin) and thromboxane A_2 (TXA$_2$) apparently
play a key role in the control of platelet aggregation and deposition within
the blood circulation. PGI$_2$ was shown by Vane and co-workers (4,12,14) to
originate from arterial rings or microsomes and inhibit platelet aggregation. It
was hypothesized that arterial walls were protected against deposition of platelets
by PGI$_2$. Subsequently, it was shown in several species that endothelial cells
lining the blood vessels were the major source of PGI$_2$. This was also demonstrated with cultured endothelial cells from bovine or pig aortas and human
umbilical veins (8,9,15). TXA$_2$ aggregates platelets, and they synthesize it in
response to stimuli. It is also a potent vasoconstrictor (6). The presence of
TXA$_2$ was demonstrated in the lung, kidney, heart, brain, and recently in cultured human lung fibroblasts WI-38 (7).

We report here the formation of PGI$_2$ and/or TXA$_2$ by fibroblasts from
different origins and the specificity of PGI$_2$ formation by bovine aortas or heart
endothelial cells.

RESULTS

Eight cell lines were tested for cyclooxygenase products of arachidonic acid
by specific radioimmunoassays. PGI$_2$ and TXA$_2$ were estimated by measuring
their breakdown products 6-keto-PGF$_{1\alpha}$ and TXB$_2$, respectively. The results,
summarized in Table 1, show that all cell types except 3T3 and BHK synthesized
PGI$_2$. 3T3 produced mainly PGE$_2$ [77% of total cyclooxygenase products measured (TCP)], while BHK had a poor cyclooxygenase enzyme activity (CLO);
nonetheless, TXB$_2$ was detected as the major product of these cells (65% TCP).
The endothelial cells from adult bovine aorta (ABAE) and fetal bovine heart
(FBHE) produced a significantly higher proportion of TCP as PGI$_2$ (95 and
75%, respectively) but failed to produce TXB$_2$, though limited amounts of PGE
and PGF$_\alpha$ were formed. The observation was made that human skin fibroblasts
(KD) and malignant fibrosarcoma cells (BP-6-T) formed considerable amounts

TABLE 1. *Comparison of PG and TX production by various cell lines in culture[a]*

Cell line	6-Keto-PGF$_{1\alpha}$	PGE	PGF$_\alpha$	TXB$_2$	Total (ng/ml)
ABAE	12.8 ± 0.97	ND[b]	0.59 ± 0.03	ND	13.4
SHE	5.65 ± 0.32	4.4 ± 0.15	1.63 ± 0.09	1.45 ± 0.2	13.1
KD	3.35 ± 0.28	1.95 ± 0.17	0.81 ± 0.13	ND	6.11
FBHE	2.83 ± 0.100	0.44 ± 0.02	0.51 ± 0.03	ND	3.78
10T½	2.0 ± 0.23	1.16 ± 0.54	ND	ND	3.16
BP-6-T	1.5 ± 0.22	1.45 ± 0.28	0.61 ± 0.04	ND	3.56
3T3	ND	9.2 ± 0.24	2.45 ± 0.29	0.34 ± 0.2	11.99
BHK	ND	ND	0.70 ± 0.19	1.31 ± 0.3	2.0

[a] Means ± SEM (ng/ml) are shown. $N = 4$.
[b] ND, not detected.

of PGI$_2$ (55 and 42% TCP, respectively). Production of PGI$_2$ was confirmed by radiochromatographic analysis and bioassay.

Monolayers of established mouse embryo fibroblast cell line (10T½), FBHE, or ABAE converted ^{14}C-arachidonate and ^{14}C-PGH$_2$ into labeled metabolites which migrated with marker ^{3}H-6-keto-PGF$_{1\alpha}$ in thin-layer chromatography system A IX (5). This conversion was inhibited by incubation of indomethacin or tranylcypromine.

Aggregation of human platelets in platelet-rich plasma (PRP) was utilized to test directly the production of PGI$_2$ by cultured cells. Aggregation induced by arachidonic acid was prevented when culture media (10–50 μl/4 ml) in which cells were grown or incubated with arachidonate were added to fresh PRP.

DISCUSSION

Cultured endothelial cells derived from bovine or pig aortas or human umbilical veins (8,9,15) synthesize PGI$_2$. Our results show that in addition to ABAE and FBHE, a number of fibroblast lines generate PGI$_2$ at rest or from exogenous substrate PGH$_2$ or arachidonate. Contrary to the current belief by many workers that fibroblasts and smooth muscle cells produce no PGI$_2$, with some lines such as 10T½, KD, or Syrian hamster embryo cells (SHE), PGI$_2$ is the major product of arachidonate metabolism via cyclooxygenase pathway. ABAE and FBHE produced only PGI$_2$ but no TXB$_2$ and frequently small amounts of PGE and PGF$_\alpha$. This supports the view that endothelial cells are specialized (under normal conditions) to produce the thrombolytic PGI$_2$ to protect the circulation against intraarterial thrombosis.

SHE cells produced both PGI$_2$ and TXB$_2$ in considerable amounts. This is the first report of a cell population producing both PGI$_2$ and TXB$_2$. A physiological balance between PGI$_2$ and TXA$_2$ may regulate biochemical events within the same cell. For example, adenyl cyclase has been reported to be altered by PGI_2 and TXA_2 in different systems (1–3,10,13,14).

Thus we have shown that some fibroblasts can produce PGI_2 and/or TXA_2 in significant amounts. These cells may be useful model systems for the study of factors that regulate PGI_2 and TXA_2 synthetase enzymes.

REFERENCES

1. Best, L. C., Martin, T. J., Russell, R. G. G., and Preston, F. E. (1977): *Nature,* 267:850–851.
2. Gorman, R. R., Bunting, S., and Miller, O. V. (1977): *Prostaglandins,* 13:377–388.
3. Gorman, R. R., Hamilton, R. D., and Hopkins, N. K. (1979): *J. Biol. Chem.* 254:1671–1676.
4. Gryglewski, R. J., Bunting, S., Moncada, S., Flower, R. J., and Vane, J. R. (1976): *Prostaglandins,* 12:685–713.
5. Hamberg, M., and Samuelsson, B. (1966): *J. Biol. Chem.,* 241:257–263.
6. Hamberg, M., Svensson, J., and Samuelsson, B. (1975): *Proc. Natl. Acad. Sci. USA,* 72:2994–2998.
7. Hopkins, N. K., Sun, F. F., and Gorman, R. R. (1978): *Biochem. Biophys. Res. Commun.,* 85:827–836.
8. MacIntyre, D. E., Pearson, J. D., and Gordon, J. L. (1978): *Nature,* 271:549–551.
9. Marcus, A. J., Weksler, B. B., and Jaffe, E. A. (1978): *J. Biol. Chem.,* 253:7138–7141.
10. Miller, O. V., and Gorman, R. R. (1976): *J. Cyclic Nucleotide Res.,* 2:79–87.
11. Moncada, S., Gryglewski, R. J., Bunting, S., and Vane, J. R. (1976): *Nature,* 263:663–665.
12. Moncada, S., Higgs, E. A., and Vane, J. R. (1977): *Lancet,* 1:18–21.
13. Rosen, P., and Schror, K. (1979): *Naunyn Schmiedebergs Arch. Pharmacol.,* 306:101–103.
14. Tateson, J., Moncada, S., and Miller, O. V. (1977): *Prostaglandins,* 13:389–399.
15. Weksler, B. B., Marcus, A. J., and Jaffe, E. A. (1977): *Biology,* 74:3922–3926.

Advances in Prostaglandin and Thromboxane Research,
Vol. 6, edited by B. Samuelsson, P. W. Ramwell,
and R. Paoletti. Raven Press, New York © 1980.

Regeneration of Prostacyclin Synthetase Activity in Cultured Vascular Cells Following Aspirin Treatment

K. F. Salata, J. D. Whiting, and J. M. Bailey

Department of Biochemistry, The George Washington University, School of Medicine and Health Sciences, Washington, D.C. 20037

Several investigators have reported the synthesis of prostacyclin (PGI_2) or PGI_2-like compounds from arachidonic acid or prostaglandin (PG) endoperoxides by vascular tissue (2,3), endothelial cells in culture (4), and human aortic smooth muscle cells (1). This paper presents evidence that cultured smooth muscle cells isolated from the rat thoracic aorta produce PGI_2 as the major product of arachidonic acid metabolism. In addition, aspirin was found to inhibit the synthesis of PGI_2 by these cells, but these cells have the ability to recover quickly from the aspirin inhibition.

Initial studies demonstrated that confluent cultures of rat smooth muscle cells superfused with arachidonic acid in serum-free medium produced a potent inhibitor of platelet aggregation. The instability of the inhibitory activity to heat and low pH and the spontaneous loss of inhibitory activity at room temperature with a half-life of about 12 min suggested that the active compound was PGI_2. In order to identify the arachidonic acid metabolites produced in these cells, [1-^{14}C]arachidonic acid was superfused on confluent cultures for 5 min. The resulting products were extracted into acidified ethyl acetate and separated by thin-layer chromatography. The major radioactive product was found to cochromatograph with 6-keto-$PGF_{1\alpha}$, the stable breakdown product of PGI_2 (Fig. 1). Additional radioactive products cochromatographed with PGE_2 and PGD_2. Aspirin at a concentration of 0.2 mM was found to be very effective in inhibiting the formation of all these arachidonate products. The final chemical identification of the major arachidonic acid metabolite from the cells was accomplished using gas chromatography–mass spectrometry of the tetratrimethylsilyl-hydroxime methyl ester derivative. The mass spectrum of this product contained characteristic ions which were in the same ratios as those observed in the authentic 6-keto-$PGF_{1\alpha}$ derivative.

In order to determine whether aspirin caused irreversible inhibition of PGI_2 in these cells, confluent cultures of rat smooth muscle cells were incubated at 37°C in serum-free medium with or without 0.2 mM aspirin. After 30 min,

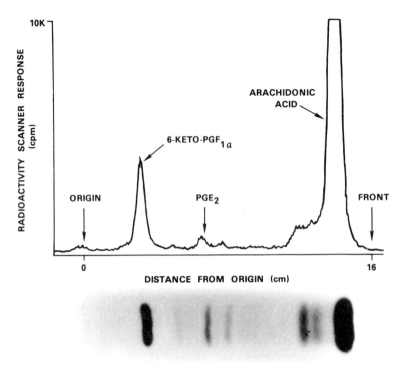

FIG. 1. Thin-layer radiochromatogram and autoradiograph of the superfusate of [1-¹⁴C]arachidonic acid metabolites from cultured smooth muscle cells.

the aspirin medium was removed and 3 ml of medium with serum was added to each culture. At various times, duplicate flasks were washed and superfused with 0.75 μCi [1-¹⁴C]arachidonic acid for 5 min. The resulting superfusate was acidified, extracted with ethyl acetate, and the organic soluble material was applied to silica gel G plates that were incubated in a humid chamber for 30 min prior to development in the organic phase of ethyl acetate/iso-octane/acetic acid/water (11:5:2:10). The position of the radioactive products was determined using a radioactivity scanner, the radioactive bands were scraped from the plate, and the radioactivity determined by liquid scintillation counting.

Figure 2 shows the radioactive product profiles from control and aspirin-treated cells. Immediately after aspirin treatment, the PGI₂ synthetic activity (measured as the formation of 6-keto-PGF$_{1\alpha}$) was almost completely inhibited. However, within 1 hr, the synthetic activity returned to normal and continued to increase to about 2.5 times the control value by 4 hr. By 24 hr, the synthetic activity had decreased to about 20% of control values. The time course of the recovery of PGI₂ biosynthetic activity after aspirin treatment is shown in Fig. 3. The addition of 20 μ/ml cycloheximide to the aspirin-treated cells completely inhibited the recovery of PGI₂ biosynthesis, indicating that the recovery of activity probably involves synthesis of new enzyme.

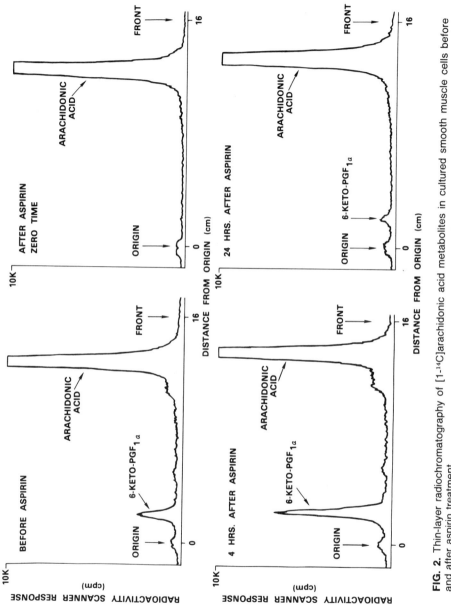

FIG. 2. Thin-layer radiochromatography of [1-^{14}C]arachidonic acid metabolites in cultured smooth muscle cells before and after aspirin treatment.

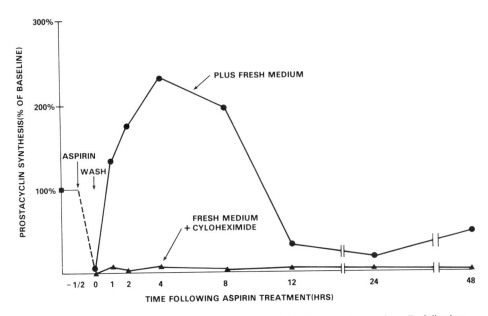

FIG. 3. Time–course of recovery of PGI₂ synthetic activity in smooth muscle cells following aspirin treatment. Dependence on protein synthesis.

Our results prove that intact smooth muscle cells can convert arachidonic acid to PGI₂. Aspirin is effective in inhibiting the production of PGI₂ in these cells, but the aspirin inhibition is short-lived, with the PGI₂ biosynthetic activity returning to normal levels within 1 hr. Jaffe and co-workers (4) have shown that human endothelial cells also possess the ability to recover from the aspirin inhibition of PGI₂ biosynthesis, but the biosynthetic levels do not return to normal for about 36 hr in these cells. The three aspirin-sensitive components of the vascular system—platelets, endothelial cells, and smooth muscle cells—have now been shown to vary in their *in vitro* response to aspirin inhibition of cyclooxygenase.

It can be shown that the cycloheximide-sensitive recovery of PGI₂ synthetase activity in smooth muscle cells following aspirin treatment probably represents a 10- to 20-fold increase in the biosynthesis of the enzyme. The nature of the control mechanisms whereby the rapid induction of the enzyme synthesis is produced is the subject of further investigation.

REFERENCES

1. Baenziger, N. L., Dillender, M. J., and Majerus, P. W. (1977): *Biochem. Biophys. Res. Commun.,* 78:294–301.
2. Bunting, S., Gryglewski, R., Moncada, S., and Vane, J. R. (1976): *Prostaglandins,* 12:897–913.
3. Moncada, S., Herman, A. G., Higgs, E. P., and Vane, J. R. (1977): *Thromb. Res.,* 11:323–344.
4. Weksler, B. B., Marcus, A. J., and Jaffe, E. D. (1977): *Proc. Natl. Acad. Sci. USA,* 74:3922–3926.

Advances in Prostaglandin and Thromboxane Research,
Vol. 6, edited by B. Samuelsson, P. W. Ramwell,
and R. Paoletti. Raven Press, New York © 1980.

Endogenous Prostaglandin E₂ Production Inhibits Proliferation of Polyoma Virus-Transformed 3T3 Cells: Correlation with Cellular Levels of Cyclic AMP

Hans-Erik Claesson, Jan Åke Lindgren, and Sven Hammarström

Department of Chemistry, Karolinska Institutet, S-104 01 Stockholm, Sweden

Previous studies have shown that polyoma virus (py) 3T3 fibroblasts produce high levels of prostaglandin (PG) E_2 compared to regular 3T3 fibroblasts (6). Endogenously produced PGE_2 also raises the cellular levels of adenosine-3':5'-monophosphate (cyclic AMP) in py 3T3 cells (2). Since cyclic AMP inhibits growth of various cells (9–11), the effect of the PG production on proliferation of py 3T3 cells *in vitro* was investigated. Indomethacin, a potent inhibitor of PG synthesis, was used for these experiments. PG synthesis inhibitors have previously been shown to stimulate growth of IMR90, (12), HeLa, L-929, and HEP-2 cells *in vitro* (12,13).

The present results show that the PG synthesis inhibitor decreases the levels of cyclic AMP and stimulates cell growth and that these effects are due to inhibition of PGE_2 biosynthesis.

METHODS

Polyoma virus-transformed Balb/c 3T3 fibroblasts were grown under standard conditions in Dulbecco's modified Eagle's medium containing 5% calf serum (2). Cells were counted in a Coulter counter (Coulter Electronics Ltd., Harpenden, Hertfordshire, United Kingdom). Concentrations of PGE_2 in culture media were analyzed by radioimmunoassay after $NaBH_4$ reduction of PGE_2 to $PGF_{2\alpha}$ and $PGF_{2\beta}$ (8). The cellular cyclic AMP concentrations were measured by the protein-binding technique of Gilman (5). DNA contents were assayed according to Burton (1).

RESULTS

Indomethacin, at a concentration of 1 μM, completely inhibited PGE_2 biosynthesis in py 3T3 (Fig. 1A). The levels of cyclic AMP were also markedly reduced in indomethacin-treated cultures (Fig. 1B). A lower inhibitor concentra-

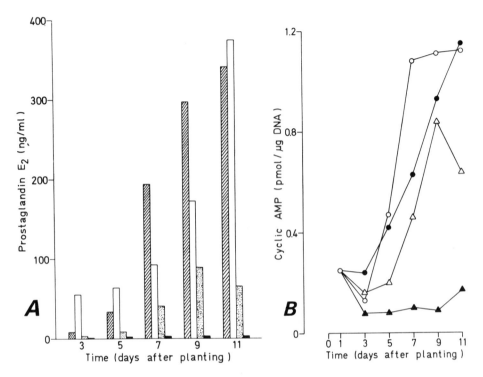

FIG. 1. PGE₂ **(A)** and cyclic AMP **(B)** production in control and indomethacin-treated py 3T3 cultures. py 3T3 cells were planted at a density of 3,200 cells/cm² on 90-mm culture dishes. Twenty-four hr later, the cultures were divided into four groups. The media were removed and fresh media with or without additions were added: fresh media without additions [control:⧅ **(A)**, ○ **(B)**] or fresh media containing 10 nM indomethacin (**A:** ⊞; **B:** △); 1 μM indomethacin (**A:** ■; **B:** ▲), or 1 μM indomethacin plus PGE₂ (**A:** □; **B:** ●). Subsequently, the media were changed every second day. Different amounts of PGE₂ were added to group four every day (10,75,75,25,120,30,180,85,300, and 250 ng/ml on days 1–10, respectively) to mimic the PGE₂ biosynthesis in control cultures. Each point represents the mean value from duplicate (PGE₂) or triplicate (cyclic AMP) determinations on each of six (controls) or four culture dishes.

tion (10 nM) decreased the PGE₂ synthesis by 60 to 80% (Fig. 1A) and cyclic AMP levels by 25 to 60% (Fig. 1B). Both 10 nM and 1 μM indomethacin retarded growth of these cells between days 1 and 3 (Table 1, Fig. 2). No noticeable effect was observed between days 3 and 5. Subsequently, the growth rate was increased in cultures treated with 1 μM indomethacin. Consequently, the cell number per culture dish also increased in these cultures (Fig. 3). No stimulation of cell proliferation was observed in cultures incubated with 10 μM indomethacin (Table 1, Fig. 2). To mimic the PGE₂ production occurring in control cultures, PGE₂ was added daily to cultures grown in the presence of 1 nM indomethacin (Figs. 1 and 2, Table 1). This raised the levels of cyclic AMP and prevented the stimulation of cell growth caused by the inhibitor.

TABLE 1. DNA content per culture dish in py 3T3 cells[a]

Addition	Day 1 DNA (μg/dish)	Day 3 DNA (μg/dish)	Day 3 Increase (%)	Day 3 p[b]	Day 5 DNA (μg/dish)	Day 5 Increase (%)	Day 5 p
None (control)	9.4	27.3 ± 0.65	190		64.4 ± 2.6	136	
Indomethacin (10 nM)		24.1 ± 1.3	156	xx ↓	60.6 ± 3.5	151	ns
(1 μM)		22.9 ± 2.2	144	x ↓	60.5 ± 1.5	164	ns
Indomethacin (1 μM) + PGE$_2$		21.8 ± 2.0	132	xx ↓	51.4 ± 2.6	136	xxx ↓

Addition	Day 7 DNA (μg/dish)	Day 7 Increase (%)	Day 7 p	Day 9 DNA (μg/dish)	Day 9 Increase (%)	Day 9 p	Day 11 DNA (μg/dish)	Day 11 Increase (%)	Day 11 p
None (control)	97.3 ± 3.5	51		128.4 ± 4.2	32		143.6 ± 3.9	12	
Indomethacin (10 nM)	96.0 ± 1.6	58	ns	127.0 ± 4.4	32	ns	146.9 ± 2.0	16	ns
(1 μM)	103.3 ± 1.6	71	xx ↑	148.7 ± 2.6	44	xxx ↑	182.0 ± 6.0	22	xxx ↑
Indomethacin (1 μM) + PGE$_2$	88.2 ± 1.8	72	xx ↓	115.4 ± 3.0	31	xx ↓	132.9 ± 3.0	15	xx ↓

[a] For experimental procedures, see legend to Fig. 1. Each DNA value is the mean of two determinations on six (controls) or four culture dishes. The increase in DNA content per group during 48 hr was used as a measure of growth rate.

[b] Statistical analyses were performed using a modified Student's t-test: x, $0.05 > p > 0.01$; xx, $0.01 > p > 0.001$: xxx, $p < 0.001$ (differences in DNA contents, μg/dish) compared to control cultures. ↓ negative effect, ↑ positive effect.

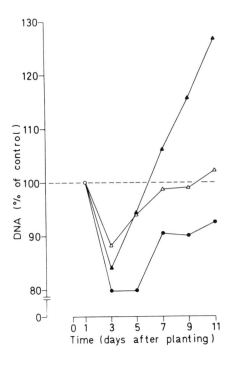

FIG. 2. Growth of indomethacin-treated py 3T3 cultures as measured by percent DNA of control: 10 nM indomethacin (△), 1 μM indomethacin (▲), 1 μM indomethacin plus PGE₂ (●). (For experimental procedure, see legend to Fig. 1.)

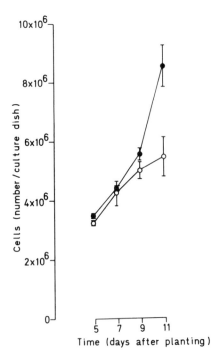

FIG. 3. Cell proliferation in control (○) and indomethacin-treated (1 μm, ●) py 3T3 cultures. Each value represents the mean ± SD of four different dishes (For experimental procedure, see legend to Fig. 1.)

DISCUSSION

The results show that the concentrations of PGE_2 in media and the cellular levels of cyclic AMP increased when the py 3T3 cells became confluent (Fig. 1, Table 1). Inhibition of PG synthesis by indomethacin lowered the levels of cyclic AMP in these cells (Fig. 1). Between days 1 and 3 the growth rate was decreased in indomethacin-treated cultures (Table 1, Fig. 2). Later, as proliferation retarded in untreated cells, growth was stimulated in cultures incubated with 1 μM indomethacin. A similar biphasic effect of PG synthesis inhibitors on proliferation has been reported for human diploid fibroblasts (12). The initial inhibitory effect might be due to inhibition of $PGF_{2\alpha}$ synthesis, since this PG appears to stimulate cell growth of various cells (3). The decrease of cyclic AMP levels and the stimulation of cell growth by indomethacin were completely reversed by addition of PGE_2 at concentrations produced in the absence of inhibitor (Figs. 1 and 2, Table 1). This suggests that the effects of indomethacin were not caused by the inhibitor itself, but indirectly by inhibition of PGE_2 biosynthesis. Incomplete (70–80%) inhibition of PGE_2 biosynthesis by 10 nM indomethacin decreased the cyclic AMP levels by 25 to 60% but did not stimulate growth (Figs. 1 and 2, Table 1). This indicates that the levels of cyclic AMP have to be further lowered before stimulation of growth occurs.

The results presented indicate that endogenously produced PGE_2 decrease cell growth by stimulating cyclic AMP formation. In spite of this, indomethacin and aspirin have been shown to retard growth of mast cell ascites tumor *in vivo* (7). It is possible that PGE_2 *in vivo* has additional effects, e.g., inhibition of lymphocyte cytotoxicity (4).

ACKNOWLEDGMENTS

We thank Margareta Hovgard and Kerstin Johansson for expert technical assistance. This work was supported by grants from the Swedish Cancer Society (1503-B80-01X) and the Swedish Medical Research Council (project 03X-217).

REFERENCES

1. Burton, K. (1956): *Biochem. J.*, 62:315–323.
2. Claesson, H. E., Lindgren, J. Å., and Hammarström, S. (1977): *Eur. J. Biochem.*, 74:13–18.
3. Jimenez de Asua, L. J., Clingan, D., and Rudland, P. S. (1975): *Proc. Natl. Acad. Sci., USA*, 72:2724–2728.
4. Droller, M. J., Lindgren, J. A., Claesson, H.-E., and Perlman, P. (1979): *Cell Immunol.*, 47:261–273.
5. Gilman, A. G. (1970): *Proc. Natl. Acad. Sci. USA*, 67:305–312.
6. Hammarström, S. (1977): *Eur. J. Biochem.*, 74:7–12.
7. Hial, V., Horakova, Z., Shaff, R. E., and Beaven, M. A. (1976): *Eur. J. Pharmacol.*, 37:367–376.
8. Lindgren, J. Å., Kindahl, H., and Hammarström, S. (1974): *FEBS Lett.*, 48:22–25.
9. Otten, J., Johnson, G. S., and Pastan, I. (1972): *J. Biol. Chem.*, 247:7082–7087.
10. Ryan, W. L., and Heidrick, M. L. (1968): *Science*, 162:1484–1485.
11. Sheppard, J. R. (1971): *Proc. Natl. Acad. Sci., USA*, 68:1316–1320.
12. Taylor, L., and Polgar, P. (1977): *FEBS Lett.*, 79:69–72.
13. Thomas, D. R., Philpott, G. W., and Jaffe, B. M. (1974): *Exp. Cell. Res.*, 84:40–46.

Advances in Prostaglandin and Thromboxane Research,
Vol. 6, edited by B. Samuelsson, P. W. Ramwell,
and R. Paoletti. Raven Press, New York © 1980.

Prostacyclin Potently Resorbs Bone *In Vitro*

A. Bennett, D. Edwards, N. N. Ali, D. Auger, and M. Harris

*Department of Surgery, King's College Hospital Medical School, and Department of Oral
Surgery, Eastman Dental Institute, London, England*

Some PGs potently resorb bone *in vitro,* and they may contribute to skeletal destruction in various benign and malignant diseases (2). We now report that prostacyclin causes osteolysis of mouse-isolated calvaria.

MATERIALS AND METHODS

PGI_2 is unstable at physiologic pH, so that sodium PGI_2, PGE_2, or 6-keto-$PGF_{1\alpha}$ for infusion were dissolved in BGJ(b) medium which had been made without sodium bicarbonate and adjusted to pH8.4 with 0.1 M sodium hydroxide. Groups for four calvaria from mice 5 to 6 days old were incubated (5% CO_2 in air, 37°C, 24 hr) in 5ml BGJ(b) medium (3) supplemented by 5% heat-inactivated rabbit serum (Wellcome Reagents, Ltd.), heparin 10 U/ml, sodium penicillin 60 μg/ml, and streptomycin sulfate 125 μg/ml. The incubation medium was then replaced with 5 ml fresh solution alone or containing 200 ng/ml PGE_2 or 6-keto-$PGF_{1\alpha}$, 41° or 41 μg/ml PGI_2, or 69 μg/ml 6-keto-$PGF_{1\alpha}$ to maintain the original PG concentrations. The half-life of PGI_2 was assumed to be about 2 min, but any inactivation of PGE_2 or 6-keto-$PGF_{1\alpha}$ was ignored. 6-Keto-$PGF_{1\alpha}$ 69 μg/ml matched the amount obtained after infusing PGI_2 200 ng/ml for 12 hr. To limit the accumulation of PGI_2 breakdown products, the media were replaced every 12 hr.

Calcium was measured by an autoanalyzer, and the amounts released by control bones were deducted from test values for each 12-hr period.

RESULTS

PGI_2 or PGE_2 at the nominal concentration of about 200 ng/ml caused substantial bone resorption, whereas 6-keto-$PGF_{1\alpha}$ exerted only a weak effect. In contrast, 69 μg/ml stimulated calcium uptake by the calvaria (Table 1). The pH of the medium removed at each 12-hr period was 7.2–7.4.

DISCUSSION

The exact potency of PGI_2 is difficult to determine because its half-life is not known precisely, and because the infused material degrades to 6-keto-$PGF_{1\alpha}$

TABLE 1. *Stimulation of bone resorption by low concentrations of prostanoids*

Prostanoid	Concentration ng/ml approx	Cumulative change in media calcium (mg/100 ml)			
		12 hr	24 hr	36 hr	48 hr
PGE$_2$	200	0.29 ± 0.134	0.97 ± 0.222	1.71 ± 0.410	2.89 ± 0.542
PGI$_2$	200	0.25 ± 0.067	0.63 ± 0.117	1.18 ± 0.126	2.12 ± 0.145
PGI$_2$	20	0.14 ± 0.083	0.47 ± 0.136	0.84 ± 0.195	1.31 ± 0.268
6-keto-PGF$_{1\alpha}$	200	0.238 ± 0.142	0.563 ± 0.178	0.60 ± 0.094	0.875 ± 0.161
6-keto-PGF$_{1\alpha}$	69,000	−0.17 ± 0.237	−0.08 ± 0.423	−0.64 ± 0.393	−1.12 ± 0.532

PGE$_2$, PGI$_2$, and 200 ng/ml 6-keto-PGF$_{1\alpha}$ stimulated bone resorption. The high concentration of 6-keto-PGF$_{1\alpha}$ 69 µg/ml increased uptake of calcium by the calvaria. $n = 5$ for each experiment except that $n = 4$ for 6-keto-PGF$_{1\alpha}$ 200 ng/ml.
1 vs 2, $p > 0.2$; 2 vs 4, $p < 0.001$; 2 vs 3, $p < 0.05$; 3 vs 4, $p > 0.2$; 4 vs 5, $p < 0.01$; Students' *t*-test for unpaired data.

which weakly stimulates bone resorption in low concentrations but causes inhibition in very high concentrations. Fuller details of the problem of calculating potency are given by Ali et al. (1), who calculate that if the half-life of PGI$_2$ is 2 min, the average concentration must be about 290 ng/ml; if the half-life is 3 min, the concentration must be about 430 ng/ml. Thus, the concentration of PGI$_2$ was probably greater than that of PGE$_2$, particularly since some degradation of PGE$_2$ occurs during incubation, and PGE$_2$ is probably somewhat more potent than PGI$_2$ in resorbing bone.

The role of PGI$_2$ in bone resorption is not known, but its breakdown product 6-keto-PGF$_{1\alpha}$ occurs in extracts of synovial fluid from patients with rheumatoid arthritis (3). Because PGI$_2$ survives passage through the pulmonary circulation (4), excessive release might contribute to bone resorption.

ACKNOWLEDGMENTS

We thank the Arthritis and Rheumatism Council, the Cancer Research Campaign, the Medical Research Council, and The Wellcome Foundation for support, and Upjohn Limited and The Wellcome Foundation for prostanoids.

REFERENCES

1. Ali, N. N., Auger, D. W., Bennett, A., Edwards, D. A., and Harris, M. (1979): In: *Prostacyclin,* edited by J. R. Vane and S. Bergstrom, pp. 179–185. Raven Press, New York.
2. Bennett, A. (1979): In: *Practical Applications of Prostaglandins and their Synthesis Inhibitors,* edited by S. M. M. Karim, pp. 149–188. MTP Press, Lancaster, England.
3. Biggers, J. D., Gwatkin, R. B. L., and Heyner, S. (1961): *Exp. Cell. Res.,* 25:41–58.
4. Moncada, S., Korbut, R., Bunting, S., and Vane, J. R. (1978): *Nature (London),* 273:767–768.

Advances in Prostaglandin and Thromboxane Research,
Vol. 6, edited by B. Samuelsson, P. W. Ramwell,
and R. Paoletti. Raven Press, New York © 1980.

Essential Fatty Acid Requirements and Metabolism of Cells in Tissue Culture

J. Martyn Bailey

*Department of Biochemistry, George Washington University, School of Medicine,
Washington, D.C. 20037*

The purpose of this chapter is twofold. In the first part, the requirements for essential fatty acids (EFAs) at the level of the individual cell are examined. Two experimental models have been used to study this problem. In one model, the behavior of transplanted tumors, growing as essentially pure cell cultures in the peritoneal cavity of EFA-deficient mice has been studied. In the other experimental approach, the growth of individual cell types maintained in EFA-deficient media in tissue culture was examined.

In the second part of this chapter, the conversion of arachidonic acid to compounds of the prostaglandin (PG) family by defined cell types growing in continuous cell culture is described. In these investigations, it will be demonstrated that in addition to cells which synthesize PGs, a specific cell line has been identified whose primary metabolic product is thromboxane A_2 (TXA_2) and another the principal product of which is prostacyclin (PGI_2). Some of the experimental procedures which can be used to induce or regulate TX and PGI_2 synthesis in these cell types will be described.

It is well established that EFAs are required in the diet for normal growth and development of mammals (5). Groups of CF1 mice were weaned onto a lipid-free diet. After 26 weeks, EFA levels in blood lipids had fallen to less than 1% of the total, and the mice displayed the classical symptoms of EFA deficiency (2). This type of mouse was used to measure the effects of EFA deficiency on the growth of experimental tumors transplanted into the peritoneal cavity and growing in the ascitic form as single-cell suspensions. Two types of tumors were used: Ehrlich ascites carcinoma as an example of a cell of epithelial origin, and sarcoma 180 as a cell of fibroblastic origin. Numbers of mice were inoculated intraperitoneally with identical aliquots (1–4 million tumor cells), and groups of mice were sacrificed at daily intervals. The tumor cells growing in the peritoneal cavity were aspirated quantitatively and counted using hemacytometer chambers or a Coulter electronic counter. Samples of each cell population were also extracted and the EFA composition of the tumor cell lipids was analyzed by gas liquid chromatography.

As shown in Fig. 1 for sarcoma 180, EFA composition, represented by the

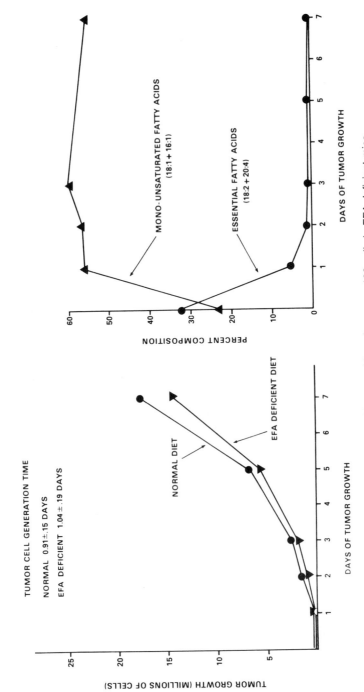

FIG. 1. Growth and fatty acid composition of sarcoma 180 cells in EFA-deficient mice.

sum of linoleic (18:2) and arachidonic acids (20:4), dropped rapidly from a total of 32% of the cell lipids in the tumor inoculum to less than 1% at the end of the 7-day period of tumor growth.

The EFAs were replaced largely by the monounsaturated acids palmitoleic (16:1) and oleic (18:1), which increased from 23% to about 60% of the total. Despite this almost complete absence of EFAs, there was no striking change in the growth rate of the sarcoma, the cell doubling time being increased from only 0.91 ± 0.15 days in the normal to 1.04 ± 0.19 days in the deficient animal, a difference which is not statistically significant. In similar studies with Ehrlich mouse carcinoma depicted in Fig. 2, although some initial decrease in the growth rate of the tumor was observed, as shown in the right-hand panel, the EFA-deficient tumor cells, following harvesting, transplanted and grew equally well in both normal and EFA-deficient mice.

Although the results of these experiments provided reasonably conclusive evidence that EFA were not required at the level of the individual growing tumor cells, there was still the possibility that the mice were supplying the tumor with EFA derivatives from some endogenous host source. The tumor cells were therefor adapted to growth in tissue culture in Eagles minimal medium supplemented with either 10% fetal calf serum for control cells or in an EFA-free medium supplemented with delipidized serum protein.

The fatty acid profile of both cell types as determined by gas liquid chromatography of the fatty acid methyl esters is illustrated in Fig. 3, in which the EFAs are shown as cross-hatched bars. Despite the almost complete absence of EFAs in cells grown in lipid-free medium, the cell doubling time of 18.0 ± 1.3 hr was not significantly different from that of normal cells (17.9 ± 1.4 hr).

Experiments similar to these have since been carried out with over 20 cell lines of various types, all of which have been successfully adapted to growth in synthetic or semisynthetic lipid-free media (3,8). All of these cell lines appear to grow normally and, where tested, have normal metabolic and morphological characteristics, including membrane and organelle morphology and mitochondrial respiration and function (3).

The conclusion from results such as these seems to be that isolated cell cultures do not need EFAs (and hence presumably PGs) for normal growth and metabolism. This is not to imply that endogenously produced PGs may not be found to regulate some cellular functions. However, it does suggest that any such endogenous functions are not essential to the cellular replication process.

There is no doubt, however, that EFAs, and by implication the PGs, are required for normal function in the intact mammalian organism. These findings taken together provide considerable support for the concept that the PG family of compounds are primarily involved in intercellular communication and integration of function at the multicellular level.

The second main topic to be described is the further metabolism of the EFAs by selected cell types in tissue culture. The studies described here have been carried out principally using two different cell types, the WI38 strain of normal

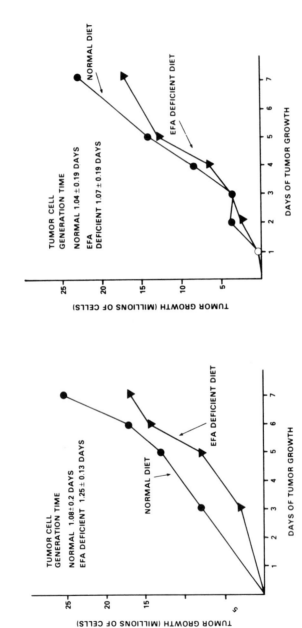

FIG. 2. Growth and transplantation characteristics of Ehrlich mouse carcinoma cells in EFA-deficient mice.

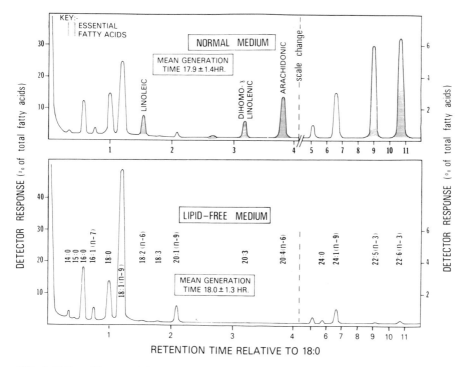

FIG. 3. Fatty acid composition and growth rate of normal and EFA-deficient Ehrlich ascites carcinoma cells in tissue culture.

diploid human lung fibroblasts and the RB strain of rat aorta smooth muscle cells.

Monolayers of cultured WI38 fibroblasts were superfused briefly for 2 to 5 min with Eagles medium containing ^{14}C-labeled arachidonic acid, and the products were extracted into acidified ether and chromatographed using previously described procedures (5). A typical chromatographic profile is shown in Fig. 4. The upper panel shows the radiochromatogram scanner profile of the thin-layer plate and the lower panel the radioautograph made by exposing the plate to X-ray film for 2 days. The center panel contains known PG standards. As indicated here, PGE$_2$ was identified as one of the products, but two other compounds, labelled X and Y, were made which could not be identified as any of the known PGs. We were aware, however, that Vargaftig (6) had reported that guinea pig lung perfused with arachidonic acid produced rabbit aorta contracting substance (RCS) and that this had subsequently been identified by Hamberg et al. as a TX (6).

Superfusates of the cultured lung fibroblasts were therefore examined in the rabbit aorta test system. Monolayers of the WI38 cells produced a potent contractile substance for rabbit aorta which had a half-life similar to that of TXA$_2$. It is significant that similar cultures of human diploid skin fibroblasts treated

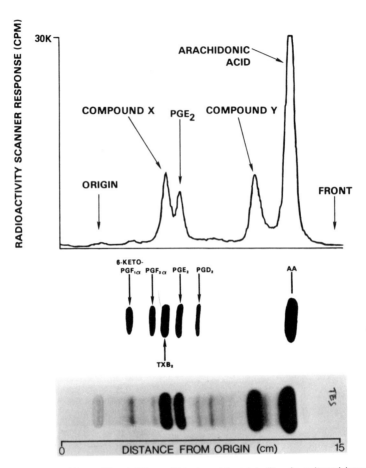

FIG. 4. Chromatographic profile of ^{14}C-arachidonic acid metabolites in cultured human lung fibroblasts.

with arachidonic acid in the same manner did not produce RCS activity, and subsequent examination of the supernatant fluid from skin fibroblasts showed it to contain PGE$_2$ as the major metabolite (4).

TXB$_2$ was prepared from platelets by the procedure of Hamberg et al. (6). for use as a reference standard. The mass spectrum of the trimethylsilyl methyl ester derivative of the platelet-derived material is shown in Fig. 5, together with the indicated fragmentation pattern of the molecule which leads to the formation of the major characteristic ions at m/e values of 510, 439, 366, and 256.

In Fig. 6 the simultaneous ion-monitoring chromatographic trace of the cell-derived material monitored at these four characteristic ion masses is illustrated; and it confirms the identity of the cell material as TXB$_2$. In a similar manner,

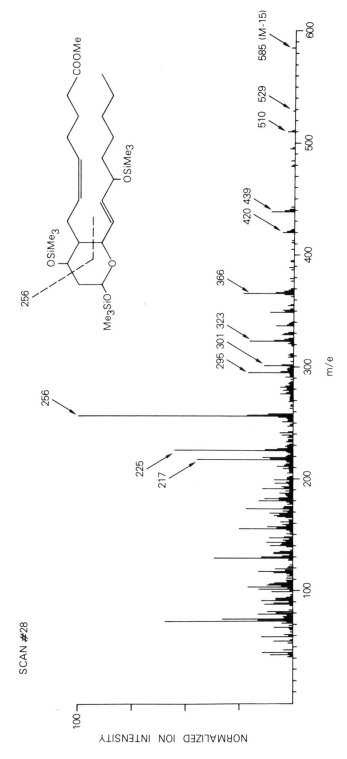

FIG. 5. Mass spectrum of Tris-trimethyl silyl methyl ester derivative of TXB₂ from human platelets.

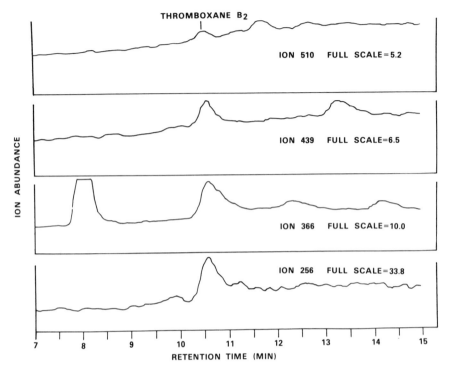

FIG. 6. Simultaneous ion-monitoring gas chromatographic-mass spectroscopy of TXB$_2$ from cultered lung fibroblasts.

the second major radioactive product of arachidonate metabolism in the cultured lung cells was identified by its mass spectrum as hydroxyheptatrienoic acid (4).

The further study of factors affecting TX production in cultured lung cells is providing some interesting insights into the control and maturation of the cyclooxygenase pathway in these cells. TX synthesis appears to be biphasic, with a rapid initial pulse lasting about 2 min followed by a slow continual release during the subsequent 24 to 48 hr or until the arachidonate substrate is exhausted. If the cultures are allowed to mature in the quiescent contact-inhibited state without refeeding them, an increase in the ability to make TXB$_2$ relative to PGE$_2$ occurs (Fig. 7). Of particular interest is the finding depicted in the lower panels of Fig. 7 that VA13A cells, the SV40 virus-transformed counterpart of WI38, do not develop the rapid response to arachidonate, although they do display a slow synthesis of TX when measured over 24- to 48-hr periods. The significance of these findings to the phenomenon of growth regulation by contact inhibition and to the possible maturation and differentiation of cells in culture is being further investigated.

The second cell type we have studied extensively is the RB rat aorta smooth

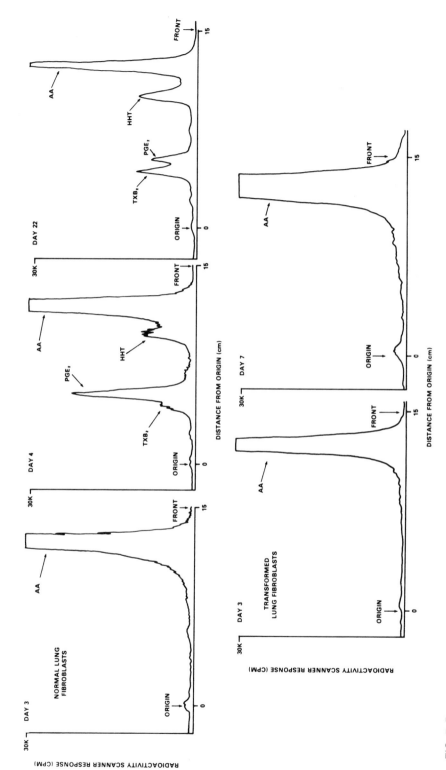

FIG. 7. Pattern of TXB$_2$ formation in growing and quiescent WI38 human diploid lung fibroblasts and their SV40 virus-transformed VA13A counterparts.

muscle cell isolated by Dr. Ann Brown of the National Institutes of Health. When challenged with arachidonic acid, this cell line produces the profile of products as illustrated in Fig. 1, Salata et al. *(this volume, this section).* The major products, as indicated in the radiochromatogram scan and on the radioautograph of the thin-layer plate below, chromatograms as 6-keto-PGF$_{1\alpha}$, the stable breakdown product of PGI$_2$.

As indicated in Fig. 8, superfusates of these cells treated briefly with arachidonic acid were potent inhibitors of platelet aggregation whose activity decayed with a half-time of 9 min, which is characteristic of PGI$_2$ under these experimental conditions. Further confirmation of the identity was obtained by converting the material to the tetratrimethyl silyl hydroxime methyl ester derivative and examination by gas chromatography–mass spectrometry. As indicated in Fig. 9, the mass spectrum of the cell-derived material was essentially identical to that of authetic 6-keto-PGF$_{1\alpha}$.

The smooth muscle cells have proved to be an interesting model for studying inactivation of the cyclooxygenase system by drugs such as aspirin and the manner in which it recovers when the drug is removed. Aspirin irreversibly inhibits the enzyme by acetylating groups in the active site. In contract to platelets, however, cultured cells possess intact protein-synthesizing machinery and hence have the potential to replace the inactivated enzyme.

In cells preincubated with 5 mg % aspirin for 30 min and then washed, the PGI$_2$-synthesizing ability was completely destroyed. When fresh growth medium was added and the cells were retested after 4 hr, the PGI$_2$ synthetase had more than completely recovered and was about 2.5 times higher than control cultures. When tested after a further 24 hr, however, the enzyme level had fallen back to about 25% of control values.

The time course of this phenomenon was followed in more detail, and furthermore, an inhibitor of protein synthesis, cycloheximide, was added to some cultures to determine the nature of the recovered enzyme activity. Recovery of enzyme was extremely rapid, control levels being attained within 1 hr. Closer examination of these early intervals has shown that some PGI$_2$ synthesis can be detected as early as 20 min after removal of aspirin, the half-life for replacement of the enzyme being about 40 min. This recovery in enzyme activity involved the synthesis of new protein, since it was completely blocked by cycloheximide. A subsequent overshoot in enzyme activity is followed by a prolonged decrease below base-line levels, full enzyme activity in the cultures not being attained until about 72 hr after the aspirin treatment. The nature of the complex control mechanisms which must underlie these fluctuations in enzyme activity is being further investigated.

One of the most interesting developments concerning these cultured vascular smooth muscle cells has been the finding that PGI$_2$ release is stimulated by thrombin. When the cell phospholipids are prelabeled by growth in ^{14}C-arachidonate for 24 hr, the cells do not respond to the normal manipulations of a change of medium, washing, etc. (Fig. 10, panels 2 and 3), but as shown in

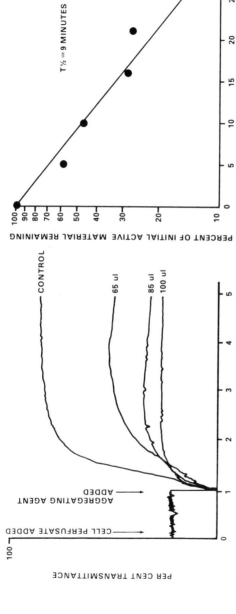

FIG. 8. Inhibition of platelet aggregation by perfusates of cultured vascular smooth muscle cells.

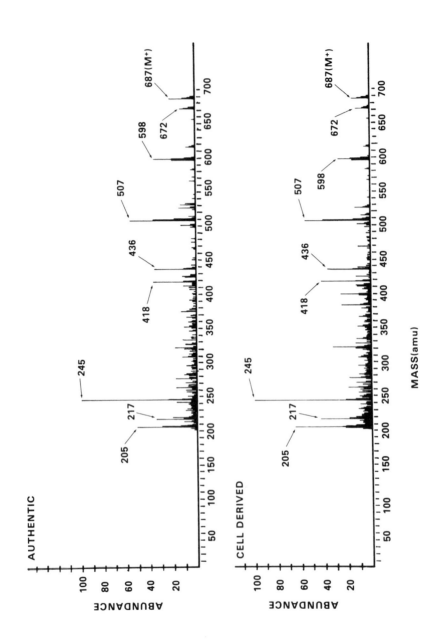

FIG. 9. Mass spectrum of 6-keto-PGF$_{1\alpha}$ from cultured vascular smooth muscle cells.

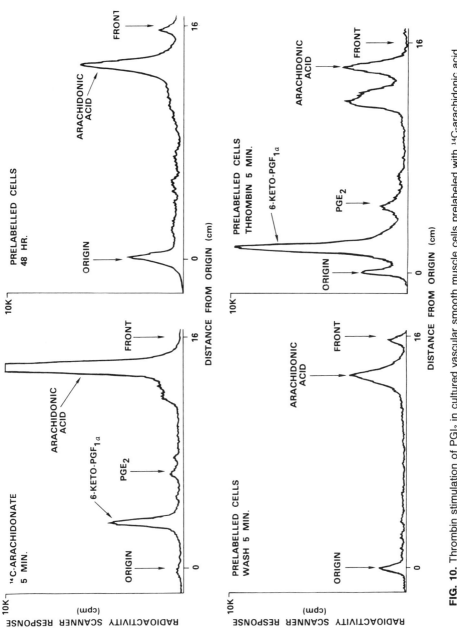

FIG. 10. Thrombin stimulation of PGI$_2$ in cultured vascular smooth muscle cells prelabeled with ^{14}C-arachidonic acid.

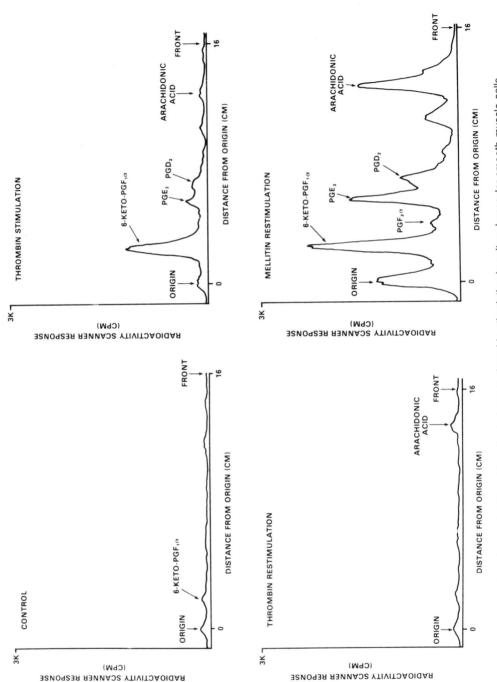

FIG. 11. Development of thrombin refractoriness to thrombin stimulation in cultured vascular smooth muscle cells.

the 4th panel, addition of a small amount of thrombin (0.5 U) to the medium elicits an immediate and large pulse of PGI_2 release. This thrombin sensitivity has a number of interesting features, including the fact that it displays the phenomenon of refractoriness, characteristic of many hormonally stimulated reactions. For example, as illustrated in Fig. 11, following a preliminary challenge with thrombin during which a large pulse of PGI_2 was released, a similar challenge 15 min later fails to elicit a second response. That this is not due to depletion of the cellular arachidonic acid substrate nor to the insufficiency or inactivation of the cellular PGI_2 synthetase enzyme system is demonstrated by the results shown in the last panel. A further large pulse of PGI_2 release was elicited from the thrombin-refractory cells by the nonspecific bee venom peptide mellitin.

As is well known, thrombin also plays a key role in the initiation of platelet aggregation during tissue injury and thrombus formation. The rapid production of the potent antiplatelet substance PGI_2 by vascular smooth muscle cells in response to thrombin suggests that this system may operate *in vivo* as a protective mechanism in blood vessel walls.

As depicted schematically in Fig. 12, thrombin activation in response to localized vascular damage or release of tissue factor would normally serve as a focus for platelet aggregation and thrombus formation. The ability of vascular smooth muscle to respond to thrombin release by producing PGIs would thus serve as a self-limiting protective mechanism against vascular thrombosis. This mechanism may thus complement that suggested by Moncada et al. (7) in explaining the well-known resistance of blood vessel walls to formation of platelet aggregates.

Finally, Fig. 13 summarizes the pathways of arachidonate metabolism which have now been identified in cultured cells. Most tissue cells appear to have the cyclooxygenase enzyme system, and this system is thus well conserved during passage in tissue culture (with the possible exception of some transformed cells). In some cells, the classical PGs are the major products of metabolism. In others, as we have seen, TXs or PGIs may be the major products of EFA metabolism.

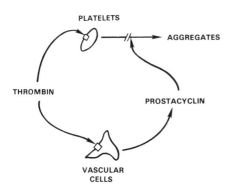

FIG. 12. Self-regulation of thrombin-induced platelet aggregation by thrombin-stimulated PGI_2 release in vascular cells.

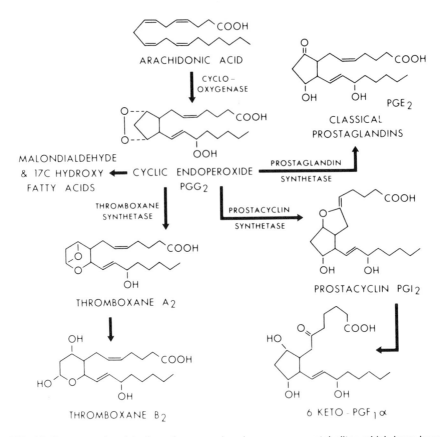

FIG. 13. Summary of metabolic pathways and cyclooxygenase metabolites which have been demonstrated in various cell types in tissue culture following incubation with ^{14}C-arachidonic acid.

The earlier experiments reported here seem to indicate that isolated cells in culture do not require EFAs for normal growth and metabolism. The later experiments, however, indicated that cultured cells retain active systems for synthesizing PGs from the EFAs and respond to specific stimuli which in all probability have considerable functional significance. It is to be expected that further progress in this area will be directed towards identifying the nature and functions of these specific stimuli. Only then will we be in a position to define fully the complex roles that EFA metabolites play in the overall process of intercellular communication and regulation in mammalian systems.

REFERENCES

1. Bailey, J. M., Bryant, R. W., Feinmark, S. J., and Makheja, A. N. (1977): *Prostaglandins,* 13:479–492.

2. Bailey, J. M., and Dunbar, L. M. (1971): *Cancer Res.*, 31:91–97.
3. Bailey, J. M., and Dunbar, L. M. (1973): *Exp. Mol. Pathol.*, 18:142–161.
4. Bryant, R. W., Feinmark, S. J., Makheja, A. N., and Bailey, J. M. (1978): *J. Biol. Chem.*, 253:8134–8142.
5. Burr, G. O., and Burr, M. M. (1959): *J. Biol. Chem.*, 82:325–355.
6. Hamberg, M., Svensson, J., and Samuelsson, B. (1975): *Proc. Natl. Acad. Sci. USA*, 72:2994–2998.
7. Moncada, S., Gryglewski, R., Bunting, S., and Vane, J. R. (1976): *Nature*, 263:663–665.
8. Takaoka, T., and Katsuta, H. (1971): *Exp. Cell. Res.*, 67:295–300.
9. Vargaftig, B. B., and Rao, N. (1971): *Pharmacology*, 6:99–108.

Advances in Prostaglandin and Thromboxane Research,
Vol. 6, edited by B. Samuelsson, P. W. Ramwell,
and R. Paoletti. Raven Press, New York © 1980.

Improved Anticancer Effect by Combining Cytotoxic Drugs with an Inhibitor of Prostaglandin Synthesis

D. A. Berstock, J. Houghton, and A. Bennett

Department of Surgery, King's College Hospital Medical School,
London SE5 8RX, United Kingdom

Tumors can usually form more prostaglandins than the normal tissues from which they arise (1,9), and this production may be related to tumor spread (1) and bone destruction (1,3,8). Nonsteroidal anti-inflammatory drugs which inhibit prostaglandin synthesis have beneficial effects on mice with malignant tumors. These drugs reduce tumor growth (2,6,8,10), and the prostaglandin synthesis inhibitor flurbiprofen in combination with chemotherapy and/or radiotherapy greatly reduces tumor growth compared to the response without flurbiprofen (2).

We now report that flurbiprofen given with chemotherapy in mice following removal of the primary tumor prolonged survival and lessened the incidence of local recurrence. Preliminary experiments indicate that flurbiprofen does not act by displacing methotrexate from plasma binding sites, nor does it increase the toxicity of the chemotherapeutic drugs.

MATERIALS AND METHODS

Ninety-seven female WHT/Ht mice were inoculated subcutaneously into the left flank with approximately 10^6 cells of NC adenocarcinoma. This tumor, which originally arose spontaneously in a mouse mammary gland, appears to be of low immunogenicity (4), is easily transplanted, and metastasizes to lungs, mediastinum, and viscera.

The primary tumors were excised with a wide rim of healthy surrounding tissue 14, 21, or 24 days after inoculation, and the mice were randomized into four treatment groups. As previously described (2), drugs were given orally in 0.1 ml of raspberry syrup, which the mice take readily. The four treatment groups were as follows: control (raspberry syrup alone); chemotherapy (melphalan, 1.4 mg/kg, and methotrexate, 2 mg/kg, daily on days 1–3, 8–10, and 15–17 after tumor excision); flurbiprofen (2.5 mg/kg twice daily); and chemotherapy together with flurbiprofen.

Treatment with flurbiprofen or syrup alone was continued until the animals died or were killed either on humane grounds (2) or on day 178, when the experiment was terminated. The incidence of recurrent disease was assessed at post-mortem examination.

In other experiments, healthy female WHT/Ht mice were given methotrexate, melphalan, and flurbiprofen (2.0, 1.4, and 5 mg/kg, respectively) for 3 days. Blood was removed 3 hr after the last dose and the serum was examined by radioimmunoassay (Dr. W. Aherne) for free and total methotrexate.

Experiments to determine the effect of flurbiprofen, 2.5 mg/kg twice daily, on chemotherapeutic toxicity were carried out on healthy male WHT/Ht mice given large daily doses of methotrexate and melphalan.

RESULTS

Early tumor excision tended to increase survival, but this was not statistically significant. Survival time was similar in controls and mice treated with either chemotherapy or flurbiprofen; but with chemotherapy and flurbiprofen no mouse died until day 40 after tumor excision, whereas about 40% had already died in the other treatment groups. Median survival time in this group was increased by approximately 50% ($p < 0.001$, log rank test; Table 1).

All mice that survived until the end of the experiment (1 control, 3 chemotherapy, 4 flurbiprofen, 4 chemotherapy + flurbiprofen group) appeared to be disease-free at postmortem examination.

Recurrence at the tumor excision site was less in the combined treatment ($p < 0.01$, Fisher's exact probability test), but the incidence of distant recurrence seemed similar (Table 1).

The serum levels of free methotrexate were similar in flurbiprofen-treated and control mice (66 and 64% of recovered methotrexate, respectively).

Melphalan and methotrexate, 5.6 and 8 mg/kg, respectively, caused 50% mortality after 2 weeks of treatment compared with 31% when flurbiprofen was also given. With double the doses of chemotherapeutic drugs, the median survival times were respectively 10 and 6 days in the control and flurbiprofen-

TABLE 1.

Treatment group	n	Survival in days[a]		Mice with local recurrence
Syrup controls	22	42	(31–52)	17
Chemotherapy	25	46	(29–67)	17
Flurbiprofen	26	44	(36–70)	17
Flurbiprofen + chemotherapy	24	66.5	(48–123)[b]	6[c]

[a] Medians and semiquartiles.
[b] $p < 0.01$.
[c] $p < 0.001$.

treated groups, but this difference was not statistically significant. Further ᴅ bling of the chemotherapy dose resulted in a median survival of 6 days ι both groups.

The prolongation of survival time using chemotherapy combined with flurbi-profen is interesting, particularly because flurbiprofen does not increase the toxicity of the chemotherapeutic drugs. The combined therapy also protected the mice against local recurrence. Absence of an effect on distant metastases may have been due at least partly to the longer survival, which allowed more time for the metastases to grow.

Although the NC tumor is of low immunogenicity, depression of the immune system by prostaglandins may be a contributory factor (6). Perhaps prostaglan-dins released by the action of cytotoxic agents (5) add to the immunodepression. Flurbiprofen does not seem to increase the plasma levels of methotrexate by displacing it from protein binding sites, as occurs with aspirin (11), but we do not know the effect on melphalan. However, toxicity of melphalan and methotrex-ate is not altered in normal mice by flurbiprofen. Furthermore, the reduction of tumor growth was greater when flurbiprofen was given with radiotherapy (2), which presumably demonstrates an effect of flurbiprofen which does not involve protein binding. Prostaglandins can protect gastrointestinal epithelial cells from damage (7), and this protective effect might occur with other cells.

ACKNOWLEDGMENTS

We thank the Cancer Research Campaign and the Medical Research Council for support, and The Boots Company Limited, Nottingham, England, for supply-ing the flurbiprofen.

REFERENCES

1. Bennett, A., Charlier, E. M., McDonald, A. M., Simpson, J. S., Stamford, I. F., and Zebro, T. (1977): *Lancet*, 2:624–626.
2. Bennett, A., Houghton, J., Leaper, D. J., and Stamford, I. F. (1979): *Prostaglandins*, 17:179–191.
3. Galasko, C. S. B., and Bennett, A. (1976): *Nature*, 263:508–510.
4. Hewitt, H. B., Blake, E. R., and Walder, A. S. (1976): *Br. J. Cancer*, 33:241–259.
5. Ohuchi, K., and Levine, L. (1978): *Prostaglandins*, 15:723.
6. Plescia, O. J., Smith, A. M., and Grinwich, K. (1975): *Proc. Natl. Acad. Sci. USA*, 72:1848–1851.
7. Robert, A. (1977): In: *Prostaglandins and Thromboxanes*, edited by F. Berti, B. Samuelsson, and G. P. Velo, pp. 287–313. Plenum Press, New York.
8. Strausser, H., and Humes, J. (1975): *Int. J. Cancer*, 15:724–730.
9. Sykes, J. A. C., and Maddox, I. S. (1972): *Nature [New Biol.]*, 237:59–61.
10. Tashjian, A. H., Voelkel, E. F., Goldhaber, P., and Levine, L. (1973): *Prostaglandins*, 3:515–524.
11. Taylor, J. R., and Halprin, K. M. (1977): *Arch. Dermatol.*, 113:588–591.

ou-
in

Advances in Prostaglandin and Thromboxane Research,
Vol. 6, edited by B. Samuelsson, P. W. Ramwell,
and R. Paoletti. Raven Press, New York © 1980.

Human Breast Carcinomas Release Prostaglandin-Like Material Into the Blood

I. F. Stamford, J. MacIntyre, and A. Bennett

Department of Surgery, King's College Hospital Medical School, London SE5 8RX England

Reports on the release of prostaglandin-like material (PG-lm) into the blood from human or animal malignant tumors reach conflicting conclusions, even with endocrine tumors that secrete hormones into the circulation (see ref. 1). Part of the problem has been the sampling of peripheral venous blood, since many PGs are rapidly metabolized in pulmonary and other vascular beds. With regard to human nonendocrine tumors, Mortel et al. (3) overcame the problem of inactivation by measuring PGE in blood from the internal iliac vein of patients with gynecological tumors. They claimed that there was no significant PG release from the tumors, but recalculation of their data indicates that at least some tumors release PG-lm into the blood. Powles et al. (4) found raised levels of 13,14-dihydro-15-keto PGE$_2$ in peripheral venous blood of patients with breast cancer, but this does not identify the source of PG. Other data below show elevated amounts of PG-lm in the blood draining some breast carcinomas but the amounts did not correlate with the ability of the excised tumors to synthesize PG-lm during homogenization.

METHODS

In 12 patients (aged 38 to 77 years) undergoing surgery for breast cancer (11 primary, 1 secondary), a needle was inserted into a vein directly draining the tumor or, in two cases, into the axillary vein. Ten-ml blood samples were withdrawn and transferred immediately to a lithium-heparin tube containing 100 μg indomethacin. A similar collection was made from the antecubital vein in the contralateral arm. Blood was centrifuged within a few minutes of sampling, plasma extracted (5), and PG-lm assayed against authentic PGE$_2$ on the rat stomach strip preparation (2). Samples of tumor were homogenized in acid ethanol to indicate "basal" amounts of PG-lm or in Krebs solution which allows PG synthesis from endogenous precursors released during homogenization (2). The amounts extracted from the homogenates in Krebs solution are referred to as 'total PG-lm' (i.e., "basal" + "synthesized").

RESULTS

In many cases, the amount of PG-lm extracted from blood draining the tumor was greater than from venous blood from the contralateral arm (Table 1; $P = 0.024$, Wilcoxon matched pairs test). However, the amounts did not correlate with measurements of tumor PG-lm.

DISCUSSION

Our results indicate that some malignant breast tumors either release PG-lm into the venous blood or stimulate blood elements to release PG-lm. The amounts extracted from venous blood from the contralateral antecubital vein were often less, probably because much of the released PG-lm was inactivated in the pulmonary circulation and elsewhere, and the residual amounts were diluted with blood not draining the tumor.

The mobilization of the carcinoma prior to blood sampling may have contributed to PG release, but the local venepuncture itself was probably no more damaging than antecubital venepuncture. The finding by Powles et al. (4) of raised plasma PGE_2 metabolite levels in breast cancer patients are consistent with a release of PGE_2 from the primary tumor, but it does not exclude release from secondary tumors or other sites. Taken together with our present findings, and the ability of breast tumors to synthesize PG-lm (1), it seems likely that at least some breast carcinomas release PGs into the bloodstream.

Mortel et al. (3) reported that the amounts of PGE sampled from the iliac veins of patients with benign or malignant gynecological tumors were not significantly different. The respective values (PGE pg/ml) were benign 56,31,55,42, and 51; malignant 83,50,75,70,64,48,92,56,360,82, and 70. Since the data do not seem to be normally distributed they should either be normalized or analyzed

TABLE 1. *PG-lm in extracts of blood and breast carcinomas*

Plasma PG-lm (pg/ml)		Tumor PG-lm (ng/g)		
Draining tumor	Peripheral	Total	Basal	Synthesized
320	430	98		
<10	<10	4	3	1
480	100	41	12	29
<10	<10	92	15	77
<10	<10	13	6	7
2,600	<10	10	0	10
13	<10	4	3	1
590	530	5	2	3
12	<10	16	11	5
4,500	200	13	5	8
110	<10	24	8	16
1,000	590	34	7	27

by a nonparametric statistical test for unpaired results. The Mann-Whitney U-test indicates that the levels of PG were higher in the blood from patients with malignant disease (P = 0.0174), so that these nonendocrine tumors also seem capable of releasing PG-lm into the bloodstream or stimulating its release from blood.

REFERENCES

1. Bennett, A. (1979): In: *Practical Applications of Prostaglandins and their Synthesis Inhibitors,* edited by S. M. M. Karim. MTP Press Ltd., Lancaster, pp. 149–188.
2. Bennett, A., Stamford, I. F., and Unger, W. G. (1973): *J. Physiol. (Lond.),* 229:349–360.
3. Mortel, R., Allegra, J. C., Demers, L. M., Harvey, H. A., Trautlein, J., Nahhas, W., White, D., Gillin, M. A., and Lipton, A. (1977): *Cancer,* 39:2201–2203.
4. Powles, T. J., Coombes, R. C., Neville, A. M., Ford, H. T., Gazet, J. C., and Levine, L. (1977): *Lancet,* 2:138.
5. Unger, W. G., Stamford, I. F., and Bennett, A. (1971): *Nature (Lond.),* 233:336–337.

ACKNOWLEDGMENT

We thank the Cancer Research Campaign and Medical Research Council (London) for support.

Advances in Prostaglandin and Thromboxane Research,
Vol. 6, edited by B. Samuelsson, P. W. Ramwell,
and R. Paoletti. Raven Press, New York © 1980.

Prostaglandin Production and Metabolism in Human Breast Cancer

Pierre H. Rolland, Pierre M. Martin, Jocelyne Jacquemier,
Anne M. Rolland, and M. Toga

Laboratoire des Récepteurs et des Stéroides Hormonaux, Institut Paoli-Calmettes,
F 13273 Marseille Cedex 2, France

It has been reported that human tumors may contain or secrete excessive amounts of prostaglandin (PG) materials. In particular, synthesis of PGs has been found to occur primarily in human breast cancers revealing hypercalcemia and bone metastasis; both PGE_2 and $PGF_{2\alpha}$ were found to be produced in large quantities in homogenates and in whole tissue of mammary carcinomas (1,3). Having examined the metabolism of PG in tumors in order to determine a screening test of PG production, we present a report on PG production in a representative sample of human breast carcinomas.

PG METABOLISM IN HUMAN BREAST TUMOR

To determine the assay's conditions of a PG production screening test in human breast tumor specimens, PGE_2 and $PGF_{2\alpha}$ productions were investigated in microsomal preparations, since both PGs were found to be produced in homogenates and whole tissue. From results presented in Fig. 1, it is apparent that PGE_2 is the main product and that a biphasic production is observed to occur for PGE_2. In contrast, $PGF_{2\alpha}$ occurs during a 1- to 2-min period of incubation which corresponds to the first phase of PG biosynthesis. Indomethacin at 10^{-6}M final concentration is able to suppress PG production (data not shown). To examine the source of endogenous $PGF_{2\alpha}$ production and the PGE_2 metabolism, *in vitro* experiments were carried out with the cytosol fraction from human breast tumors. Products from the incubation of ^{3}H-labeled PGE_2 with cytosol are shown in Fig. 2. Two radioactive peaks were observed on thin-layer chromatography (TLC). One corresponded to the original PGE_2 and the other had an R_f value corresponding to that of $PGF_{2\alpha}$. The identities of both compounds were confirmed by radioimmunoassay. These findings support the idea that the cytosol has an enzymatic activity capable of converting PGE_2 into $PGF_{2\alpha}$, i.e., a PG-9-keto-reductase activity. In addition, these identities were confirmed by TLC of ^{3}H-arachidonate products of incubation with microsomes in which

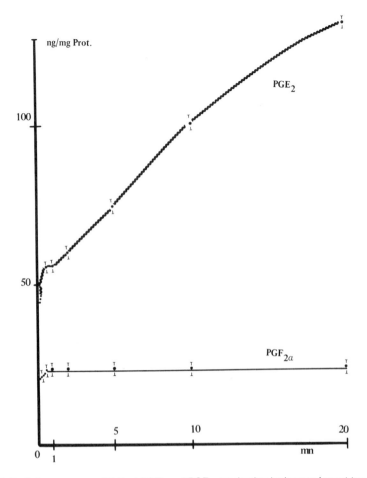

FIG. 1. Radioimmunoassay (RIA) of PGE_2 and $PGF_{2\alpha}$ production by human breast tumor micro-some preparations. Microsomal fractions (0.1 ml, 50 mg protein/ml) were incubated with $10^{-6}M$ arachidonate in a final volume of 1 ml 0.1 M MES buffer, pH 7.4, containing 2 mM $CaCl_2$, 1 mM $MgCl_2$, 1 mM monothioglycerol, and 2% glycerol (w/v) in the presence of 1 mM reduced glutathione and 1 mM epinephrine for 10 min at 37°C. PG material was extracted with ethyl ether and separated by silicic acid chromatography before RIA.

only two peaks were observed: one corresponded to PGE_2 and the other was in the area of the hydroxy free fatty acids (data not shown).

These findings show that PGE_2 is the predominant primary PG produced by an enzymatic activity located in the microsomal fraction of human breast cancer. In contrast, $PGF_{2\alpha}$ is mainly produced from PGE_2 by a cytosolic PG-9-keto-reductase. One could conclude from these results that PGE_2 production at the microsomal level will reflect the PG synthetase activity of a given tumor specimen.

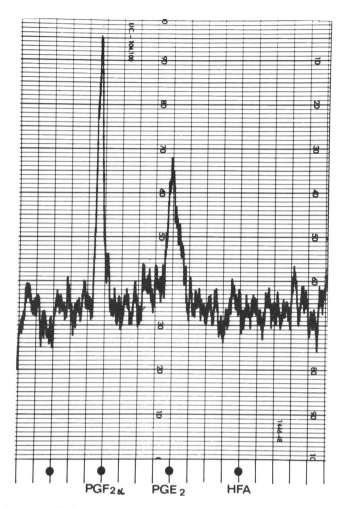

FIG. 2. Radiographic thin-layer chromatogram of products from incubation of ^{3}H-PGE$_2$ with cytosols from human breast tumor. Cytosol (0.1 ml, 3 mg protein/ml) was incubated in a final volume of 1 ml MES buffer (see legend Fig. 1) with ^{3}H-PGE$_2$ (final specific activity, 10 Ci/mmole, 10^6 cpm for each experiment) in the presence of 5 mM nicotinamide-adenine dinucleotide (NAD) and 5 mM NAD phosphate. Silica gel plates were developed in chloroform/methanol/acetic acid (180:12:10,v/v) and radioscanned.

PG PRODUCTION IN HUMAN BREAST TUMOR

A representative sample of human breast carcinomas was constituted. The selection was based on the histopathology of lesions in such a way that the histological profile of the present series was made similar to that of our general population of breast tumors (6,7). PG production by breast carcinoma was

TABLE 1. *Relationship between the clinical extension of the primary carcinoma and results of PG production analysis of tissue[a]*

	Clinical extension of lesions			
	T1	T2	T3	T4
No. specimens	11	32	24	4
PG production	$1,022 \pm 481$	$1,197 \pm 275$	919 ± 316 $(n=24)$	401 ± 201
			638 ± 154 $(n=23)$	
T1 + T2		$1,150 \pm 236$ $(n=43)$		
T3 + T4			594 ± 134 $(n=28)$	

[a] The clinical extension of the tumor was determined according to the IUAC TNM classification of breast tumors (2). A representative population of tumors was made on the basis of their histopathology. A high-speed centrifuge pellet (0.2 ml, 0.5 mg protein/ml) from human breast tumor homogenate was incubated for 10 min at 37°C in a shaking water bath with 0.8 ml MES buffer (see legend to Fig. 1) containing 1.25 mM reduced gluathione, 1.25 mM epinephrine, and 1.25×10^{-6} M sodium arachidonate. PGE_2 production was evaluated by radioimmunoassay. Results are expressed as pmoles PGE_2/50 mg protein at 10 min (means ± S.E.M.). In T3 lesions, the results are presented for the whole T3 sample $(n=24)$ and after the withdrawal of the high-value specimen of 7,358 pmoles $(n=23)$.

investigated in relation to the clinical extension and histological differentiation of the lesions. The results in Table 1 make it apparent that there is an inverse relationship between PG synthesis activity and the size of lesions, provided results from T1 and T2 tumors are added ($p < 0.001$). With respect to the clinical extension and consequently the size of lesions, these findings suggest

TABLE 2. *Relationship between histological differentiation of carcinoma and results of PG production analysis[a]*

Carcinoma type	No. specimens	PG production
1. Atypical + 0% polymorphic differentiation	25	741 ± 136
2. Polymorphic, <10% differentiation	15	$2,176 \pm 470$
3. Polymorphic, <50% differentiation	12	760 ± 177
4. Polymorphic, >50% differentiation	5	535 ± 268
5. Well-differentiation + 100% polymorphic differentiation	7	444 ± 347
Average of 3–5		622 ± 119 $(n=24)$

[a] Following to the acinoductal differentiation and prognostic value of the lesions, we recorded carcinoma histological types as those commonly found (atypical, polymorphic, and well-differentiated) and as special types. Only the commonly found types are reported here. Classification follows that used in ref. 3. See footnote to Table 1 for conditions of PG production for analysis.

that PG synthesis occurs early in the course of tumor evolution. PG production is correlated to the histological differentiation of lesions in Table 2. Lesions with less than 10% differentiation showed a greater capacity for PG synthesis than all other classes of tumor ($p < 0.005$). Both histologically differentiated and atypical tumors, on the other hand, produced lower amounts of PG. These results show that PG production is low in neoplastic tissue that has retained the morphological characteristics of the normal mammary tissue. Yet the PG synthesis capacity represented a drop in the case of atypical lesions, whereas it was at a high level in poorly differentiated lesions.

DISCUSSION

The findings reported in this paper strongly suggest that PG production in human breast cancer mainly consists of PGE_2 synthesis at the enzyme level whereas $PGF_{2\alpha}$ was produced within the cytosol. Similar to what has been suggested for thyroid cancers (4), the presence of a PG-9-keto-reductase activity could result in PGE_2 inactivation, taking the place of 15-OH-PG dehydrogenase. The absence of less polar metabolites of PGE_2 gives further support for this hypothesis. Tumor PG production was found to have an inverse relationship with histological differentiation. These findings could presumably be related to our previous work (5) on thyroid cells in culture, in which PG production increases in the absence of stimulation by thyroid-stimulating hormone, while histological differentiation is decreased. However, this could not explain why atypical lesions were found to produce lower amounts of PG than poorly differentiated tumors.

PG production appears to be an event occurring early in the course of tumor evolution. Paralleling the growth of the tumors, the development of distant metastasis is a major part of the natural course of breast cancer. It is tempting to speculate about the association of PG with tumor spread to explain the lowering of PG production in both large lesions and atypical carcinomas. Many questions remain unclear; in particular, it would be of importance to know whether the decline in PG production with tumor growth is a local phenomenom or whether PG-producing cells are involved in the tumor spread.

ACKNOWLEDGMENT

Dr. Rolland is a fellow of the Ligue Nationale Française de Lutte contre le Cancer.

REFERENCES

1. Bennet, A., Charlier, E. M., McDonald, A. M., Simpson, J. S., Stamford, I. F., and Zebro, T. (1977): *Lancet,* 2:624–627.
2. Denoix, P. (1970): *Recent Results Cancer Res.,* 31.

3. Easty, G. C., and Easty, D. M. (1976): *Cancer Treat. Rev.,* 3:217–225.
4. Friedman, Y., Levasseur, S., and Burke, G. (1976): *Biochim. Biophys. Acta,* 431:615–623.
5. Margotat, A., Rolland, P. H., Charrier, B., and Mauchamp, J. (1978): *FEBS Lett.,* 95:347–351.
6. Martin, P. M., Rolland, P. H., Jacquemier, J., Rolland, A. M.,and Toga, M. (1979): *Cancer Chemother. Pharmacol.,* 2:107–113.
7. Martin, P. M., Rolland, P. H., Jacquemier, J., Rolland, A. M., and Toga, M. (1979): *Cancer Chemother. Pharmacol.,* 2:115–120.

Advances in Prostaglandin and Thromboxane Research,
Vol. 6, edited by B. Samuelsson, P. W. Ramwell,
and R. Paoletti. Raven Press, New York © 1980.

Human Benign Breast Disease: Relationships Between Prostaglandin E₂, Steroid Hormones, and Thermographic Effects of the Inhibitors of PG Biosynthesis

*Pierre H. Rolland, *Pierre M. Martin, †Marielle Bourry,
*Anne M. Rolland, and † Henri Serment

*Laboratoire des récepteurs et des stéroides hormonaux, Institut Paoli-Calmettes, 232
Bd Sainte-Marguerite, F 13273 Marseille Cedex 2; and †Clinique Gyneco-obstétricale,
Hopital de la Conception, Marseille, France

It has been suggested that women suffering from benign mastopathies have an inadequate corpus luteum, resulting in a reduction in the ratio between progesterone and estrogen (3). This, coupled with the fact that estrogen regulates prostaglandin (PG) synthesis in the uterus (1), stimulated us to explore the relationship between blood levels of PGE_2 and the progesterone/estrogen ratio (P/E2) in patients with benign breast disease. In an attempt to establish the importance of circulating PG in women with mastopathies, we looked at the effects of inhibitors of PG biosynthesis on breast thermography, since thermography has been reported to be useful in the study of breast modifications accompanying hormonal variations (4). In this work, 22 women between 23 and 38 years of age suffering form benign mastopathies and from mastodynia for all or part of the cycle and 5 normal women without breast disease were studied. The length of cycle varied between 25 and 32 days. Thermographic examinations and blood collection for PG and steriod analysis were simultaneously performed twice between days 10 and 12 and twice between days 18 and 22 of the cycle.

PG AND STEROID ANALYSIS

Although not statistically significant, mean plasma levels of E2 and P were found to be lower in patients with benign mastopathies than in control women. In comparing steroid levels of patients in the luteal phase with those of controls, we found a greater difference in P levels ($4,981 \pm 606$ pg/ml, $n = 34$, vs. $13,156 \pm 2,221$ pg/ml, $n = 10$) than in E2 levels (98 ± 11 pg/ml, $n = 34$, vs. 205 ± 34, $n = 10$). Also, these results are compatible with the concept that there is a relationship between benign mastopathies and an inadequate corpus luteum

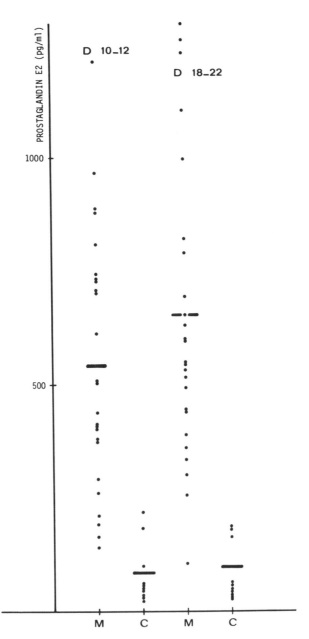

FIG. 1. PGE$_2$ plasma levels in 22 patients with mastopathies (M) and in 5 control women (C). Samples were collected twice at days 10–12 and twice at days 18–22 of the cycle. After acidification of plasma (pH 3.0) and addition of tracer amounts of ^{3}H-PGE$_2$ to evaluate procedural losses, PG was extracted with diethyl ether. The dried organic extracts were submitted to chromatography on a minicolumn of silicic acid. Radioimmunoassay of PGE$_2$ was performed on benzene/ethyl acetate/methanol (6:4:0.3, v/v) fraction of elution. Means of the levels are shown.

function, which corresponds to a relative excess of E2 as the potential for steroid hormone secretion is diminished.

The results presented in Fig. 1 demonstrate that in both phases of the cycle, PGE_2 blood levels were significantly higher ($p < 0.005$) in patients with benign mastopathies (days 10–12: 548 ± 57 pg/ml, $n = 34$; days 18–22: 638 ± 74 pg/ml, $n = 33$) than in control patients (days 10–12: 70 ± 21 pg/ml, $n = 10$; days 18–22: 83 ± 30 pg/ml, $n = 10$). In both groups, Mean plasma PGE_2 levels were not different between the phases of the cycle.

The results presented here demonstrate that patients suffering form benign mastopathies have higher blood levels than normal women. Furthermore, the patients have a reduced P/E2 ratio. A cause and effect relationship between PG synthesis and estrogenic influence could presumably be the case for breast tissue of patients suffering from benign mastopathies. On the other hand, a uterine contribution to PGE_2 blood level cannot be ruled out.

CORRELATIONS BETWEEN THERMOGRAPHIC RESPONSE AND HORMONE LEVELS

Patients underwent repeated thermographic examinations before and after (2–3 hr) administration of aspirin (1 g) or indomethacin (0.1 g). The results shown in Table 1, demonstrate that aspirin and indomethacin do result in a reduction in temperature in at least some of the patients suffering from mastopathies. Thermographic responses (TRs) were constant in both phases of the cycle and were recorded as positive in 4 cases, partly positive in 3, and negative in 3. The respondent patients presented a steroid defect of variable magnitude without a P/E2 ratio imbalance. In patients with a negative TR, the opposite was true. E2 levels were within the same range in both positive and negative

TABLE 1. *Relationships between mammary TR and steroid and PG levels according to the phase of the menstrual cycle of 10 patients[a]*

Cycle phase	Response to PG biosynthesis inhibitors		E_2 (pg/ml)	P (pg/ml)	P/E_2	PGE_2 (pg/ml)
Follicular	+	($n = 4$)	134 ± 16	57 ± 18	0.415 ± 0.12	481 ± 36
	+/−	($n = 3$)	75 ± 22	149 ± 49	2.03 ± 0.29	669 ± 160
	−	($n = 3$)	75 ± 18	35 ± 6	0.49 ± 0.05	638 ± 87
Luteal	+	($n = 4$)	99 ± 12	$7,135 \pm 934$	71.6 ± 2.4	534 ± 83
	+/−	($n = 3$)	53 ± 9	$5,351 \pm 843$	102.6 ± 11	653 ± 135
	−	($n = 3$)	84 ± 5	$3,402 \pm 1009$	39.6 ± 9.4	745 ± 168

[a] E_2 and P were assayed by radioimmunoassay after ethylether extraction and liquid–liquid chromatography on Celite support. A contact thermography apparatus was used to perform thermographic examinations. TR was classified as positive (+) when an objective cooling was recorded, partly positive (+/−) when unclear, and negative (−) when no thermographic variation was recorded.

TR patients, but P was significantly lower in TR negative patients than in TR positive women ($p < 0.02$). Furthermore, TR patients had a highly unbalanced E2/P ratio (P/E2 = 39.6 vs. 65 ± 6 in controls). There were no significant differences between groups with respect to PGE_2 plasma levels. However, a trend towards increasing levels of PGE_2 was found in the nonresponders. The cause and effect relationship between inhibition of PG synthesis and cool TR was studied in two cases: in the luteal phase, 2 TR positive patients had a drop in PGE_2 levels after treatment. Before aspirin administration, the PGE_2 levels were 340 and 710 pg/ml, and 2 hr after treatment they were 74 and 50 pg/ml, respectively.

CONCLUSIONS

In patients exhibiting TR, PGE_2 levels presumably reflect a variable phenomenom and/or has a variable effect, depending how great the P/E2 ratio variation from normal is. On the other hand, one could speculate that these will be magnified in nonresponders. The biological significance of PGE_2 in breast remains unclear. But the involvement of PGE_2 as an expression of a "precancer" state is conceivable, since patients with very low P/E2 ratios are much prone to breast cancer, first, because it is well-known that benign mastopathies represent a high-risk factor for breast cancer and, second, because estrogen-associated neoplasms have been reported (2).

ACKNOWLEDGMENT

Dr. Rolland is a fellow of the Ligue National Française contre le Cancer.

REFERENCES

1. Ham, E. A., Cirillo, V. J., Zanetti, M. E., and Kuehl, F. A. (1975): *Proc. Natl. Acad. Sci. USA,* 72:1420–1424.
2. MacDonald, J. S., Lippman, M. E., Wooley, P. V., Petrucci, P. P., and Schein, P. S. (1978): *Cancer Chemother. Pharmacol.,* 1:135–138.
3. Sitruk-Ware, L. R., Sterkers, N., Mowszowicz, I., and Mauvais-Jarvis, P. (1977): *J. Endocrinol. Metab.,* 44:771–774.
4. Verzini, L., Romani, F., and Talia, B. (1977): *Acta Thermogr.,* 2:143–149.

Advances in Prostaglandin and Thromboxane Research,
Vol. 6, edited by B. Samuelsson, P. W. Ramwell,
and R. Paoletti. Raven Press, New York © 1980.

Perioperative Behavior of Prostaglandin E_2 and 13,14-dihydro-15-keto-PGF$_{2\alpha}$ in Serum of Bronchial Carcinoma Patients

*L. Fiedler, †H. P. Zahradnik, and *G. Schlegel

*Departments of Surgery and †Gynecology and Obstetrics, University of Freiburg,
D-78 Freiberg, Federal Republic of Germany

Certain human tumors contain or secrete excessive quantities of prostaglandins (PGs). These compounds seem to be involved in carcinomas of the mammary gland (2), the colon and rectum (1), renal cell (3), and thyroid (7). In this connection the well-supported theory that PGs are causally related to the genesis of hypercalcemia and development of skeletal metastases is of special interest (6). Hardly any reports have yet been published concerning the behavior of PGs in bronchial malignancies (4).

PATIENTS

Twelve patients were on trial after lung resection for bronchial carcinomas of different histological types. Twenty patients were examined after lung resection for benign diseases (12 tuberculosis, 8 various diseases of the lung: 3 hamartoma, 2 chronic bronchitis, 2 lung fibrosis, 1 neurofibroma). In 7 patients thoracic wall operations were done for pleural empyema and pneumothorax. Nine healthy controls were included in the study. Blood sampling was performed before surgery and 2 weeks postoperative from peripheral veins into prechilled tubes. For further information concerning perioperative PGE$_2$ and 13,14-dihydro-15-keto (DHK)-PGF$_{2\alpha}$ levels after tumor removal, 3 tuberculosis and 4 bronchial carcinoma patients were followed preoperatively, just before clamping of the first tumor draining vessel and at 5,15,30,60, min, 24 hr, and 2 weeks postoperatively. Blood was collected from a central venous catheter.

METHODS

PG levels were determined by radioimmunoassay (RIA) after extraction, which was performed in accordance with Keirse and Turnbull (5). The recovery rates of labeled PGs were calculated as 74.7% for PGE$_2$ and 84.3% for DHK-PGF$_{2\alpha}$. High specific antibodies (anti-PGE$_2$, Institut Pasteur Paris; anti-DHK-

PGF$_{2\alpha}$, The Upjohn Co., Kalamazoo, Mich.; kindly supplied by Dr. J. Pike) were used. For RIA control purposes, intra- and interassay precisions were determined. Statistical evaluation was done by variance analysis for symmetric models.

RESULTS

PGE$_2$ significantly decreased from 66 pg/ml preoperative to 28 pg/ml postoperative in bronchial carcinoma patients and DHK-PGF$_{2\alpha}$ from 384 pg/ml preoperative to 228 pg/ml postoperative. Both preoperative values were significantly elevated in comparison with healthy controls. Serum values of patients undergoing lung surgery for benign lesions, whether with or without resection procedures, did not differ from normal values and did not postoperatively. The perioperative follow-up of 3 tuberculosis and 4 cancer patients showed a rapid decline in serum concentration after tumor removal within 30 min and normalization 24 hours later. No changes could be detected after resection of tuberculosis-destroyed lung tissue. No correlation between the amount of resected lung tissue and PG levels could be demonstrated. PG-mediated hypercalcemia could not be evaluated because of the lack of bone metastases in all patients on trial.

CONCLUSIONS

Determination of PGE$_2$ and DHK-PGF$_{2\alpha}$ might be a possible method of evaluating the postoperative course of lung surgery for bronchial malignancy. These preliminary results must be extended to a longer follow-up period. The correlation between PG levels and tumor size still needs to be evaluated. Further analysis of PG metabolite-mediated effects on tumors, bone, and circulation might clarify specific mechanisms and open new therapeutic advances.

REFERENCES

1. Bennett, A., Del Tacca, M., Stamford, I. F., and Zebro, T. (1977): *Br. J. Cancer,* 35:881.
2. Bennett, A., McDonald, A. M., Simpson, J. S., and Stamford, I. F. (1975): *Lancet,* 1:1218.
3. Cummings, K. B., Wheelis, R. F., and Robertson, R. P. (1975): *Surg. Forum,* 26:572.
4. Demers, L. M., Allegra, J. C., Harvey, H. A., Lipton, A., Luderer, J. R., Mortel, R. and Brenner, D. E. (1977): *Cancer,* 39:1559.
5. Keirse, M. I. N. C., and Turnbull, A. C. (1973): *Prostaglandins,* 4:607.
6. Seyberth, H. W., Raisz, L. G., and Oates, J. A. (1978): *Am. Rev. Med.,* 29:23–29.
7. Williams, E. D., Karim, S. M. M., and Sandler, M. (1968): *Lancet,* 1:22.

Advances in Prostaglandin and Thromboxane Research,
Vol. 6, edited by B. Samuelsson, P. W. Ramwell,
and R. Paoletti. Raven Press, New York © 1980.

Interactions of Cytotoxic and Anti-Inflammatory Agents on Normal and Neoplastic Tissue

*T. J. Powles, G. J. Frank, and *J. L. Millar

*Chester Beatty Institute for Cancer Research, Royal Marsden Hospital, Sutton, Surrey; and The Boots Company Limited, Nottingham, United Kingdom

Two factors determine the ultimate effect of cytotoxic agents on normal or malignant tissue—First, the number of cells killed by the agent and, second, the ability of the surviving cells to recover, divide, and thereby repair the tissue.

There is abundant evidence that prostaglandins (PGs) are involved in the mechanisms of cell replication. Generally, it seems that PGE inhibits cell division and, conversely, that inhibition of PG synthesis by nonsteroidal anti-inflammatory (NSA) drugs stimulates cell division. It is, therefore, possible that these agents might influence recovery of tissues. The antitumor activity of most cytotoxic agents is limited by the maximum dose which can be tolerated by normal tissues, particularly the gut and bone marrow. Therefore, agents which enhance normal tissue recovery without enhancement of tumor recovery would be valuable as a supplement to anticancer therapy.

The ability of normal bone marrow to produce white cells and platelets depends on the number of parent or stem cells present and the rate of division and maturation of their daughter cells. Cytotoxic chemotherapy may prevent the bone marrow from producing hemopoietic cells by reducing the number of stem cells and/or by inhibiting the maturation of dividing cells. Cytotoxic agents can stimulate PG synthesis, and inhibition of PG synthesis would be expected to enhance recovery.

Most experimental studies on factors influencing hemopoiesis have used standard stem cell assays which depend on the ability of hemopoietic cells removed from a mouse to divide and give rise to colonies of cells either in the spleens of irradiated recipient mice or in organ cultures. Bone marrow removed from animals which have been heavily irradiated or given high doses of cytotoxic agents develop into very few colonies in the spleens of donor animals, indicating considerable damage to the stem cells. Few colonies develop even if the bone marrow is removed 1 week after drug or irradiation, indicating little recovery. However, if the animals are treated with NSA agents such as indomethacin or flurbiprofen, there is a substantial increase in the number of colonies which develop 1 week after irradiation, indicating enhanced recovery of the marrow. (Table 1)

TABLE 1. *Survival and recovery of stem cells per mouse femur after whole-body irradiation (900 R)*

Day	Control	Flurbiprofen[a]	Indomethacin[b]
1	<1	—	<1
7	4.1 (0.6)	56 (6.0)	54 (4.0)

[a] Dose: 14 mg/kg/day.
[b] Dose: 6 mg/kg/day for 3 days.

A similar stem cell assay is not available for rats, but measurement of the recovery of the peripheral white count after a single large dose of chlorambucil indicates enhanced recovery of the bone marrow (Table 2).

Gut toxicity with ulceration and perforation occurs after high-dose cytotoxic therapy or heavy irradiation. This presumably reflects damage to the crypt cells from which other cells in the gut arise. If a high dose of an alkylating agent such as melphelan (20 mg/kg) is given to mice, death occurs within 5 days from gut toxicity in 36 of 39 animals. Survival depends on the extent of the gut damage and the ability of remaining cells to repair the damage. Only 17 of 30 mice given indomethacin (4.25 mg/kg/day) and 3 of 8 mice given flurbiprofen (12 mg/kg/day) for 3 days died when also given high-dose melphelan, indicating that these agents will protect animals against a lethal dose of melphelan, presumably by enhanced recovery from gut toxicity.

Reduction of gut or marrow toxicity is of no therapeutic benefit, if there is reduced anticancer activity. The *in vitro* sensitivity of tumor cells remains unaffected by flurbiprofen and in most animal tumor models which we have examined, there has been no reduction in the anticancer activity of cytotoxic drugs. In fact, in one model we used there was apparently an enhanced cytotoxic effect. Using the specially developed chemoresistant Walker tumor cell line, death from malignant ascites occurs within 9 days of intraperitoneal injection of 10^7 tumor cells (4/4) and remains unaffected by administration of chlorambucil (0/8), indomethacin (0/8), or flurbiprofen (0/8). Enhanced survival occurs with animals treated with chlorambucil and flurbiprofen (4/8) or indomethacin (2/8). This may reflect enhanced cytotoxic activity on these chemoresistant tumor cells. More likely, it may reflect enhanced recovery of the bone marrow-depen-

TABLE 2. *Peripheral leukocyte count in rats 8 days after a single injection of chlorambucil, 10 mg/kg, and flurbiprofen 21 mg/kg/day for 3 days at the time of injection*

Drug	Leukocyte count (% of initial count)
Chlorambucil	33 ± 3
Chlorambucil + flurbiprofen	55 ± 7

dent immune system after chemotherapy, which may be of importance in this allogenic system.

It may, therefore, be possible to improve the therapeutic index of anticancer agents by manipulation of PG synthesis with anti-inflammatory drugs.

ACKNOWLEDGMENTS

We thank the Boots Company Ltd., United Kingdom, for supplying Flurbiprofen.

Advances in Prostaglandin and Thromboxane Research,
Vol. 6, edited by B. Samuelsson, P. W. Ramwell,
and R. Paoletti. Raven Press, New York © 1980.

Reduction by Flurbiprofen of Primary Tumor Growth and Local Metastasis Formation in Mice

D. J. Leaper, B. French, and A. Bennett

Departments of Surgery and Morbid Anatomy, Westminster and King's College Hospitals, London, England

Our previous studies with the NC transplantable mouse mammary tumor indicate beneficial effects of the PG synthesis inhibitor flurbiprofen. Doses of 5 mg/kg daily orally in 0.1 ml raspberry syrup reduced tumor growth, and substantially reduced the size of established tumors when used in conjunction with radiotherapy ± chemotherapy. Survival time after primary tumor resection was also prolonged provided that drug treatment was started just prior to tumor transplantation (1).

In this chapter, we investigate the effects of a lower dose of flurbiprofen (2.5 mg/kg daily) on the histologic changes associated with a reduction of tumor growth, and on the formation of local metastases and scar recurrences following excision of the primary tumor.

MATERIALS AND METHODS

WHT/Ht mice (equal numbers of males and females) were injected sc with NC carcinoma and given vehicle alone (raspberry syrup) or flurbiprofen 2.5 mg/kg by mouth daily. Three weeks later, the primary tumors were excised with a narrow rim of macroscopically normal tissue under ether anesthesia. Sections from 32 out of 56 tumors from each group were stained (hematoxylin, eosin, van Geison's stain) and blindly assessed histologically for tumor grade (3) necrosis, lymphocytic infiltration, and fibroblastic reaction. Histologic evaluation was satisfactory in 61 of the 64 tumors.

Following tumor resection, the mice were put into various groups for treatment with radiotherapy and/or chemotherapy to determine the effects on local metastasis formation and scar recurrence. Only the effects of flurbiprofen are discussed here: the effects of radiotherapy and chemotherapy are reported by Leaper et al. (5).

RESULTS

The primary tumors excised at 3 weeks from mice treated with flurbiprofen 2.5 mg/kg daily were smaller than controls (0.12 ± 0.02 g and 0.22 ± 0.02 g

TABLE 1. *Lymphocytic infiltration of tumors*

	Slight	Intermediate	Prominent
Flurbiprofen-treated	21	5	5
Controls	27	3	0

TABLE 2. *Local metastases and scar recurrences following primary tumor excision*

Week after tumor excisior	Local metastases				Scar recurrence			
	% incidence		Mean vol (cm³)		% incidence		Mean vol (cm³)	
	F	C	F	C	F	C	F	C
4	45	77	1.30	4.57	73	77	0.22	0.27
5	45	77	3.05	5.74	73	77	0.78	0.50

respectively, means $\pm$ sem, $p < 0.001$). All tumors were poorly differentiated and the only difference between test and control tumors was a tendency ($0.1 > p > 0.05$, Fisher's exact probability test) for a greater lymphocytic infiltration in tumors from flurbiprofen-treated mice (Table 1).

Scar recurrences and local metastases (satellite growths connected by invaded lymphatic vessels to a primary tumor or its scar) were easily measured with calipers from 4 weeks onwards after primary tumor excision (volume $= \pi$ W²L/6, where L and W are the two largest diameters). There were initially 11 flurbiprofen-treated mice (F) and 13 controls (C). Flurbiprofen had no significant effect on scar recurrence, and caused only a nonsignificant tendency to reduce local metastatic spread and growth (Table 2).

Values at 6 or more weeks after tumor excision are not given because some mice died during this time. The full results are presented by Leaper et al. (5).

DISCUSSION

The NC tumor is thought to be of low immunogenicity (4). However, the tendency for flurbiprofen to increase the lymphocytic infiltration of the tumor may indicate a restoration of the immune defense by the host (6). Alternatively, more lymphocytes may be attracted to the tumor because of greater cell death.

Berstock et al. (2) reported that flurbiprofen reduced scar recurrences following resection of primary NC tumors, but they did not observe satellite metastases. However, they excised the tumors with a wide rim of healthy tissue, unlike the narrow rim used here, and perhaps any satellite metastases present became fused in the excision scar.

CONCLUSION

These results, together with the beneficial effects of flurbiprofen on the response of mice to treatment with conventional therapeutic agents, help lay a basis for testing flurbiprofen, and possibly other inhibitors of PG synthesis, as adjuncts to treatment of human cancers.

ACKNOWLEDGMENTS

We thank the Cancer Research Campaign and Medical Research Council for support, and the Boots Company Ltd., Nottingham, England for flurbiprofen.

REFERENCES

1. Bennett, A., Houghton, J., Leaper, D. J., and Stamford, I. F. (1979): *Prostaglandins,* 17:179–191.
2. Berstock, D. A., Houghton, J., and Bennett, A. (1979): *Cancer Treat. Rev., (in press).*
3. Bloom, H. J., and Richardson, W. W. (1957): *Br. J. Cancer,* 11:359–377.
4. Hewitt, H. B., Blake, E. R., and Walder, A. S. (1976): *Br. J. Cancer,* 33:241–259.
5. Leaper, D. J., French, B. T., and Bennett, A. (1979): *Br. J. Surg. (in press).*
6. Plescia, D. J., Smith, A. H., and Grinwick, K. (1975): *Proc. Natl. Acad. Sci. USA,* 72:1848–1851.

Advances in Prostaglandin and Thromboxane Research,
Vol. 6, edited by B. Samuelsson, P. W. Ramwell,
and R. Paoletti. Raven Press, New York © 1980.

Prostaglandins and Their Relationships to Malignant and Benign Human Breast Tumors

A. Bennett, D. A. Berstock, *M. Harris, B. Raja, *D. J. F. Rowe,
I. F. Stamford, and J. E. Wright

*Department of Surgery, King's College Hospital Medical School, London SE5 8RX; and
*Department of Oral and Maxillo-Facial Surgery, Eastman Dental Hospital,
London WC1, United Kingdom*

There is substantial evidence that many human and animal malignant tumors can produce more prostaglandins (PGs) than the normal tissues from which they arise (1). Human malignant breast tumor homogenates usually contained large amounts of PG-like material (PG-lm), whereas those of benign tumors or normal breast tissue contained much smaller amounts (2,3,5). These results show a correlation between the amounts of PG-lm extracted from malignant tumors and their spread, especially to the skeleton, as indicated by bone scans, and away from the primary tumor as judged histologically. Others too have found high PG production by human malignant breast tumors, but they also obtained substantial release from benign breast tumors (8,10,12). In this paper we first demonstrate that the different findings with benign tumors are due to methodology. We then report that the ability of human malignant tumors to produce PG-lm correlates inversely with patient survival.

METHODS

Benign and malignant breast tumors were obtained at surgery and processed within 1 hr of removal. After being cut into small pieces and washed with Krebs solution, samples were then either homogenized or incubated. The homogenization was carried out at room temperature for 30 sec in acidified aqueous ethanol to indicate "basal" amounts of PG-lm, or in Krebs solution to allow synthesis of PGs from precursors released during disruption of the tissue (6). The amount extracted from homogenates in Krebs solution is called "total" PG-lm and "synthesized" PG-lm is calculated as total–basal.

Cut pieces of tumor were incubated in BGJ medium alone or medium containing 5% heated human serum for 48 hr at 37°C. The PG-lm in the homogenates or incubates was extracted (15) and bioassayed on the rat stomach strip preparation against PGE_2 (6).

Patient survival was measured to the nearest half month from the date of operation until death from cancer.

Results are expressed as medians, with semiquartile ranges in parentheses, and analyzed statistically using the Wilcoxon matched-pairs test, the Mann-Whitney U-test, or Spearman's rank correlation as appropriate.

RESULTS

PG-lm from Benign and Malignant Human Breast Lesions

Studies were made on 13 benign lesions (7 fibroadenomas, 6 mammary dysplasias) and 25 carcinomas. The results with the two types of benign lesions were similar and are therefore combined. Malignant tumors homogenized in Krebs solution or acid ethanol yielded more PG-lm than did samples from benign lesions (Table 1). In contrast, samples from the same benign lesions incubated in BGJ medium for 48 hr tended to release more PG-lm than did malignant tumors (Table 2). The amount extracted from the incubates was very much higher than from homogenates, showing that the material was newly synthesized rather than stored.

Relationship Between Malignant Tumor PG and Patient Survival

This study concerns 25 women who died of breast cancer, 92 others still alive after breast cancer surgery, and 3 dead patients whose tumors were measured only for total PG-lm. The 25 women of the first group (age range, 42–87 years; median, 60 at the time of surgery) died 1.5 to 36 (median, 15) months postoperatively. The highest levels of PG-lm were extracted from the resected tumors of the patients who died the earliest ($p < 0.01$ to $p < 0.05$ for total, basal, and synthesized PG-lm).

The results from all the women (age range, 28–96 years; median, 54 at the time of surgery) had to be analyzed differently. Tumor PG-lm was compared

TABLE 1. *PG-lm extracted from homogenates of human malignant and benign breast tumors*

	PGE$_2$ equivalents/g (ng)		
	Malignant	Benign	*p*
Total	30(18–60)	8.8(2–15)	0.0016
Basal	9(2–28)	1.5(0–5)	0.0074
Synthesized	21(7–42)	5(2–11)	0.077

Total basal and synthesized amounts of PG-lm were higher in homogenates of malignant than of benign human breast tumors.

TABLE 2. *PG-lm extracted from incubates of human malignant and benign breast tumors*

PGE$_2$ eq/g (ng)		
Malignant	Benign	p
400 (245–865)	943 (115–2020)	0.187

The amounts of PG-lm released from incubated benign human breast tumors tended to be higher than from malignant tumors.

in women living less than 6 months with those living at least 6 months, and similar comparisons were made at 12, 18, and 24 months (Table 3). The tumor PG-lm tended to be higher in the patients who had died by the end of each 6 month period than in patients who were still alive. For example, the median total PG-lm in the 5 patients living 6 months or less compared with the 115 living at least 6 months was 210 and 42 ng PGE$_2$/g, respectively (Table 3). The differences in total and basal tumor PG-lm were often statistically significant, but synthesized PG-lm was significantly different only at 12 months. Tumor PG measurements correlated with the early death of some patients who, on the basis of clinical staging had been thought to have good prognoses.

DISCUSSION

The amount of PG-lm obtained from human benign breast tumors *in vitro* depends on the methodology. Homogenization of fibroadenomas or mammary dysplasias yielded amounts substantially lower than obtained from malignant breast tumors, whereas the yield from incubated unhomogenized benign tumors was at least as high as with carcinomas. The reason for the different results with homogenized or incubated benign tumors is not known, but it might involve substantial degradation of PGs during homogenization. Seyberth et al. (13) found that supernatant from homogenized normal rabbit lung or kidney metabolized PGE$_2$. The failure of VX2 tumor supernatant to metabolize PGE$_2$ (13) may be the reason why malignant tumors yield substantial amounts of PG-lm with either method. Our findings therefore explain the difference between various reports, and confirm the results of Dowsett et al. (8) and Robinson (12), who found high PG-lm production by incubated benign breast tumors. The amount which Greaves (10) obtained from benign breast tumors was somewhat less, but he first cut the tumors with scissors and then homogenized the tissue without washing away any PG formed as a result of cutting. Thus his procedure is to some extent a combination of incubation and homogenization.

We have previously correlated PG amounts in malignant breast tumors with the spread of the tumor locally and to the skeleton (2,3,5). Since benign tumors

TABLE 3. Relationship between tumor PG-lm and patient survival time

Survival[a] (months)	n	PGE₂ equivalents/g tumor (ng)				
		Total	n	Basal	n	Synthesized
<6	5	210 (88–250)[b]	5	63 (46–170)[c]	5	147 (42–232)
>6	115	42 (16–80)[b]	95	12 (4–28)[c]	95	22 (9–51)
<12	11	120 (80–300)	10	55 (19–140)	10	128 (35–260)
>12	109	40 (14–80)[c]	92	11 (3–27)[c]	92	22 (8–47)[c]
<18	17	88 (18–210)	16	19 (4–63)	16	39 (7–147)
>18	83	42 (16–80)	70	12 (4–32)	70	22 (10–43)
<24	23	88 (39–190)	20	19 (4–69)	20	34 (8–147)
>24	48	38 (11–75)	40	10 (2–32)[d]	40	22 (9–51)

[a] Patients whose malignant breast tumors yielded most PG-lm often died soonest (e.g., compare median total PG-lm of 210 ng PGE₂ equivalents/g in the 5 patients surviving <6 months with the 42 ng in the 115 patients surviving >6 months).
[b] $p < 0.05$.
[c] $p < 0.01$.
[d] $p < 0.1$.

can produce substantial amounts of PG-lm during incubation, the relevance of PGs to the spread of cancer might seem to be in question. This is not so, because benign tumors tend to be encapsulated and do not spread. Carcinomas rarely have a capsule, and malignant cells are readily shed into lymphatics and blood vessels.

The finding that breast carcinomas produce substantial amounts of PG-lm during homogenization or incubation probably means that either method is suitable for determining the ability to synthesize PGs.

Correlation of breast carcinoma PGs with patient survival following local surgery is of importance for several reasons. Prognosis greatly influences the choice of therapy, and a preliminary analysis suggests that the PG measurements may identify patients with a poor prognosis who on clinical staging would be expected to do well. It remains to be seen whether or not the indication of prognosis by PG measurements is better than by other techniques such as counting the number of involved regional lymph nodes removed during breast surgery (9).

An even more exciting possibility is that PGs contribute to tumor growth and/or spread (1). Various studies have supported the observation first made by Tashjian et al. (14) that indomethacin reduces the growth of tumors in mice and the finding of Powles et al. (11) that inhibitors of PG synthesis reduce destruction of bone caused by tumors (1). Our own studies in mice with NC tumors show several striking effects of the PG synthesis inhibitor flurbiprofen. When given daily starting at the time of tumor transplantation, the drug reduces tumor growth and can prolong survival time following primary tumor excision (4). With established, previously untreated tumors, flurbiprofen produces a dramatic reduction of tumor growth when combined with local radiotherapy and/or chemotherapy (4). In another experiment which mimics clinical practice more closely, the survival of mice is prolonged by treatment with flurbiprofen and chemotherapy compared with chemotherapy alone (7). This increased response is not associated with increased damage to normal cells by chemotherapeutic drugs, since flurbiprofen does not increase the toxicity of melphalan and methotrexate.

Cancer therapy can cause so severe a distress in patients as to prevent optimal treatment. PGs may be involved in these unwanted effects, since radiotherapy or chemotherapy can increase the amount of PGs in tissues (1). For these and other reasons discussed in Ref. 1, trials with flurbiprofen and possibly other nonsteriodal anti-inflammatory drugs are warranted in the treatment of cancer patients.

ACKNOWLEDGMENTS

We thank the Cancer Research Campaign and Medical Research Council for support, and Upjohn Limited for supplies of PGs.

REFERENCES

1. Bennett, A. (1979): In: *Practical Application of Prostaglandins and Their Synthesis Inhibitors,* edited by S. M. M. Karim, pp. 149–188. MTP Press Ltd., Lancaster.
2. Bennett, A., Charlier, E. M., MacDonald, A. M., Simpson, J. S., and Stamford, I. F. (1976): *Prostaglandins,* 11:461–463.
3. Bennett, A., Charlier, E. M., MacDonald, A. M., Simpson, J. S., Stamford, I. F., and Zebro, T. (1977): *Lancet,* 2:624–626.
4. Bennett, A., Houghton, J., Leaper, D. J., and Stamford, I. F. (1979): *Prostaglandins,* 17:179–191.
5. Bennett, A., MacDonald, A. M., Simpson, J. S., and Stamford, I. F. (1975): *Lancet,* 1:1218–1220.
6. Bennett, A., Stamford, I. F., and Unger, W. G. (1971): *J. Physiol.,* 229:349–360.
7. Berstock, D. A., Houghton, J., and Bennett, A. (1979): *Cancer Treat. Rev. (Suppl)* 6:69–71.
8. Dowsett, M., Gazet, J. C., Powles, T. J., Easty, G. C., and Neville, A. M. (1976): *Lancet,* 1:970–971.
9. Fisher, B., and Slack, N. H. (1970): *Surg. Gynaecol. Obstet.,* 131:79–88.
10. Greaves, M. (1978): M.D. Thesis, University of Sheffield.
11. Powles, T. J., Clark, S. A., Easty, D. M., Easty, G. C., and Neville, A. M. (1973): *Br. J. Cancer,* 28:316–321.
12. Robinson, D. R. (1976): Breast Cancer Task Force Program and Related Projects, p63, Division of Cancer Biology and Diagnosis. U.S. National Cancer Institute, Bethesda.
13. Seyberth, H. W., Hubbard, W. C., Oelz, O., Sweetman, B. J., Watson, J. T., and Oates, J. A. (1977): *Prostaglandins,* 14:319–331.
14. Tashjian, A. H., Voelkel, E. F., Goldhaber, P. and Levine, L. (1973): *Prostaglandins,* 3:515–524.
15. Unger, W. G., Stamford, I. F., and Bennett, A. (1971): *Nature,* 233:336–337.